Nursing Theorists
AND THEIR *Work*

Nursing Theorists
AND THEIR Work

FOURTH EDITION

Ann Marriner Tomey, PhD, RN, FAAN
Professor
School of Nursing
Indiana State University
Terre Haute, Indiana

Martha Raile Alligood, PhD, RN
Professor
College of Nursing
University of Tennessee
Knoxville, Tennessee

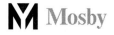
Mosby

St. Louis   Baltimore   Boston
Carlsbad   Chicago   Naples   New York   Philadelphia   Portland
London   Madrid   Mexico City   Singapore   Sydney   Tokyo   Toronto   Wiesbaden

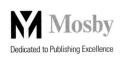
Mosby

Dedicated to Publishing Excellence

A Times Mirror Company

Publisher Nancy L. Coon
Editor Loren S. Wilson
Developmental Editor Brian Dennison
Project Manager Dana Peick
Production Editor Dan Begley
Editing and Production Top Graphics
Book Design Amy Buxton
Cover Art Wolf Communications
Manufacturing Manager Karen Boehme

FOURTH EDITION

Copyright © 1998 by Mosby–Year Book, Inc.

Previous editions copyrighted 1986, 1989, and 1994

Printed in the United States of America
Composition by Top Graphics
Printing/binding by R.R. Donnelley & Sons Company

Mosby–Year Book, Inc.
11830 Westline Industrial Drive
St. Louis, Missouri 63146

Library of Congress Cataloging in Publication Data

Nursing theorists and their work / [edited by] Ann Marriner Tomey,
    Martha Raile Alligood. — 4th ed.
        p.   cm.
    Includes bibliographical references and index.
    ISBN 0-8151-4421-0
    1. Nursing—Philosophy.   2. Nursing models.   I. Marriner Tomey,
Ann.   II. Alligood, Martha Raile.
    [DNLM: 1. Nursing Theory.   2. Nurses—biography.   WY 86 N9738
1998]
RT84.5.N9   1998
610.73′01—dc21
DNLM/DLC
for Library of Congress   97-11533
                                                                CIP

98 99 00 01 02 / 9 8 7 6 5 4 3 2 1

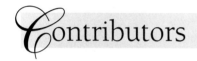Contributors

Mary Lee Ackermann

Sr. Judith E. Alexander

Martha Raile Alligood

Gloria S. Artigue

Jill K. Baker

Deborah A. Barnhart

Carolyn J. Beagle

Sarah J. Beckman

Alberta M. Bee

Quilla Bell

Patricia M. Bennett

Sue Marquis Bishop

Carolyn L. Blue

Debra A. Borchers

Sanna Boxley-Harges

Sallie Anne Brink

Gail H. Brophy

Victoria M. Brown

Karen M. Brubaker

Cheryl Bruick-Sorge

Kaye Bultemeier

Pam Butler

Jane A. Caldwell-Gwin

Elizabeth T. Carey

Lisa A. Carr

Patricia Chapman-Boyce

Elizabeth Chong Choi

Jo Anne Clanton

Debra Trnka Cochran

Sydney Coleman-Ehmke

Angela Compton

Sharon S. Conner

Donna J. Crawford

Terri Creekmur

Joann Sebastian Daily

Marguerite Danko

Janet DeFelice

Karen R. de Graaf

Deborah Wertman DeMeester

Snehlata Desai

Marilyn Sue Doub

Deborah A. Dougherty

Phyllis MacDonald du Mont

Dorothy Kay Dycus

Jeanne Donohue Eben

Sarah Emerson

Margaret E. Erickson

Carolyn H. Fakouri

Julia M.B. Fine

Susan Fisher

Karen J. Foli

Barbara Freese

Nergess N. Gashti

Alta J.H. Gochnauer

Marcy Grandstaff

S. Brook Gumm

Mary Gunther

Cheryl A. Hailway

Tamara D. Halterman

Linda S. Harbour

Brenda Kay Harmon

Susan Matthews Harris

Karen Hartman

Terrence J. Heidenreiter

DeAnn M. Hensley

Mary E. Hermiz

Deborah Hissa

William H. Hobble

Anne Hodel

Beulah A. Hofmann

Chérie Howk

Nancy E. Hunt

Connie Rae Jarlsberg

Tamara Johnson

Cathy Greenwell Jones

Rhonda G. Justus

Karla G. Kaltofen

Juanita Fogel Keck

M. Jan Keffer

Susan L. Keller

Kimberly A. Kilgore-Keever

Martha J. Kirsch

Jill Vass Langfitt

Theresa Lansinger

Tamara Lauer

Rickard E. Lee

Denise Legge

Jude A. Magers

Judith E. Marich

Ann Marriner Tomey

Judy Sporleder Maupin

Elizabeth A. McClure

Judy McCormick

Cynthia A. McCreary

Nancy J. McKee

Mary M. Meighan

Mary Meininger

Kathleen Millican Miller

Deborah I. Mills

Jullette C. Mitre

Sandra L. Moody

Cynthia L. Mossman

Cathy A. Murray

Margaret J. Nation

Susan E. Neal

John Noll

Kathryn W. Noone

Sherry B. Nordmeyer

Stephanie Oetting

Nancy Orcutt

Katherine R. Papazian

Tracey J.F. Patton

Jean A. Peacock

Gwynn Lee Perlich

Kim Tippey Peskoe

LaPhyllis Peterson

Cheryl Y. Petty

Susan A. Pfettscher

Kenneth D. Phillips

Kathleen D. Pickrell

Mary Carolyn Poat

LaDema Poppa

Beverly D. Porter

Debra L. Price

Beth Bruns Prusinski

Rosalyn A. Pung

Sheila Rangel

LyNette Rasmussen

Cynthia M. Riester

Karen D. Andrews Robards

Martha Carole Satterly

Marcia K. Sauter

Karen Moore Schaefer

Donna N. Schmeiser

Denise L. Schnell

Larry P. Schumacher

Bryn Searcy

Christina L. Sieloff

Maribeth Slebodnik

Rebecca S. Sloan

Cathy R. Smith

Mary Ann Sobiech

Kathleen C. Solotkin

Nancy L. Stark

Sandra E. Steinkeler

Margery Stuart

Flossie M. Taggart

Susan G. Taylor

Elizabeth Godfrey Terry

Lucy Anne Tillett

Prudence Twigg

Catherine Velotta

Therese L. Wallace

Judith K. Watt

Alice Z. Welch

Cynthia A. Wesolowski

Sandy Williams

Roberta Woeste

Roseanne Yancey

Lorraine A. Yeager

Susan T. Zoretich

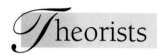heorists

Faye Glenn Abdellah
Graduate School of Nursing
The Uniformed Services of the
  Health Sciences
4301 Jones Bridge Road
Bethesda, MD 20814-4799
(301) 295-1993

Evelyn Adam
Professor Emeritus
University of Montreal
6950 Côte Saint-Lue
Montreal, Quebec H4V 2Z9
(514) 484-0217

Kathryn E. Barnard
University of Washington
  School of Nursing
T-303 H.S.B., SC-72
Seattle, WA 98195
(206) 543-4152

Patricia Benner
University of California
  at San Francisco
School of Nursing
San Francisco, CA 94143
(415) 476-4313

Helen C. Erickson
University of Texas
Austin, TX 78701
(512) 471-7311

Joyce J. Fitzpatrick
Case Western Reserve University
Frances Payne Bolton School
  of Nursing
2121 Abington Road
Cleveland, OH 44106
(216) 368-2544

†Lydia E. Hall

†Virginia Henderson

Dorothy E. Johnson
(Retired)
325 Citrus Open Drive
New Smyrna Beach, FL 32168
(904) 423-2007

Imogene King
(Retired)
7400 Sun Island Drive
South Pasadena, FL 33707
(813) 360-1943

Madeleine Leininger
1121 Woolworth Plaza
Omaha, NE 68144-1875
(402) 691-0791

†Myra Estrin Levine

Winifred W. Logan (Gordon)
East Grange
St. Andrews
Scotland
United Kingdom KY16 8LL
  0133-447-4196

†Deceased.

ix

Ramona T. Mercer
(Retired)
1809 Ashton Avenue
Burlingame, CA 94010
(415) 697-2324

Betty Neuman
Box 488
Beverly, OH 45715
(614) 749-3322

Margaret A. Newman
289 E. Fifth #511
St. Paul, MN 55101
(612) 292-0437

†Florence Nightingale

Dorothea E. Orem
Orem & Shields, Inc.
55 Dear Run
Savannah, GA 31411
(912) 598-1759

Rosemarie Rizzo Parse
Nursing Science Quarterly
320 Fort Duquesne Blvd.
Suite 25J
Pittsburgh, PA 15222
(412) 391-8471

Ida Jean Orlando (Pelletier)
111 Waverly
Belmont, MA 02178
(617) 489-0348

Nola J. Pender
University of Michigan
School of Nursing
400 North Ingalls Building
Ann Arbor, MI 48108-0482
(313) 764-7188

Hildegard E. Peplau
(Retired)
14024 Ostego Street
Sherman Oaks, CA 91403
(818) 783-2272

†Martha E. Rogers

Nancy Roper
70 Polwarth Gardens
Edinburgh, Scotland
United Kingdom EH11 1LL
0131-229-4748

Sister Callista Roy
Boston College
Cushing Hall
140 Commonwealth Avenue
Chestnut Hill, MA 02167
(617) 552-8811

Joan Riehl-Sisca
P.O. Box 24405
Los Angeles, CA 90024

Mary Ann P. Swain
Office of Academic Affairs
University of Michigan
Ann Arbor, MI 48109
(313) 764-0151

Alison J. Tierney
Department of Nursing Studies
University of Edinburgh
Adam Ferguson Building
40 George Square
Edinburgh, Scotland
United Kingdom EH 8 9LL
0131-650-1000

†Deceased.

Evelyn M. Tomlin
P.O. Box 128
Big Rock, IL 60511
(312) 556-3087

†*Joyce Travelbee*

Jean Watson
University of Colorado
Health Sciences Center
School of Nursing
4200 E. Ninth Avenue
Denver, CO 80262
(303) 384-7754

Ernestine Wiedenbach
(Retired)
926 Eastridge Village Drive
Miami, FL 33157
(305) 235-5931

†Deceased.

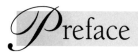

Preface

This book is a tribute to nursing theorists. It identifies major thinkers in nursing; reviews some of their important ideas; and lists their publications, what has been written about them, and the major sources they used. The first chapter is a brief overview of the book and is appropriate for the baccalaureate level. The other chapters in Unit I define terminology and discuss the history and philosophy of science, logical reasoning, the theory development process, and the evolution of nursing theory development at a graduate level.

The theorists are clustered into three categories. Nightingale, Wiedenbach, Henderson, Abdellah, Hall, Watson, and Benner wrote philosophies. Orem; Levine; Rogers; Johnson; Roy; Neuman; King; and Roper, Logan, and Tierney designed conceptual models, or grand theories. Peplau; Orlando; Travelbee; Riehl-Sisca; Erickson, Tomlin, and Swain; Mercer; Barnard; Leininger; Parse; Fitzpatrick; Newman; Adam; and Pender wrote middle-range nursing theories.

The following are identified for each theorist: credentials and background, theoretical sources for theory development, use of empirical data, major concepts and definitions, assumptions, theoretical assertions, logical form, acceptance by the nursing community, further development, and a critique of the work. Critical Thinking Activities have been added, and bibliographies are updated. Baccalaureate students may be most interested in the concepts, definitions, and theoretical assertions. Graduate students will be interested in logical form, acceptance by the nursing community, the theoretical sources for theory development, and the use of empirical data. The extensive bibliographies should be particularly useful to graduate students for locating primary and secondary sources.

Many of the scholars identified in this book do not consider themselves theorists and never intended to develop theory. Is it fair to evaluate them as theorists and their work as theory? Probably not, but their thoughts are important contributions to the development of nursing theory. It is now our responsibility to analyze and synthesize their work, generate new ideas, and continue theory development.

I would like to thank the theorists for critiquing the original chapters about themselves so that the content could be current and accurate. So that their omission does not appear to have been an oversight, it must be noted that the work of Paterson and Zderad has not been included in this volume at their request.

Thanks to all the people working behind the scenes and to administrative and office assistants Eileen Anderson, Kaye Blackburn, Sherri Beaver, Tami Hubble, and Linda Moore for facilitating the work on this book. Thanks also go to research assistant Marie Hockersmith. Dr. Martha Raile Alligood reordered the chapters, served as a contributing author, and edited for consistency with the new organization for the third edition. After Dr. Alligood co-edited *Nursing Theory: Utilization and Application,* and based on her expertise in nursing science theory, I invited her to become a co-editor as well as a contributing author for this fourth edition.

I thank my loving husband, H. Keith Tomey, for enriching my private life while supporting my professional activities.

Ann Marriner Tomey

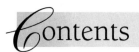

Contents

UNIT THREE

Conceptual Models: Grand Theories

UNIT FOUR

Middle-Range Nursing Theories

UNIT

1

Analysis of Nursing Theories

- *Analysis includes such activities as examination, inquiry, investigation, study, test, appraisal, estimation, evaluation, and judgment.*

- *Its purpose in education is to lead the student to new understanding through the process of organized review and critical thinking.*

- *Analysis of theoretical works utilizes knowledge of the theory development process, history and philosophy of science, logic, the nature of science within the discipline, and the state of progress in the various theoretical endeavors.*

- *The works of the nursing theorists analyzed in this text represent various types of theory that have been formalized as philosophies, conceptual frameworks, and theories.*

Introduction to Analysis of Nursing Theories

Ann Marriner Tomey

REASONS FOR THEORY

Theory helps provide knowledge to improve practice by describing, explaining, predicting, and controlling phenomena. Nurses' power is increased through theoretical knowledge because systematically developed methods are more likely to be successful. In addition, nurses will know why they are doing what they are doing if challenged. Theory provides professional autonomy by guiding the practice, education, and research functions of the profession. The study of theory helps develop analytical skills, challenge thinking, clarify values and assumptions, and determine purposes for nursing practice, education, and research.[15,16,22 77,83]

MAJOR CONCEPTS AND DEFINITIONS OF THEORY DEVELOPMENT

Philosophy

Philosophy is the science comprising logic, ethics, aesthetics, metaphysics, and epistemology. It is the "investigation of causes and laws underlying reality" and is "inquiry into the nature of things based on logical reasoning rather than empirical methods."[55:985]

Science

Science is "the observation, identification, description, experimental investigation, and theoretical explanation of natural phenomena."[55:1162] It is a "body of knowledge."[13:72]

Knowledge

"Knowledge is an awareness or perception of reality acquired through learning or investigation."[15:72]

Fact

A fact is "something known with certainty."[55:469]

Model

"A model is an idea that explains by using symbolic and physical visualization."[90:62] Symbolic models may be verbal, schematic, or quantitative. They no longer have a recognizable physical form and are a higher level of abstraction than physical models are. Verbal models are worded statements. Schematic models may be diagrams, drawings, graphs, or pictures. Quantitative models are mathematical symbols. Physical models may look like what they are supposed to represent, for example, body organs, or they may become more abstract while still keeping some of the physical properties, like ECG.[37] Models can be used "to facilitate thinking about concepts and relationships between them"[13] or to map out the research process.[14]

Conceptual Model

Conceptual models are made up of abstract and general ideas (concepts) and propositions that specify their relationships.[22]

Paradigm

A paradigm is "a conceptual diagram."[90:62] It can be a large structure used to organize theory.

Theory

A theory is "a set of concepts, definitions, and propositions that project a systematic view of phenomena by designing specific interrelationships among concepts for purposes of describing, explaining, and predicting."[15:79]

Concept

A concept is a "complex mental formulation of an object, property, or event that is derived from individual perceptual experience."[15:202] It is "an idea, a mental image, or a generalization formed and developed in the mind."[2:116] Concepts label phenomena.

Abstract concept. Abstract concepts are completely independent of time or place. Temperature, for example, is an abstract concept.[78:49]

Concrete concept. A concrete concept is specific to time and place, such as the body temperature of a specific person, at a specific time, on a specific day.[78:49]

Phenomenon

A phenomenon is "any occurrence or fact that is directly perceptible by the senses."[78:983] It is reality on "what exists in the real world."[34:7]

Definitions

Definitions are statements of the meaning of a word, phrase, or term.[55:346]

Theoretical definitions. Theoretical definitions convey the general meaning of the concept in a manner that fits the theory.[15:207]

Operational definitions. Operational definitions specify "the activities of 'operations' necessary to measure a construct or a variable."[88:62]

Assumptions

Assumptions are statements supposed to be true without proof or demonstration.[42:80] They may be explicit or implicit.[15:126]

Theoretical Statements

Theoretical statements describe a relationship between two or more concepts.

Law. A law is "a statement that describes a relationship in which scientists have so much confidence they consider it an absolute 'truth.'"[78:78]

Axiom. Axioms are "a basic set of statements, each independent of the others (they say different things), from which all other statements of the theory may be logically derived."[78:78] Axioms are often associated with plane geometry.

Proposition. Propositions are theorems or statements derived from axioms. The term is often used interchangeably with hypotheses to mean "any idea or hunch that is presented in the form of a scientific statement."[78:78]

Hypothesis. A hypothesis is a relationship statement to be tested.[78:78]

Empirical generalization. Empirical generalizations are patterns "of events found in a number of different empirical studies."[78:79]

Existence statement. Existence statements establish a topology by indicating a concept exists.[78:76]

Relational statement. Relational statements indicate that values of one concept are associated or correlated with values of another. Relationships may be linear or curvilinear. Linear relationships may be either positive ("when one concept occurs, or is high, the other concept occurs, or is high, or vice versa") or negative ("when one concept occurs or is high, the other concept is low, and vice versa") or no relationship may exist (when "the occurrence of one concept gives no information about the occurrence of the other concept and vice versa").[78:70] Curvilinear relationships are characterized by curved lines (when one concept is high and low, the other concept is high or low).

Causal statement. One concept is believed to cause the occurrence of another concept if they have a causal relationship.[78:71] Correlation is not causation.

Deterministic statement. Dependent variables are determined by independent variables.[78:74]

Probabilistic statement. Probability predicts both nonoccurrence and occurrence of something.[78:75]

Research

"Research is application of systematic methods to obtain reliable and valid knowledge about empirical reality."[15:82] Research may generate theory with an inductive approach or test it by a deductive approach.

Range of Theories

"Subject matter for a theory may be very broad and all inclusive or very narrow and limited."[34:13]

Grand theory. Grand theories are broad in scope and complex. "In most instances, grand theories require further specification and partitioning of theoretical statements for them to be empirically tested and theoretically verified. Grand theorists state their theoretical formulations at the most general level of abstraction, and it is often difficult to link these formulations to reality."[34:13] Grand theories contain summative concepts that incorporate smaller range theories.

Middle-range theory. Middle-range theory has a narrower focus than grand theory and a broader focus than micro theory. The scope is not so large as to be relatively useless for summative concepts and not so narrow that it cannot be used to explain complex life situations.[54:68]

Micro theory. Micro theories are the least complex and most specific. They are "a set of theoretical statements, usually hypotheses, that deal with narrowly defined phenomena."[34:13]

DEVELOPMENT OF THEORY
Theory Development Process

Theory development is a process that primarily involves induction, deduction, and retroduction.

Induction. Induction is "a form of reasoning that moves from the specific to the general. In inductive logic, a series of particulars is combined into a larger whole or set of things. In inductive research, particular events are observed and analyzed as a basis for formulating general theoretical statements, often called grounded 'theory.'"[15:204] This is a research-to-theory approach.

Deduction. Deduction is a form of logical reasoning that progresses from general to specific. This process involves a sequence of theoretical statements derived from a few general statements or axioms. Two or more relational statements are used to draw a conclusion. Abstract theoretical relationships are used to derive specific empirical hypotheses. This is a theory-to-research approach.[15:202]

Retroduction. Retroduction combines induction and deduction.[15:205]

Forms of Theory

Theories may be organized according to their form into three categories. These categories include set-of-laws, axiomatic, and causal process.

Set-of-laws. Set-of-laws is an inductive approach that seeks patterns in research findings. Research findings are selected and sorted according to degree of empirical support into categories of laws, empirical generalizations, and hypotheses. It may be difficult to organize and interrelate these generalizations. Because the statements are not interrelated, support for one statement does not support another statement. Consequently, research efforts must be extensive.[78]

Axiomatic. The axiomatic form is an interrelated logical system of concepts, definitions, and relationship statements arranged in hierarchical order. Abstract axioms are at the top of the hierarchy, with derived propositions being lower. Required research is less extensive because empirical support for one relational statement also supports the theory.[78]

Causal process. The causal process increases understanding through relationship statements that specify cause between independent and dependent variables. This form also requires concepts, definitions, and relationship statements. It explains how something happens.[78,88]

CRITERIA FOR EVALUATION OF THEORY

Although many authors use different terms to describe criteria for evaluating theory, issues often discussed are clarity, simplicity, generality, empirical precision, and derivable consequences.

Clarity

Semantic and structural clarity and consistency are important. To assess these, one should identify the major concepts and subconcepts and identify definitions for them. Words should be invented only if necessary, and they should be carefully defined. Sometimes words have multiple and competing meanings within and across disciplines. Therefore words should be borrowed cautiously and defined carefully. Diagrams and examples may provide more clarity and should be consistent. The logical development should be clear, and assumptions should be consistent with the theory's goals.[14:133-137]

Reynolds refers to intersubjectivity when he says, "there must be shared agreement of the definitions of concepts and relationships between concepts within a theory."[78:13] Hardy refers to meaning and logical adequacy when stating that "concepts and relationships between concepts must be clearly identified and valid."[28:106] Stevens also speaks of clarity and consistency.[85] Ellis refers to the criterion of terminology to evaluate theory and addresses the danger of lost meaning when terms are borrowed from other disciplines and used in a different context.[18:221] Walker and Avant say, "Logical adequacy of a theory is the logical structure of the concepts and statements independent of the meaning of those concepts or statements."[89:119]

Simplicity

Chinn and Jacobs state, "In nursing, practitioners need simple theory to guide practice."[14:138] Argyris

and Schon indicate that a theory "should be maximally comprehensive and concrete, and it should do so with the fewest concepts and the simplest relations of concepts."[6:198] In contrast, Ellis believes a theory must have complexity to be significant.[18:219] Reynolds suggests that simply counting the number of concepts is not sufficient. He says the most useful theory provides the greatest sense of understanding.[78:135] Walker and Avant refer to parsimony as "elegant in its simplicity, even though it may be broad in content."[89:130]

Generality

To determine the generality of a theory, the scope of concepts and goals within the theory are examined. The more limited the concepts and goals, the less general the theory. Ada Jacox says, "There is no pressing need to develop a 'grand theory' that supposedly includes everything that nurses need to know."[85:65] Chinn and Jacobs believe situations to which the theory applies should not be limited.[14:139-140] Ellis says, "The broader the scope, the greater the significance of the theory."[18:219] Stevens suggests that both broad and narrow scopes are necessary and that their complexity or simplicity should be determined by the complexity of the subject matter.[85:65-66]

Empirical Precision

Empirical precision is linked to the testability and ultimate use of a theory and refers to the "extent that the defined concepts are grounded in observable reality."[14:144] Hardy states that "how well the evidence supports the theory is indicative of empirical adequacy" and agrees there "should be a match between theoretical claims and the empirical evidence."[28:105] Reynolds refers to empirical relevance and the trait that "anyone be able to examine the correspondence between a particular theory and the objective empirical data.[78:18] He notes that other scientists should be able to evaluate and verify results of themselves. Walker and Avant say, "If theory cannot generate hypotheses, it is not useful to scientists and does not add to the body of knowledge."[89:131] In contrast, Ellis states that the testability of a theory can be sacrificed in favor of scope, complexity, and clinical usefulness.

Elegance and complexity of structure are preferred to precision in the meaning of concepts.[18:220] She maintains that theories should be clearly recognized as tentative and hypothetical. Chinn and Jacobs believe "if research, theory, and practice are to be meaningfully related, then theory in nursing should lend itself to research testing, and research testing should guide practice."[15:145]

Derivable Consequences

Chinn and Jacobs state, "Nursing theory ought to guide research and practice, generate new ideas, and differentiate the focus of nursing from other professions."[15:145] Ellis indicates that to be considered useful, "it is essential for theory to develop and guide practice. . . . Theories should reveal what knowledge nurses must, and should, spend time pursuing."[15:220] Hardy believes the nursing profession should "make use of existing theory to predict certain outcomes and control events in such a way that desired outcomes are achieved."[28:106]

NURSING THEORISTS' WORKS

There are various ways in which theoretical works might be organized, such as using broad classifications that are also used by other disciplines, as was done in the first two editions of this text. However, by the third edition of the text, progress had been made in nursing so that the works could be categorized according to a structure of nursing knowledge that differentiated nursing models from nursing theories.[23] In addition, by this time very early works, as well as several more recent works, were noted to be philosophical in nature.[4] Therefore, beginning with the third edition, the works of the nursing theorists were organized into one of three types of knowledge based on their predominant characteristics as a type of theoretical work in nursing. These categories continue to be used in this fourth edition.

Philosophies

The early work used analysis, reasoning, and logical argument to identify nursing phenomena and predated nursing theory. In the late 1980s and early 1990s the philosophy of humanistic nursing resurfaced. Nightingale, Wiedenbach, Henderson, Abdellah, Hall, Watson, and Benner are grouped together because of their views about humanistic nursing as both an art and a science.

Florence Nightingale believed every woman would be responsible for someone's health at some time and, consequently, would be a nurse. She thought disease was a reparative process and the nurse should manipulate the environment to facilitate the process. Her directions regarding ventilation, warmth, light, diet, cleanliness, and noise are recorded in her *Notes on Nursing.*[64,65]

Ernestine Wiedenbach, a maternity nurse, was stimulated by Orlando to think about the use of self and how thoughts and feelings affect a nurse's actions and by Dickoff and James about theory development.[17] She identifies and defines many concepts in her book *Clinical Nursing: A Helping Art.*[93] Concepts and subconcepts include patient, need-for-help, nurse, purpose, philosophy, practice (knowledge, judgment, and skills), ministration, validation, coordination (reporting, consulting, conferring), and art (stimulus, preconception, interpretation, and actions—rational, reactionary, and deliberative). Nurses need to identify the patient's need-for-help by (1) observing behaviors consistent or inconsistent with comfort, (2) exploring the meaning of patient's behavior with him, (3) determining the cause of the discomfort or incapability, and (4) determining if the person can resolve his problem or has a need-for-help. Next the nurse administers the help needed and validates that the need-for-help was met.

Virginia Henderson has made enormous contributions to nursing in her more than 60 years of service as a nurse, teacher, author, and researcher. She has published prolifically throughout those years. Her definition of nursing first appeared in 1955 in the fifth edition of *Textbook of the Principles and Practice of Nursing* by Hauner and Henderson.[29] Henderson indicates, "The unique function of the nurse is to assist the individual, sick or well, in the performance of those activities contributing to health or its recovery (or to peaceful death) that he would perform unaided if he had the necessary strength, will, or knowledge and to do this in such a way as to help him gain independence as rapidly as possible."[31:7]

In *The Nature of Nursing: A Definition and Its Implications for Practice, Research, and Education* (1991), she also identified the following 14 basic needs of patients that comprise the components of nursing care: (1) breathing, (2) eating and drinking, (3) elimination, (4) movement, (5) rest and sleep, (6) suitable clothing, (7) body temperature, (8) clean body and protected integument, (9) safe environment, (10) communication, (11) worship, (12) work, (13) play, (14) learning.[31:16-17] She identified three levels of nurse-patient relationships in which the nurse is a (1) substitute for the patient, (2) helper to the patient, and (3) partner with the patient.[31:16] She supports empathetic understanding and says the nurse needs to "get inside the skin of each of her patients in order to know what he needs."[30:63] Henderson believes many nurses' and physicians' functions overlap. She says the nurse works in interdependence with other health professionals, and she compares the health team to wedges on a pie graph. The sizes of pie vary, depending on the patient's needs. The goal is to have the patient represented by most of the pie as he gains independence.[31:22-23]

In *The Nature of Nursing: Reflections After 25 Years* (1991), Henderson added addendums to each chapter of the 1966 edition to present changes in her views and to explain her opinions.[32]

Faye Glenn Abdellah has written prolifically since the early 1950s about a variety of subjects. She and others conceptualized 21 nursing problems based on systematic use of research data to teach and evaluate students. The typology of 21 nursing problems first appeared in the 1960 edition of *Patient-Centered Approaches to Nursing.*[1]

Lydia E. Hall used her philosophy of nursing to design and develop the Loeb Center for Nursing at Montefiore Hospital in New York. She served as administrative director of the Loeb Center from its opening in 1963 until her death in 1969. Most of her work was published in the 1960s. Her model for nursing was presented in 1964 in "Nursing: What Is It?" in *The Canadian Nurse*[26] and discussed in 1969 in "The Loeb Center for Nursing and Rehabilitation" in the *International Journal of Nursing Studies.*[27] She believed nursing functions differently in the three interlocking circles that constitute aspects of the patient. She labeled the circles the body (the care), the disease (the cure), and the person (the core). Nursing functions in all three circles but shares them with other providers to different degrees. Hall believed that more professional nursing care and teaching are needed as less medical care is needed and that professional nursing care will hasten recovery.

Jean Watson started publishing in the mid-1970s. Her book *Nursing: The Philosophy and Science of Caring* was published in 1979.[90] The content was further refined in *Nursing: Human Science and Health Care* in 1985.[91] In an effort to reduce the dichotomy between theory and practice, Watson proposed a philosophy and science of caring. She identified the following 10 carative factors: (1) the formation of a humanistic-altruistic system of values; (2) the instillation of faith-hope; (3) the cultivation of sensitivity to self and to others; (4) the development of a helping-trust relationship; (5) the promotion and acceptance of the expression of positive and negative; (6) the systematic use of the scientific problem-solving method for decision making; (7) the promotion of interpersonal teaching-learning; (8) the provision for a supportive, protective, or corrective mental, physical, sociocultural, and spiritual environment; (9) assistance with the gratification of human needs; and (10) the allowance for existential-phenomenological forces. Watson believes nurses should develop health promotion through preventive actions such as recognizing coping skills and adaptation to loss, teaching problem-solving methods, and providing situational support. Jean Watson extended her previous work on caring to transpersonal caring in *Nursing: Human Science and Human Care: A Theory of Nursing* in 1988.[92]

Patricia Benner validated the Dreyfus model of skill acquisition in nursing practice by systematic description of the five stages—novice, advanced beginner, competent, proficient, and expert. In *From Novice to Expert: Excellence and Power in Clinical Nursing Practice* (1984), she provided many exemplars and described nursing practice at each stage.[9] Seven domains of nursing practice were derived from the descriptions of the cases, and a list of 31 nursing competencies was generated. From Benner's description of nursing practice, a phenomenological theory describing caring evolved and is presented in Benner and Wrubel's 1989 book, in which they examine the relationships among caring, stress and coping, and health. They declare that caring is primary in *The Primacy of Caring: Stress and Coping in Health and Illness*, which was published in 1989. Further work has been published in Benner's 1994 publication, *Interpretative Phenomenology: Embodiment, Caring and Ethics in Health and Illness*[10] and in Benner, Tanner, and Chesla's 1996 publication, *Expertise in Nursing Practice: Caring, Clinical Practice, and Ethics.*[11]

Conceptual Models

The grand theorists often included aspects of human beings, their environment, and health in the nursing conceptual models. Orem; Levine; Rogers; Johnson; Roy; Neuman; King; and Roper, Logan, and Tierney are clustered together because they developed conceptual models that helped direct theory development.

Dorothea E. Orem had a spontaneous insight in 1958 about the concept of nursing. She has been publishing since the 1950s about nursing practice and education. She identifies her Self-Care Deficit Theory of nursing as a general theory composed of the following three related theories: (1) the Theory of Self-Care, (2) the Theory of Self-Care Deficit, and (3) the Theory of Nursing Systems. Orem identifies the following three types of nursing systems: (1) wholly compensatory—doing for the patient, (2) partly compensatory—helping the person do for himself, and (3) supportive-educative—helping the person learn to do for himself. The theories are discussed more fully in her book *Nursing: Concepts of Practice.* She believes nurses share some functions with other health care providers.[66]

Myra Estrin Levine started publishing in the mid-1960s and has written about numerous topics. Never intending to develop theory, she wrote *Introduction to Clinical Nursing*[45,47] as a textbook to teach medical-surgical nursing to beginning students. Journal articles containing information about holism and the four conservation principles of nursing include "Adaptation and Assessment: A Rationale for Nursing Intervention,"[43] "The Four Conservation Principles of Nursing,"[41] "For Lack of Love Alone,"[42] "The

Pursuit of Wholeness,"[44] and "Holistic Nursing."[46] More recently, Levine has given presentations about the conservation principles at nurse theory conferences, some of which have been audiotaped. Wholism, holism, integrity, and conservation are major concepts. The nurse is to use the principles of conservation of (1) energy, (2) structural integrity, (3) personal integrity, and (4) social integrity to keep the holism of the individual balanced. Levine also identified four levels of organismic response—fear, inflammatory response, response to stress, and sensory response—and recommended trophicognosis, a scientific approach to determine nursing care, as an alternative to nursing diagnosis.

Levine substantially changes and clarifies her theory in her chapter, "Four Conservation Principles: Twenty Years Later," in Riehl-Sisca's 1989 book, *Conceptual Models for Nursing Practice.*[80] She indicates that adaptation is the essence of conservation and elaborates on how redundancy characterizes availability of adaptive responses when stability is threatened. Adaptation processes establish a body economy to safeguard the individual's stability.

Levine admits that research must focus on discrete issues but stresses the importance of acknowledging all four conservation principles to sustain wholeness of a person in her chapter in *Levine's Conservation Model: A Framework for Nursing Practice* (1991), edited by Schaefer and Pond.[48]

Martha E. Rogers, considered one of the most creative thinkers in nursing, has published widely since the early 1960s. Her work regarding Unitary Human Beings is published in *An Introduction to the Theoretical Basis of Nursing.*[81] She characterizes life process by wholeness, openness, unidirectionality, pattern and organization, sentience, and thought. She also works with energy fields, open systems, and four-dimensionality. The principles are (1) complementarity, mutual and simultaneous movement of human and environmental fields; (2) resonancy, wave patterns that change from lower frequency to higher frequency patterns; and (3) helicy, field changes characterized by increasing diversity of field patterns. Rogers has stimulated a number of other scholars including Fitzpatrick, Newman, and Parse. In 1986, Dr. Malinski's *Explorations on Martha*

Rogers's Science of Unitary Human Beings provided evidence of pure and applied research extending Dr. Rogers's conceptual systems.[49] *Visions of Rogers's Science-Based Nursing* by Barrett in 1990 represented evolutionary movement in Rogerian science.[8]

Dorothy E. Johnson published from the mid-1940s to the early 1970s, with most of her work published during the 1960s. Many of her unpublished works are housed at Vanderbilt University. Johnson presented her behavioral system model in Riehl and Roy's book, *Conceptual Models for Nursing Practice*.[33] She identified the following six subsystems of the behavioral system: (1) attachment-affiliation, (2) achievement, (3) sexual, (4) ingestive-eliminative, (5) aggressive, and (6) dependency. Each subsystem can be analyzed in terms of structure and functional requirements. The four structural elements are (1) drive, or goal; (2) set, a predisposition to act; (3) choice, alternatives for action; and (4) behavior. The functional requirements are protection, nurturance, and stimulation. A need for nursing intervention exists if there is a state of instability in the behavioral system. The nurse needs to identify the source of the problem in the system and take appropriate nursing actions to maintain or restore the behavioral system balance.

Sister Callista Roy has been publishing prolifically since the late 1960s. She developed her adaptation model after being challenged by Johnson to develop a conceptual model for nursing. It is discussed at length in Roy's book, *Introduction to Nursing: An Adaptation Model*,[83,84] and in *Essentials of the Roy Adaptation Model* by Andrews and Roy.[5] Major concepts include system, adaptation, stimuli, regulator, cognator, and adaptive modes—physiological, self-concept, role performance, and interdependence. Man's self and his environment are sources of focal, residual, and conceptual stimuli that create needs for adaptation. The four interrelated adaptive modes are physiological needs, self-concept, role function, and interdependence. The adaptation mechanisms are the regulator and the cognator. Adaptation maintains integrity. Roy believes people constantly scan the environment for stimuli so they can respond and adapt. The nurse is to help the person adapt by managing the environment.

Betty Neuman developed her first teaching-practice model for mental health consultation in the late 1960s. She designed the Systems Model in 1970 to help graduate students evaluate nursing problems. It was first published in *Nursing Research* in 1972[59] and further refined in *The Neuman Systems Model* in 1982, 1989, and 1995.[56-58] Major concepts include the following: total persons approach, holism, open-system, stressors, energy resources, lines of resistance, lines of defense, degree of reaction, interventions, levels of prevention, and reconstitution. By 1989, the spiritual variable was explicitly added to the Neuman Systems Model and created-environment was added to the typology as a safety mechanism for the system. Neuman believes the nurse should use purposeful interventions and a total person approach to help individuals, families, and groups reach and maintain wellness.

Imogene King has been publishing since the mid-1960s. *Toward a Theory for Nursing* was published in 1971,[35] and *A Theory for Nursing* was published in 1981.[36] Many of her publications have dealt with conceptual framework, models, theory, and specifically her theory of goal attainment. King's conceptual framework specifies the following three interacting systems: personal system, interpersonal system, and social system. The concepts of the personal system are perception, self, body image, growth and development, and time and space. The concepts of the interpersonal system are role, interaction, communication, and transaction and stress. The concepts of the social system are organization, power-authority status, and decision making and role. From her major concepts—interaction, perception, communication, transaction, role, stress, growth and development, and time and space—she derived her theory of goal attainment. She suggests that the patient's and the nurse's perceptions, judgments, and actions lead to reaction, interaction, and transaction, which she describes as the process of nursing.

Nancy Roper started publishing about the principles of nursing in the 1960s. She has since asked Winifred W. Logan and Alison J. Tierney to work with her to refine a Model for Nursing based on a Model for Living. The latest edition of *The Elements* of Nursing: A Model for Nursing Based on a Model for Living[82] was published in 1996. These European theorists have refined a model with five major concepts: (1) 12 activities of living (ALs), (2) life span, (3) dependence-independence continuum, (4) factors influencing ALs, and (5) individuality. The 12 ALs include maintaining a safe environment, communicating, breathing, eating and drinking, eliminating, personal cleansing and dressing, controlling body temperature, mobilizing, working and playing, expressing sexuality, sleeping, and dying. Life span ranges from birth to death, and the dependence-independence continuum ranges from total dependence to total independence. The five groups of factors influencing the ALs are biological, psychological, sociocultural, environmental, and politicoeconomic. The individuality in living is the way the individual attends to the ALs given the individual's place on the life span, place on the dependence-independence continuum, and as influenced by biological, psychological, environmental, and politicoeconomic factors.

Nursing Theories

Middle-range theories are more precise than grand theories and focus on developing theoretical statements to answer questions about nursing. Peplau, Orlando, Travelbee, Riehl-Sisca, Erickson, Tomlin, Swain, Mercer, Barnard, Leininger, Parse, Fitzpatrick, Newman, Adam, and Pender are middle-range theorists.

Hildegard E. Peplau's contributions to nursing in general and the specialty of psychiatric nursing specifically have been enormous. She has been publishing prolifically since the early 1950s, beginning with her book *Interpersonal Relations in Nursing.*[77] She teaches psychodynamic nursing and stresses the importance of the nurse's understanding his or her own behavior in order to help others identify perceived difficulties. She identifies the following four phases of the nurse-patient relationship: (1) orientation, (2) identification, (3) exploitation, and (4) resolution. Peplau describes the following six nursing roles: (1) stranger, (2) resource person, (3) teacher, (4) leader, (5) surrogate, and (6) counselor. She discusses four psychobiological experiences—needs,

frustrations, conflicts, and anxieties— that compel destructive or constructive responses.

Ida Jean Orlando (Pelletier) first described her discipline's Professional Response Theory in *The Dynamic Nurse-Patient Relationship* in 1961,[67] which was reissued by the National League for Nursing in 1990.[69] Related research is reported in *The Discipline and Teaching of Nursing Process.*[68] Her theory stresses the reciprocal relationship between the nurse and the patient. Each is affected by what the other says and does. Orlando emphasizes the importance of exploring perceptions, thoughts, and feelings with the other party for verification. This process, discipline, or exploration validates the patient's need for help, which the nurse then meets directly or indirectly. Deliberative nursing actions purposefully identify and meet the patient's immediate need for help. If nursing actions are not deliberative, they are automatic and may not meet the patient's need for help.

Joyce Travelbee published predominantly in the mid-1960s. She died in 1973 at a relatively young age. Travelbee promoted her Human-to-Human Relationship Model in her book, *Interpersonal Aspects of Nursing.*[86,87] She wrote about illness, suffering, pain, hope, communication, interaction, therapeutic use of self, empathy, sympathy, and rapport. She believed nursing was accomplished through human-to-human relationships that began with (1) the original encounter and then progressed through stages of (2) emerging identities, (3) developing feelings of empathy, and (4) later of sympathy, until (5) the nurse and patient attained a rapport in the final stage.

Joan Riehl-Sisca began publishing in the mid-1970s. Her work on symbolic interactionism is presented in Riehl and Roy's book, *Conceptual Models for Nursing Practice.*[79] According to Symbolic Interactionism Theory, people interpret each other's actions based on the meaning attached to the action before reacting. Human interaction is mediated by symbols, interpretation, and meaning and is a process of interpretation between the stimulus and response.

Helen C. Erickson, Evelyn M. Tomlin, and *Mary Ann P. Swain's* book, *Modeling and Role-Modeling: A Theory and Paradigm for Nursing*[20] was published in 1983 and 1990,[21] and Erickson published *Modeling and Role-Modeling: Theory, Practice and Research*[19] with Kinney in 1990. Modeling is developing an understanding of the client's world. Role-modeling is the nursing intervention, or nurturance, that requires unconditional acceptance. Erickson, Tomlin, and Swain believe that while people are alike because of their holism, lifetime growth and development, and affiliated individualism, they are also different because of inherent endowment, adaptation, and self-care knowledge.

Ramona T. Mercer has researched and published prolifically since the 1970s. She systematically researched the field of maternal role attainment and developed a complex model about factors impacting on maternal role development over time. Mercer's work culminates in her 1986 book *First-Time Motherhood: Experience from Teens to Forties.*[50] With Elizabeth G. Nichols and Glen Caspers Doyle, Mercer published a study of transitions in the life cycle of 80 women in *Transitions in a Woman's Life: Major Life Events in Developmental Context* in 1989.[53] Mercer's book *Parents at Risk* was published in 1990[51] and *Becoming a Mother: Research on Maternal Role Identity Since Rubin* was published in 1995.[52]

Kathryn E. Barnard[7] is an active researcher who has published extensively about infants and children since the mid-1960s. She started by studying mentally and physically handicapped children and adults, moved into studying activities of the well child, and then expanded her work to include methods of evaluating growth and development of children and mother-infant relationships. She was also concerned about disseminating research and consequently developed the Nursing Child Assessment Satellite Training Project. While Barnard never intended to develop theory, the longitudinal nursing child assessment study provided the basis for her Child Health Assessment Interaction Model. Barnard believes that the parent-infant system is influenced by individual characteristics of each member and that those characteristics are modified to meet the needs of the system by adaptive behavior.[7]

Madeleine Leininger has published prolifically about a variety of topics since 1960. Although she has written several books about transcultural nursing and caring, the most complete account of Transcultural Care Theory was found in her 1984 book *Care:*

The Essence of Nursing and Health.[38] Some of the major concepts are care, caring, culture, cultural values, and cultural variations. Leininger has generated many hypotheses and hopes to stimulate further ethnoscience research by nurses in ethnonursing. Her more recent books are *Culture Care Diversity and Universality: A Theory of Nursing*[39] (1991), *Transcultural Nursing: Concepts, Theories, Research and Practices*[40] (1995), and *Caring: The Compassionate Healer* (1991) with Gaut.[25]

Rosemarie Rizzo Parse drew from the work of Martha Rogers and the existential-phenomenologists for the development of *Man-Living-Health: A Theory of Nursing.*[70] Major concepts include imaging, valuing, languaging, revealing-concealing, enabling-limiting, connecting-separating, power, originating, and transforming. Parse stresses humanism. She described research methods for studying her theory in *Nursing Research: Qualitative Methods.*[72] She presented her theory and others in *Nursing Science: Major Paradigms, Theories, and Critiques.*[71]

Joyce J. Fitzpatrick derived her Life Perspective Model from Rogers's work. The major concepts are nursing, person, health, environment, temporal patterns, motion patterns, consciousness patterns, and perceptual patterns. She began publishing in 1970 and has written about aging, suicidology, temporal experience, and motor behavior.[24]

Margaret A. Newman started publishing in the mid-1960s. She has drawn from several fields of inquiry and was influenced by Johnson and Rogers. Her model appeared in *Theory Development in Nursing*[60] and has been explained further in subsequent chapters of various books and in her 1986 book *Health as Expanding Consciousness.*[61] More recently she has published *Health as Expanding Consciousness* (1994) and *A Developing Discipline: Selected Work of Margaret Newman* (1995).[62,63] The major concepts in her model of health are movement, time, space, and consciousness. They are all interrelated. "Movement is a reflection of consciousness. Time is a function of movement. Time is a measure of consciousness. Movement is a means whereby space and time become a reality."[60]

Evelyn Adam started publishing in the mid-1970s. Much of her work focuses on development models and theories on the concept of nursing. She uses a model she learned from Dorothy Johnson. In her book, *To Be a Nurse*,[2] she applies Virginia Henderson's definition of nursing to the model and identifies the assumptions, beliefs and values, and major units. In the latter category she includes the goal of the profession, the beneficiary of the professional service, the role of the professional, the source of the beneficiary's difficulty, the intervention of the professional, and the consequences. She expands her work in the second edition.[3]

Nola Pender began the foundation for studying how individuals made decisions about their own health in her article, "A Conceptual Model for Preventive Health Behavior."[73] In her book, *Health Promotion in Nursing Practice*, she suggests that optimal health supersedes disease prevention. Her health promotion model identifies cognitive-perceptual factors and modifying factors that influence participation in health-promoting behavior. Importance of health, perceived control of health and self-efficacy, definition of health, perceived health status, benefits of health promoting behaviors, and barriers to health-promoting behaviors are cognitive-perceptual factors. Modifying factors include demographic characteristics, biological characteristics, interpersonal influences, situational factors, and behavioral factors. The interaction of cognitive-perceptual factors and modifying factors influences the likelihood of engaging in health-promoting behaviors.[74,75] The third edition of *Health Promotion in Nursing Practice*,[76] published in 1996, added three new variables that influence people to engage in health promotion activities: activity-related affect, commitment to a plan of action, and immediate competing demands and preferences.

EVALUATION OF THEORY DEVELOPMENT

Early nursing scholars dealt with the philosophy, definition, and art of nursing. Interpersonal communications received considerable attention during the 1960s. By the end of the decade the focus had shifted to the science of nursing. Humanism and nursing as an art and a science gained popularity during the 1980s.

The published works share some common themes. There is also evidence that scholars use the same or similar terms differently and have divergent views of nursing, environment, health, and person. Authors have also changed their views over time as their historical perspective changed. It is appropriate to analyze the previous work for themes, similarities, and differences to generate more ideas. Several middle- and micro-range theories are emerging to direct our nursing practice. As we develop generalizable theories about humanism, other disciplines have begun to borrow theory from nursing as we have borrowed theories from other disciplines.

REFERENCES

1. Abdellah, F.G., Beland, I.L., Martin, A., & Matheney, R.V.(1960). *Patient-centered approaches to nursing*. New York: Macmillan.
2. Adam, E. (1980). *To be a nurse*. Philadelphia: W.B. Saunders.
3. Adam, E. (1991). *To be a nurse*. Montreal: W.B. Saunders Company Canada Ltd.
4. Alligood, M.R. (1994). Evolution of nursing theory development. In Ann Marriner-Tomey (Ed.), *Nursing theorists and their work* (pp. 58-69). St. Louis: Mosby.
5. Andrews, H., & Roy, C. (1986). *Essentials of the Roy adaptation model*. Norwalk, CT: Appleton-Century-Crofts.
6. Argyris, C., & Schon, D. (1974). *Theory in practice*. San Francisco: Jossey-Bass.
7. Barnard, K.E. (1978). *Nursing child assessment and training: Learning resource manual*. Seattle: University of Washington.
8. Barrett, E.A.M. (Ed.). (1990). *Visions of Rogers's science-based nursing*. New York: National League for Nursing.
9. Benner, P. (1984). *From novice to expert: Excellence and power in clinical nursing practice*. Menlo Park, CA: Addison-Wesley.
10. Benner, P. (1994). *Interpretive phenomenology: Embodiment, caring and ethics in health and illness*. Thousand Oaks, CA: Sage.
11. Benner, P., Tanner, C., & Chesla, C. (1996). *Expertise in nursing practice: Caring, clinical practice, and ethics*. New York: Springer.
12. Benner, P., & Wrubel, J. (1989). *The primacy of caring: Stress and coping in health and illness*. Menlo Park, CA: Addison-Wesley.
13. Bush, H.A. (1979). Models for nursing. *Advances in Nursing Science, 1* (2), 13-21.
14. Chinn, P., & Jacobs, M.K. (1979). A model for theory development in nursing. *Advances in Nursing Science, 1* (1), 1-11.
15. Chinn, P.L., & Jacobs, M.K. (1987). *Theory and nursing: A systematic approach*. St. Louis: Mosby.

16. DeTornyay, R. (1977, Nov.-Dec.). Nursing research: The road ahead. *Nursing Research, 26*, 404-407.

17. Dickoff, J., James, P., & Wiedenbach, E. (1968). Theory in a practice discipline, Part I. Practice oriented theory. *Nursing Research, 17* (5), 415-435.

18. Ellis, R. (1968). Characteristics of significant theories. *Nursing Research, 17* (5), 217-222.

19. Erickson, H., & Kinney, C. (Eds.). (1990). *Modeling and role-modeling: Theory, practice and research.* Austin: Society for Advancement of Modeling and Role-Modeling.

20. Erickson, H.C., Tomlin, E.M., & Swain, M.A. (1983). *Modeling and role-modeling: A theory and paradigm for nursing.* Englewood Cliffs, NJ: Prentice-Hall.

21. Erickson, H.C., Tomlin, E.M., & Swain, M.A. (1990). *Modeling and role-modeling: A theory and paradigm for nursing.* Englewood Cliffs, NJ: Prentice-Hall (EST Company Original Publication, 1983).

22. Fawcett, J. (1980, June). A declaration of nursing independence: The relation of theory and research to nursing practice. *Journal of Nursing Administration*, 10, 36-39.

23. Fawcett, J. (1993). *Analysis and evaluation of nursing theories.* Philadelphia: F.A. Davis.

24. Fitzpatrick, J., & Whall, A. (1983). *Conceptual models for nursing: Analysis and application.* Bowie, MD: Robert J. Brady.

25. Gaut, K., & Leininger, M. (1991). *Caring: The compassionate healer.* New York: National League for Nursing Press.

26. Hall, L.E. (1964, Feb.). Nursing: What is it? *The Canadian Nurse, 60*, 150-154.

27. Hall, L.E. (1969). The Loeb Center for nursing and rehabilitation. *International Journal of Nursing Studies, 6*, 81-95.

28. Hardy, M.E. (1978). Perspectives on nursing theory. *Advances in Nursing Science, 1*, 37-48.

29. Hauner, B., & Henderson, V. (1955). *Textbook of the principles and practice of nursing.* New York: Macmillan.

30. Henderson, V. (1964, Aug.). The nature of nursing. *American Journal of Nursing, 64*, 62-68.

31. Henderson, V. (1966). *The nature of nursing: A definition and its implications for practice, research, and education.* New York: Macmillan.

32. Henderson, V.A. (1991). *The nature of nursing: Reflections after 25 years.* New York: National League for Nursing Press.

33. Johnson, D.E. (1980). The behavioral system model for nursing. In J.P. Riehl & C. Roy (Eds.), *Conceptual models for nursing practice* (2nd ed.). New York: Appleton-Century-Crofts.

34. Kim, H.S. (1983). *The nature of theoretical thinking in nursing.* Norwalk, CT: Appleton-Century-Crofts.

35. King, I. (1971). *Toward a theory for nursing: General concepts of human behavior.* New York: John Wiley & Sons.

36. King, I. (1981). *A theory for nursing: Systems, concepts, process.* New York: John Wiley & Sons.

37. Lancaster, W., & Lancaster, J. (1981). Models and model building in nursing. *Advances in Nursing Science, 3*, 31-42.

38. Leininger, M. (Ed.). (1984). *Care: The essence of nursing and health.* Thorofare, NJ: Charles B. Slack.

39. Leininger, M. (1991). *Culture care diversity and universality: A theory of nursing.* New York: National League for Nursing Press.

40. Leininger, M. (1995). *Transcultural nursing: Concepts, theories, research and practices* (2nd ed.). New York: McGraw-Hill.

41. Levine, M. (1967). The four conservation principles of nursing. *Nursing Forum, 6*, 45.

42. Levine, M. (1967, Dec.). For lack of love alone. *Minnesota Nursing Accent, 39*, 179.

43. Levine, M.E. (1966). Adaptation and assessment: A rationale for nursing intervention. *American Journal of Nursing, 66*(11), 2450-2453.

44. Levine, M.E. (1969, Jan.). The pursuit of wholeness. *American Journal of Nursing, 69*, 93.

45. Levine, M.E. (1969). *Introduction to clinical nursing.* Philadelphia: F.A. Davis.

46. Levine, M.E. (1971, June). Holistic nursing. *Nursing Clinics of North America, 6*, 253.

47. Levine, M.E. (1973). *Introduction to clinical nursing* (2nd ed.). Philadelphia: F.A. Davis.

48. Levine, M.E. (1991). The conservation principles: A model for health. In F.M. Schaefer & J.B. Pond (Eds.), *Levine's conservation model: A framework for nursing practice.* Philadelphia: F.A. Davis.

49. Malinski, V.M. (1986). *Explorations on Martha Rogers's science of unitary human beings.* Norwalk, CT: Appleton-Century-Crofts.

50. Mercer, R.T. (1986). *First-time motherhood: Experiences from teens to forties.* New York: Springer.

51. Mercer, R.T. (1990). *Parents at risk.* New York: Springer.

52. Mercer, R.T. (1995). *Becoming a mother: Research on maternal role identity since Rubin.* New York: Springer.

53. Mercer, R.T., Nichols, E.G., & Doyle, G.C. (1989). *Transitions in a woman's life: Major life events in developmental context,* New York: Springer.

54. Merton, R. (1968). *Social theory and social structure.* New York: The Free Press.

55. Morris, W. (Ed.). (1978). *The American heritage dictionary of the English language.* Boston: Houghton Mifflin.

56. Neuman B. (1982). *The Neuman systems model: Application to nursing, education, and practice.* Norwalk, CT: Appleton-Century-Crofts.

57. Neuman, B. (1989). *The Neuman systems model: Application to nursing, education, and practice.* Norwalk, CT: Appleton-Century-Crofts.

58. Neuman, B. (1995). *The Neuman systems model* (3rd ed.). Norwalk, CT: Appleton-Lange.

59. Neuman, B.M., & Young, R.J. (1972, May-June). A model for teaching total person approach to patient problems. *Nursing Research, 21*, 264-269.

60. Newman, M. (1980). *Theory development in nursing.* Philadelphia: F.A. Davis.

61. Newman, M.A. (1986). *Health as expanding consciousness.* St. Louis: Mosby.

62. Newman, M.A. (1994). *Health as expanding consciousness* (2nd ed.). New York: National League for Nursing Press.

63. Newman, M.A. (1995). *A developing discipline: Selected work of Margaret Newman.* New York: National League for Nursing Press.

64. Nightingale, F. (1957). *Notes on nursing.* Philadelphia: J.B. Lippincott. (Originally published in 1859.)

65. Nightingale, F. (1992). *Notes on nursing: What it is, and what it is not.* Philadelphia: J.B. Lippincott.

66. Orem, D. (1985). *Nursing: Concepts of practice.* New York: McGraw-Hill.

67. Orlando, I. (1961). *The dynamic nurse/patient relationship.* New York: G.P. Putnam's Sons.

68. Orlando, I. (1972). *The discipline and teaching of nursing process.* New York: G.P. Putnam's Sons.

69. Orlando, I.J. (reissued 1991). *The dynamic nurse-patient relationship.* New York: National League for Nursing.

70. Parse, R.R. (1981). *Man-living-health: A theory of nursing.* New York: John Wiley & Sons.

71. Parse, R.R. (1987). *Nursing science: Major paradigms, theories, and critiques.* Philadelphia: W.B. Saunders.

72. Parse, R.R., Coyne, A.B., & Smith, M.J. (1985). *Nursing research: Qualitative methods.* Bowie, MD: Robert J. Brady.

73. Pender, N.J. (1975). A conceptual model for preventive health behavior. *Nursing Outlook, 23*(6), 385-390.

74. Pender, N.J. (1982). *Health promotion in nursing practice.* New York: Appleton-Century-Crofts.

75. Pender, N.J. (1987). *Health promotion in nursing practice* (2nd ed.). New York: Appleton & Lange.

76. Pender, N.J. (1996). *Health promotion in nursing practice* (3rd ed.). Norwalk, CT: Appleton & Lange.

77. Peplau, H. (1952). *Interpersonal relations in nursing.* New York: G.P. Putnam & Sons.

78. Reynolds, P.D. (1971). *A primer for theory construction.* Indianapolis: Bobbs-Merrill.

79. Riehl, J.P., & Roy, C. (Eds.). (1980). *Conceptual models for nursing practice* (2nd ed.). New York: Appleton-Century-Crofts.

80. Riehl-Sisca, J.P. (Ed.). (1989). *Conceptual models for nursing practice.* New York: Appleton-Century-Crofts.

81. Rogers, M.E. (1970). *An introduction to the theoretical basis of nursing.* Philadelphia: F.A. Davis.

82. Roper, N., Logan, W.W., & Tierney, A.J. (1996). *The elements of nursing: A model for nursing based on a model for living.* San Francisco: Churchill Livingstone.

83. Roy, C. (1976). *An introduction to nursing: An adaptation model.* Englewood Cliffs, NJ: Prentice-Hall.

84. Roy, C. (1984). *An introduction to nursing: An adaptation model* (2nd ed.). Englewood Cliffs, NJ: Prentice-Hall.

85. Stevens, B.J. (1984). *Nursing theory: Analysis, application, evaluation.* Boston: Little, Brown.

86. Travelbee, J. (1966). *Interpersonal aspects of nursing.* Philadelphia: F.A. Davis.

87. Travelbee, J. (1971). *Interpersonal aspects of nursing.* (2nd ed.) Philadelphia: F.A. Davis.

88. Turner, J.H. (1982). *The structure of sociological theory.* Homewood, IL: The Dorsey Press.

89. Walker, L., & Avant, K. (1983). *Strategies for theory construction in nursing.* Norwalk, CT: Appleton-Century-Crofts.

90. Watson, J. (1979). *Nursing: The philosophy and science of caring.* Boston: Little, Brown.

91. Watson, J. (1985). *Nursing: Human science and health care.* Norwalk, CT: Appleton-Century-Crofts.

92. Watson, J. (1988). *Nursing: Human science and human care: A theory of nursing.* New York: National League for Nursing.

93. Wiedenbach, E. (1964). *Clinical nursing: A helping art.* New York: Springer.

Terminology of Theory Development

Juanita Fogel Keck

Terms associated with theory and theory development have been used inconsistently in the nursing literature. Establishing the meanings of terms used in this book will enable the reader to gain a better understanding of the material covered. The definitions of terms used in this chapter represent those definitions accepted by a consensus of nursing theorists and noted philosophers of science.

In the interest of professionalism nursing leaders have suggested the discipline needs an identified body of knowledge that can be used to guide nursing practice. The terms *science, philosophy, theory,* and *paradigm* all relate to the development of an identified body of knowledge that can be recognized as associated with a particular scientific discipline.

SCIENCE

Science is defined as both a unified body of knowledge concerned with specific subject matter and the skills and methodologies necessary to provide such knowledge. Therefore nursing science is that knowledge germane to the discipline of nursing, plus the processes and methodologies used to gain that knowledge. A goal of science is the identification of truths or facts about the subject matter of a discipline—ascertaining the what, where, when, who, and how of phenomena of interest to the discipline.

KNOWLEDGE

The term *knowledge* suggests that science is composed of what one knows about the subject matter of a discipline. A distinction is made between what is *known* to be (fact) and what is *believed* to be. Knowledge is based on factual information. One derives a fact through the use of sound logic or empirical testing. Fact is truth supported by repeated observation and replication.[1]

Science is empirically based. Feigl[3] suggested a characteristic of science is that it is replicable by scientists using the appropriate scientific methodologies within a discipline. Replication requires that the components of phenomena studied to provide knowledge be observable and measurable. One acquires knowledge about things and events comprising the subject matter of interest through experience. Experiencing things or events requires the involvement of one or more of the human senses of sight, hearing, touch, taste, and smell. An empirical entity is that which can be experienced through the human senses.

PHENOMENA

Phenomena comprise the subject matter of a discipline. A *phenomenon* is defined as an object or aspect known through the senses rather than by thought or intuition, "a fact or event of scientific interest susceptible to scientific description and explanation."[18:1696]

PHILOSOPHY

Philosophy is concerned with judgments about components of science. Philosophical concerns are not empirically based. Components of a discipline that are not amenable to empirical testing are within the realm of philosophy. The "this we believe" statements associated with nursing practice contribute to the philosophy of the discipline. Statements that reflect values, goals, or opinions contribute to philosophy. It is the philosopher who suggests the methodologies by which scientific knowledge is obtained. Philosophical statements are based on opinion. They are by their very nature untestable because there is no definitive truth about them to discover. They cannot be tested for their correctness. They are accepted in a discipline through public affirmation. The prevailing philosophy of a discipline is the one shared by the greatest number of members in terms of accepting the beliefs, values, goals, and opinions of the philosophy.

THEORY

Although it is facts about phenomena of interest to the discipline that comprise the knowledge germane to the discipline, a mass of uncollated facts provides little guidance to the members of the discipline as they attempt to use that knowledge. The facts need to be ordered in a cohesive entity that will result in an organized body of knowledge. This will allow one to explain past events, provide a sense of understanding about current events, predict future events, and provide the potential for controlling them. If one can predict events, one has the basis for control of those

events. Nursing intervention is served through the ability to predict and ultimately to control phenomena associated with health and health care.

It is through the construction of theories that such ordering occurs. Theories are models of empirical real world phenomena that identify the components or elements of the phenomena and the relationships between them. Theories are comprised of hypothetical propositions that are not necessarily based on empirical data.[18]

A degree of uncertainty is inherent in theories. The concepts may be tentative and the propositions may be predictions of what reality is believed to be like rather than a set of known, undeniable facts.[8]

The functions of theory include summarization of knowledge, explanation of phenomena of interest to the discipline employing the theory, and provision of the means to predict and ultimately to control phenomena.[11;14] In fact, Theobald[16] suggested that only through theory is explanation or prediction possible. Hoover[8] suggested that theory contributes to the scientific base of a discipline by (1) providing a basis for interpreting observations and data about phenomena, (2) linking the results of research together, leading to cumulative scientific knowledge, (3) providing frameworks by which to study concepts and variables, allowing them to acquire special significance in terms of phenomena studied, and (4) providing a framework that allows interpretation of research findings beyond the specific data collection situation, thereby expanding the knowledge base of the discipline.

Numerous definitions of theory exist in the literature. Most reflect an understanding of theory consistent with the following: Theory is a logically consistent set of propositions that presents a systematic view of a phenomenon. A proposition is composed of the elements of the phenomenon and the relationships between them. The elements, or components, of a phenomenon are the concepts necessary to understand the phenomenon. The concepts are linked by specific statements identifying how two or more concepts are related to each other to provide understanding about the phenomenon. Therefore theories are composed of statements that state specific relationships between two or more concepts.

CONCEPTS

Concepts are the subject matter of theory. When concepts are employed in research efforts, they are symbolic representations of the things or events of which phenomena are composed. Concepts represent some aspect of reality that can be quantified. They are abstract and are derived from impressions the human mind receives about phenomena through sensing the environment.[15] In addition, Guba suggested that a concept has meaning only in the context of the theory to which it contributes.[4]

An example of concepts necessary to explain phenomenon is found in Hoffman's Beginning Theory of Altruism.[7] Altruism is the phenomenon Hoffman has attempted to explain. One of the propositions of the theory is that helping behavior and empathy are related in a curvilinear manner. Both low and high levels of empathy are associated with low levels of helping behavior. Moderate empathy is associated with a high level of helping. *Helping behavior* and *empathy* are the concepts comprising the proposition. To be able to ultimately explain altruism by means of this theory, one must include empathy and helping behavior (Fig. 2-1).

Dubin[2] categorized concepts into five groups— enumerative, associative, relational, statistical, and summative.

Enumerative Concepts

Enumerative concepts are characteristics of a phenomenon that are always present. The concept of *age* is an enumerative unit. Everyone to whom a theory incorporating age is generalizable is characterized by an age. The concept is universal to all persons in the population to which the theory applies. Age is always present in the phenomenon being explained. An enumerative concept cannot have a zero value. There is no such thing as an individual with zero age. As soon as an individual exists, his or her age can be ascertained.

Associative Concepts

Associative concepts are those concepts that can exist in only some conditions within the phenomenon.[2] Associative concepts can have a zero value. Persons to whom a theory composed of the concepts applies can exist with none of the concepts. Examples include income, presence of disease, and anxiety. It is possible to identify persons with no income in the population to which a theory incorporating income applies. Associative and enumerative units are the simplest, least complex forms of concepts.

Relational Concepts

Relational concepts are those characteristics of phenomenon that can be understood only through the combination or interaction of two or more enumerative or associative concepts.[2] *Elderly* is a concept that cannot be understood without an understanding of the combination of age and *longevity. Mother* cannot exist without the interaction of *man, woman,* and *birth.* Therefore both *elderly* and *mother* are relational concepts.

Statistical Concepts

Statistical concepts are those that relate the property of the thing being represented in terms of its distribution in the population.[2] *Average blood pressure* is an example of a statistical unit.

Summative Concepts

Summative concepts are the most complex. Dubin[2] suggested summative concepts were global units that

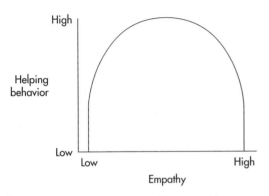

Fig. **2-1** Hoffman's Beginning Theory of Altruism.

represented an entire complex entity or phenomenon. Four concepts—nursing, man, health, and environment—have been identified by numerous nurse authors and theorists as the concepts of primary concern for the discipline of nursing. They are readily identifiable as summative concepts because each represents a global and extremely complex entity.

Dubin[2] suggested many problems exist when summative concepts are used within a theory. An entire phenomenon is explained by the use of one or two words. Each summative concept is composed of numerous enumerative, associative, and relational concepts and their interactions, but none are named or defined. One can only assume which of these less complex concepts contribute to the summative unit, how they interact, and under what conditions they contribute to the phenomenon.

Dubin[2] said that summative concepts have little use in theory development because the concepts cannot be adequately defined and the interactions between them are not readily ascertainable. For a theory to be useful in aiding the attainment of the goals of science, it must contribute to understanding, explanation, prediction, and ultimately control. Before prediction and control are possible, the theory must be testable. One can only predict future events if the proposed relationships between concepts have been repeatedly supported by empirical findings. In other words, the real world correlates of the concepts have been measured and the relationships between them verified. If such relationships have been repeatedly verified in the past, one can predict the relationship between the concepts will hold true in the future.

Summative units are not measurable. How would one measure environment as a totality? One is usually interested in individual components of environment and their interactions with some specific attributes of human beings. One may be interested in a theory that states a person's recovery from illness is related to environment. However, the theory is not useful to one concerned with a specific attribute of humans, such as *recovery,* unless specific aspects of the environment that influence recovery and their interactions are stated. A useful theory then would be composed of the less complex concepts that refer to the specific environmental attributes rather than the

totality of the environment. Concepts must be clearly definable and measurable to be of use to the practicing nurse in the clinical setting.

DEFINITIONS

Concepts are abstract symbols of the real world. They are mental representations constructed in language terms. The concepts of a theory reflect the theorist's own individual perception and definition of reality that the concept is supposed to represent. The concept may be open to many interpretations. Different individuals may hold differing understandings of the meanings of the words used to convey conceptual aspects of the real world. Definitions supplied by the theorist are needed so the user of theory can know what the theorist means by the concept. It is the theorist's meaning that must be used in the theory he or she developed. Therefore the user of theory must know the meaning intended by the author.

Two classifications of definitions are associated with theory. *Conceptual definitions* relate the general meaning of the concept. *Operational definitions* identify an empirical referent for the concept. For example, *pain* may be conceptually defined as a subjective experience perceived as unpleasant, initiated by potentially damaging stimuli but influenced by affective variables. It may be operationally defined as the score obtained on a 10 cm visual analogue scale in which 0 represents no pain and 10 represents the worst pain imaginable.

0	10
No pain	Worst pain imaginable

Scores are obtained by asking subjects to place a mark on the line to represent the severity of their pain. The resulting score is observable and is therefore an empirical referent for the subject's pain. The score is the operational definition for pain.

An additional classification of definitions may be considered. Definitions may be classified as either denotative or connotative. *Denotative definitions* define concepts in terms of what the concept is or represents. A denotative definition of father is *male parent.* Father is the male parent. A *connotative defini-*

tion suggests or implies associations one might make with the concept. A connotative definition suggests what one might think when considering the term *father*. A connotative definition of father is *strong, provider, disciplinarian,* that is, terms that are associated with *father.*

RELATIONSHIP STATEMENTS

Concepts alone do not create theory. A theory does not exist until the specific relationships between concepts comprising the theory are expressed in relationship statements. Several labels for relationship statements may be found in the literature related to theory. Relationship statements may be classified as propositions, hypotheses, empirical generalizations, laws, axioms, or theorems. Nursing and philosophical theorists essentially agree that all relationship statements, regardless of classification, indicate specific relationships between two or more concepts. Examples of relationship statements include the following:

> *If* one has a family history of Alzheimer's disease, *then there is a specific probability that* one will develop Alzheimer's disease.
> Tissue damage *is the antecedent of* pain perception.
> Learning ability *varies* with anxiety *in a curvilinear relationship.*
> Job satisfaction *is a function of* the fit between the job environment and the individual's personality.
> Anxiety and accurate information about a diagnostic procedure *are negatively related.*

The goals of science are to aid in understanding, explaining, predicting, and controlling phenomena. These goals are achieved through the relationships proposed by theory. Meeting these goals requires that *specific* relationships between concepts be clearly stated. Simply stating that anxiety and learning ability are related is insufficient. For the theory to be useful one needs to understand how and under what conditions they are related. Stating there is a curvilinear relationship between anxiety and learning provides the practitioner with information that may allow the prediction of situations in which one is most or least able

to learn. The practitioner responsible for developing and implementing a teaching program for home care following myocardial infarction would be directed to implement the program during periods of moderate anxiety for the recipients of the program rather than during periods of low or high anxiety.

Laws

Differences between classifications of relationship statements appear to reflect the abstractness of the concepts that are included in the statements and the amount of empirical support derived through testing the proposed relationship. Laws, empirical generalizations, and hypotheses are classifications of statements that include relatively concrete concepts. [4,5,12,17] The concepts incorporated in these statements represent things or events observable in the real world. Because they are observable, they can provide measures that are valid indicators of the concept. Laws and empirical generalizations are found primarily in disciplines such as chemistry and physics that deal with readily observable and measurable phenomena. They differ in the amount of empirical support that has been generated for the proposition. Laws are associated with a great deal of empirical support and are considered true statements about empirical reality. They have universal applicability, always true in every situation in which the law applies.[6] Boyle's law states that when temperature is held constant, the volume of a gas is inversely proportional to the pressure exerted on it. The statement suggests volume is influenced by the variables of temperature and pressure. To determine the influence of pressure alone, one must control for the influence of temperature. Because current technology makes temperature and pressure readily manipulatable, a researcher can control for the influence of temperature by holding temperature constant. Then by measuring volume and pressure he or she determines the influence of pressure changes on volume. If volume repeatedly and invariably decreases when pressure is increased, a law regarding the influence of pressure on gas volume becomes tenable. A great deal of empirical support can be generated for the proposition.

Laws differ from theories in several ways. Theories incorporate components that are to some degree unobservable; laws incorporate only the observable. Therefore laws can be directly tested; theories cannot. Theories tend to be more general than laws.

Laws are more often single statements about relationships among concrete components; theories are sets of abstract statements detailing idealistic compositions of systems and phenomena.[4]

Empirical Generalizations

Empirical generalizations differ from laws only in the amount of empirical support generated for the proposed relationship statements. Laws have overwhelming support; empirical generalizations have moderate support. The problem in classifying statements is deciding when moderate support becomes overwhelming support. The decision is a philosophical one and is arrived at through agreement among scientists in a discipline.

Hypotheses

Hypotheses differ from empirical generalizations and laws again in the amount of empirical support generated. Hypotheses are the first tentative suggestions that a specific relationship exists. As a hypothesis is repeatedly confirmed, it progresses to an empirical generalization and ultimately to a law. The words used in the proposition may not change. Boyle's law was Boyle's hypothesis and Boyle's empirical generalization before being accepted as a law within disciplines using the relationship.

Axioms and Theorems

Axioms and theorems are relationship statements that include abstract concepts—concepts that relate mental images of entities not readily observable. Theories emanating from the social sciences contain primarily axioms and theorems. Concepts such as anxiety, job satisfaction, learning ability, and personality are abstractions in the real world. They are neither directly observable nor measurable. Therefore they would be amenable to incorporation in either a theorem or an axiom.

Axioms and theorems differ in the degree of generality incorporated in the relationship. Axioms state the most general relationship between concepts. Theorems emanate from axioms. An example of a statement that could be an axiom is "Anxiety is negatively related to accurate information about a diagnostic procedure." That statement allows for the full range of possible values associated with each concept. A theorem suggests that a specific range of values of one concept is associated with a specific range of values of the other. An example of a possible theorem would be "Low levels of anxiety are associated with a high degree of accurate information about a diagnostic procedure."

Relationship statements become an axiom or theorem through the mechanism of empirical support. A statement is not referred to as an axiom unless it has been subjected to considerable testing and repeatedly supported. However, neither axioms nor theorems are directly testable. They have no directly observable empirical referent to be measured. Hypotheses provide the mechanism for testing them. Previously it was suggested that a hypothesis is a statement of relationship between concrete measurable entities for which little empirical support has been generated. Hypotheses must also be the antecedents of axioms and theorems. The abstract concepts must be operationalized to provide an empirical referent for each. Relationships are then tested by means of the empirical referent. A previous example included a visual analogue scale to measure pain. The scale and the resulting score provide an empirical referent for the abstract concept *pain*. One cannot directly observe pain, but one can see the scale and the score used to represent it. Hypotheses are used to test propositions incorporating abstract concepts regardless of the previous empirical support for the proposed relationships among concepts.

The discussion concerning differing classifications of relationship statements is provided to explain terms often used in the literature germane to theory development. They differ primarily in degree of abstractness and amount of empirical support. The components of the statements, concepts, and specified relationships between them may not differ. One can conclude that although the classification of relationship statements may differ among scientists, there is general agreement as to the structure of the statements. Relationship statements must include appropriate concepts that have been clearly defined, and the specific relationships among those concepts must also be clearly stated.

ASSOCIATIONAL OR CAUSAL STATEMENTS

Relationship statements are generally considered to be of two types, associational and causal process.

Associational Relationship Statements

Associational relationship statements assert that values of one concept are associated with values of another. Linear and curvilinear are the two general types of associational relationships. If the relationship is linear, three possibilities exist. There may be a positive relationship, a negative relationship, or no relationship among the concepts.[12] In a linear relationship, the direction of the relationship is established in the relationship statement. If the relationship is curvilinear, such is stated in the relationship statement. An example of an associational relationship statement is "Anxiety is negatively related to the degree of accurate information one has about a diagnostic procedure." If one knows a category of values for one variable, one can infer a category of values for another. Relationship statements found in the social sciences are primarily of the associational form.

Causal Relationship Statements

Causal relationship statements assert that one concept is the cause of another. Boyle's law is an example of a causal relationship statement. When temperature is held constant, a change in pressure causes an inverse change in the volume of gas. For every value of pressure there is an exact value for volume. If one knows the value for pressure, one can determine the exact value for volume.

ASSUMPTIONS

Assumptions are beliefs about phenomena one must accept as true in order to accept a theory about the phenomena as true. They are not tested but are assumed to represent reality. An example of assumptions can be found in Selye's Theory of Human Stress.[13] Selye proposed a theory of stress based on animal studies. The theory was to operate within the realm of human stress and was to reflect the totality of the stress experience. The theory requires several assumptions before one can accept it as an explanation of the totality of human stress. One must first accept the assumption that results of animal studies are completely generalizable to humans and that the stress measured in rodents is the same as the stress experienced by humans. In addition, the theory suggests that human stress is mediated by stress energy that enables one to handle that stress. A major assumption of the theory is that everyone is born with a finite amount of stress energy and death ensues when the energy is depleted. The assumption is not testable because the amount of stress energy one might have throughout life is not measurable; it is a belief one must accept before accepting Selye's theory as an appropriate and adequate explanation of total human stress.

MODELS AND CONCEPTUAL FRAMEWORKS

The terms *model* and *conceptual frameworks* are often used in nursing literature. A model is a schematic representation of some aspects of reality. Theories are models of some phenomenon. Models fall into two broad classifications, theoretical and empirical. *Empirical models* are replicas of observable reality. A plastic model of the heart is an empirical model. *Theoretical models* are representatives of the real world expressed in language or mathematic symbols. Theories are theoretical models of reality, often a reality that is not directly observable. Models are useful in theory development because they aid in the selection of relevant concepts necessary to represent a phenomenon of interest and the determination of the relationships among the concepts. Models also allow manipulation of concepts on paper before actual testing occurs. In addition, models aid theory users by providing an observable explanation of theory components. Although all theories are models, not all models are theories.

Guba distinguishes between two definitions of models. The logician defines a model as a "set of entities that constitutes an interpretation of all axioms and theorems of a system and in which those axioms and theorems hold true,"[4:354] in other words, a model of the system. As such, this definition suggests that a model is synonymous with well-developed and supported theory, and the model cannot exist until the formal theory has been generated. This definition of a model was also suggested by Hoover.[8] The second consideration of models holds that theories may in fact be identical to models but may be viewed as different among members of the discipline depending on acceptability of the concepts and relationship statements.[4] Thus a model is a set of relationship statements with less acceptability than a set of such statements defined as a theory. The model represents the early theoretical formulations existing prior to generation of adequate empirical support. Models evolve into theories on the generation of empirical support for the relationship statements.

Conceptual frameworks tend to be used by nurses to refer to beginning theoretical constructions that have little empirical support. In these terms, conceptual frameworks would differ little from a beginning theoretical model described by Guba for which testing has been sparse.

The distinctions among theories, models, and conceptual frameworks may be less obvious than the similarities. The discussion here suggests that if the entities differ, they do so by how tentative the relationship statements are, the amount of support for the components of the abstractions, and the degree of acceptability of the abstractions by the discipline, not by the components themselves. In general, theories, models, and conceptual frameworks are identical in structure. They are composed of sets of relationship statements which attempt to describe or explain phenomena and systems.

RANGE OF THEORIES

Theories differ in complexity and scope along a continuum from micro theories to grand theories. *Micro theories* are the least complex. They contain the least complex concepts and refer to specific, easily defined phenomena. They are narrow in scope because they attempt to explain a small aspect of reality and are primarily composed of enumerative or associative concepts. *Grand theories* are the most complex and broadest in scope. They attempt to explain broad areas within a discipline. They are composed of summative concepts and incorporate numerous narrower range theories. Middle-range theories fall somewhere in between. They are primarily composed of relational concepts. The domain represented by middle-range theory is not so large as to be useless to the user as summative concepts are useless. Middle-range theories, however, do not represent such a narrow aspect of reality that they cannot be used in the more complex realm of real life.

Partial theories are theories in the development stage. In a partial theory some concepts necessary to explain a phenomenon have been identified and some relationships have been identified between them, but the theory is not complete. A criterion of a complete theory is that the concepts and proposed relationships must be exhaustive. That is, every thing or event comprising the phenomenon is represented in the theory. Theories derived from the social sciences, including nursing, are probably exclusively partial theories because there are few, if any, phenomena that have been totally and completely explained.

PARADIGM

Science, philosophy, and theory are all components of the domain of any scientific discipline. *Paradigm* is a term used to denote the prevailing network of science, philosophy, and theory accepted by a discipline. Current interest in paradigmatic issues stems from the work of Kuhn.[9] Kuhn defined a *paradigm* to reflect his belief that a paradigm was synonymous with the scientific community or community of individuals comprising a discipline. The term was meant to refer to what members of the community have in common.[4,10] Included in the matrix shared by the scientific community are the knowledge, philosophy, theory, educational experience, practice orientation, research methodology, and literature identified with the discipline. The prevailing paradigm directs the activities of a discipline. As such, it is accepted by the majority of individuals within the discipline and suggests the areas of study of interest to the discipline and the means to study them. Nursing literature includes numerous references to conceptual models and frameworks. I believe these terms are synonymous with *paradigm*. Suppe and Jacox[15] defined conceptual framework similarly, stating that paradigmatic conceptual frameworks (such as grand theories explaining nursing) provide "a broad perspective within which specific theories can be developed and tested" (p.249). As such, conceptual frameworks "spawn" specific theories. This definition is consistent with the descriptions of a paradigm identified by Kuhn.[10]

SUMMARY

This chapter has been concerned with the terminology associated with theory development. Science, theory, philosophy, and paradigm have been addressed. In addition, terms necessary for a clearer understanding of these terms have been included. Fact, phenomenon, concepts, definitions, categories of concepts, relationship statement, law, empirical generalization, theorem, axiom, hypothesis, associational relationship statement, causal process relationship statement, assumption, model, and range of theories have been considered. I hope this discussion will allow a clearer understanding of the theoretical work addressed in the rest of this book.

REFERENCES

1. Brodbeck, M. (1953). The nature and function of the philosophy of science. In H. Feigl & M. Brodbeck (Eds.), *Readings in the philosophy of science.* New York: Appleton-Century-Crofts.
2. Dubin, R. (1978). *Theory building* (Rev. ed.). New York: The Free Press.
3. Feigl, H. (1953). The scientific outlook: naturalism and humanism. In H. Feigl & M. Brodbeck (Eds.), *Readings in the philosophy of science.* New York: Appleton-Century-Crofts.
4. Guba, E. (1990). *The paradigm dialog.* Newbury Park, CA: Sage.
5. Hardy, M.E. (1973). The nature of theories. In M. Hardy (Ed.), *Theoretical foundation for nursing.* New York: MSS Corp.
6. Hempel, C.G., & Oppenheim, P. (1988). Studies in the logic of explanation. In J.C. Pitt (Ed.), *Theories of explanation.* New York: Oxford University Press.
7. Hoffman, M.L. (1981). Is altruism part of human nature? *Journal of Personality and Social Psychology, 40,* 126-131.
8. Hoover, K.R. (1988). *The elements of social scientific thinking* (4th ed.). New York: St. Martin's Press.
9. Kuhn, T.S. (1970). *The structure of scientific revolutions.* Chicago: University of Chicago Press.
10. Kuhn, T.S. (1974). Second thoughts on paradigms. In F. Suppe (Ed.), *The structure of scientific theories.* Urbana, IL: University of Illinois Press.
11. Mehlberg, H. (1962). The theoretical and empirical aspects of science. In E. Nagel, P. Suppes, & A. Tarski (Eds.), *Logic, methodology and philosophy of science.* Stanford, CA: Stanford University Press.
12. Reynolds, P.D. (1971). *A primer in theory construction.* Indianapolis: Bobbs-Merrill.
13. Selye, H. (1956). *The stress of life.* New York: McGraw-Hill.
14. Suppe, F. (1989). *The semantic conception of theories and scientific realism.* Urbana, IL: University of Illinois Press.
15. Suppe, F., & Jacox, A.K. (1985). Philosophy of science and the development of nursing theory. *Annual Review of Nursing Research, 3,* 214-267.
16. Theobald, D.W. (1968). *An introduction to philosophy of science.* London: Methuen.
17. Wartofsky, M.W. (1968). *Conceptual foundations of scientific thought and introduction to the philosophy of science.* New York: Macmillan.
18. *Webster's third new international dictionary unabridged* (1986). Springfield, MA: Merriam-Webster, Inc.
19. Wolman, B.J. (1965). Toward a science of psychological science. In B.J. Wolman (Ed.), *Scientific psychology: principles and approaches.* New York: Basic Books.

*H*istory and Philosophy of Science

Sue Marquis Bishop

*M*odern science is a relatively new intellectual activity. Established as recently as 400 years ago, it has occupied only a short span of time in the history of humankind.[4] Scientific activity has persisted because it has improved the quality of life while satisfying human needs for creative work, a sense of order, and the desire to understand the unknown.[4,14,30] If we are interested in understanding, predicting, or controlling a given phenomenon or in describing what we know in science, we are seeking a theory.[33,47] The development of science thus requires the *formalization of the phenomena and events* with which each science is concerned.[45] The construction of nursing theories is the formalization of attempts to describe, explain, predict, or control states of affairs in nursing (i.e., nursing phenomena).

HISTORICAL VIEWS OF THE NATURE OF SCIENCE

If we are interested in formalizing the science of nursing, we must consider such basic questions as: What is science? What is to be regarded as knowledge? What is truth? What are the methods by which scientific knowledge can be produced? These are philosophical questions. The term *epistemology* is concerned with the theory of knowledge in philosophical inquiry. The particular philosophical perspective selected to answer these questions will influence how scientists choose to carry out scientific activities, how they interpret outcomes, and even what they regard as science and knowledge.[5:8] Although philosophy as an activity has been documented for 3000 years, formal science is a relatively new human pursuit.[13] Only recently has scientific activity itself become the object of investigation.[5]

Two competing theories of science have evolved (with several variations) in the era of modern science—*rationalism and empiricism.*[14] Gale[14] labeled these alternative epistemologies as centrally concerned with the "power of reason" and the "power of sensory experience." He noted some similarity in the divergent views of science in the time of the classical Greeks. For example, Aristotle believed advances in biological science would develop through systematic observation of objects and events in the natural world, whereas Pythagorus believed knowledge of the natural world would develop from mathematical reasoning.[5,14]

RATIONALISM

Rationalist epistemology emphasizes the importance of a priori reasoning as the appropriate method for advancing knowledge. The scientist in this tradition approaches the task of scientific inquiry by developing a systematic explanation (theory) of a given phenomenon.[14] This conceptual system is analyzed by addressing the logical structure of the theory and the logical reasoning involved in its development. Theoretical assertions, derived by *deductive reasoning,* are then subjected to experimental testing to corroborate the theory. Reynolds[33] labeled this approach the "theory-then-research" strategy. If the research findings fail to correspond with the theoretical assertions, additional research is conducted or modifications are made in the theory and further tests devised, or the theory is discarded in favor of an alternative explanation.[14,47]

Popper[31] argued that science would evolve more rapidly through the process of conjectures and refutations in which new ideas are formulated and research is devised to attempt to refute them.

The rationalist view is most clearly evident in the work of the theoretical physicist Einstein, who made extensive use of mathematical equations in developing his theories. The theories Einstein *constructed* offered an "imaginative framework" which has directed research in numerous areas.[6] As Reynolds[33] noted, if one believes that science is a process of "inventing descriptions of phenomena," the appropriate strategy for theory construction is the theory-then-research strategy. In Reynolds's view[33:145]:

> As the continuous interplay between theory construction (invention) and testing with empirical research progresses, the theory becomes more precise and complete as a description of nature and, therefore, more useful for the goals of science.

EMPIRICISM

The empiricist view is based on the central idea that scientific knowledge can only be derived from sensory experience. Francis Bacon (c. 1620) is given credit for popularizing the basis for the empiricist approach to inquiry.[14] Bacon believed scientific truth was discovered by the generalization of observed facts in the natural world. This approach, which has been called the *inductive* method, is based on the idea that collection of facts precedes attempts to formulate generalizations, the "research-then-theory" approach.[33]

The strict empiricist view is reflected in the work of the behaviorists Watson and Skinner. In a 1950 paper, Skinner[37] asserted that advances in the science of psychology could be expected if scientists would focus on the collection of empirical data. He cautioned against the drawing of premature inferences and proposed a moratorium on theory building until further facts were collected. Skinner's approach to theory construction was clearly an inductive one. His view of science and the popularity of behaviorism have been credited with influencing the shift in emphasis in psychology between the 1950s and 1970s from theory construction to fact gathering.[38] The difficulty with the inductive mode of inquiry is that the world presents an infinite number of possible observations.[40] Therefore the scientist must "bring ideas to experiences" to decide what to observe and what to exclude.[40] Although in his early writings Skinner disclaimed to be developing a theory, Bixenstine[2:465] noted:

> Skinner is startlingly creative in applying the conceptual elements of his let's be frank theory to a wide variety of issues, ranging from training pigeons in the guidance of missiles, to developing teaching machines, to constructing a model society.

During the first half of this century, philosophers focused on the analysis of the structure of theories, whereas scientists focused on empirical research.[5] There was minimal interest in the history of science, the nature of scientific discovery, or the similarities between the philosophical view of science and scientific methods.[5] *Positivism,* a term first used by Comte, emerged as the dominant view of modern science.[14] Modern logical positivists believed empirical research and logical analysis were the two approaches that would produce scientific knowledge. The system of symbolic logic, published from 1910 to 1913 by Whitehead and Russell, was hailed by the logical positivists as an appropriate approach to discovering truth.[5]

The logical empiricists, offering a more lenient view of logical positivism, argued that theoretical propositions must be able to be tested through observation and experimentation.[5] This perspective is rooted in the idea that empirical facts exist independently of theories and offer the only possible basis for objectivity in science.[5] In other words, objective truth exists in the world, independent of the researcher. In this view, the task of science is to discover it. The empiricist view shares similarities with Aristotle's view of biological science and Bacon's inductive method as the true method of scientific inquiry.[14] Gale[14] argued that this view of science is often presented in methodology courses as the "single orthodox view" of the scientific enterprise. In his words, this view is taught in the following manner:

> The scientist first sets up an experiment; observes what occurs . . . ; reaches a preliminary hypothesis to describe the occurrence; runs further experiments to test the hypothesis [and] finally corrects or modifies the hypothesis in light of the results.[14:13]

The increasing use of computers permitting the analysis of large data sets may have contributed to the acceptance of the positivist approach to modern science.[38] In the 1950s, however, the literature began to reflect an increasing challenge to the positivist view, thereby ushering in a new view of science.[4]

EMERGENT VIEWS OF SCIENCE AND THEORY

In recent years, several authors have presented analyses challenging the positivist position, thus offering the basis for a new perspective of science.[13,16,20,42] In 1977, Brown[5] argued that there was a new intellectual revolution in philosophy that emphasized the *history of science,* replacing formal logic as the major analytical tool in the philosophy of science. One of the major perspectives in the new philosophy was the focus on science as a *process of continuing research,* as opposed to the emphasis on accepted findings. In this emergent epistemology, the *emphasis was on understanding scientific discovery* and the processes involved in changes in theories over time. In 1966, Foucault[13] published his analysis (in French) of the

epistemology of human sciences from the seventeenth to the nineteenth centuries. His major thesis was that empirical knowledge was arranged in different patterns at a given time and in a given culture. He found changes over time in the focus of inquiry, in what was regarded as scientific knowledge, and in how knowledge was organized. Further, he concluded that humans only recently emerged as objects of study. Schutz,[35] in his *Phenomenology of the Social World,* argued that scientists seeking to understand the social world cannot cognitively know an external world, independent of their own life experiences.

Empiricists argue that for science to maintain objectivity, data collection and analysis must be independent of theory.[5] This assertion is based on the position that objective truth exists in the world, waiting to be discovered. Brown[5] argues that the new epistemology challenged the empiricist view of perception by acknowledging that theories play a significant role in determining what the scientist will observe and how it will be interpreted. A story related to me by my grandmother illustrates Brown's thesis that observations are "concept-laden"; that is, what one observes is influenced by ideas in the mind of the observer:

> A husband and wife are sitting by the fire silently watching their firstborn son asleep in the cradle. The mother looks at her infant son and imagines him learning to talk and then to walk. She continues her reverie by imagining him playing with friends, coming home from school, and then going to college. She ends her daydreaming by visualizing him elected president of the United States. She smiles and glances up at her husband, who also had been staring intently at their son, "What are you thinking, honey?" The husband replies, "I was just thinking that I can't imagine how anyone could build a fine cradle like this, sell it for $12.98, and still make a profit."

Brown[5] presented the example of a chemist and a child walking together past a steel mill. The chemist perceived the odor of sulfur dioxide, while the child smelled rotten eggs. Each of them responded to the same observable data with distinctly different cognitive interpretations. In teaching nurses to be family therapists, I frequently use videotapes of family therapy sessions for students to analyze as we progress through the study of different approaches to family therapy. Novice student therapists tend to focus on the content of family interaction (what one member says to another) or the behavior of individual family members. After studying the systems view of families, which uses examples of patterned transactions among family members, during the second viewing, students can "see" and describe transactions among family members that they did not perceive during the first viewing (for example, the son withdrawing when his parents argue or the wife gritting her teeth when her husband talks). Concepts and theories create boundaries for selecting phenomena to observe and for reasoning about specific patterns. For example, the "social network" concept may be more fruitful for studying social relations than the "group" concept because it focuses attention on a more complex set of relationships, beyond the boundaries of any one setting.[1,18]

If, however, scientists perceive patterns in the empirical world based on their presupposed theories, how can new patterns ever be perceived or new discoveries be formulated? Gale[14] answered this question by arguing that the scientist is able to perceive "forceful intrusions" from the environment that challenge his or her "a priori mental set," thus raising questions in regard to the current theoretical perspective. Brown[5] maintained that while a presupposed theoretical framework influences perception, theories are not the single determining factor of the scientist's perception. He identified three different views of the relationships of theories to observation:

1. Scientists are merely passive observers of occurrences in the empirical world. Observable data are objective truth waiting to be discovered.
2. Theories structure what the scientist perceives in the empirical world.
3. Presupposed theories and observable data interact in the process of scientific investigation.[5:298]

Brown's argument[5] for an *interactionist's perspective* coincides with scientific consensus in the study of pattern recognition in human information processing.

Two distinct mini theories have directed research efforts in this area: the Data-Driven, or Bottom-Up, Theory and the Conceptually Driven, or Top-Down, Theory.[26] In the former, cognitive expectations (what is known or ways of organizing meaning) are used to select input and process incoming information from the environment. The second theory asserts that incoming data are perceived as unlabeled input and analyzed as raw data with increasing levels of complexity until all the data are classified. Current research evidence suggests human pattern recognition progresses by an interaction of both data-driven and conceptually driven processes, using sources of information in both currently organized cognitive categories and stimuli from the sensory environment.[26] The interactionist's perspective also is clearly reflected in Piaget's theory of human cognitive functioning:

> Piagetian man actively selects and interprets *environmental* information in the construction of his own knowledge rather than passively copying the information just as it is presented to his senses. While paying attention to and taking account of the structure of the environment during knowledge seeking, Piagetian man reconstrues and reinterprets that environment [according to] his own mental framework. . . . The mind neither copies the world . . . nor does it ignore the world [by] creating a private mental conception of it out of whole cloth. . . . The mind meets the environment in an extremely active, self-directed way.[11:6]

If we are to accept the thesis that no objective truth exists and that science is an interactive process between "invented" theories and empirical observations, how are scientists to determine truth and scientific knowledge? In the new epistemology, science is viewed as an ongoing process, and much importance is given to the idea of *consensus among scientists*. As Brown[5] concluded, we must forgo the myth that science can establish "final truths" and accept the notion that tentative consensus based on reasoned judgments about the available evidence is the most that can be expected.

In this view of science, scientific knowledge is what the community of scientists in any given historical era regard as such. The truth of a given theoretical statement is determined by current consensus among scientists as to whether it presents an "adequate description of reality."[5] This consensus is possible through the collaboration of many scientists, in making their work available for public review and debate and building on previous inquiries.[32] "The individual (scientist) *introduces* ideas, the scientific community *appraises* them" by its objective criteria.[32:59]

Science, in any given era and in any given discipline, is structured by an accepted set of presuppositions that define the phenomena to study and the appropriate methods for data collection and interpretation.[5] These presuppositions set the boundaries for the scientific enterprise in a particular field. In Brown's[5] view of the transactions between theory and empirical observation:

> Theory determines what observations are worth making and how they are to be understood, and observation provides challenges to accepted theoretical structures. The continuing attempt to produce a coherently organized body of theory and observation is the driving force of research, and the prolonged failure of specific research projects leads to scientific revolutions.[5:167]

The presentation and acceptance of a revolutionary theory may alter the existing presuppositions and theories, thereby creating a different set of boundaries and procedures. The result is a new set of problems or a new way to interpret observations, that is, a new picture of the world.[20] It is crucial that the emphasis in this view of science be on *ongoing research* rather than on established findings.

THEORY AND RESEARCH

Traditionally, theory building and research have been presented to students in separate courses. This separation has often resulted in problems for students in understanding the nature of theories and in comprehending the relevance of research efforts.[46] The acceptance of the positivist view of science may have influenced the sharp distinction between theory and research methods.[14] Although theory and research can be viewed as distinct operations, they are more appropriately regarded as interdependent compo-

nents of the scientific process.[9] In constructing a theory, the theorist must be knowledgeable about available empirical findings and attempt to take these into account, since theory is in part concerned with the formalization of available knowledge.[47] The theory also is subject to revision if the hypotheses fail to correspond to empirical findings, or the theory may be abandoned in favor of an alternative explanation that accounts for the new information.[5,9,20]

In contemporary theories of science, the scientific enterprise has been described as a series of phases, with emphasis on the discovery and verification (or acceptance) phases.[14,15] Gale[14] described these phases as primarily concerned with the presentation and testing of new ideas. Discovery is the phase during which new ways of thinking about phenomena or new data are introduced to the scientific community. The focus during this time is on presenting persuasive argument that the new conceptions represent an improvement over previous conceptions.[14] Verification is characterized by efforts in the scientific community to critically analyze and test the new conceptions in an attempt to refute them. During this time, the new views are "put through the trial by fire."[14] Brown[5] argued, however, that discovery and verification cannot really be viewed as sharply distinct phases because a new conception is not usually accepted by the scientific community until it has "passed enough tests to warrant acceptance as a new discovery."

At this point it should be clear that in a scientific discipline it is not appropriate to judge a theory on the basis of "authority, faith, or intuition."[32] A theory should be judged on the basis of *scientific consensus*.[32] For example, if a specific nursing theory is to be determined acceptable, this judgment should not be made because a respected nursing leader advocates the theory. Neither should personal feelings about the theory, such as "I like this theory" or "I don't like this one," provide the basis for the judgment. The only defensible reason for judging a theory acceptable is on the basis of logical and conceptual or empirical grounds. These judgments are made by the scientific community.[4]

The advancement of science is a collaborative endeavor in which many researchers evaluate and build on one another's work. For evidence to be cumulative, theories, procedures, and findings from empirical studies must be made available for critical review by scientists. In this way, the same procedures can be used to support or refute a given analysis or finding.[32] A theory is accepted when the consensus of scientists is that the theory provides an "adequate description of reality."[5] The acceptance of a scientific hypothesis depends on the appraisal of the *coherence* of theory, which involves questions of logic, and the *correspondence* of the theory, which involves efforts to relate the theory to observable phenomena through research.[41] Gale[14] labeled these criteria epistemological and metaphysical concerns.

The consensus of correspondence of the theory with reality is not based on a single study. Repeated testing is crucial, replicating the study under the same conditions and exploring the theoretical assertions under different conditions, or with different measures. Consensus is therefore based on accumulated evidence.[15] Even when the theory does not appear to be supported by research, it is not necessarily rejected by the scientific community. Rather than an automatic agreement that there is a problem with the theory itself, there may be judgments made about the validity or reliability of the measures used in testing the theory or in the appropriateness of the research design. These possibilities are considered in critically evaluating attempts to test a given theory.

Dubin[9] identified the following three areas in which scientific consensus is necessary in regard to any given theory: (1) agreement on the boundaries of the theory, that is, the phenomenon it addresses and the phenomena it excludes (criterion of coherence[41]); (2) agreement on the logic used in constructing the theory, so meanings can be understood from a similar perspective (criterion of coherence[41]); (3) agreement that the theory fits the data collected and analyzed through research (criterion of correspondence[41]). Consensus in these three areas essentially constitutes agreement among scientists to "look at the same 'things', to do so in the same way, and to have a level of confidence certified by an empirical test."[9:13] Therefore the theory must be capable of being operationalized for testing in order to check the theory against reality. In the process of science, retro-

ductive, deductive, and inductive forms of reasoning may be used as science progresses by building theoretical descriptions and explanations of reality, attempting to account for available findings, deriving testable hypotheses, and evaluating theories from the perspective of new empirical data.[41]

Most research can be considered to fall into the category Kuhn[20] described as *normal science*. Scientific inquiry in normal science involves testing a given theory, developing new applications of theory, or extending a given theory. Occasionally, a new theory with different assumptions is developed that seeks to replace previous theories. Kuhn[20] described this as *revolutionary science*, and the theory with different presuppositions as a *revolutionary theory*. A change in the accepted presuppositions creates a set of boundaries and procedures that suggest a new set of problems or a new way to interpret observations.[20]

Currently, there is some challenge in the social and behavioral sciences to the assumptions underlying accepted methods of experimental design, measurement, and statistical analysis that emphasize the search for universal laws and the use of procedures for random assignment of subjects across contexts.[23] Mishler[23] argued that scientists should develop methods and procedures for studying behavior as dependent on context for meaning, rather than eliminating context by searching for laws that hold across contexts. This critique of the methods and assumptions of research is emerging from phenomenological and ethnomethodological theorists who view the scientific process from a very different paradigm.[3,17,23,28,43]

The proper focus of research is not to attempt to prove a theory or hypothesis, but to attempt to set up research to refute a given hypothesis.[31] Failure of repeated attempts at refutation lends support to the theory and acceptance of the theory by the scientific community.[9] The emphasis, however, is always on ongoing research rather than established findings.[5] In the future, new information or a new, compelling way to view the same evidence may lead to a reappraisal of the theory. One previously accepted theory may be abandoned for another theory if it fails to correspond to empirical findings or if it no longer presents clear directions for further research. The theory selected as an alternative is judged by the scientific community to account for available data and to suggest further lines of inquiry.[5]

Popper[31] observed that, unfortunately, refutations of a given theory are frequently viewed as a failure of the theorist or of the theory. In his view:

> Every refutation should be regarded as a great success; not merely as a success of the scientist who refuted the theory, but also of the scientist who created the refuted theory and who thus . . . suggested, if only indirectly, the refutation experiment.[31:243]

There is no one science and no single scientific method; there are several sciences, each with its own phenomena and structure and methods for inquiry.[39] The various sciences are at different stages of development. Physics is considered the most exacting of the sciences (not including mathematics); the life sciences (e.g., botany) are not as well developed scientifically, and the social sciences even less so.[39] The commonality among sciences, however, concerns the efforts made by scientists to "separate truth from conjecture"[39] to advance knowledge. Questions about the structure of knowledge in a given science, what is to be regarded as scientific knowledge, and the methods of inquiry are decided by the consensus of scientists in the discipline.[5,14]

ISSUES IN NURSING SCIENCE DEVELOPMENT

In comparison to other developing sciences, nursing science is in the early stages of scientific development. Until the late 1950s, the use of the term nursing science in the literature was rare.[7] Consensus has emerged in the field of nursing that the knowledge base for nursing practice is "inadequate and incomplete" and that the development of a scientific base for nursing practice is a high priority for the discipline.[34] In 1985, Meleis concluded:

> Theory is no longer a luxury in nursing. There was a time when theory use was equated with the development of a conceptual framework, to be used only as a guide to curriculum development. Theory now is part and parcel of the nursing lexicon in education, administration, and practice.[22:2]

Meleis[22] characterized the years of progress of the discipline of nursing in the following four stages: (1) practice, (2) education and administration, (3) research, and (4) the development of nursing theory. In 1952, Peplau developed the first theory for the practice of nursing in her book, *Interpersonal Relations in Nursing.*[29] The journal *Nursing Research* was published the same year, providing a source for dissemination of research findings in nursing. During the 1950s and the early 1960s, other formulations of nursing were developed (see Chapter 6).

During the late 1960s and 1970s, nurse theorists analyzed and debated a variety of metatheoretical issues, and the first issue of the journal *Advances in Nursing Science* was published. *Metatheoretical issues* relate to issues of theory development or philosophy of science issues (i.e., theories about theories). Nursing scholars questioned: What is a theory? How should nursing theory be developed? Should theories be borrowed from other fields? How should theories be critiqued? What is nursing knowledge? For example, in 1976, Carper[7] conceptualized four fundamental patterns of knowledge in nursing—empirical knowledge (nursing science), esthetic knowledge (nursing art), moral knowledge (ethics in nursing), and personal knowledge (therapeutic use of self). This period was characterized by the acceptance by nurse theorists of the necessity to devise nursing theories and a focus on developing directions for the field to continue progress in theory development. (Refer to Meleis[22] for an analysis of the milestones in theory development in nursing from 1955 to 1985.)

During the 1980s, further acceptance of nursing theory was evidenced by continued theory development in nursing and the increased incorporation of nursing theories into nursing curricula. The nursing theory literature during this period increasingly addressed the analysis and use of nursing theories in clinical practice.[22] The number of nursing journals publishing articles on theory and research increased significantly. Consensus was achieved on the "domain concepts" of nursing—person, environment, health, and nursing—as defining the major concepts central to nursing.[10]

In the 1990s, philosophical debate continues in the literature over whether nursing science is a basic science, an applied science, or a practical science.[19] Further, while the numbers of educational and practice settings adopting a single nursing theory approach to curriculum and nursing practice increased in the 1980s, the "one theory approach" has not achieved consensus in the field. A number of scholars in nursing are emphasizing "pluralism in nursing theories."[22] For example, Nagle and Mitchell[24] argued for "theoretic diversity," the use of multiple theory approaches in the practice setting. Meleis[22] asserted that in a discipline that deals with human beings, it is perhaps not feasible that only one theory should explain, describe, predict, and change all the discipline's phenomena.[20:64-65] "This blanket acceptance of one (single theory) approach smothers creativity, scholarly inquiry and growth."[24:24]

The nursing literature in the early 1990s continued to address the meaning of the "domain concepts," in particular, the need to establish interconnections among these central nursing concepts; "such unconnected concepts do not raise philosophic issues or scientific questions that stimulate inquiry."[25:2] Current nursing literature also reflects increasing concern with the methods of inquiry to be utilized in developing nursing knowledge, with several scholars stressing the importance of diversity of methods in research and qualitative as well as quantitative methods.[3,8,28]

In the mid-1990s nursing scholars are addressing the development of an epistemology of nursing therapeutics,[21] enhancing the connectedness between nursing science and art (e.g., see reference 36), and arguing for pluralism in nursing theories and research methods (e.g., see references 12 and 27). "No one view may be sufficient to embrace or drive nursing knowledge in its totality."[27:x] It has been argued that evolutionary changes underway in society associated with the information age are changing nurses' views of "possible realities" and creating a philosophical shift in nursing.[36] This shift was viewed as shifting the focus from an exclusive philosophical focus on epistemological questions about knowing, to ontological questions of meaning, being, and reality.[36]

How the nurse uses expert knowledge to administer complex chemotherapy treatments is as important as how the nurse uses artistry of being to help a young mother find meaning in her impending death. Often the two converge. . . . The gap between nursing science and art has begun to close, generating a creative synthesis of the two . . . the "science-art" of nursing.[36:12, 11]

The postpositivist and interpretive paradigms have achieved a current degree of acceptance in nursing as paradigms to guide knowledge development.[12] Postpositivism focuses on discovering patterns that may describe, explain, and predict phenomena, and it rejects older traditional positivist views of an ultimate objective knowledge observable only through the senses (see references 12 and 44 for more discussion). The interpretive paradigm tends to promote understanding by addressing the meanings of social interaction by the participants that emphasize situation, context, and the multiple cognitive constructions individuals create of everyday events.[12] The critical paradigm for knowledge development in nursing has been described as an emergent postmodern paradigm that provides the framework for inquiring about the interaction between social, political, economic, gender, and cultural factors and the experiences of health and illness.[12] A broad conception of postmodernism includes the particular philosophies that challenge the "objectification of knowledge," such as phenomenology, hermeneutics, feminism, critical theory, and poststructuralism.[27:91]

SCIENCE AS A SOCIAL ENTERPRISE

The process of scientific inquiry may be viewed as a social enterprise.[23] In Gale's words, "Human beings do science.[14:290] It therefore might be anticipated that the scientific enterprise may be influenced by social, economic, or political factors.[5] For example, the popularity of certain ideologies may influence how phenomena are viewed and what problems are selected for study.[17] In addition, the availability of funds for research in a specified area may precipitate a flurry of research activity in that area. Science, however, does not depend on the "personal characteristics" or persuasions of any given scientist, or group of scientists, but is powerfully self-correcting within the community of scientists.[32] Science thus progresses by *"reasoned judgments on the part of scientists and through debate within the scientific community."*[5:167] The evidence is that nursing scholars are fully engaged in this process to develop nursing science.

REFERENCES

1. Bishop, S.M. (1984). Perspectives on individual-family-social network interrelations. *Interrelational Journal of Family Therapy, 6*(2), 124-135.
2. Bixenstine, E. (1964). Empiricism in latter-day behavioral science. *Science, 145,* 465.
3. Bowers, L. (1992). Ethnomethodology I: An approach to nursing research. *International Journal of Nursing Studies, 29*(1), 59-67.
4. Bronowski, J. (1979). *The visionary eye: Essays in the arts, literature and science.* Cambridge, MA: The MIT Press.
5. Brown, H. (1977). *Perception, theory and commitment: The new philosophy of science.* Chicago: The University of Chicago Press.
6. Calder, N. (1979). *Einstein's universe.* New York: Viking.
7. Carper, B. (1978). Fundamental patterns of knowing in nursing. *Advances in Nursing Science, 1*(1), 13-23.
8. Cull-Wilby, B., & Pepin, J. (1987). Towards a coexistence of paradigms in nursing knowledge development. *Journal of Advanced Nursing, 12,* 515-521.
9. Dubin, R. (1978). *Theory building.* New York: The Free Press.
10. Fawcett, J. (1984). The metaparadigm of nursing: Present status and future refinements. *Image, 16*(3), 84-87.
11. Flavell, J.H. (1977). *Cognitive development.* Englewood Cliffs, NJ: Prentice-Hall.
12. Ford-Gilboe, M., Campbell, J., & Berman, H. (1995). Stories and numbers: Coexistence without compromise. *Advances in Nursing Science, 18*(1), 14-26.
13. Foucault, M. (1973). *The order of things: An archaeology of the human sciences.* New York: Vintage Books.
14. Gale, G. (1979). *Theory of science: An introduction to the history, logic and philosophy of science.* New York: McGraw-Hill.
15. Giere, R.N. (1979). *Understanding scientific reasoning.* New York: Holt, Rhinehart & Winston.
16. Hanson, N.R. (1958). *Patterns of discovery.* Cambridge: Cambridge University Press.
17. Hudson, L. (1972). *The cult of the fact.* New York: Harper & Row.
18. Irving, H.W. (1977). Social networks in the modern city. *Social Forces, 55,* 867-880.
19. Johnson, J. (1991). Nursing science: Basic, applied, or practical? *Advances in Nursing Science, 14*(1), 7-16.
20. Kuhn, T.S. (1962). *The structure of scientific revolutions.* Chicago: The University of Chicago Press.
21. Liaschenko, J. (1995). Ethics in the work of acting for patients. *Advances in Nursing Sciences, 18*(2), 1-12.
22. Meleis, A. (1985). *Theoretical nursing: Development and progress.* Philadelphia: J.B. Lippincott.
23. Mishler, E.G. (1979). Meaning in context: Is there any other kind? *Harvard Educational Review, 49,* 1-19.
24. Nagle, L., & Mitchell, G. (1991). Theoretic diversity: Evolving paradigmatic issues in research and practice. *Advances in Nursing Science, 14*(1), 17-25.
25. Newman, M., Sime, A.M., & Cororan-Perry, S. (1991). The focus of the discipline of nursing. *Advances in Nursing Science, 14*(1), 1-6.
26. Norman, D.A. (1976). *Memory and attention: An introduction to human information processing.* New York: John Wiley & Sons.
27. Omery, A., Kasper, C.E., & Page, G.G. (1995). *In search of nursing science.* Thousand Oaks, CA: Sage.
28. Pallikkathayil, L., & Morgan, S. (1991). Phenomenology as a method for conducting clinical research. *Applied Nursing Research, 4*(4), 195-200.
29. Peplau, H. (1952). *Interpersonal relations in nursing.* New York: G.P. Putman's Sons.
30. Piaget, J. (1970). *The place of the sciences of man in the system of sciences.* New York: Harper & Row.
31. Popper, K. (1962). *Conjectures and refutations.* New York: Basic Books.
32. Randall, J.H. (1964). *Philosophy: An introduction.* New York: Barnes & Noble.
33. Reynolds, P. (1971). *A primer in theory construction.* Indianapolis: Bobbs-Merrill.
34. Schlotfeldt, R. (1992). Why promote clinical nursing scholarship? *Clinical Nursing Research, 1*(1), 5-9.
35. Schutz, A. (1967). *The phenomenology of the social world.* Evanston, IL: Northwestern University Press.
36. Silva, M.C., Sorrell, J.M., & Sorrell, C.D. (1995). From Carper's patterns of knowing to ways of being: An ontological philosophical shift in nursing. *Advances in Nursing Science, 18*(1), 1-13.
37. Skinner, B.F. (1950). Are theories of learning necessary? *Psychological Review, 57,* 193-216.
38. Snelbecker, G. (1974). *Learning theory, instructional theory, and psychoeducational design.* New York: McGraw-Hill.
39. Springagesh, K., & Springagesh, S. (1986). Philosophy and scientific approach. *Contemporary Philosophy, 11*(6), 18-20.
40. Steiner, E. (1977). *Criteria for theory of art education* [Monograph] Presented at Seminar for Research in Art Education, Philadelphia. Unpublished.
41. Steiner, E. (1978). *Logical and conceptual analytic techniques for educational researchers.* Washington, DC: University Press.

42. Toulmin, S. (1961). *Foresight and understanding.* New York: Harper & Row.

43. Turner, J. (1978). *The structure of sociological theory.* Homewood, IL: The Dorsey Press.

44. Weiss, S.J. (1995). Contemporary empiricism. In A. Omery, C.E. Kasper, & G.G. Page (Eds.), *In search of nursing science.* Thousand Oaks, CA: Sage.

45. Werkmeister, W. (1959). Theory construction and the problem of objectivity. In L. Gross (Ed.), *Symposium of sociological theory.* Evanston, IL: Row, Peterson, & Co.

46. Winston, C. (1974). *Theory and measurement in sociology.* New York: John Wiley & Sons.

47. Zetterberg, H.L. (1966). *On theory and verification in sociology.* Totowa, NJ: The Bedminister Press.

Logical Reasoning

Sue Marquis Bishop

theory may be evaluated by using the criterion of *logical development.* This requires that the development of the series of theoretical statements follow a logical form of reasoning; that is, the premises justify the conclusions. *Logic* is a branch of philosophy concerned with the analysis of inferences and arguments.[10] An *inference* involves the forming of a conclusion based on some evidence. Although the common meaning of argument implies a disagreement, in logic an *argument* consists of a conclusion and its supportive evidence. The evidence supporting a conclusion may involve one or more theoretical statements, or premises. The tools of logic permit the analysis of the reasoning from the premises to the conclusion.[8]

Theories can be developed and tested through deductive, inductive, or retroductive forms of reasoning. Traditionally these approaches have been explicitly presented in the literature as systematic procedures for devising theory. An in-depth discussion of these forms is beyond the scope of this chapter, and the reader is referred to Geach,[2] Giere,[3] Pospesel,[8], Salmon,[9,10] and Steiner[15] for further study.

It is important, however, to grasp the basic differences between these forms of reasoning in order to understand how a given theorist may choose to approach the task of theory building.

DEDUCTION

Deduction is a form of logical reasoning in which specific conclusions are inferred from more general premises or principles. Reasoning thus proceeds from the general to the particular.[14] The deductively developed theory usually involves a lengthy sequence of theoretical statements derived from a relatively few broad axioms or general statements.[9] Conclusions thus derived may offer predictions that can be tested empirically. The *deductive argument* usually takes the form of a syllogism with general premises and a conclusion. In logical analysis, letters may be substituted for concepts, since emphasis on the analysis of the argument is focused on the *form of the argument.*[9] Example A presents a valid deductive argument with letter notation.

EXAMPLE A

Premise: All victims of abuse have low self-esteem. (**All S are M**)
Premise: Martha and Tom are victims of abuse. (**All P are S**)
Conclusion: Therefore Martha and Tom have low self-esteem. (***Ergo,* all P are M**)

EXAMPLE B

Premise: All victims of abuse have low self-esteem.
Premise: Martha has low self-esteem.
Conclusion: Therefore Martha is a victim of abuse.

In Example A, the conclusion follows from, or was deduced from, the general premises. There may be a lengthy number of premises in a given argument preceding the conclusion. Note that in the above example there is no new information presented in the conclusion that is not at least implied in the premises. The deductive form of reasoning is defined as:

1. If A were true, then B would be true.
2. A is true.
3. Hence B is true.[15:9]

As you study the nursing literature, you will not often find arguments presented in the form demonstrated in Example A with the premises and conclusions placed in order and clearly labeled. But with practice you can sharpen your skills in identifying arguments and labeling the premises and conclusions from your reading of narrative text.[10] You may find the conclusion may be presented at the beginning or end, or even in the middle of an argument.[10] Salmon[10] suggests that certain words or phrases are clues that specific statements are offered as premises or conclusions. Examples of terms that often precede a premise include *since, for,* and *because.* Examples of terms that often precede a conclusion are *therefore, consequently, hence, so,* and *it follows that.*[10]

Arguments may be evaluated in two different ways: (1) the validity of the argument may be assessed as to whether the conclusion logically follows from the premises and (2) the content of the premises may be assessed in terms of the truth or falsity of the statements.[8] The *validity* of a deductive argument refers to the logic involved in reasoning from the premises to the conclusion in such a way that, if the premises are true, the conclusion must necessarily be true.[8,10,15] A deductive argument may contain all true statements or one or more false statements and be considered either valid or invalid. This judgment is made on the basis of whether the conclusion is supported by the premises. For example:

Although Martha may very well be the victim of abuse, the truth or falsity of the conclusion (or any of the statements) is not an issue when evaluating the validity of an argument. In Example B, the conclusion that Martha is a victim of abuse is not established by the supporting evidence in the premises. The conclusion goes beyond the explicit and implicit information in the premises. This is not a valid argument. (Compare the reasoning in Examples A and B.)

Whereas *validity* refers to the forms of the deductive argument, *truth* refers to the content of a given theoretical statement. It is therefore inappropriate to label a single theoretical statement valid or an argument true.[10]

In a valid deductive argument, if the premises are true, it necessarily follows that the conclusion must be true. (This combination is marked *[R]* In Fig. 4-1.) It is therefore impossible for the conclusion to be false. (This combination is marked *[S]* in Fig. 4-1.) If, however, one or more of the premises is false,

		The conclusion is:	
		True	False
If the premises are:	All true	Necessary (R)	Impossible (S)
	Not all true	Possible (Y)	Possible (X)

(R) If the premises are true, it *necessarily follows* that the conclusion be true.
(S) If the premises are true, it is therefore *impossible* for the conclusion to be false.
(Y), (X) If one or more of the premises are false, it is *possible* the conclusion may be *either* true or false.

Fig. **4-1 Potential outcomes of a valid deductive argument.** *Modified from Giere, R.N. (1979).* Understanding scientific reasoning. *New York: Holt, Rinehart & Winston.*

two outcomes are possible: the conclusion may be either true or false.

Example C presents a deductively valid argument that leads from false premises to a false conclusion. (This combination is marked *[X]* in Fig. 4-1.)

EXAMPLE C

Premise: The dime is larger than the nickel. (**False**)
Premise: The nickel is larger than the Susan B. Anthony dollar. (**False**)
Conclusion: Thus the dime is larger than the Susan B. Anthony dollar. (**False**)

As Fig. 4-1 suggests and Example D illustrates, it is also possible that a valid argument can lead from one or more false premises to a true conclusion. (This combination is marked *[Y]* in Fig. 4-1.)

EXAMPLE D

Premise: The nickel is larger than the Susan B. Anthony dollar. (**False**)
Premise: The Susan B. Anthony dollar is larger than the dime. (**True**)
Conclusion: Thus the nickel is larger than the dime. (**True**)

It may be helpful to study Examples C and D to understand how the conclusions are derived from the information given in the premises. (Note in these examples that "larger than" refers to physical size, not to the value of the coins.) In science, deductive arguments can be a powerful form of reasoning for deriving new conclusions by making explicit the implied information contained in what is known. These derived conclusions can then be subjected to empirical test.

INDUCTION

Induction is a form of logical reasoning in which a generalization is induced from a number of specific observed instances. Inductive reasoning has been less well developed than deductive reasoning.[8] The form of the inductive argument follows:

1. A is true of $b_1, b_2 \ldots b_n$.
2. $b_1, b_2 \ldots b_n$ are some members of class B.
3. Hence A is true of all members of class B.[15:9]

The inductive form is based on the assumption that members of any given class share common characteristics. Therefore what is true of any randomly selected members of the class is accepted as true for all members of the class.[15] Suppose a sample of the population of victims of abuse has been selected for study. Example E presents an argument in the inductive form that may be developed based on this hypothetical study.

EXAMPLE E

Premise: Every victim of abuse that has been observed has low self-esteem.
Conclusion: All victims of abuse have low self-esteem.

The premise in Example E states observations from a number of instances, that is, a limited number of subjects. The conclusion states a generalization extending beyond the observations to the whole class of victims of abuse.

The inductive generalization also may be stated in terms of a mathematical quantity.[10] For example, assume a researcher decides to survey a sample of 400 nurses to determine their opinions as to whether nurses would establish independent private practices. Results indicate 65% of nurses in the sample support independent private practice activities in nursing. The inductive statement may be stated as follows:

EXAMPLE F

Premise: Sixty-five percent of nurses in the sample support independent private practice activities in nursing.
Conclusion: Sixty-five percent of all nurses support independent private practice in nursing.

Whereas, in a deductive argument, if the premises are true, the conclusion must necessarily be true, the inductive argument can have true premises and yet produce a false conclusion.

An inductive conclusion based on limited or biased evidence can clearly lead to a fallacious argument and perhaps a false conclusion.[10] Suppose the argument in Example E was developed by one nurse's experience with observing five victims of abuse. The conclusion that victims of abuse have low self-esteem may or may not be true. However, this conclusion is not warranted based on the number of observed instances. There is too little evidence in this case to justify the conclusion about all victims of abuse.

Even if the sample size is appropriately sufficient (or based on several studies), the sample may be biased. Assume in Example F that the sample of nurses was drawn from faculty in schools of nursing. The opinions of this select group of nurses may be expected to be different in some respects and may not reflect the opinions of all nurses. It may be that a greater proportion of nursing faculty members are engaged in private practice activities than the proportion of all nurses. Considering a number of factors in selecting representative samples can help avoid introducing bias into observations. This reasoning is the basis for the random selection of subjects in research projects. Descriptive and inferential statistics are used to characterize the sample of population and help with decisions about the strength of the evidence.[3] The inductive inference thus has been termed the statistical inference.[15,18]

A distinguishing characteristic of inductive arguments is that the inferred conclusion goes beyond the implicit and explicit information in the premises. In Example E not all victims of abuse have been observed. This conclusion is inferred on the basis of selected instances. In a deductive argument, the conclusion can be considered true if the argument is structured so that implicit information in the premises is made explicit.[10] The inductive argument, on the other hand, goes beyond the information in the premises. The inductive argument thus expands on the information presented. Giere[3] has argued this characteristic permits the justification of scientific conclusions that may not be justifiable by deductive reasoning, since they contain information beyond the premises. An example would be a scientific hypothesis about the future based on observations in the present.[3]

Although deductive arguments are considered to be either valid or invalid, the concept of validity does not apply to inductive arguments. The correctness of inductive arguments is not viewed in either/or terms

but on degrees of strength, measured in terms of the *probability* with which the premises lead to a given conclusion.[10] The inferred conclusion then can be determined to have low, medium, or high probability.[10] Statistical procedures can be used for making these judgments.

In Example A, the only possibility for the conclusion's being false is if one or more of the premises are false, that is, if all victims of abuse do not have low self-esteem, or if Martha and Tom are not victims of abuse. If these are true, the conclusion must necessarily be true. However, in Example E the reasoning suggests that all victims of abuse have low self-esteem. But the premises state that only selected victims of abuse have been observed. The premises may lend some support for the conclusion. The fact that no victims of abuse without low self-esteem have been observed may be considered some evidence but will not preclude the possibility that a victim with high self-esteem will not be observed in the future.[10]

Deductive arguments are considered "truth preservers," whereas inductive arguments can be a source of new information.[3,10] Scientific generalizations about instances not observed in the present or projections about the future are examples. Although this form of reasoning is useful in advancing science, the very nature of induction may introduce error into the scientific process.[4] Even if we could be sure the premises were accurate, we could not be absolutely certain of the accuracy of the conclusion. In Giere's view,[3] if we assume the premises are true:

> The difference between a *good inductive argument* and a *valid deductive argument* is that the deductive argument guarantees the *truth* of its conclusion while the inductive argument guarantees only an *appropriately high probability* of its conclusion.[3:37-38]

RETRODUCTION*

Whereas deduction and induction may explicate and evaluate ideas, retroduction originates ideas.[14] The retroductive form of reasoning is an approach to inquiry using analogy as a method for devising theory. In 1878, Pierce described three kinds of reasoning as comprising the major steps of inquiry: retroduction, deduction, and induction.[15] Pierce viewed retroductive reasoning as the first stage in the search for understanding some "surprising phenomenon" in which a viewpoint offering a possible explanation is identified. Pierce stated that once a viewpoint that held the promise of explanation for the observed phenomenon was identified, deductive reasoning was used to develop the explanation. Pierce considered the final stage of inquiry in terms of induction with the focus on checking out the devised hypotheses in experience.[15] The theory models approach using retroductive inference was further developed by Steiner* as a method for devising theory. The form of the retroductive inference follows:

1. The surprising fact, C, is observed.
2. But if A were true, C would be a matter of course.
3. Hence there is reason to suspect that A is true.[15:9]

An analysis of the preceding form reveals that the theory models (or retroductive) approach does not establish truth. Its function is to originate ideas about selected phenomena that can be developed further and tested. The theory models approach is most useful as a strategy for devising theory in a field in which there are few available theories, and innovation is indicated to advance knowledge in describing and understanding selected observations.[15,17]

The retroductive theorist approaches the development of wanted theory by identifying a source theory in another field that may have potential for developing the wanted theory. The theory models approach is based on the use of analogy and metaphor between two sets of phenomena. This requires considerable creativity on the part of the theorist and an intuitive knowledge of the phenomena of interest.[13] The theory models approach is represented as follows[14,15]:

$$THEORY_1 \quad \rightarrow \quad THEORY \rightarrow THEORY_2$$
$$MODEL$$

(Source theory)   (Wanted theory)

Thus theory models are not "models of" but are "models for" devising representations of selected phenomena.[13] The theory model is essentially a metamodel, which serves as a model to develop theory.[14]

To devise a theory using retroductive inference, the theorist seeks out a source theory to form a theory model from which the wanted theory will be devised. The source theory is selected on the basis of a "suspected similarity in the structure of form or pattern of relations" between the two sets of phenomena.[15] The selected source theory is perceived to present ideas that may be useful for developing a theory about the observations of interest. These ideas are selected from theory $_1$ and formed into a point of view or theory model that will serve as the framework for developing theory$_2$. This approach is based on the assumption that new conjectures, or ideas, in a given field may be devised from other conjectures in theories in other fields.[4,5,15] The ideas selected from theory$_1$ for the theory model may involve any combination of concepts, hypothesized relationships, or theory structures. The viewpoint presented by the theory model is used to develop theory$_2$ by adding *content* to theory model and by *altering concepts and relationships to fit with the phenomenon of interest* for theory$_2$. It should be clear that this process of theory building is not simply borrowing a theory from one field and applying it unchanged to another.[12] The deliberate selection of aspects of theory $_1$ to form the theory model, the addition of new information, and the alteration of concepts and relationships for congruence with different phenomena in a new context, result in a new theory. Of course a theory devised by this method must meet the criteria for adequacy of a theory[12] (see Chapter 1). As Steiner (Maccia)[5,14,15] argued, the theory models approach cannot be considered reductive since theory$_1$ is not equivalent to theory$_2$. To be reductive, the theorist would simply borrow concepts and hypotheses and use them as formulated in a new context. Neither can this approach be considered deductive, since theory$_2$ was not developed by deduction from theory$_1$. The hy-

*References 4, 5, 12, 13. Elizabeth Steiner-Maccia's earlier work on theory models was published under her married name of *Maccia.*

potheses in theory$_2$ cannot be derived from theory$_1$.[14,15]

The use of analogy to develop theory has been a common occurrence in the development of a number of scientific fields. In Sigmund Freud's day, the machine model was a popular advanced model of the times. Freud used the notion of machine operations to develop his theoretical assertions about psychological tension-reduction relationships in his theory of psychosexual development. Three or more decades ago basic texts in human anatomy and physiology used the telephone switchboard as an analogy for explaining the functioning of the brain. Currently, the computer is often used as a model for thinking about the brain and in developing theories of human information processing.[6,11] In nursing, general systems theory has been used as a model for developing nursing theory.[7] Steiner's development of the theory models approach provides guidelines for using this strategy in theory building.

Table **4-1**

Deduction, induction, and retroduction summary		
TYPE	**QUESTION**	**TECHNIQUES**
DEDUCTION	Given that the premises are true, what other propositions may be inferred as necessary conclusions from the premises?[13:67]	Logical and conceptual analysis[13]
INDUCTION	Given that the premises are true, what is the strength of the link between them and the conclusion?[13:87]	Logical and conceptual analysis based on statistical analysis[12,16]
RETRODUCTION	Given a surprising observation, what explanation would result in the expectation that the observation would be a matter of course?[13]	Logical and conceptual analysis[12]

Stevens[16] has argued that one of the reasons much of nursing research has so little impact on nursing practice is that nursing research is often based on the "categories and characteristics" of borrowed theories. A borrowed theory tends to be used unchanged in the new context. Although theories in other fields may suggest a possible framework for addressing phenomena in the field of nursing, this framework may need to be contextualized within nursing. That is, aspects of the "borrowed theory" may need to be altered to reflect the appropriate categories and characteristics within nursing. Walker and Avant's "derivation strategy" for theory construction[17] draws from the theory models approach developed by Steiner. Walker and Avant[17] present a number of examples of using the derivation strategy to "shift and reformulate" concepts, theoretical statements, and theories from other fields to nursing. The theory models approach permits the translation and expansion of ideas within the milieu of nursing and may result in the development

DEFINITION	EXAMPLE	FUNCTION
	Premises	*Explicates and derives further truths[12:9]*
1. If A were true, then B would be true. 2. A is true. 3. Hence B is true.[15:9]	All victims of abuse have low self-esteem. Marty and Tom are victims of abuse. *Conclusion* Marty and Tom have low self-esteem.	If premises are true, establishes truth of something else by derivation.[12:9]
	Premise	*Evaluates and expands information[3]*
1. A is true of $b_1, b_2 \ldots b_n$. 2. $b_1, b_2 \ldots b_n$ are members of some class B. 3. Hence A is true of all members of class B.[15:9]	$b_1, b_2 \ldots b_n$ victims of abuse who have been observed have low self-esteem. *Conclusion* All victims of abuse have low self-esteem.	Based on probability of observed cases. Does not establish truth. Establishes probability of certainty. New data may change conclusion.[3,9,12]
	Proposition 1	*Originates ideas[12:9]*
1. The surprising fact C is observed. 2. But if A were true, C would be a matter of course. 3. Hence there is reason to suspect that A is true.[15:9]	The role of expecting *reward* determines a relation between *student* and *teacher* that establishes a path for influence of the teacher on the *student.*[5:121] *Proposition 2* The role of expecting *care* and *comfort* determines a relation between *patient* and *nurse* that establishes a path for influence of *nurse* on the *patient.*	Does not establish truth. Suggests lines of thought worthy of exploration and testing.[12:9]

of a new nursing theory. A nursing theory devised by this method can be further developed through the use of deductive strategies.

A summary of deductive, inductive, and retroductive forms of reasoning is presented in Table 4-1.

In contrast to reasoning based on traditional logical assumptions presented in this chapter, scholarly work is also ongoing with other unconventional approaches to logic, such as *fuzzy set theory* and *fuzzy logic theory*, which provides a model for modes of reasoning that are approximate rather than exact. For example, Bosque[1] uses fuzzy logic in nursing to devise a theoretical perspective of nurse and machine symbiosis in the design of a new neonatal pulse oximeter alarm.

REFERENCES

1. Bosque, E.M. (1995). Symbiosis of nurse and machine through fuzzy logic: Improved specificity of neonatal pulse oximeter alarm. *Advances in Nursing Science, 18*(2), 67-75.
2. Geach, P.T. (1979). *Reason and argument.* Los Angeles: University of California Press.
3. Giere, R.N. (1979). *Understanding scientific reasoning.* New York: Holt, Rinehart & Winston.
4. Maccia, E.S., & Maccia, G. (1966). *Construction of educational theory derived from three educational theory models* (Project No. 5-0638). Washington, DC: U.S. Department of Health, Education, and Welfare.
5. Maccia, E.S., Maccia, G., & Jewett, R. (1963). *Construction of educational theory models* (Cooperative Research Project No. 1632). Washington, DC: Office of Education, U.S. Department of Health, Education, and Welfare.
6. Norman, D.A. (1976). *Memory and attention: An introduction to human information processing.* New York: John Wiley & Sons.
7. Nursing Theories Conference Group (1980). *Nursing theories: The base for professional nursing practice.* Englewood Cliffs, NJ: Prentice-Hall.
8. Pospesel, H. (1974). *Propositional logic.* Englewood Cliffs, NJ: Prentice-Hall.
9. Salmon, W.C. (1967). *The foundations of scientific inference.* Pittsburgh: University of Pittsburgh Press.
10. Salmon, W.C. (1973). *Logic.* Englewood Cliffs, NJ: Prentice-Hall.
11. Shepherd, G.M. (1974). *The synaptic organization of the brain.* New York: Oxford University Press.
12. Steiner, E. (1976). *Logical and conceptual analytic techniques for educational researchers.* Paper presented at the American Educational Research Association, San Francisco. © Copyright Elizabeth Steiner. All rights reserved.
13. Steiner, E. (1976). *The complete act of educational inquiry.* © Copyright Elizabeth Steiner. All rights reserved.
14. Steiner, E. (1977). *Criteria for theory of art education.* Paper represented at the Seminar for Research in Art Education, Philadelphia. © Copyright Elizabeth Steiner. All rights reserved.
15. Steiner, E. (1978). *Logical and conceptual analytic techniques for educational researchers.* Washington, DC: University Press.
16. Stevens, B. (1979). *Nursing theory: Analysis, application, evaluation.* Boston: Little, Brown.
17. Walker, L., & Avant, K. (1983). *Strategies for theory construction in nursing.* Norwalk, CT: Appleton-Century-Crofts.
18. Weiner, P. (1958). *Values in universe of chance.* New York: Doubleday.

Theory Development Process

Sue Marquis Bishop

*N*ursing theory development is not a mysterious, magical activity. Many nurses have been developing their own private ideas about nursing since their first day in the field (or perhaps before) and have continued to develop private assumptions based on their readings and experiences. These private notions may include such generalizations as "A clean, smooth bed allows for greater rest and less need for pain medication for a patient" or "Encouraging the patient to have some say in his or her care leads to greater cooperation with treatment procedures." Nurses usually do not talk explicitly about their *private theories*, although these theories may influence the nursing activities they choose to implement and the manner in which they practice.

If in fact all nurses are evolving private theories of nursing, why all the fuss about studying published theories? The major reason is the nurses' private conceptions of nursing may be "incomplete, inconsistent, or muddled."* This leads to considerable problems in

using the private theory as a sound basis for practice. Further, an incomplete, inconsistent, or muddled theory may be difficult to use in studying clinical nursing situations that would advance our knowledge of nursing. If we agree that the availability of more systematic theories would provide a clearer understanding of nursing and would enable us to explore whether this understanding corresponds with activities in the nursing environment, then we also must agree with Hardy[9] and other researchers that rigorous development of nursing theory is a priority. The systematic development of scientific nursing theories has a better chance of advancing nursing and may lead to the basis for advancing nursing science.

It is important to grasp the concept of *systematic development*. Approaches to the construction of theory differ. One aspect they have in common, however, is the agreement among scientists to approach theory development in a systematic fashion and to make the stages in development explicit so that others can review the logical processes and test the hypotheses presented. The nurse who systematically devises a theory of nursing and presents it for public review by the nursing community is engaging in the process essential to advancing theory development.

---

*I wish to acknowledge my indebtedness to Nicholas Mullins, one of my former teachers, for his discussion of private and public theories and for communicating both the complexity and creative playfulness in theoretical work.

THEORY COMPONENTS

Hage[8] identified six components of a complete theory and specified the contribution each makes to the whole theory (Table 5-1). He argued that the failure to include one or more of the components resulted in the elimination of that particular contribution to the total theory. These six aspects of a theory are discussed as a basis for understanding the *function* of each element in the theory building process.

Concepts

Concepts, the building blocks of theories, classify the phenomena with which we are concerned.[11] It is crucial in any separate discussion of concepts to recognize that concepts must not be considered separately from the theoretical system in which they are embedded and from which they derive their meaning.[3] Concepts may have completely different meanings in different theoretical systems. Because scientific progress is based on the critical review and testing of a researcher's work by others in the scientific community, consensus regarding the meaning of scientific concepts is important.[3,8]

Concepts may be classified as *abstract* or *concrete*. Abstract concepts are independent of a specific time or place, whereas concrete concepts relate to a particular time or place.[8,18]

Abstract concepts	*Concrete concepts*
Social system	The Vaughn Family; University of North Carolina at Charlotte
Debate	Dole-Clinton Debate

In the above example, the Vaughn family is an instance of the more general abstract concept of social system.

Concepts also may be classified as *discrete* or *continuous*. This system of labels differentiates concepts that vary along a continuum from concepts that specify categories of phenomena.

A *discrete concept* identifies *categories or classes* of phenomena, such as, patient, nurse, or environment. For example, one can be a nurse or a non-nurse, but not a partial nurse. Phenomena are thus identified as belonging to or not belonging to a given class (either/or). Discrete concepts have therefore been called

Table **5-1**

Theory components and their contributions to the theory

THEORY COMPONENTS	CONTRIBUTIONS
Concepts	Description and classification
Theoretical statements	Analysis
Definitions	
Theoretical	Meaning
Operational	Measurements
Linkages	
Theoretical	Plausibility
Operational	Testability
Ordering of concepts and definitions into primitive and derived terms	Elimination of overlap (tautology)
Ordering of statements and linkages into premises and equations	Elimination of inconsistency

Modified from Hage, J. (1972). *Techniques and problems in theory construction in sociology.* New York: John Wiley & Sons.

nonvariable concepts.[8] The sorting of phenomena into nonvariable discrete categories carries the assumption that the reality associated with the given phenomenon is "captured by the classification."[8] The "amount" or "degree" is not an issue. The discrete concept of bureaucracy was devised by Max Weber as an ideal type to characterize organizations.[13] Organizations can then be classified as *bureaucratic* or *nonbureaucratic.*

The definition of the discrete concept is critical in knowing how to classify the phenomenon. Theories may be developed using a series of nonvariable discrete concepts (and subconcepts) to build typologies.[18] *Typologies* consist of a systematic arrangement of the concepts.

A *continuous concept* permits the classification of *dimensions* or gradations of a phenomenon *on a continuum,* such as degree of marital conflict. For example, marital couples may be classified across a range representing the amount of marital conflict in their relationships.

The use of variable concepts based on a range or continuum tends to be focused on one dimension without the assumption that a single dimension "captures all the reality" connected with the phenomenon.[8] Additional dimensions may be devised to measure further aspects of the phenomenon. In contrast to the nonvariable term *bureaucracy,* variable concepts such as rate of conflict, ratio of professional to nonprofessional staff, and communication flow may be used to characterize organizations.[8] Although nonvariable concepts are useful in classifying phenomena in theory development, it has been argued that major breakthroughs have occurred in several fields when the focus shifted from nonvariable to variable concepts.[8] Variable concepts permit scoring the full range of the phenomenon on a continuum.[8]

The development of theoretical concepts thus permits the *description and classification* of phenomena.[8] The labeled concept suggests boundaries for selecting phenomena to observe and for reasoning about the phenomena of interest. New concepts may focus attention on new phenomena or may facilitate thinking about and classifying phenomena in a different way.[8]

Theoretical Statements

Although concepts are considered the building blocks of theory, they must be *connected* in some way with a set of theoretical statements to devise theory.[2,3,6,13,20] The development of theoretical statements asserting a connection between two or more concepts introduces the possibility of *analysis.*[8]

Statements in a theory can be classified into the following three general categories: *existence statements, definitions,* and *relational statements.*[18,27] Existence statements and definitions relate to specific concepts. Whereas definitions provide descriptions of the concept, existence statements simply assert that a given concept exists and is labeled with the concept name. Relational statements assert relationships between the properties of two or more concepts (or variables). Various types of relational state-

ments have been described in the literature.[16,18,27] Discussion in this chapter is limited to an introduction to probabilistic statements and necessary and sufficient conditional statements. These types of statements are important in understanding scientific reasoning.[7]

In the connections between variables, one variable may be assumed to influence a second variable. In this instance, the first variable may be labeled an *antecedent* (or determinant) variable and the second variable a *consequent* (or resultant) variable.[7,24,29] In this instance, the first variable may be viewed as the independent variable and the second as the dependent variable.[7] Because of its complexity, nursing presents a situation in which multiple antecedents and consequences may be involved in studying a selected phenomenon. Zetterberg[29] concluded, however, that the development of two-variate theoretical statements may be an important intermediate step in the development of a theory. These statements later can be reformulated as the theory evolves or as new information is made available.

Relational statements may be expressed as a necessary and/or sufficient condition. These labels characterize the conditions that help explain the nature of the relationship between the two variables in the theoretical statements.

An example of a relational statement expressed as a *sufficient condition* is, "If nurses react with approval of patients' independent behaviors, patients increase their efforts in self-care activities." This is a type of compound statement linking antecedent and consequent variables. The statement does not assert the truth of the antecedent. Rather, the assertion is made that *if* the antecedent is true, then the consequent also is true.[7] In addition, there is no assertion in the statement explaining *why* the antecedent is related to the consequent.[8] In symbolic notation form, the above statements can be expressed as:

$$NA \longrightarrow PSC$$
(Nurse Approval)   (Patient Self-Care)

This statement asserts that nurse approval of a patient's independent behaviors is sufficient for the occurrence of the patient's self-care activities. However, patient assumption of self-care activities resulting from other factors such as the patient's health status and personality variables is not ruled out. In other words, there could be other antecedents that are sufficient conditions for the patient's assumption of self-care activities.

A statement in the form of a *necessary condition* asserts that one variable is required for the occurrence of another variable.[7,17,20] For example:

> Without the motivation to get well (MGW), patients will not adhere strictly to their prescribed treatment regimen (PTR).
> MGW ⟶ PTR

This means PTR never occurs when MGW does not occur.[7,17] No assertion is made that patients' strict adherence to the prescribed treatment regimen follows from their motivation to get well. It is asserted, however, that if motivation to get well is absent, patients will not assume strict adherence to their treatment regimen. The motivation to get well is thus a necessary, but not a sufficient, condition for the occurrence of this consequent.

The term *if* is generally used to introduce a sufficient condition, whereas *only if* and *if . . . then* are used to introduce necessary conditions.[7] In most instances conditional statements are not both necessary and sufficient.[7] It is possible, however, for a statement to express both conditions. In such instances the term *if and only if* is used to imply that the conditions are both necessary and sufficient for one another.[7] In this case (1) the consequent never occurs in the absence of the antecedent and (2) the consequent always occurs when the antecedent occurs.[7,17]

Although *causal statements* (one variable causes another) may be expressed as a conditional statement, not all conditional statements are causal.[7] For example, the statement "If this month is March, then the next month is April" does not assert that March causes April to occur. Rather the sequence of months suggests that April follows March.[7] (For an extensive discussion of conditional and unconditional causal statements see Nowak.[17])

Probabilistic statements are generally derived from statistical data and express connections that do not always occur but are likely to occur based on some estimate of probability.[27] Walker and Avant[27] used as an example the statement "Cigarette smoking will most likely lead to cancer of the lung." It is clear that cigarette smoking does not always lead to lung cancer since some persons who smoke do not develop this disease. However, the probability of developing cancer of the lung is increased for cigarette smokers. In symbolic notation[18]:

> IF CS ⟶ P LC

The development of relational statements asserting connections between variables provides for analysis and establishes the basis for explanation and prediction.[8]

Definitions

The development of science is a collaborative endeavor in which the community of scientists critique, test, and build on one another's work.[3] It is therefore crucial that concepts be as clearly defined as possible to reduce ambiguity in understanding a given concept or set of concepts. Although it is not possible to entirely eliminate perceived differences in meaning, these differences can be minimized by setting forth explicit definitions. In the development of a complete theory, both theoretical and operational definitions provide meaning for the concept and a basis for searching for empirical indicators.[8] *Theoretical definitions* also permit consideration of the relationships of a given concept to other theoretical ideas, but a clear meaning for concepts is not sufficient.

If theories are to be tested against reality, then concepts also must be measurable.[8] *Operational definitions* relate the concepts to observable phenomena by specifying empirical indicators.[8] Hage[8] asserted that the concept name and the theoretical and operational definitions establish reference points for "locating the concept," that is, viewing the concept as related to both theoretical systems and the observable environment.

Linkages

The specification of linkages is an important part of the development of theory.[8] Although the theoretical statements assert connections between concepts, the rationale for the stated connections needs to be developed. The development of *theoretical linkages* offers a reasoned explanation of why the variables in the theory may be connected in some manner, that is, the theoretical reasons for asserting particular interrelationships.[8] This rationale contributes *plausibility* to the theory.[8]

Operational linkages, on the other hand, contribute the element of *testability* to the theory by specifying how variables are connected.[8] Although operational definitions provide for measurability of the concepts, operational linkages provide for testability of the assertions. The operational linkage contributes a perspective for understanding the nature of the relationship between concepts, such as whether the relationship between concepts is negative or positive, linear or curvilinear.[8]

Ordering

Finally, Hage[8] concluded that a theory may be considered "fairly complete" if it presents the elements of *concepts, definitions, statements,* and *linkages.* Complete development of the theory, however, requires the organization of concepts and definitions into primitive and derived terms and the organization of statements and linkages into premises and equations.[8] As the theory evolves, concepts and theoretical statements multiply, and the need arises to establish some logical arrangement or *ordering* of the theoretical components to bring conceptual order to the theory.[8] Hage stated the concepts should be ordered if the theory contains more than two variables. He also recommended that concepts and definitions be ordered into *primitive* and *derived* terms. *Primitive terms* are not defined within the theory. This process of ordering may point up any existing overlap between concepts and definitions.[8] The conceptual arrangement of statements and linkages into premises and equations may reveal areas of inconsistency.[8] Premises (or axioms) are regarded as the more general assertions from which the hypotheses are derived in the form of equations. Hage suggested that the ordering of statements and linkages is indicated when the theory contains a large number of theoretical statements.[8]

FORMS OF THEORY ORGANIZATIONS*

A formal theory is a systematically developed conceptual system that addresses a given set of phenomena. There are different ideas about how this conceptual system should be organized so as to constitute a theory. Three forms for organizing theory are set-of-laws, axiomatic, and causal process.

Set-of-Laws Form

The set-of-laws approach attempts to organize findings from empirical research.[18] The theorist first reviews the research literature in an area of particular interest. Empirical findings from available research are identified and selected from the literature for evaluation. Findings are evaluated and sorted into categories based on the degree of empirical evidence supporting each assertion.[18] The available categories are *laws, empirical generalizations,* and *hypotheses.*[18]

Since construction of the set-of-laws form of theory requires the selection and evaluation of research findings in terms of degree of empirical support, several limitations emerge as a result of this approach to constructing theory. Reynolds[18] discussed these limitations as disadvantages to the set-of-laws approach to theory building.

First, the nature of research requires focusing on relationships between a limited set of variables, often two variables. Therefore attempts to develop a set-of-laws theory from statements of findings may result in a lengthy number of statements that assert relationships between two or more variables. This lengthy set of generalizations may be difficult to organize and interrelate.

Second, for research to be conducted, concepts must be operationally defined so as to be measurable. Concepts in the statements of empirical findings are therefore most likely to be measurable and operational concepts. This procedure eliminates other more highly abstract or theoretical concepts that might be useful in developing an understanding of the phenomenon of interest.

*This section is largely based on Reynolds's discussion[18] of these forms.

Reynolds[18] concluded that although the set-of-laws form may provide for classification of phenomena or predictions of relationships between selected variables, it does not permit a "sense of understanding" crucial for the advancement of science. Finally, Reynolds[18] noted that each statement in the set-of-laws form is considered to be independent in that the various statements have not been interrelated into a system of description and explanation (Fig. 5-1). Therefore each statement must be tested. Because the *statements are not interrelated,* research support for one statement does not provide support for any other statement. Research efforts must therefore be more extensive.

The set-of-laws approach to theory building is consistent with the view that scientific knowledge consists of empirical findings and that science is advanced by conducting research and then looking for patterns in the data.[18] Patterns do not, of their own accord, arise from empirical data.[24] The theorist must bring "ideas to experience" to conceptualize and order theoretical relationships.[24] Reynolds[18] stated that this may be difficult to do with a "lengthy catalogue" of empirical findings in the set-of-laws form.

Axiomatic Form

In contrast to the set-of-laws forms, the axiomatic form of theory organization is an interrelated logical system. Specifically, an axiomatic theory consists of a set of concepts, explicit definitions, a set of existence statements, and a set of relationship statements arranged in hierarchical order.[18,26,29] The concepts include highly *abstract concepts, intermediate concepts,* and *more concrete concepts.* The set of existence statements describes situations in which the theory is applicable.[18,26,27] Statements helping delineate the boundaries of the theory are referred to as *describing the scope conditions of the theory.*[5,8,18] *The relational statements consist of axioms and propositions.* The highly abstract theoretical statements, called *axioms,* are organized at the top of the hierarchy.[26] All other propositions are developed through logical deduction from the axioms or from other more abstract propositions[26] (Fig. 5-2).

The axiomatic theory is determined to be integrated when there are no propositions in Set B that cannot be logically derived from Set A.[28] This results in a highly interrelated explanatory system. An essential criterion for the axiomatic form is that the theoretical statements may not be contradictory.[28] A basic

---

SET-OF-LAWS FORMS

Laws (overwhelming empirical support)
1.
2.
3.
Empirical generalizations (some empirical support)
1.
2.
3.
4.
Hypotheses (no empirical support)
1.
2.
3.
4.
5.

Fig. **5-1 Set-of-laws forms.** *From Reynolds, P. (1971). A primer in theory construction. Indianapolis: Bobbs-Merrill.*

principle of logic asserts that when two statements are contradictory, one or both of the statements must be false.[20,28] Thus axiomatic theorists seek to avoid this problem by developing a conceptual system with a few broad axioms from which a set of propositions can be derived.[28] As science progresses and new empirical data become known, the general axioms may be modified or extended. If, however, these additions to the logical system produce contradictions in the theory, the theory must be rejected for one without contradictions.[28] New theories often subsume portions of previous theories as special cases.[3,28] For example, Einstein's Theory of Relativity incorporated Newton's law of gravitation as a special case within the theory.

Axiomatic theories are not common in the social and behavioral sciences but are clearly evident in the fields of physics and mathematics. For example, Euclidean geometry is an axiomatic theory.[28,29]

Developing theories in axiomatic form has several advantages.[18,20] First, since theory is a *highly interrelated set of statements, some of which are derived from others,* all concepts do not need to be operationally defined.[18] This allows the theorist to incorporate some highly abstract concepts that may be unmeasurable but provide for explanation. The interrelated axiomatic system may also be more efficient for explanation than the lengthy number of theoretical statements in the set-of-laws form. In addition, *empirical support for one theoretical statement may be judged to provide support for the theory,* thus permitting less extensive research than the requirement to test each statement in the set-of-laws form. Finally, Reynolds[18] concluded that in certain instances the axiomatic theory may be organized in a causal process form to increase understanding.

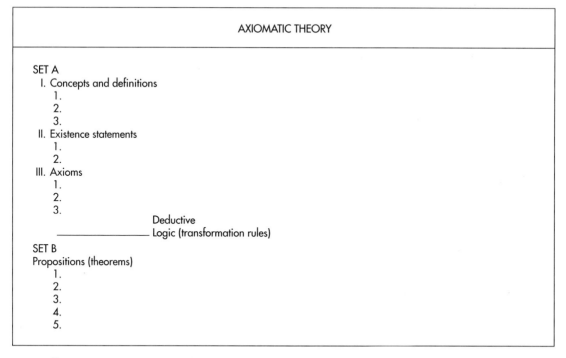

Fig. **5-2 Axiomatic theory represented in schematic form.** *Developed from Werkmeister, W. (1959). Theory construction and the problem of objectivity. In L. Gross (Ed.),* Symposium of sociological theory. *Evanston, IL: Row, Peterson, & Co. [schemata]; and Reynolds, P. (1971).* A primer in theory construction. *Indianapolis: Bobbs-Merrill [terminology].*

Causal Process Form

The distinguishing feature of the causal process form of theory is the development of theoretical statements specifying *causal mechanisms* between independent and dependent variables.[17,18] This form of theory organization consists of a set of concepts, a set of definitions, a set of existence statements, and a set of theoretical statements specifying causal process.[18] Concepts include abstract as well as concrete ideas. Existence statements function as in axiomatic theories to describe the scope conditions of the theory—the situations to which the theory applies.[5,8,18] In contrast to the hierarchial arrangement in the axiomatic theory, causal process theories contain a set of statements describing the causal mechanisms or effects of one variable on one or more other variables.[16,18] Causal process theories may be limited to a few variables or may be quite complex, having several variables (Fig. 5-3).

The causal statements specify the hypothesized effects of one variable on one or more variables. In complex causal process theories, feedback loops and paths of influence through several variables may be hypothesized in the set of interrelated causal statements.[16,17] Reynolds[18] concluded that the causal process form of theory provides for an explanation of "how something happens." He identified several advantages of the causal process form of organization. First, it provides for highly abstract theoretical concepts, as does axiomatic theory. Second, also like axiomatic theory, this form with its *interrelated theoretical statements* permits more efficient research testing. Finally, the causal process statements provide a sense of understanding about the phenomenon of interest not possible with other forms. However, Turner[26] observed that causal process theories may not necessarily include highly abstract concepts, since a number of available theories simply contain

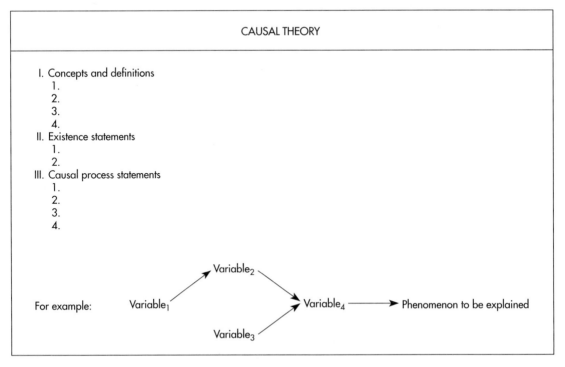

Fig. **5-3** Elements of causal theory. *Developed from Reynolds, P. (1971). A primer in theory construction. Indianapolis: Bobbs-Merrill; and Turner, J. (1978). The structure of sociological theory. Homewood, IL: The Dorsey Press.*

"descriptions of causal connections among events." This approach does permit the development of a causal explanation of the sequence of events that may affect the phenomenon of interest.[26]

CREATIVITY IN THEORY BUILDING

Although a number of strategies for developing theory have been presented in the literature, the theorist who attempts to approach theory construction in a mechanical way by applying structured procedures may have limited success. Theory building involves discovery and creativity. A scientific theory is clearly "a creation of the human mind."[2] Bronowski[2] has written about the similarities in the processes of constructing theories and designing works of art; each requires a high level of imagination. In his view, "There is no difference in the use of such words as 'beauty' and 'truth' in the poem and such symbols as 'energy' and 'mass' in the equation."[2:21]

Although it is possible to teach specific techniques and content, we don't really know how to facilitate creativity and originality in students. In Rosenberg's words, "You can teach someone how to look, but not how to see, how to search, but not how to find."[19:2] Bronowski[2] suggests a sense of "imagination, playfulness, and participation" is essential not only for the theorist but for the reader who seeks to understand theories:

> If science is a form of imagination, if all experiment is a form of play, then science cannot be dry-as-dust. Science, or art, every creative activity is fun. If a theorem in science seems dull to you, that is because you are not reading it with the same active sense of participation (and imagination) which you bring to the reading of a poem.[2:22-23]

In addition to imagination, developing and presenting theories requires personal discipline. Innovative ideas tend to occur in a "vague, disconnected, and tenuous form."[14] Self-discipline is required to work with the idea, develop it, and express it in written form for others to review.[10] Rosenberg[19] stated that, although "critical acumen" and creativity cannot be taught, they can be "nourished, enhanced, and matured." The individual's role is to attain familiarity with the phenomenon of interest and "practice, practice, practice."[19]

NURSING THEORIES

In the 1990s, there is less preoccupation in nursing with the question of whether nursing formulations are "really theories." In 1980, Flaskerud and Halloran noted that, although nurses identify formulations in nursing as "simply models or conceptual frameworks," they are not reluctant to label frameworks from other fields, such as psychology or sociology, as "theories."[6] They argued that this depreciated available efforts to systematize nursing. Meleis[12] characterized the early 1980s as the period of acceptance of the need to further develop nursing theory to advance the discipline of nursing as well as a time of lingering "confusion" in regard to the semantics of how theories were characterized. In 1985, she asserted the view of several other nurse scholars, for example, Stevens in 1979:

> The differences between the different labels (theory, metaparadigm, conceptual frameworks, and so forth) are differences in emphasis rather than substance and are not worth the debate. . . . Why continue to unwittingly downgrade nursing theory by relegating it to a conceptual frameworks status when other conceptualizations (in other fields) have been called theory. . . . A theory in process should not be considered a conceptual framework; it is simply in an expected stage in the process of development.[25:28]

The use of rigorous criteria for a scientific theory to critique nursing formulations will surely result in nursing theories being found deficient since theory construction in nursing is currently still in the early stages. However, does the negation of theory work in nursing (that is, saying that there are no nursing theories) lead to the desired outcome?

The debate about whether nursing formulations are theories is often based on the conceptual sorting of theories into two either-or categories: *Theories* (T) and *not-theories* ($\cancel{T}$).

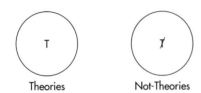

Theories   Not-Theories

COMPLETE THEORIES	INCOMPLETE THEORIES	NOT-THEORIES
High	Medium	Low

In using these conceptual classes for analysis, there are two categories for classifying nursing formulations. If the T category (theory) is defined on the basis of rigorous criteria for a scientific theory, most and perhaps all nursing formulations would fall into the Ŧ category. The result may be that all nursing formulations would occupy only one category. What has been gained, in terms of advancing knowledge of nursing, by the time spent on the analysis of whether nursing formulations are or are not *theories,* especially if analysis ends at this point? Turner[26] labeled this approach the "game" of "criticize-the-discipline."

Suppose, hypothetically, we have two distinct sets of nursing formulations, X and Y. Assume that we determine X meets the rigorous criteria for the theory class, whereas Y is incompletely developed and does not. However, further suppose that the formulations in X do not address the phenomenon we are interested in describing, understanding, or predicting. It is also possible that X does not even address anything we find particularly interesting. On the other hand, Y, which is now labeled *not-theory,* addresses a domain of interest that fits our particular concerns in our practice area. What do we do? Develop the incomplete Y theory further!

In our efforts to prepare a new generation of nurse scholars to advance theory building in nursing, it may be more fruitful to give less attention to whether a given nursing formulation is a theory and concentrate on analyzing how much of a theory it is.[8] In this perspective, the category of theory is defined so a range of theoretical formulations can be considered (see Mullins,[16] Hage[8]). We have therefore expanded the conceptual categories from two, in which all nursing formulations tend to fall into the T category, to the notion of a continuum in the theory category. In this sorting system, sets of nursing formulations can be evaluated in terms of their relative completeness, according to where they fall in the following schematic:

Once a nursing theory that fits our area of interest has been identified, several questions arise, such as: How complete is it? What components or relationships are missing? Is it internally consistent? What is its correspondence with available empirical findings? Is it operationally defined for testing? Analyses of this nature logically leads to the question: What are the next steps in the further development of this theory? In Turner's view[26:12-13]:

> As soon as the question becomes one of potential for theory building, critical analysis must move beyond the mechanical comparisons of a particular theoretical perspective with the canons of scientific theory. While such comparisons . . . are an important and appropriate concern . . . , their polemic intent often gets in the way of the productive analysis of a particular conceptual perspective.

Turner recommended for his own discipline of sociology that any analysis of theory should begin with the "blunt admission" that theory construction "has a long way to go" to identify and address current inadequacies in available theories. Hage's similar conclusions about sociological knowledge are quoted below. *Nursing* has been substituted for *sociology* to illustrate relevance for states of affairs in nursing.

> The major difficulty in discussing whether there is any (nursing) knowledge is that many individuals think about this issue in either-or terms. . . . We do not want an either-or conception of knowledge. Because we are used to reasoning in this way, we are prevented from perceiving that perhaps there is some knowledge in (nursing), albeit it is incomplete.[8:182]

The goal ahead is to direct our attention and energies to the critical analysis of existing incomplete theories in terms of their potential for further development.

However, it is only through repeated and rigorous research that scientific evidence can accumulate to support or refute theoretical assertions, or provide the basis for suggesting modifications in a nursing theory. Theory-testing research also may lead to the decision to abandon one nursing theory in favor of another theory that more adequately explains available research data. Yet, in an analysis of 720 nursing practice studies in six research journals from 1977-1986, Moody et al. found that only 3% of the studies were designed to test theory from an explicit theoretical framework.[15] It is critical that theory-testing research in nursing receive greater emphasis in the 1990s if nursing science is to advance. Current nursing literature reflects this priority need; several nursing scholars have presented their ideas for guidelines and criteria for evaluating theory-testing research in nursing (for example, see Silva[22] and Acton, Irvin, and Hopkins[1]). These criteria emphasize the importance of utilizing a nursing theory to design the purpose and focus of the study and to derive hypotheses as well as the necessity to relate the significance of the findings back to the nursing theory.

In addition to the call for more rigorous theory-testing research in nursing, both nursing scholars and practitioners are arguing for the need for increased attention to the relationships between theory and practice (for example, Chinn and Kramer,[4] Hoffman and Bertus,[10] Schlotfeldt,[21] Sparacino[23]). Priorities include (1) continued development of nursing theories that are relevant to specialty practice engaged in by nurses, (2) increased use of nursing theories in clinical decision making, (3) increased collaboration between scientists and practitioners, (4) efforts by nurse researchers to communicate findings from research to relevant practitioners, and (5) increased emphasis on clinical research. In 1992, in the first issue of the journal *Clinical Nursing Research*, Schlotfeldt states:

> It will be nursing's clinical scholars . . . that will identify the human phenomena that are central to nurses' practice . . . and that provoke consideration of the practice problems about which knowledge is needed but is not yet available. It is nursing's clinical scholarship that must be depended on to generate promising theories for testing that will advance nursing knowledge and insure nursing's continued essential services to humankind.[21:9]

REFERENCES

1. Acton, G., Irvin, B., & Hopkins, B. (1991). Theory-testing research: Building the science. *Advances in Nursing Science, 14* (1), 52-61.
2. Bronowski, J. (1979). *The visionary age: Essay with arts, literature, and science.* Cambridge, MA: The MIT Press.
3. Brown, H. (1977). *Perception, theory and commitment: The new philosophy of science.* Chicago: The University of Chicago Press.
4. Chinn P., & Kramer, M. (1991). *Theory and nursing: A systematic approach* (3rd ed.). St. Louis: Mosby.
5. Dubin, R. (1978). *Theory building.* New York: The Free Press.
6. Flaskerud, J., & Halloran, E. (1980). Area of agreement in nursing theory development. *Advances in Nursing Sciences, 3,* 1-7.
7. Giere, R.N. (1979). *Understanding scientific reasoning.* New York: Holt, Rhinehart, & Winston.
8. Hage, J. (1972). *Techniques and problems in theory construction in sociology.* New York: John Wiley & Sons.
9. Hardy, N. (1983). Metaparadigm and theory development. In N. Chaska (Ed.), *The nursing profession: A time to speak.* New York: McGraw-Hill.
10. Hoffman, A., & Bertus, P. (1991). Theory and practice: Bridging scientists' and practitioners' roles. *Archives of Psychiatric Nursing, 7* (1), 2-9.
11. Kaplan, A. (1964). *The conduct of inquiry: Methodology for behavioral science.* New York: Chandler.
12. Meleis, A. (1985). *Theoretical nursing: Development and progress.* Philadelphia: J.B. Lippincott.
13. Merton, R., et al. (Eds.). (1952). *Reader in bureaucracy.* New York: The Free Press.
14. Mills, C.W. (1959). On intellectual craftsmanship. In L. Gross (Ed.), *Symposium on sociological theory.* Evanston, IL: Row, Peterson, & Co.
15. Moody, L., Wilson, M., Smyth, K., Schwartz, R., Tittle, M., & VanCott, M.L. (1988). Analysis of a decade of nursing research: 1977-1986. *Nursing Research, 27* (6), 374-379.
16. Mullins, N. (1971). *The art of theory: Construction and use.* New York: Harper & Row.
17. Nowak, S. (1975). Causal interpretations of statistical relationships in social research. In H. Blalock, et al. (Eds.), *Quantitative sociology: International perspectives on mathematical and statistical modeling.* New York: Academic Press.
18. Reynolds, P. (1971). *A primer in theory construction.* Indianapolis: Bobbs-Merrill.
19. Rosenberg, J. (1978). *The practice of philosophy.* Englewood Cliffs, NJ: Prentice Hall.
20. Salmon, W.D. (1973). *Logic.* Englewood Cliffs, NJ: Prentice Hall.
21. Schlotfeldt, R. (1992). Why promote clinical nursing scholarship? *Clinical Nursing Research, 1* (1), 5-8.

22. Silva, M. (1986). Research testing nursing theory: State of the art. *Advances in Nursing Science, 9* (10), 1-11.

23. Sparacino, P. (1991). The reciprocal relationship between practice and theory. *Clinical Nurse Specialist, 5* (3), 138.

24. Steiner, E. (1978). *Logical and conceptual analytic techniques for educational researchers.* Washington, DC: University Press.

25. Stevens, B. (1979). *Nursing theory: Analysis, application and evaluation.* Boston: Little, Brown.

26. Turner, J. (1978). *The structure of sociological theory.* Homewood, IL: The Dorsey Press.

27. Walker, L., & Avant, K. (1983). *Strategies for theory construction in nursing.* Norwalk, CT: Appleton-Century-Crofts.

28. Werkmeister, W. (1959). Theory construction and the problem of objectivity. In L. Gross (Ed.), *Symposium of sociological theory.* Evanston, IL: Row, Peterson, & Co.

29. Zetterberg, H.L. (1966). *On theory and verification in sociology.* New York: John Wiley & Sons.

Evolution of Nursing Theory Development

Martha Raile Alligood, Elizabeth Chong Choi

*N*ursing has been practiced as a profession for more than a century, and theory development in nursing has evolved rapidly over the past four decades to finally be recognized as an academic discipline with a substantive body of knowledge.[4,5] In the mid-1800s, Nightingale[38] expressed her firm conviction that nursing knowledge was distinct from medical knowledge. She described a nurse's proper function—as putting the patient in the best condition for nature to act upon him—and set forth the idea that nursing was based on knowledge of persons and their environment, a different knowledge base than that used by physicians for their practice. In spite of this edict from Nightingale, it was not until after the 1950s that members of the nursing profession began serious discussion about the need to develop, articulate, and test nursing theory.[11,60] Until the emergence of nursing as a science in the 1950s, nursing practice was based on principles and traditions passed on through an apprenticeship form of education and a common-sense type of wisdom that came with years of experience.[5]

Although there were nurses with high aspirations for nursing to develop as a profession and an academic discipline, nursing practice continued to reflect the vocational heritage of nursing more than the professional vision. The development from vocation to profession included successive eras in the search for a body of substantive knowledge on which to base nursing practice. While the curriculum era emphasized course selection and content for nursing programs, it gave way to the research era, which focused on the research process and the goal of developing new knowledge. In the mid-1970s, the evaluation of 25 years of nursing research revealed that nursing lacked conceptual connections and theoretical frameworks. This awareness of the need for concept and theory development coincided with two other milestones that are significant to the evolution of nursing theory: the standardization of curricula for nursing master's education through the National League for Nursing accreditation criteria and the decision that doctoral education for nurses should be in nursing.[5]

Out of the debates and discussion of the 1960s regarding the proper direction and appropriate discipline for nursing knowledge development emerged the nursing theory era and a new awareness of nursing as a profession and an academic discipline in its own right. This new awareness was evidenced by an explosive proliferation of nursing doctoral programs and nursing theory literature.[36,37,59] Thus the transition in the 1970s from vocation to profession was a major turning point for nursing because nurses asked the question, "Will nursing be other-discipline based or nursing based?" and answered that nursing practice will be based on nursing science.[5:6-7] This progress in nursing theory is a most significant aspect of scholarly evolution and the cornerstone of the nursing discipline, according to Meleis.[31]

In the 1980s developments in nursing theory characterized a transition from the preparadigm to the paradigm period.[25] The prevailing paradigms (models) provided various perspectives for nursing practice, administration, education, research, and further theory development. The proposal of global metaparadigm concepts for nursing in the 1980s introduced another aspect of the organizing structure for nursing knowledge development into the nursing literature.[14] The classification of nursing models as paradigms, which address the metaparadigm concepts of person, environment, health, and nursing, views nursing works in a manner that improves the comprehension of knowledge development, gives the theorists' works a larger context, and facilitates our understanding of the growth of nursing science within these paradigm perspectives.[14,15]

The body of nursing science—as well as methods for research, education, administration, and practice—continues to expand through nursing scholarship. National and international conferences, newsletters, journals, and books are written by the community of scholars who base their practice and research on a particular model or theory (paradigm perspective). These observations of nursing science development bring Kuhn's ideas of normal science to life. Clearly Kuhn's philosophy of science has helped us understand the evolution of nursing theory through paradigm science.[25]

It is important to remember that theory emerged through the individual efforts of various nursing leaders across the country and that it was in retrospect that we viewed them collectively in a process of knowledge development. What we refer to as theory development emerged from the scholarship that was a product of the professional growth process of nurse leaders, administrators, educators, and practitioners who sought higher education and saw the limitations of theory from other disciplines, such as medicine, to describe, explain, or predict nursing outcomes. These leaders sought to establish a sound scientific basis for nursing management, curricula, practice, and research. Because of the function of theory in these processes as an organizing structure, over time there was a convergence of ideas resulting in the emergence of what we refer to today as the nursing theory era.[5,36,37]

The accomplishment of normal science ushers in the utilization phase of the theory era—that is, the time when the emphasis shifts from development to utilization and application of what is known.[6] For the discipline of nursing the utilization phase restores the centrality of nursing practice with the recognition of theory and research as tools of practice rather than ends in themselves. The reader is referred to Alligood and Marriner-Tomey's book, *Nursing Theory: Utilization and Application,* for a comprehensive discussion of this new phase of the theory era and examples of applications of the nursing models and their theories in nursing practice.[6]

Each of the works of the nursing theorists has been organized into one of three types of knowledge based on its predominant characteristics as a theoretical work in nursing. Classifying the works in this manner not only adds specificity to the discussion of them, but also, and more important, it adds context so they can be considered in relation to a structure of nursing knowledge.[3,15]

Three general kinds of works are brought together in this text. The first type is nursing philosophy. Philosophy sets forth the meaning of nursing phenomena through analysis, reasoning, and logical argument. These include early works that predate or lead into the nursing theory era and have contributed to knowledge development in nursing by providing direction or forming a basis for later developments and later works that reflect more recent expansion in the areas of human science and its methods.[9,62]

The second type, nursing conceptual models, are the works of those often referred to as the *grand the-*

orists or pioneers in nursing. As one author explains, "A conceptual model provides a distinct frame of reference for its adherents . . . that tells them how to observe and interpret the phenomena of interest to the discipline."[15:3]

The works of the grand theorists are comprehensive of nursing and tend to include the aspects of human beings, their environment, and their health with which the discipline is concerned, and they provide propositional direction for members of the profession in a scientific field.[15]

The third type are nursing theories and *middle-range theories.* These theories of nursing may have been derived from works in other disciplines related to nursing, from earlier nursing philosophies and theories, from nursing grand theories, or from nursing conceptual models.[3,15] Middle-range theory has a narrower focus than grand theory and is more concrete in terms of its level of abstraction.[15] Therefore middle-range theories are more precise and focus on answering specific nursing practice questions. They specify such factors as the age group of the client, the family situation, the health condition, the location of the client, and, most important, the action of the nurse.[4] Middle-range theories address the specifics of nursing situations within the perspective of the model or theory from which they are derived.[3,4]

This chapter introduces the work of a large number of theorists. These works can be viewed in various ways for different purposes. To trace the evolution of theory development in nursing, the theorists and their work are presented chronologically in terms of their historical sequence and are classified as philosophies, conceptual models, and theories (Box 6-1).

FLORENCE NIGHTINGALE

The first author to be examined is Florence Nightingale.[38] Her work is closely related to her philosophical orientation of the patient-environment interaction and the principles and rules on which nursing practice was founded. Nightingale's emphasis on environment reflected a predominant concern of the late 1800s, when sanitation was a major health problem. Nightingale believed that disease was a reparative process. The manipulation of the external environment—through ventilation, warmth, light, diet, cleanliness, and noise—would contribute to the reparative process and the patient's well-being. She did not believe in the germ theory that was being postulated during her lifetime.[42] Nightingale's beliefs about nursing, what it is and what it is not, distinguished nursing from the work of domestic servants and formed the foundation for professional nursing.[38] Her contribution to theory development was in explicating nursing's focus as the patient-environment relationship and in pioneering statistical analysis for health and professional nursing. Nightingale's writings represent a philosophy of nursing.

ERNESTINE WIEDENBACH

Ernestine Wiedenbach[64] concentrated on the art of nursing, focusing on the needs of the patient. Wiedenbach's work grew from 40 years of experience, primarily in maternity nursing, and her definition of nursing reflects that background. She said, "People may differ in their concept of nursing, but few would disagree that nursing is nurturing or caring for someone in a motherly fashion."[64:1] Wiedenbach's orientation is a philosophy of nursing. It tells the nurse what to do, which is a philosophy of art. According to Wiedenbach, clinical nursing has the following four elements: (1) philosophy, (2) purpose, (3) practice, and (4) art. Clinical nursing is directed toward the fulfillment of a specific purpose. The nurse's goal is to meet the perceived need-for-help that the patient is experiencing.[64:15] Wiedenbach's philosophy of practice is influenced by her conception of nursing as an art. Her vision of nursing reflects the period of nursing history during which considerable emphasis was placed on the art of nursing. She follows Orlando's theory of deliberate rather than automatic nursing and incorporates the steps of the nursing process. Wiedenbach's work may be considered a philosophy of nursing.

VIRGINIA HENDERSON

Virginia Henderson[18] viewed the patient as an individual requiring help toward independence. She envisioned the practice of nursing as independent from that of physicians. Henderson acknowledged her interpretation of the nurse's function as a synthesis of many influences. Her philosophy is based on Thorndike's work, her experience in rehabilitation nursing, and Orlando's work regarding the conceptualization of deliberate nursing action.[2] Henderson emphasized the art of nursing and identified 14 basic human needs of patients on which nursing care builds. Her contributions include defining nursing, delineating autonomous nursing functions, stressing goals of interdependence for the patient, and creating self-help concepts, the last of which influenced the works of Abdellah and Adam. Henderson's work is a philosophy of nursing.

FAYE GLENN ABDELLAH

Faye Glenn Abdellah's work, which is based on the problem-solving method, had a great impact on nursing curriculum development.[1] Problem solving was the vehicle for delineating nursing (client) problems as the client moved toward a healthy outcome. According to Abdellah,[1] nursing is both an art and a science; as such, it molds the attitude, intellectual competencies, and technical skills of the individual nurse into the desire and ability to help people cope with their health needs whether they are ill or not. She believed that nursing actions were carried out under general or specific medical direction. Abdellah formulated 21 nursing problems based on research studies. Her work seems to be based on Henderson's 14 basic human needs and on research studies to establish the classification of nursing problems.[11] A major difference between Henderson and Abdellah is that Abdellah's problems are formulated in terms of nursing-centered services, which are used to determine the client's needs. Abdellah's contribution to nursing theory development was the systematic analysis of research data to formulate and validate the 21 nursing problems that served as an early guide for comprehensive nursing care. Abdellah's work is a philosophy of nursing.

LYDIA E. HALL

Lydia E. Hall[17] stressed the autonomous function of nursing. She proposed three overlapping circles that comprise nursing: (1) the therapeutic use of self (the core aspect), (2) treatment within the health team (the cure aspect), and (3) the nurturing component (the care aspect). Her work is a philosophy of nursing influenced by Carl Rogers and other psychologists. Hall's conceptualization encompasses adult patients who have passed the acute stage of illness. The goal for the patient is rehabilitation and feelings of success in self-actualization and self-love. Her contribution to theory development was the utilization of her philosophy of nursing care at The Loeb Center in New York and her encouragement of professional nurses to make a contribution to patient outcomes. Hall's work is a philosophy of nursing.

JEAN WATSON

Jean Watson's work [62,63] emphasizes caring, as does Leininger's theory, but Watson borrows the existential phenomenologist's view of psychology and the humanities and proposes nursing as a human science. Nursing concerns itself with promoting and restoring health, preventing illness, and caring for the sick. Clients require holistic care that promotes humanism, health, and quality living. Caring is a universal social phenomenon that is effective only when practiced interpersonally. Watson sets forth 10 "carative factors" that represent both feelings and actions pertaining to the nurse, the client, and the professional and include things to be felt, experienced, communicated, expressed, and promoted by nurses.[63] Watson's work contributes by sensitizing individual practitioners to humanistic aspects and caring. Her work may be classified as a philosophical theory of nursing.

PATRICIA BENNER

Benner's work[9] describes caring in the context of nursing practice with rich meaning and a broad understanding of personhood. She borrowed Dreyfus and Dreyfus's Model of Skill Acquisition[12] and developed and validated this model in nursing practice by systematic descriptions of the five stages of skill development of nurses. Benner provided many exemplars describing nursing practice at each stage—

novice, advanced beginner, competent, proficient, and expert. Seven domains of nursing practice were derived from the descriptions with a list of 31 nursing competencies. From Benner's description of nursing practice, Benner and Wrubel's (1988) theory, presented in *The Primacy of Caring: Stress and Coping in Health and Illness*, evolved.[10] This phenomenological work describes caring as a common bond of persons situated in meaning, a state of being that is essential to nursing. Benner's work is classified as a philosophical theory of nursing.

DOROTHEA E. OREM

Dorothea E. Orem[39] explicated self-care as a human need and nursing as a human service, emphasizing nursing's special concern for a person's need for the provision and management of self-care actions on a continuous basis to sustain life and health or to recover from disease and injury.[39] She has generated three theories that are used together to design and guide the delivery of nursing care. Orem's contribution to theory development is the continued evolution of her original ideas in her scholarship to further delineate nursing function, self-care needs, and nursing systems and her emphasis on empirical support through research. Her book *Nursing: Concepts of Practice* is in its fifth edition.[39] Orem's work is a conceptual model of nursing with three nursing theories.

MYRA ESTRIN LEVINE

Myra Estrin Levine used the sciences, such as psychology, sociology, and physiology, to analyze various nursing practices and described detailed nursing skills and activities.[28,29] Levine's Nursing Activity Analysis resulted in the formulation of four conservation principles to help clients adapt to their environment. She presented the person as holistic and the center of nursing activities. In spite of Levine's emphasis on the ill person in the health care setting and the fact that she was writing a textbook to teach medical-surgical nursing to beginning students, she developed a model that has proved useful in health promotion as well as in illness care. Levine's model building was influenced by the use of borrowed theory as well as analyses of nursing practice.[56] Levine's work is categorized as a conceptual model of nursing with three theories: conservation, redundancy, and therapeutic intention.[3:36]

MARTHA E. ROGERS

Martha E. Rogers's *Science of Unitary Human Beings*[51] was influenced by general system theory and field theory. She clearly emphasized the science and the art of nursing in her delineation of the unitary human being and environment as central to the discipline of nursing.[50] Rogers was a clear voice calling for the development of nursing as a basic scientific discipline over the years. Rogers's model has had a significant influence on current scientific inquiry and professional nursing practice. In addition, the model has served as a basis for the explication of other nursing theories, including those of Newman, Parse, and Fitzpatrick. Rogers's model has promoted much research that has influenced the scientific community of nursing scholars who have investigated its utility in research, practice, education, and administration.[8,30,50,51] Rogers's work is categorized as a conceptual model of nursing with "many theories."[3:38]

DOROTHY E. JOHNSON

Dorothy E. Johnson[19,22] developed the Behavioral System Model for nursing practice, education, and research. Her model is influenced by ethological theory and general system theory. Johnson[22:212] considered attachment, or the affiliative subsystem, the cornerstone of social organizations. Her behavioral system also includes the dependency, achievement, aggressive, ingestive, eliminative, and sexual subsystems. In Johnson's words, "Nursing problems arise because there are disturbances in the structure or function of the subsystems of the system, or because the level of behavioral functioning is less than desirable."[22:214] Other than her model, Johnson's contributions to nursing theory development are her writings related to philosophical issues and knowledge development and her influences on students, such as Roy, Neuman, and Adam, who have subsequently developed nursing theory.[20,21] Johnson's work is a conceptual model of nursing with several theories.

SISTER CALLISTA ROY

Sister Callista Roy[53,54] based her work on Helson's Adaptation Theory. Her model is an example of how borrowed knowledge becomes unique to nursing.[53] Roy synthesizes different (borrowed) theories, such as system, stress, and adaptation, into a collective view for explication of a person interacting with the environment. According to Roy, humans are biopsychosocial beings who exist within an environment. Environment and self provide three classes of stimuli—focal, residual, and contextual. Stimuli impact humans and create needs in one or more interrelated adaptation modes, such as physiological self-concept, role function, and interdependence. Through two adaptative mechanisms, regulator and cognator, an individual demonstrates adaptive responses or ineffective responses that require nursing intervention. Roy's Adaptation Model[55] has been developed consistently. Although the model was developed for education, continued work in practice and research has led to broader use, testing, and numerous publications.[55] Roy's work is a conceptual model of nursing with several theories.

BETTY NEUMAN

Betty Neuman's model[33] uses Gestalt, stress, and system theory as well as levels of prevention. Her conceptualization of the total-person approach to client care helps individuals, families, and groups attain and maintain an optimal level of wellness by purposeful interventions.[35] Nursing intervention is aimed at prevention through the reduction of stress factors and adverse conditions that potentially or actually impact on optimal client functioning. Neuman's model is used in practice, education, and research. Her work is a conceptual model of nursing with two theories: optimal client stability and prevention as intervention.[3:37]

IMOGENE KING

Imogene King's systems framework[23,24] has a personal, interpersonal, and social system. The nurse and the patient perceive each other, judge the situation, and then act, react, interact, and transact. King[23] defined nursing as a process of human interaction between nurses and clients, who communicate to set goals, explore means for achieving the goals, and then agree on the means to attain the goals. King's work is categorized as a conceptual model of nursing from which she has derived the Theory of Goal Attainment.[24]

NANCY ROPER, WINIFRED W. LOGAN, AND ALISON J. TIERNEY

Roper, Logan, and Tierney[52] are European theorists who are new to this fourth edition. A Model of Living originated from research conducted in the 1970s to discover the "core of nursing" in response to the use of qualifiers for naming nursing practice according to the ideas of medical practice. Three decades of study of the elements of nursing by Roper (and Logan and Tierney, who joined her efforts) evolved into a Model of Living with five main components (concepts).

Twelve *activities of living (ALs)* describe the person, the central focus, in the complex process of living from the perspective of an amalgam of activities. *Lifespan* is the concept of continuous change from birth to death. *Dependence/independence continuum,* the third conceptual component, relates closely to the first two and ranges from being incapacitated in ALs to having the capacity to achieve ALs. Both occur at anticipated points across the lifespan, as well as at unanticipated times throughout life. *Factors influencing ALs,* the fourth component, are grouped as biological, psychological, sociocultural, environmental, and politicoeconomic. The person experiences this complex process as an individual, so variances in the four conceptual components are both an expression and a reflection of the person's *individuality.* This model has been used as a guide for nursing practice, research, and education.

HILDEGARD E. PEPLAU

Hildegard E. Peplau's work[47] is a theory for the practice of nursing. Peplau was greatly influenced by Sullivan's interpersonal relationship theories and reflects the view of the contemporaneous psychoanalytical model. Peplau is the earliest author to borrow theory from other scientific fields and synthesize a theory for nursing. Her work was praised by Sills as a second-order change in the area of theory development.[58] Peplau's work is categorized as a theory of nursing.[47]

IDA JEAN ORLANDO

Ida Jean Orlando[40,41] used the interpersonal nurse-patient relationship as the basis for her work. She focused on the patient's verbal and nonverbal expressions of needs and the nurse's reactions to the patient's behavior, emphasizing attention to both meaning of the distress and what would alleviate the distress. Three elements—patient behavior, nurse reaction, and nursing actions—comprise a nursing situation. Orlando differentiated *automatic actions* from *deliberate actions.* She stressed the importance of nurses testing their inferences about patients. Orlando used the nursing process to meet the patient's need with deliberate action and thus alleviate distress. Her contribution as a theorist advanced nursing beyond personal and automatic responses to disciplined and professional responses.[57] Orlando's work is categorized as a theory of nursing.

JOYCE TRAVELBEE

Joyce Travelbee's theory[61] extended Peplau's and Orlando's interpersonal relationship theories, but her unique synthesis of their ideas differentiated her work in terms of the therapeutic human relationship between nurse and patient. Travelbee's emphasis on caring stressed empathy, sympathy, and rapport and the emotional aspects of nursing. The work is categorized as a nursing theory.

JOAN RIEHL-SISCA

Joan Riehl-Sisca's theory of nursing interaction[48] is a synthesis of works by Mead, Rose, and Blumer that uses symbolic interaction as the focus of nurse-client interaction. Her Symbolic Interaction Theory was developed to explain nursing interaction in terms of communication, a major ingredient of symbolic interaction.[49] Riehl-Sisca's work is borrowed from sociology, synthesized for nursing, and categorized as a theory of nursing.

HELEN C. ERICKSON, EVELYN M. TOMLIN, AND MARY ANN P. SWAIN

Erickson, Tomlin, and Swain's Modeling and Role-Modeling Theory[13] is a synthesis of the works of Erikson, Maslow, Selye, Engel, and Piaget. From the synthesis of multiple theories related to basic needs, developmental tasks, object attachment, and adaptive coping potential, they developed their Modeling and Role-Modeling Theory. Modeling and role-modeling provides a framework for understanding the way clients structure their world. Erickson, Tomlin, and Swain view nursing as self-care based on the client's perception of the world and adaptations to stressors. This is a theory that promotes the client's growth and development while recognizing individual differences according to the client's world view and inherent endowment. Erickson, Tomlin, and Swain's work can be categorized as a theory of nursing.

RAMONA T. MERCER

Mercer's theory[32] is focused on parenting and maternal role attainment in diverse populations. The Maternal Role Attainment Theory is a middle-range theory with close linkages between theory, research, and practice. This theory follows a traditional social science approach to theory development. Mercer's early research was based on Goffman's systems theory. Mercer systematically researched the area of maternal role attainment and developed a complex theory to explain the factors impacting the development of the maternal role over time. The application of Mercer's theory has predictable outcomes for nursing practice in women's health and maternal child health. Mercer's work is categorized as a theory of nursing.

KATHRYN E. BARNARD

Kathryn E. Barnard's middle-range theory[7] borrows from psychology and human development and fo-

cuses on mother-infant interaction with the environment. Her theory is based on research that uses scales developed to measure feeding, teaching, and environment. Barnard's theory is descriptive and follows traditional science. Continuous research refined the theory, providing a closer link between practice and the theory. Barnard provides a role model for nurse researchers in clinical practice who engage in theory development for furthering the science of nursing. Barnard's work is a theory of nursing.

MADELEINE LEININGER

Madeleine Leininger[26,27] set forth caring as the central theme in nursing care, nursing knowledge, and nursing practice. Caring includes assistive, supportive, or facilitative acts toward an individual or a group with evident or anticipated needs. Caring serves to ameliorate or improve human conditions and life ways (life processes). Her methodology is borrowed from anthropology, but it synthesizes the concept of caring as an essential characteristic of nursing practice. Leininger is credited with the foundation of transcultural nursing and the resultant nursing research, education, and practice in this subfield of nursing. Leininger's work is a theory of nursing.

ROSEMARIE RIZZO PARSE

Rosemarie Rizzo Parse[43,44] derives her theory from Rogers's principles and concepts and synthesizes these ideas with the existential phenomenology of Heidegger, Ponty, and Sartre. Parse's view of nursing is based on humanism. Even though Parse developed her work largely from that of Rogers, Parse's subsequent work has explicated each concept in existentialist relevancy to nursing. The strength of Parse's theory may be a more humanistic approach as opposed to a physiological basis for nursing. Parse's work is categorized as a theory of nursing derived from Rogers's conceptual model.

JOYCE J. FITZPATRICK

Joyce J. Fitzpatrick's Life Perspective Rhythm Theory[16] was derived from Rogers's conceptual model. Fitzpatrick uses Rogers's conceptualization of unitary man as a building block for her Life Perspective Rhythm Theory.[50,51] She proposes that human development occurs within the context of continuous person-environment interaction.[16:300] Fitzpatrick's major concepts relate to the development of persons as indexes of temporal, motion, and consciousness patterns. She proposes that the meaning attached to life, as the basic understanding of human existence, is a central concern of nursing science and the nursing profession.[16:301] Fitzpatrick's contribution to theory development is that she builds on earlier work—the temporal pattern—developed by other researchers. Fitzpatrick's work is a theory of nursing derived from Rogers's conceptual model.

MARGARET A. NEWMAN

Margaret Newman's theory[34] of health is derived from Rogers's model. According to Newman, the goal of nursing is not to promote wellness or to prevent illness but to help people use the power within them as they evolve toward a higher level of consciousness.[34:37] Her contributions to theory development are the replication of earlier works and further expansion of methodology for research on the interaction of time, movement, space, and consciousness in maintaining life processes. Newman also developed a text, *Theory Development in Nursing*,[35] that has helped numerous nursing scientists. Newman's work, like Rogers's, is abstract, requiring linking of concepts to operational definitions for validation or testing. Newman's work is categorized as a theory of nursing derived from Rogers's conceptual model.

EVELYN ADAM

Evelyn Adam[2] is a Canadian nurse who formalized a theory from Henderson's writings as the basis of nursing practice, research, and education. Adam's work is a good example of using a unique basis of nursing for further expansion or addition.[2] She has contributed to theory development by clarification and explication of an earlier work. Adam's work is a theory of nursing.

NOLA J. PENDER

Nola Pender defines the goal of nursing care as *the optimal health of the individual*. She began to build

the foundation for studying how individuals make decisions about their own health care in her article, "A Conceptual Model for Preventive Health Behavior."[45] In her book *Health Promotion in Nursing Practice*,[46] she developed the idea that promoting optimal health supersedes disease prevention. Pender's theory identifies cognitive-perceptual factors in the individual, such as the importance of health-promoting behaviors and perceived barriers to health-promoting behaviors. According to Pender's theory, these factors are modified by demographical and biological characteristics, interpersonal influences, and situational and behavioral factors that help predict participation in health-promoting behavior. Pender's work is a theory of nursing.

CONCLUSIONS

From this overview, one can trace the evolution of theory development in nursing. First, a philosophy for nursing evolved (Nightingale); then early nursing theories, with an emphasis on interpersonal relationships, were developed (Peplau, Orlando, Travelbee, Barnard, and Mercer). Next came more philosophies emphasizing the art of nursing (Henderson, Wiedenbach, and Hall), followed by the beginning of an emphasis on the scientific aspects of nursing (Abdellah). These were followed by the conceptual models of nursing, which reflect adaptation, behavioral field theory, and systems approaches as well as emphasis on science (Johnson; Neuman; Rogers; King; Orem; Roy; Levine; and Roper, Logan, and Tierney). Finally, there is nursing theory derived from earlier philosophies and nursing models (Parse, Newman, Fitzpatrick, and Adam). Along with these developments, nurses continue to synthesize theories from other disciplines into nursing applications (Erickson, Tomlin, Swain, and Pender) as was done earlier in nursing (Leininger and Riehl-Sisca). The late 1980s and early 1990s evidence the blending of theory and philosophy for a humanistic nursing approach that reemphasizes nursing practice (Watson, Parse, and Benner).

The future of nursing is bright and hopeful. The theorists' different conceptualizations of nursing continue to enrich the discipline and its search for knowledge. The task for the future is to test the theories in nursing research and practice and to derive new theories from the nursing conceptual models. Kuhn[25:42] states that "paradigms can guide research in the absence of rules"; however, normal science cannot progress without paradigms. The same is true for nursing practice. As theory development gives way to theory utilization, the significance of nursing models and theories becomes even more clear for nursing education.[6] As noted elsewhere:

> Kuhn has said that it is the models or paradigms of a scientific discipline that primarily prepare students for practice as members of that professional community. The paradigm (model or framework) plays a vital role in practice because without a framework all of the information that the professional encounters seems to be equally relevant. Therefore students studying to enter a professional discipline are introduced to the models or paradigms as an orientation to the approaches used in the practice of that discipline. Following an introduction and survey of the models and theories, the students are ready to choose the ones they will use in their practice. It is in studying these models and practicing with them that students learn their trade.[3:39-40]

Nurses are recognizing the rich heritage of the works of the nursing theorists—philosophies, conceptual models, and theories of nursing. These contributions represent the status of nursing as a discipline, and further developments continue to occur. What is important is that models and theories guide the critical thinking of nurses and are therefore becoming more and more accepted by the nursing community.[3] The debate is not about what each model represents but about how each represents the diverse values we are seeking. The future direction should be toward further clarification of our understanding of these works so that they can be used as frameworks for structuring nursing practice with predictable outcomes as well as for the derivation of new middle-range theories to be tested in nursing research and practice.[6]

Recognition of the significance of normal science has occurred in this era. The scholarship of this decade alone is a demonstration of that outcome, not only as nursing literature around the philosophies, models, and theories proliferates quantitatively but also as the depth of the scientific scholarship improves qualitatively.[4]

As our understanding of the nursing models has expanded and their use has increased dramatically, we have begun to see their capacity for the development of nursing knowledge. In fact, nursing models serve the purpose Kuhn predicted—as organizing structures for schools of thought or communities of scholars who share in the work. Whether the individuals working within each community of scholars are focused on theory, research, administration, education, or nursing practice, they all work together and share their experiences in the development and utilization of nursing science. This is reflected in publications, organizations, and regional, national, and international conferences centered around the work of the nursing theorists.

REFERENCES

1. Abdellah, F., Beland, I., & Martin, A.(1973). *New direction in patient-centered nursing*. New York: Macmillan.
2. Adam, E.(1980). *To be a nurse*. Toronto: W.B. Saunders.
3. Alligood, M.R. (1997). Models and theories: Critical thinking structures. In M. Alligood & A. Marriner-Tomey (Eds.), *Nursing theory: Utilization and application* (pp. 31-45). St. Louis: Mosby.
4. Alligood, M.R. (1997). Models and theories in nursing practice. In M. Alligood & A. Marriner-Tomey (Eds.), *Nursing theory: Utilization and application* (pp. 15-30). St. Louis: Mosby.
5. Alligood, M.R. (1997). The nature of knowledge needed for nursing practice. In M. Alligood & A. Marriner-Tomey (Eds.), *Nursing theory: Utilization and application* (pp. 3-13). St. Louis: Mosby.
6. Alligood, M.R., & Marriner-Tomey, A. (Eds.) (1997). *Nursing theory: Utilization and application*. St. Louis: Mosby.
7. Barnard, K.E., et al. (1977). *The nursing child assessment satellite training study guide*. Unpublished program learning manual. Seattle: University of Washington.
8. Barrett, E. (1990). *Visions of Rogers's science-based nursing*. New York: National League for Nursing.
9. Benner, P. (1984). *From novice to expert: Excellence and power in clinical nursing practice*. Menlo Park, CA: Addison-Wesley.
10. Benner, P., & Wrubel, J. (1988). *The primacy of caring: Stress and coping in health and illness*. Menlo Park, CA: Addison-Wesley.
11. Chinn, P., & Kramer, M. (1994). *Theory and nursing* (4th ed.). St. Louis: Mosby.

12. Dreyfus, H.L., & Dreyfus, S.E. (1986). *Mind over machine.* New York: The Free Press.

13. Erickson, H., Tomlin, E., & Swain, M. (1983). *Modeling and role-modeling: A theory and paradigm for nursing.* Englewood Cliffs, NJ: Prentice Hall.

14. Fawcett, J. (1984). The metaparadigm of nursing: Current status and future refinements. *Image: The Journal of Nursing Scholarship, 16,* 84-87.

15. Fawcett, J. (1995). *Analysis and evaluation of conceptual models of nursing* (3rd ed.). Philadelphia: F.A. Davis.

16. Fitzpatrick, J. (1989). A life perspective rhythm model. In J. Fitzpatrick & A. Whall (Eds.), *Conceptual models of nursing: Analysis and application* (2nd ed.). Norwalk, CT: Appleton & Lange.

17. Hall, L. (1969). The Loeb Center for Nursing and Rehabilitation. *International Journal of Nursing Studies, 6,* 81-95.

18. Henderson, V. (1966). *The nature of nursing: A definition and its implications, practice, research, and education.* New York: Macmillan.

19. Johnson, D.E. (1968). *One conceptual model of nursing.* Unpublished paper presented April 25 at Vanderbilt University, Nashville, TN.

20. Johnson, D.E. (1968). State of the art of theory development in nursing. In *Theory development: What, why, how?* New York: National League for Nursing.

21. Johnson, D.E. (1974). Development of a theory: A requisite for nursing as a primary health profession. *Nursing Research, 23* (5), 372-377.

22. Johnson, D.E. (1980). The behavioral system model for nursing. In J.P. Riehl & S.C. Roy (Eds.), *Conceptual models for nursing practice* (2nd ed.). New York: Appleton-Century-Crofts.

23. King, I. (1971). *Toward a theory for nursing.* New York: John Wiley.

24. King, I. (1981). *A theory for nursing: Systems, concepts, process.* New York: John Wiley.

25. Kuhn, T.S. (1970). *The structure of scientific revolutions.* Chicago: University of Chicago Press.

26. Leininger, M. (1978). *Transcultural nursing concepts, theories, and practice.* New York: John Wiley.

27. Leininger, M. (1991). *Culture care diversity and universality: A theory of nursing.* New York: National League for Nursing.

28. Levine, M.E. (1967). The four conservation principles of nursing. *Nursing Forum, 6,* 45-59.

29. Levine, M.E. (1973). *Introduction to clinical nursing.* Philadelphia: F.A. Davis.

30. Malinski, V. (1986). *Explorations of Martha Rogers's science of unitary human beings.* Norwalk, CT: Appleton-Century-Crofts.

31. Meleis, A. (1983). The evolving nursing scholars. In P. Chinn (Ed.), *Advances in nursing theory development.* Rockville, MD: Aspen Systems.

32. Mercer, R. (1986). *First-time motherhood: Experience from teens to forties.* New York: Springer.

33. Neuman, B. (1995). *The Neuman systems model* (3rd ed.). Norwalk, CT: Appleton & Lange.

34. Newman, M. (1986). *Health as expanding conciousness.* St. Louis: Mosby.

35. Newman, M. (1979). *Theory development in nursing.* Philadelphia: F.A. Davis.

36. Nicoll, L. (1986). *Perspectives on nursing theory.* Boston: Little, Brown.

37. Nicoll, L. (1992). *Perspectives on nursing theory* (2nd ed.). Philadelphia: J.B. Lippincott.

38. Nightingale, F. (1969). *Notes on nursing: What it is and what it is not.* New York: Dover. (Originally published, 1859).

39. Orem, D.E. (1995). *Nursing: Concepts of practice* (5th ed.). St. Louis: Mosby.

40. Orlando, I.J. (1961). *The dynamic nurse-patient relationship.* New York: G.P. Putnam's Sons.

41. Orlando, I.J. (1972). *The discipline and teaching of nursing process.* New York: G.P. Putnam's Sons.

42. Palmer, I. S. (1977). Florence Nightingale: Reformer, reactionary, researcher. *Nursing Research, 26*(2), 84-89.

43. Parse, R. (1992). Human becoming: Parse's theory of nursing. *Nursing Science Quarterly, 5*(1), 35-42.

44. Parse, R. R. (1981). *Man-living-health: A theory of nursing.* New York: John Wiley.

45. Pender, N.J. (1975). A conceptual model for preventive health behavior. *Nursing Outlook, 23*(6), 385-390.

46. Pender, N.J. (1996). *Health promotion in nursing practice.* (3rd ed.). New York: Appleton & Lange.

47. Peplau, H.E. (1952). *Interpersonal relations in nursing.* New York: G.P. Putnam's Sons.

48. Riehl, J. (1989). The Riehl-Sisca interaction model. In J. Riehl-Sisca (Ed.), *Conceptual models for nursing practice* (3rd ed.). Norwalk, CT: Appleton & Lange.

49. Riehl-Sisca, J. (1989). *Conceptual models for nursing practice* (3rd ed.). Norwalk, CT: Appleton & Lange.

50. Rogers, M.E. (1970). *The theoretical basis of nursing.* Philadelphia: F.A. Davis.

51. Rogers, M.E. (1994). The science of unitary human beings: Current perspectives. *Nursing Science Quarterly 7*(1), 33-35.

52. Roper, N., Logan, W., & Tierney, A. (1996). *The elements of nursing: A model for nursing based on a model of living* (4th ed.). New York: Churchill Livingstone.

53. Roy, C. (1984). *Introduction to nursing: An adaptation model* (2nd ed.). Englewood Cliffs, NJ: Prentice Hall.

54. Roy, C.S. (1976). *Introduction to nursing: An adaptation model.* Englewood Cliffs, NJ: Prentice Hall.

55. Roy, C., & Andrews, H. (1991). *The Roy adaptation model: The definitive statement.* Norwalk, CT: Appleton & Lange.

56. Schafer, K., Pond, J. Levine, M., & Fawcett, J. (1991). *Levine's conservation model: A framework for nursing practice.* Philadelphia: F.A. Davis.

57. Schmeiding, N.C. (1983). An analysis of Orlando's nursing theory based on Kuhn's theory of science. In P. Chinn (Ed.), *Advances in nursing theory development.* Rockville, MD: Aspen Systems.

58. Sills, G. (1978). Leader, practitioner, academician, scholar, theorist. *Perspectives in Psychiatric Care 16,* 122-128.

59. Sullivan, H.S. (1952). *The interpersonal theory of psychiatry.* New York: W.W. Norton.

60. Torres, G., & Yura, H. (1975). The meaning and functions of concepts and theories within education and nursing. In *Conceptual framework: Its meaning and function.* New York: National League for Nursing.

61. Travelbee, J. (1971). *Interpersonal aspects of nursing.* Philadelphia: F.A. Davis.

62. Watson, J. (1979). *Nursing: The philosophy and science of caring.* Boston: Little, Brown.

63. Watson, J. (1985). *Nursing: Human science and health care.* Norwalk, CT: Appleton-Century-Crofts.

64. Wiedenbach, E. (1964). *Clinical nursing: A helping art.* New York: Springer.

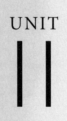

UNIT

II

Philosophies

- *Nursing philosophy sets forth the meaning of nursing phenomena through analysis, reasoning, and logical argument.*

- *Philosophies contribute to nursing knowledge by providing direction for the discipline and forming a basis for professional scholarship, which leads to new theoretical understanding.*

- *Nursing philosophies represent early works that predate the theory era and later works of a philosophical nature.*

- *Philosophies are works that provide broad understanding used to further the discipline in its professional application.*

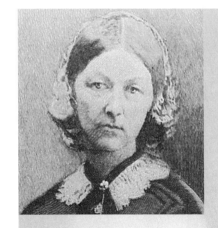

*F*lorence Nightingale

Modern Nursing

Susan A. Pfettscher, Karen R. de Graff, Ann Marriner Tomey,
Cynthia L. Mossman, Maribeth Slebodnik

CREDENTIALS AND BACKGROUND OF THE THEORIST

Florence Nightingale, the matriarch of modern nursing, was born on May 12, 1820, while her parents were on an extended European tour. Her parents, Edward and Frances Nightingale, named their daughter for her birthplace, Florence, Italy. The Nightingales were a well-educated, affluent Victorian family who maintained residences in both Derbyshire (Lea Hurst was their original home) and Hampshire (Embly Park). The latter residence was near London, allowing the family to participate in the spring and autumn social seasons there.

While the extended Nightingale family was large, the immediate family included only Florence and her elder sister Parthenope. During her childhood, Florence was educated by her father much more broadly and rigorously than were other young women of her time. Florence was tutored in mathematics, languages, religion, and philosophy (subjects that were later to influence the course of her work). While Florence participated in the usual Victorian aristocratic activities and social events during her adolescence, she developed the sense that her life should become more useful.

Much attention has been paid to the "calling" that Nightingale recorded in her diary (her private note) in 1837, when she wrote that "God spoke to me and called me to his service."[11:41] Her "calling" was unclear; however, it was finally realized in 1851, when she entered nursing training at Kaiserwerth, Germany, a protestant religious community with a hospital facility. Her stay there was for approximately 3 months at the end of which her teachers declared her to be trained as a nurse.

Following her return to England, Nightingale began to examine hospital facilities, reformatories, and charitable institutions. Soon thereafter, in 1853, she became the superintendent of the Hospital for In-valid Gentlewomen in London.

During the Crimean War, Nightingale received a request from Sidney Herbert, a family friend and Secretary of War, to go to Scutari, Turkey, where she provided trained nurses to care for wounded soldiers. She arrived there in November 1854. To achieve her mission of providing nursing care, she needed to address the environmental problems that existed, including the lack of sanitation and the presence of filth (few chamber pots, contaminated water, contaminated sheets and blankets, overflowing cesspools). In addition, the soldiers were faced with exposure, frostbite, lice infestation, and other opportunistic disease during their recovery from the wounds received in battle.

Nightingale's work in improving these deplorable conditions made her a popular, even revered, person to these soldiers. However, the support of the physicians and the military officers demonstrated less enthusiasm. Because of her ward rounds performed during the night, she was called "The Lady of the Lamp" and was immortalized in the poetry of Henry Wadsworth Longfellow. While at Scutari, Nightingale became critically ill with Crimean fever, which might actually have been typhus.

Following the war, Nightingale returned to England to great accolades, particularly from the royal family (Queen Victoria) and the soldiers who had served in the Crimea. From the funds she was awarded in recognition of this work, Nightingale established a teaching institution for nurses at St. Thomas Hospital and at King's College Hospital in London. Within a few years after it was founded, the Nightingale School began receiving requests to found new schools at hospitals worldwide. Florence Nightingale's reputation as the founder of modern nursing was established.

During her life, Nightingale devoted her energies to societal issues and causes in an attempt to create social change. She continued to concentrate on army sanitation reform, the functions of army hospitals, sanitation in India, and sanitation and health care of the poor in England. Her writings, *Notes on Matters Affecting the Health, Efficiency, and Hospital Administration of the British Army* (1858), *Notes on Hospitals* (1858), *Notes on the Sanitary State of the Army in India* (1871), and *Life or Death in India* (1874), reflect her continuing concerns about these issues, particularly for the military.

Shortly after her return to England, Nightingale confined herself to her residence, citing her continued ill health. From this environment, however, she wrote between 15,000 and 20,000 letters to friends, acquaintances, and allies in her causes, as well as to her opposition. Her written word was strong and clear, thus conveying her beliefs, observations, and desire for changes in health care; through this medium, her work was successfully achieved. In addition, she received the most powerful as visitors in her home to maintain her dialogues and to win approval and support for her causes.

Nightingale's work was recognized in her lifetime through the many awards she received from both her own country and many others. She was able to work into her eighties and died in her sleep at the age of 90 on August 13, 1910.

Modern biographies and essays have attempted to analyze Nightingale's lifework through her family relationships (notably with parents and sister), and film dramatizations have frequently and inaccurately focused on her personal relationships.[12-14] While her personal and public life holds great intrigue for many, these retrospective analyses are often either very negative and harshly critical or overly positive in their descriptions of this Victorian leader. Kalisch and Kalisch have provided a critique of these different media portrayals that may assist the reader in better understanding the presentations of Florence Nightingale.[12-14]

THEORETICAL SOURCES

Many factors influenced the development of Nightingale's theory for nursing. Individual, societal, and professional values were all integral in the development of her work. She combined her individual resources with societal and professional resources to produce change.

Nightingale's education was an unusual one for a Victorian girl. Her tutelage by her well-educated, intellectual father and her obvious interest in subjects such as mathematics and philosophy provided her with knowledge and conceptual thought that was unique for women of her time. Nightingale's Aunt Mai, her devoted relative and champion, described her as having a great mind. It remains unknown whether Nightingale was a "genius" who developed her greatness through her unique formal education; in any century, she would likely have been a leader.

The Nightingale family's aristocratic social status provided Florence with access to persons of power and influence; many, such as Stanley Herbert, were family friends who remained important to her throughout her life. She comprehended the political process of Victorian England through the experiences of her father in his short-lived political foray, and she probably used this knowledge as she successfully waged political battles for her causes.

Nightingale also recognized the societal changes of her time and their impact on the health status of individuals; the industrial age had come to England, creating new classes of society, new diseases, and new social problems. Dickens's social commentaries and novels provided English society with scathing commentaries on health care and the need for both health and social reform in England. Her alliance with Dickens undoubtedly served as a factor in her definition of nursing and health care and her theory for nursing.[14]

Similar dialogues with other intellectuals and social reformers of the day—John Stuart Mill, Benjamin Jowett, and Harriet Marineau—aided in developing Nightingale's philosophical and logical thinking, which is evident in her theory for nursing. It is likely that her belief that she should strive to change the things that she saw as unacceptable in society was derived from this aspect of her life. No nursing leader could better exemplify the statement of Chinn and Jacobs that "When individual or professional values are in conflict with and challenge societal values, there is potential for creating change in society."[3:46]

Finally, Nightingale's religious affiliation and beliefs were especially strong sources for her nursing theory. Reared as a Unitarian, she believed that action for the benefit of others is a primary way of serving God. This religious belief allowed her to define nursing as a religious calling. In addition, the Unitarian faith strongly supported the education of persons as a means of developing their divine potential and moving toward perfection in their lives and in their service to God. Nightingale's faith provided her with personal strength throughout her life and the belief that education was a critical factor in establishing the profession of nursing.

USE OF EMPIRICAL EVIDENCE

A review of Nightingale's reports describing health and sanitary conditions both in Crimea and in England identify her as an outstanding scientist and empirical researcher. Her expertise as a statistician is also evident in the reports that she generated throughout her lifetime on the varied subjects of health care, nursing, and social reform.[1,4]

Perhaps best known is Nightingale's carefully collected information to prove the efficacy of her system of hospital nursing and organization during the Crimean War. The report of her experiences and data collected, *Notes on Matters Affecting the Health, Efficiency, and Hospital Administration of the British Army,* was submitted to the British Royal Sanitary Commission, which had been organized in response to Nightingale's charges of poor sanitary conditions. These data provided a strong argument for the reforms she sought in the hospital barracks in the Crimea. According to Cohen,[4] Nightingale invented the polar-area diagram to represent dramatically the extent of needless death in the British military hospitals in the Crimea. In this article Cohen summarizes the work of Nightingale as a researcher and statistician by noting that "she helped to pioneer the revolutionary notion that social phenomena could be objectively measured and subjected to mathematical analysis."[4:128] Palmer identified Nightingale's research skills to include recording, communicating, ordering, coding, conceptualizing, inferring, analyzing, and synthesizing.[20] Observation of social phenomena at both an individual and a systems level was of special importance to Nightingale and serves as the basis of her writings. For nurses, she viewed observation and practice as concurrent activities.

MAJOR CONCEPTS & DEFINITIONS

Nightingale's theory focused on the environment. Murray and Zentner define environment as "all the external conditions and influences affecting the life and development of an organism and capable of preventing, suppressing, or contributing to disease, accidents, or death."[18:149] While Nightingale never specifically used the term *environment* in her writing, she did define and describe in detail the concepts of ventilation, warmth, light, diet, cleanliness, and noise, which are components of the environment.

Although Nightingale often defined concepts precisely, she did not specifically separate the patient's environment into physical, emotional, or social aspects; she apparently assumed that all these aspects were included in the environment. In reading *Notes on Nursing* and her other writings, it is easy to identify her emphasis on the "physical" environment.[19] In the context of the specific issues that she had identified and struggled to improve or correct in various settings (e.g., war-torn environment, workhouses) and in her time, this emphasis appears to be most appropriate.[11] Nightingale's concern about healthy surroundings included not only the hospital settings in both the Crimea and England but also extended to the private homes of patients and the physical living conditions of the poor. Nightingale believed that healthy surroundings were necessary for proper nursing care. Her theory of the five essential components of environmental health—pure air, pure water, efficient drainage, cleanliness, light—are as essential today as they were 150 years ago.

Proper ventilation for the patient seemed to be of greatest concern to Nightingale; her charge to nurses was to "keep the air he breathes as pure as the external air, without chilling him."[19:12] Notwithstanding her rejection of the germ theory, which was newly developed at the time, Nightingale's emphasis on ventilation seemed to recognize this environmental component as an aid in recovery.

The concept of light was also important in Nightingale's theory.[19:84-87] In particular, she identified direct sunlight as a specific need of patients.

She noted that "light has quite as real and tangible effects upon the human body.... Who has not observed the purifying effect of light, and especially of direct sunlight, upon the air of a room?"[19:84-85] To achieve the beneficial effects of sunlight, nurses were instructed to move and position patients so that they would be exposed to sunlight.

Cleanliness as a concept is another critical component of Nightingale's environmental theory.[19:87-93] In regard to this concept, she specifically addressed the patient, the nurse, and the physical environment. She noted that a dirty environment—floors, carpets, walls, bed linens—was a source of infection through the organic matter it contained. Even if an area were well ventilated, the presence of organic material would create a dirty area; thus appropriate handling and disposing of bodily excretions and sewage were required to prevent contamination of the environment. Finally, Nightingale advocated the bathing of patients on a frequent (even daily) basis at a time when this practice was not the norm. In addition, she required that nurses themselves bathe regularly, that their clothing be clean, and that they wash their hands frequently.[19:93-95] This concept not only held special significance for individual patient care but also was critically important to improving the health status of the poor living in crowded, environmentally inferior conditions with inadequate sewage and limited access to pure water.[19:87-93]

Nightingale included the concepts of warmth, quiet, and diet in her environmental theory. In addition to discussing the ventilation in a room or home, Nightingale provided a description for measuring the patient's body temperature through palpation of the extremities to assess for heat loss.[19:17] The nurse was instructed to manipulate the environment continually to maintain both ventilation and patient warmth through the use of a good fire, open windows, and placement of the patient in the room.

Unnecessary noise and the need for quiet was also a concept that required assessment and intervention by the nurse.[19:44-58] Nightingale believed that noise created by physical activities in the environment (room) was to be avoided by the nurse because it could harm the patient.

Nightingale was concerned with the patient's diet.[19:63-69] She instructed nurses to assess not only dietary intake but also the meal schedule and its effect on the patient. She believed that patients with chronic illnesses could be starved to death and that intelligent nurses were those who were successful in meeting a patient's nutritional needs.

Another component of Nightingale's theory was that of a definition or description of "petty" management.[19:35-44] The nurse was in control of the environment both physically and administratively. She was to control the environment to protect the patient from both physical and psychological harm (e.g., receipt of upsetting news, visitors who might negatively affect recovery, sudden disruptions in sleep). In addition, Nightingale recognized that having pets (small animals) as visitors might be of comfort to the patient. Nightingale also believed that the nurse was in charge of the environment even when she was not physically present because she was to oversee those who worked in her absence.

MAJOR ASSUMPTIONS

Nursing

Nightingale believed that every woman, at one time in her life, would be a nurse in the sense that nursing involved having the responsibility for someone else's health. Thus, *Notes on Nursing* was written to provide women with guidelines for providing nursing care and advice on how to "think like a nurse."[19:4]

Fitzpatrick and Whall described Nightingale's concept of environment as "those elements external to and which affect the health of the sick and healthy person" and as including "everything from the patient's food and flowers to the patient's verbal and nonverbal interactions with the patient."[6:16-17] Little, if anything, in the patient's world is excluded from her definition of environment.

Person

Nightingale referred to the person as a patient in most of her writings. Nurses performed tasks to and for the patient and controlled the environment in which the patient resided to enhance recovery. For the most part, these descriptions describe a passive patient in this relationship. However, there are specific references to the patient performing self-care when possible and of being involved in both the tim-

ing and the substance of meals; for example, the nurse is specifically instructed to ask the patient about his preferences. Emphasis, however, is placed on the nurse as being in control of the patient's environment as Nightingale has defined it.

Health

Nightingale defined health as being well and using to the fullest extent every power that the person has. Additionally, she saw disease as a reparative process that nature instituted because of some want of attention. Nightingale envisioned health as being maintained through the prevention of disease via environmental control; she called this "health nursing" and distinguished it from nursing of the sick patient toward recovery or at least to live better until death.

Environment

Nightingale's assumptions about societal conditions are also relevant to her theory. She believed that the "sick poor" would benefit from environmental improvements that addressed both their bodies and their minds; she believed that nurses could be instrumental in changing the social status of the poor through improvement in their living conditions.

THEORETICAL ASSERTIONS

Nightingale believed that disease was a reparative process; disease was nature's effort to remedy a process of poisoning or decay or a reaction against the conditions in which a person was placed. Nightingale did not provide a definition of "nature." It has been noted that she often capitalized the word *nature* in her writings, thus suggesting that it was synonymous with God. Her Unitarian religious belief would support this view of God as Nature; however, when used without capitalization, it is unclear whether the meaning is different and perhaps synonymous with an organic pathological process. Nightingale believed that nursing's role was to prevent the reparative process from being interrupted and to provide optimal conditions for its enhancement.

Nightingale was totally committed to nursing education (training). Although she wrote *Notes on Nursing* for all women, her primary treatise was that women were to be specifically trained to provide care for the sick person and that nurses providing preventive health care (public health nursing) required even more training. Nightingale also felt that nurses needed to be excellent at observation of their patients and the environment; this was an ongoing activity for trained nurses.[19:59-71] In addition, she believed that nurses needed to use common sense in their nursing practice coupled with observation, perseverance, and ingenuity. Finally, Nightingale believed that persons desired good health and that they would cooperate with the nurse and nature to allow the reparative process to occur or to alter their environment to prevent disease.

Although Nightingale has often been maligned or ridiculed for not embracing the "germ theory," she very clearly understood the concept of contagion and contamination through organic materials from the patient and in the environment. Many of her observations are consistent with concepts of infection and the germ theory; for example, she embraced the concept of vaccination against various diseases. She also strongly believed that appropriate manipulations of the environment would prevent disease, a concept that underlies modern sanitation activities.

Nightingale does not explicitly discuss "caring behaviors" of nurses. She wrote very little about interpersonal relationships except as they influenced the patient's reparative processes. She did describe the phenomenon of being "called" to nursing and the need for commitment to one's work. From the perspectives of Victorian England and her religious beliefs, these descriptors may well describe a caring component of her nursing theory.

Finally, Nightingale believed that nurses should be moral agents. She addressed their "professional" relationship with their patients. She instructed them on the principle of confidentiality and advocated care for the poor to improve their health and social situation. In addition, she commented on patient decision-making (a relevant modern ethical concept); she called for conciseness and clear decision-making regarding the patient, noting that indecision ("irresolution") or changing one's mind is more harmful to the patient than the patient having to make a decision for himself.[19:96]

LOGICAL FORM

Nightingale used inductive reasoning to extract laws of health, disease, and nursing from her observations and experiences. Her childhood education, particularly in philosophy and mathematics, may well have contributed to her logical thinking and her inductive reasoning abilities. For example, her observations of the conditions in the Scutari hospital led her to conclude that the contaminated, dirty, dark environment led to disease. Not only could she prevent disease from flourishing in such an environment, she also recognized that prevention of disease would be achieved through environmental controls. From her own nursing training, from her brief experience as a superintendent in London, and from her experiences in the Crimea, she was able to make her observations and form the principles for her nursing training and patient care.[22]

ACCEPTANCE BY THE NURSING COMMUNITY

Practice

Nightingale's nursing principles remain applicable today. The environmental aspects of her theory (ventilation, warmth, quiet, diet, and cleanliness) remain integral components of current nursing care. As nurses approach practice in the twenty-first century, these concepts continue to be relevant—in fact, to have increased relevance as society is facing new issues of disease control. Modern sanitation and water treatment have fairly successfully controlled traditional sources of disease, but contaminated water has again become a health issue for many communities in the United States. In addition, global travel has more dramatically altered the actual and potential spread of diseases than ever anticipated.

Other new environmental concerns have been created by modern architecture (e.g., "sick building" syndrome). Nurses need to ask whether modern environmentally controlled buildings meet Nightingale's principle of good ventilation. Disposal of waste, including toxic waste, and use of chemicals in this modern society also challenge health care professionals to reassess the concept of a healthy environment.[7]

In health care facilities, the ability to control room temperature individually for a patient is becoming increasingly difficult, and that same environment may create a high noise level through multiple activities and the technology (equipment) used to assist the patient's reparative process. Nurses are looking at these problems in a scholarly way because they continue to affect patients and our health care system.[16,21]

Monteiro provided the American public health community with a comprehensive review of Nightingale's work as a "sanitarian and social reformer," again reminding the health care community of the breadth of Nightingale's impact on health care in various settings and her concern about issues of poverty and sanitation.[17] Although such issues have been increasingly addressed by other disciplines in the United States, it is clear that there is an active role for nurses and nursing, both in providing direct patient care and in the sociopolitical arena of ensuring healthy environments for all citizens.

Although some of Nightingale's rationales have been modified or disproved by medical advances and scientific discovery, many of her concepts and portions of her theory have withstood the test of time and technological advances. In reading Nightingale's Victorian writings, remembering the uniqueness of her early life, and considering the sociopolitical na-

ture of the era, it is clear that much of her theory remains relevant for nursing today. Concepts from Nightingale's writings continue to be cited in the nursing literature—from political commentary to scholarly research.

Nightingale's "petty management" concepts and actions have also recently been analyzed by several authors, again identifying examples of the timelessness and universality of her management style.[5,10,23]

Finally, several writers have analyzed Nightingale's role in the suffrage movement and its relevance to feminist theory development. Although she has often been criticized for not actively participating in this movement, Nightingale indicated in a letter to John Stuart Mill that she felt that she could do work for women in other ways and that she did not have the time to participate in this movement actively although she supported the principle of political power for women. Scholars are reassessing Nightingale's significance in the women's movement of this modern era.[9,24]

Education

Nightingale's principles of nursing training (i.e., instruction in scientific principles and practical experience for the mastery of skills) provided a universal template for early nurse training schools, beginning with St. Thomas Hospital and King's College Hospital in London. With the Nightingale model used as a guide, three experimental schools—Bellevue Hospital in New York City, New Haven Hospital in Connecticut, and Massachusetts Hospital in Boston—were established in the United States in 1873.[2] The influence of this training system and many of its principles still can be found in today's nursing programs.

Although Nightingale advocated the nursing school's independence from a hospital so that nursing students would not be involved in the hospital's labor pool as part of their training, American nursing schools were unable to achieve such independence for many years.[2] Nightingale believed that the measurement of the "art of nursing" could not be accomplished through licensing examinations, but she used testing methods, including case studies (notes), for nursing probationers at St. Thomas Hospital.[5]

It is clear that Nightingale understood that good practice could result only from good education (training). That message resounds throughout her writings on nursing. Nightingale historian Joanne Farley responds to a modern nursing student by noting that "Training is to teach a nurse to know her business. . . . Training is to enable the nurse to act for the best . . . like an intelligent and responsible being."[5:13] It is difficult to imagine what the care of sick human beings would be like if Nightingale had not defined the educational needs of nurses and established these first schools.

Research

Nightingale's interest in scientific inquiry and statistics continues to define the scientific inquiry used in nursing research. Nightingale was exceptionally efficient and resourceful in her ability to gather and analyze data; her ability to represent data graphically was first identified in the polar diagrams, the graphic illustration style that she invented.[4] Her empirical approach to solving problems of health care delivery is obvious in the data that she often included in her numerous letters.

If Nightingale's writings are defined and analyzed as theory, they do lack the complexity and testability found in modern nursing theories. Thus her theory cannot generate the nursing research used to test modern theories. On the other hand, concepts identified by Nightingale have served as the basis for current research, which adds to modern nursing science and practice. A review of the current nursing literature suggests that nurses in the United Kingdom tend to take a more scholarly, perhaps even reverent, view of Nightingale's work than some nurses in the United States do, although there seems to be a subtle shift in the analysis of Nightingale's concepts in U.S. graduate nursing study.

Finally, it is interesting to note that Nightingale used brief case studies (possible exemplars?) to illustrate a number of the concepts that she discussed in *Notes on Nursing.* Scholarly nurses have refined this technique for inclusion in texts and research studies; such a style thus has an auspicious history in nursing literature.

FURTHER DEVELOPMENT

Nightingale's theory for nursing is stated clearly and concisely in *Notes on Nursing,* her most widely known work. Its content seems most amenable to theory analysis. Nightingale organized the chapters of this text by concept; however, continued discussion of other concepts may appear in a specific chapter as it relates to the discussion. Fitzpatrick and Whall[6] refer to this approach as a "set of laws" theory; they define laws as theoretical statements with overwhelming empirical support.

Hardy[8] proposed that Nightingale formulated a "grand theory" that explains the totality of behavior. Grand theories tend to be somewhat vague—without specific definition of terms and concepts and without full development of relationships between concepts. They often provide untestable formulations. This type of theory is an early development that relies on anecdotal situations to illustrate its meaning and support its claims. Although her work can be classified as lower level theory, Nightingale provided the foundation for the development of both nursing practice and current nursing theories.

CRITIQUE
Simplicity

Nightingale's theory contains three major relationships—environment to patient, nurse to environment, and nurse to patient. Nightingale believed that the environment was the main factor creating illness in a patient; she regarded disease as "the reactions of kindly nature against the conditions in which we have placed ourselves."[19:56] Nightingale recognized not only the harmfulness of an environment; she also emphasized the benefits of good environment in preventing disease.

The nurse's practice includes the manipulation of the environment in a number of ways to enhance patient recovery. Elimination of contamination and contagion and exposure to fresh air, light, warmth, and quiet were identified as elements to be controlled or manipulated in the environment. Nightingale began to develop relationships between some of these elements in her discussions of contamination and ventilation, light and patient position in the room, cleanliness and darkness, and noise and patient stimulation. The relationship of the sickroom to the rest of the house and of the house to its neighborhood was also described. In addition, Nightingale recognized the need to manipulate the environment to prevent disease, as evidenced by her discussion of the homes of the poor, the workhouses, and preventing exposure of children to measles.

The nurse-patient relationship is perhaps least well defined in Nightingale's writings. Yet there are suggestions of cooperation and collaboration in her discussions of eating patterns and preferences, the comfort of a loved pet to the patient, protection of the patient from emotional distress, and conservation of energy while allowing the patient to participate in self-care. Finally, it is interesting to note that Nightingale discussed the concept of observation extensively, including the use of those observations to guide the care of patients and to measure improvement or lack of response to nursing interventions. This aspect of training and practice would suggest the origins of the nursing process.

Combining the concepts that Nightingale identified does not aid in increasing their simplicity; her original statements are expressed in an economical form. Diagrams of these concepts and their relationships have been proposed, thus supporting their logic and simplicity.[15]

Nightingale provided a descriptive, explanatory theory rather than one of prediction. However, its environmental focus, with its epidemiological components, had predictive potential, but the theory was never tested in that manner by Nightingale. It is not clear that Nightingale intended to develop a theory of nursing. She did intend to define the science and art of nursing and to provide general rules with explanations that would result in good nursing care for patients. Thus her objective of setting forth general rules for the practice and development of nursing was met through this simple theory.

Generality

Nightingale's theory has been used to provide general guidelines for all nurses in all times. The universality and timelessness of her concepts (even though specific activities are no longer relevant) remain pertinent. The relation concepts—nurse, patient, and environment—are applicable in all nursing settings today. To address her audience of women who may provide care to another (not only professional nurses), the theory she proposed remains relevant. Thus it meets the criterion of generalizability.

Empirical Precision

Concepts and relationships within Nightingale's theory are frequently stated implicitly and are presented as truths rather than as tentative, testable statements. In contrast to her quantitative research on mortality performed in the Crimea, Nightingale advised nurses that their practice should be based on their observations and experiences rather than on systematic empirical research. If she were addressing the development of the "art of nursing," her admonition would suggest a role for qualitative and phenomenological research methodology in nursing.

Derivable Consequences

Nightingale's writings, to an extraordinary degree, direct the nurse to action on behalf of her patient and herself. These directives encompass the areas of practice, research, and education. Most specific are her principles that attempt to shape nursing practice. Nightingale urged nurses to provide to physicians "not your opinion, however respectfully given, but your facts."[19:122] Similarly, she advised that "If you cannot get the habit of observation one way or other, you had better give up the being a nurse, for it is not your calling, however kind and anxious you may be."[19:113] Her encouragement for a measure of independence and precision previously unknown in nursing may still guide and motivate us today as the nursing profession continues to evolve.

Nightingale's view of humanity was consistent with her theories of nursing. She believed in creative, universal humanity with the potential and ability for growth and change[20] Deeply religious, she viewed nursing as a means of doing the will of her God. Perhaps it is because of this concept of nursing as a divine calling that she relegated the patient to a relatively passive role with the patient's desires and needs provided by the nurse. The zeal and self-righteousness that come from being a reformer might explain some of Nightingale's beliefs and practices that she advocated. Finally, one must consider the historical period (Victorian England) in which she lived to better understand her views.

Nightingale's basic principles of environmental manipulation and psychological care of the patient can be applied in contemporary nursing settings. Although her rejection of the germ theory and her inability to recognize a unified body of nursing knowledge that is testable (rather than relying only on personal observation and experience) have subjected her to some ridicule, other parts of her theory and her activities are relevant to nursing's professional identity and practice.

Lack of specificity has hindered use of Nightingale's ideas for the generation of nursing research. However, her writings continue to stimulate productive thinking for the individual nurse and the nursing profession. They give nurses much food for thought—food that continues to nourish us even after nearly 150 years. It is only right that Nightingale continues to be recognized as the brilliant and creative founder of modern nursing and its first nursing theorist.

CRITICAL THINKING *Activities*

1 Analyze the setting in which you are practicing nursing (i.e., working as an employee or a student) by using Nightingale's concepts of ventilation, light, noise, and cleanliness.

2 Use Nightingale's theory to evaluate the nursing interventions you have identified for an individual patient in your facility or practice.

3 Your hospital patient is an 82-year-old woman. She has no immediate family and has been living alone in her own home. Her hospitalization was unanticipated; it followed a visit to the emergency department for a burn on her lower legs. The patient has been hospitalized for 14 days. On this day, she pleads

with you to allow her friend to bring her dog, a 16-year-old Scottish terrier, to the hospital. She tells you that none of the other nurses seemed to listen to her when she asked them about such a visit. Based on Nightingale's work, what actions would you take for this patient?

REFERENCES

1. Agnew, L.R. (1958, May). Florence Nightingale: Statistician. *American Journal of Nursing, 58,* 644.
2. Ashley, J.A. (1976). *Hospitals, paternalism, and the role of the nurse.* New York: Teachers College Press.
3. Chinn, P., & Jacobs, M. (1983). *Theory and nursing: A systematic approach.* St. Louis: Mosby.
4. Cohen, I.B. (1984, March). Florence Nightingale. *Scientific American, 250*(3), 128-137.
5. Decker, B., & Farley, J.K. (1991, May/June). What would Nightingale say? *Nurse Educator, 16*(3), 12-13.
6. Fitzpatrick, J., & Whall, A. (1983). *Conceptual models of nursing.* Bowie, MD: Robert J. Brady.
7. Gropper, E. I. (1990). Florence Nightingale: Nursing's first environmental theorist. *Nursing Forum, 25*(3), 30-33.
8. Hardy, M. (1978). Perspectives on nursing theory. *Advances in Nursing Science, 1,* 37-48.
9. Hektor, L.M. (1994, Nov.). Florence Nightingale and the women's movement: Friend or foe? *Nursing Inquiry, 1*(1), 38-45.
10. Henry, B., Woods, S., & Nagelkerk, J. Nightingale's perspective of nursing administration. *Nursing and Health Care 11*(4), 200-206.
11. Isler, C. (1970). *Florence Nightingale: Rebel with a cause.* Oradell, NJ: Medical Economics.
12. Kalisch, B.J., & Kalisch, P.A. (1983, April). Heroine out of focus: Media images of Florence Nightingale. Part I. Popular biographies and stage productions. *Nursing and Health Care, 4*(4), 181-187.
13. Kalisch, B.J., & Kalisch, P.A. (1983, May). Heroine out of focus: Media images of Florence Nightingale. Part II. Film, radio, and television dramatizations. *Nursing and Health Care, 4*(5), 270-278.
14. Kalisch, P.A., & Kalisch, B.J. (1987). *The changing image of the nurse.* Menlo Park, CA: Addison-Wesley.
15. Lobo, M.L. (1995). Florence Nightingale. In J.B. George (Ed.), *Nursing theories: The base for professional nursing practice.* Norwalk, CT: Appleton & Lange.
16. McCarthy, D.O., Ouimet, M.E., & Daun, J.M. (1991, May). Shades of Florence Nightingale: Potential impact of noise stress on wound healing. *Holistic Nursing Practice, 5*(4), 39-48.
17. Monteiro, L.A. (1985, Feb.). Florence Nightingale on public health nursing. *American Journal of Public Health, 75,* 181-186.

18. Murray, R., & Zentner, J. (1975). *Nursing concepts in health promotion.* Englewood Cliffs, N.J.: Prentice Hall.
19. Nightingale, F. (1969). *Notes on nursing: What it is and what it is not.* New York: Dover.
20. Palmer, I.S. (1977, March-April). Florence Nightingale: Reformer, reactionary, researcher. *Nursing Research, 26,* 84-89.
21. Pope, D.S. (1995, Winter). Music, noise, and the human voice in the nurse-patient environment. *Image: Journal of Nursing Scholarship, 27,* 291-295.
22. Thomas, S. P. (1993, April-June). The view from Scutari: A look at contemporary nursing. *Nursing Forum, 28*(2), 19-24.
23. Ulrich, B.T. (1992). *Leadership and management according to Florence Nightingale.* Norwalk, CT: Appleton & Lange.
24. Welch, M. (1990, June). Florence Nightingale: The social construction of a Victorian feminist. *Western Journal of Nursing Research, 12,* 404-407.

BIBLIOGRAPHY
Primary sources
Books

Nightingale, F. (1911). *Letters from Miss Florence Nightingale on health visiting in rural districts.* London: King.
Nightingale, F. (1954). *Selected writings.* Compiled by Lucy R. Seymer. New York: Macmillan.
Nightingale, F. (1956). *The institution of Kaiserwerth on the Rhine, Dusseldorf, Germany.* Anna Sticker.
Nightingale, F. (1957). *Notes on nursing.* Philadelphia: J.B. Lippincott. (Originally published, 1859).
Nightingale, F. (1969). *Notes on nursing: What it is and what it is not.* New York: Dover.
Nightingale, F. (1974). *Letters of Florence Nightingale in the history of nursing archive.* Boston: Boston University Press.
Nightingale, F. (1976). *Notes on hospitals.* New York: Gordon.
Nightingale, F. (1978). *Notes on nursing.* London: Duckworth.
Nightingale, F. (1992). *Notes on nursing.* Commemorative edition with commentaries by contemporary nursing leaders. Philadelphia: J.B. Lippincott.

Journal articles

Nightingale, F. (1930, July). Trained nursing for the sick poor. *International Nursing Review, 5,* 426-433.
Nightingale, F. (1954, May 7). Maternity hospital and midwifery school. *Nursing Mirror, 99,* ix-xi, 369.
Nightingale, F. (1954). The training of nurses. *Nursing Mirror, 99,* iv-xi.

Secondary sources
Book reviews

Nightingale, F. (1954). Selected writings. *Nursing Mirror, 100,* 846, Dec. 24, 1954.
Royal Sanitary Institute Journal, 75, 275-276, April 1955.
American Journal of Nursing, 55, 162, May 1955.

Nursing Times, 52, 502-503, 507, May 6, 1955.
Nightingale, F. (1969). *Notes on nursing: What it is and what it is not.*
Nursing Times, 66, 828, June 25, 1970.
Nursing Mirror, 131, 47, Oct. 9, 1970.
Nightingale, F. *Notes on nursing: What it is and what it is not, the science and art.*
Nursing Times, 76, 187, Oct. 23, 1980.
Nursing Mirror, 151, 41, Dec. 11, 1980.
Australian Nurses Journal 10, 29, Feb. 1981.
Nightingale, F. (1979). Cassandra: An essay.
American Journal of Nursing, 81, 1059-1061, May 1981.
Seymer. L.R. (1950). *Florence Nightingale.*
Nursing Mirror, 92, 31, Nov. 17, 1950.
Nursing Times, 46, 1285, Dec. 16, 1950.
Journal of the American Medical Association, 146, 605, June 9, 1951.
Public Health Nursing 43, 459, Aug. 1951.

Books

Aiken, C.A. (1915). *Lessons from the life of Florence Nightingale.* New York: Lakeside.
Aldis, M. (1914). *Florence Nightingale.* New York: NOPHN.
Andrews, M.R. (1929). *A lost commander.* Garden City, NY: Doubleday.
Baly, M.E. (1986). *Florence Nightingale: The nursing legacy.* New York: Methuen.
Barth, R.J. (1945). *Fiery angel: The story of Florence Nightingale.* Coral Gables, FL: Glade House.
Bishop, W.J. (1962). *A bio-bibliography of Florence Nightingale.* London: Dawson's of Pall Mall.
Boyd, N. (1982). *Three Victorian women who changed their world.* New York: Oxford.
Bull, A. (1985). *Florence Nightingale.* North Pomfret, VT: David and Charles.
Calabria, M., & Macrae, J. (Eds.). (1994). *Suggestions for thought by Florence Nightingale: Selections and commentaries.* Philadelphia: University of Pennsylvania Press.
Collins, D. (1985). *Florence Nightingale.* Milford, MI: Mott Media.
Columbia University Faculty of Medicine and Department of Nursing. (1937). *Catalogue of the Florence Nightingale collection.* New York: Author.
Cook, E.T. (1913). *The life of Florence Nightingale.* London, Macmillan.
Cook, E.T. (1941). *A short life of Florence Nightingale.* New York: Macmillan.
Cope, Z. (1958). *Florence Nightingale and the doctors.* Philadelphia: J.B. Lippincott.
Cope, Z. (1961). *Six disciples of Florence Nightingale..* New York: Pitman.
Davies, C. (1980). *Rewriting nursing history.* London: Croom Helm.
Editors of *RN.* (1970). *Florence Nightingale: Rebel with a cause.* Oradell, NJ: Medical Economics.

French, Y. (1953). *Six great Englishwomen* London: H. Hamilton.

Goldie, S. (1987). *I have done my duty: Florence Nightingale in the Crimea War, 1854-1856.* London: Manchester University Press.

Goldsmith, M.L. (1937). *Florence Nightingale: The woman and the legend.* London: Hodder and Stoughton.

Goldwater, S.S. (1947). *On hospitals.* New York: Macmillan.

Gordon, R. (1979). *The private life of Florence Nightingale.* New York: Atheneum.

Haldale, E. (1931). *Mrs. Gaskell and her friends.* New York: Appleton.

Hall, E.F. (1920). *Florence Nightingale.* New York: Macmillan.

Hallock, G.T., & Turner, C.E. (1928). *Florence Nightingale.* New York: Metropolitan Life Insurance Co.

Herbert, R.G. (1981). *Florence Nightingale: Saint, reformer, or rebel?* Melbourne, FL: Krieger.

Holmes, M. (n.d.). *Florence Nightingale: A cameo life-sketch.* London: Woman's Freedom League.

Huxley, E.J. (1975). *Florence Nightingale.* London: Putnam.

Hyndman, J.A. (1969). *Florence Nightingale: Nurse to the world.* Cleveland: World Publishing.

Keele, J. (Ed.). (1981). *Florence Nightingale in Rome.* Philadelphia: American Philosophical Society.

Lammond, D. (1935). *Florence Nightingale.* London: Duckworth.

Miller, B.W. (1947). *Florence Nightingale: The lady with the lamp.* Grand Rapids, MI: Zondervan.

Miller, M. (1987). *Florence Nightingale.* Minneapolis: MN: Bethany House.

Mosby, C.V. (1938). *Little journey to the home of Florence Nightingale.* New York: C.V. Mosby.

Muir, D.E. (1946). *Florence Nightingale.* Glasgow: Blackie and Son.

Nash, R. (1937). *A sketch for the life of Florence Nightingale.* London: Society for Promoting Christian Knowledge.

Newton, M.E. (1949). *Florence Nightingale's philosophy of life and education.* Ed.D. dissertation. Stanford, CA: Stanford University.

O'Malley, I.B. (1931). *Life of Florence Nightingale, 1820-1856.* London: Butterworth.

Pollard, E. (1902). *Florence Nightingale: The wounded soldiers' friend.* London: Partridge.

Presbyterian Hospital, School of Nursing. (1937). *Catalogue of the Florence Nightingale collection.* New York: Author.

Quiller-Couch, A.T. (1927). *Victor of peace.* New York: Nelson.

Quinn, V., & Prest, J. (Eds.). (1987). *Dear Miss Nightingale: A selection of Benjamin Jowett's letters to Florence Nightingale, 1860-1893.* Oxford: Clarendon Press.

Rappe, E.C. (1977). *God bless you, my dear Miss Nightingale.* Stockholm: Almqvist och Wiksell.

Sabatini, R. (1934). *Heroic lives.* Boston: Houghton.

St. Thomas's Hospital. (1960). *The Nightingale Training School: St. Thomas's Hospital, 1860-1960.* London: Author.

Saleeby, C.W. (1912). *Surgery and society: A tribute to Listerism.* New York: Moffat, Yard & Co.

Schmidt, M.M. (1933). *400 Outstanding women of the world and costumology of their time.* Chicago: Author.

Selanders, L.C. (1993). *Florence Nightingale: An environmental adaptation theory.* Newbury Park, CA: Sage Publications.

Seymer, L.R. (1951). *Florence Nightingale.* New York: Macmillan.

Shor, D. (1987). *Florence Nightingale.* Lexington: NH: Silver.

Smith, F.B. (1982). *Florence Nightingale: Reputation and power.* New York: St. Martin.

Stephenson, G.E. (comp.) (1924). *Some pioneers in the medical and nursing world.* Shanghai: Nurses's Association of China.

Strachey, L. (1918). *Eminent Victorians.* London: Chatto & Windus.

Tabor, M.E. (1925). *Pioneer women..* London: Sheldon.

Tooley, S.A. (1905). *The life of Florence Nightingale.* New York: Macmillan.

Turner, D. (1986). *Florence Nightingale..* New York: Watts.

Wilson, W.G. (1940). *Soldier's heroine.* Edinburgh: Missionary Education Movement.

Woodman-Smith, C. (1983). *Florence Nightingale.* New York: Atheneum.

Woodham-Smith, C.B. (1951). *Florence Nightingale, 1820-1910.* New York: McGraw-Hill.

Woodham-Smith, C.B. (1951). *Lonely crusader: The life of Florence Nightingale, 1820-1910.* New York: Whittlesey House.

Woodham-Smith, C.B. (1956). *Lady-in-chief.* London: Methven.

Woodham-Smith, C.B. (1977). *Florence Nightingale, 1820-1910.* London: Collins.

Woodsey, A. H. (1950). *A century of nursing.* New York: Putnam.

World's Who's Who in Science. Florence Nightingale (entry). (1968). Chicago: A.N. Marquis.

Wren, D. (1949). *They enriched humanity: Adventurers of the 19th century..* London: Skilton.

Book chapters

Reed, P.G., & Zurakowski, T.L. (1983 & 1989). Nightingale: A visionary model for nursing. In J. Fitzpatrick & A. Whall, *Conceptual models of nursing: Analysis and application.* Bowie, MD: Robert J. Brady.

Torres, G.C. (1980 & 1990). Florence Nightingale. In Nursing Theories Conference Group, J.B. George, Chairperson, *Nursing theories: The base for professional nursing practice.* Englewood Cliffs, NJ: Prentice Hall.

Unpublished dissertations

Hektor, L.M. (1992). *Nursing, science, and gender: Florence Nightingale and Martha E. Rogers.* Unpublished doctoral dissertation, University of Miami.

Selanders, L.C. (1992). *An analysis of the utilization of power by Florence Nightingale.* Unpublished doctoral dissertation, Western Michigan University.

Tschirch, P. (1992). *The caring tradition: Nursing ethics in the United States, 1890-1915.* Unpublished doctoral dissertations, The University of Texas Graduate School of Biomedical Science at Galveston.

Journal articles

Abbott, M.E. (1916, Sept. 14). Portraits of Florence Nightingale. *Boston Medical and Surgical Journal 1975,* 361-367.

Abbott, M.E. (1916, Sept. 21). Portraits of Florence Nightingale. *Boston Medical Surgery Journal, 175,* 413-422.

Abbott, M.E. (1916, Sept. 28). Portraits of Florence Nightingale. *Boston Medical Surgery, 175,* 453-457.

Address by the Archbishop of York. (1970, May 21). Florence Nightingale. *Nursing Times, 66,* 670.

Address given at fiftieth anniversary of founding by Florence Nightingale of first training school for nurses at St. Thomas's Hospital, London, England. (1911, Feb.). *American Journal of Nursing, 11,* 331-361.

At Embley Park and East Willow. (1937, July 24), *Nursing Times, 33,* 730-731.

Ball, O.F. (1952, May). Florence Nightingale. *Modern Hospital, 78,* 88-90, 144.

Baly, M. (1986, June 11-18). Shattering the Nightingale myth. *Nursing Times, 82*(24), 16-18.

Baly, M.E. (1969, Jan. 2). Florence Nightingale's influence on nursing today. *Nursing Times 65*(suppl.), 1-4.

Barber, E.M. (1935, July). A culinary campaign. *Journal of the American Dietetic Association, 11,* 89-98.

Barker, E.R. (1989, Oct.). Caregivers as casualties...war experiences and the postwar consequences for both Nightingale- and Vietnam-era nurses. *Western Journal of Nursing Research, 11,* 628-631.

Barritt, E.R. (1973). Florence Nightingale's values and modern nursing education. *Nursing Forum, 12,* 7-47.

Berentson, L. (1982, April-May). Florence Nightingale: Change agent. RN, *Idaho, 6*(2), 3,7.

Berman, J.K. (1974, Aug.). Florentia and the Clarabellas: A tribute to nurses. *Journal of the Indiana State Medical Association, 67,* 717-719.

Bishop, W.J. (1957, Jan.). Florence Nightingale bibliography. *International Nursing Review, 4,* 64.

Bishop, W.J. (1957, May). Florence Nightingale's letters. *American Journal of Nursing, 57,* 607.

Bishop, W.J. (1960, May). Florence Nightingale's message for today. *Nursing Outlook, 8,* 246.

Black, B.W. (1939, July). A tribute to Florence Nightingale. *Pacific Coast Journal of Nursing, 35,* 408-409.

Blanc, E. (1980, May). Nightingale remembered: Reflections on times past. *California Nurse, 75*(10), 7.

Blanchard, J.R. (1939, June). Florence Nightingale: A study in vocation. *New Zealand Nursing Journal, 32,* 193-197.

Book reviews and digests. (1920, May). *Public Health Nursing, 12,* 442-448.

Boylen, J.O. (1974, April). The Florence Nightingale–Mary Stanley controversy: Some unpublished letters. *Medical History, 18*(2), 186-193.

Bridges, D.C. (1954, April). Florence Nightingale centenary. *International Nurses Review, 1,* 3.

Brow, E.J. (1954, April). Florence Nightingale and her international influence. *International Nursing Review, (ns) 1,* 17-19.

The call to war. (1970, May). *RN, 33,* 42.

Carlisle, D. (1989, Dec. 13-19). A nightingale sings...Florence Nightingale...unknown details of her life story. *Nursing Times, 85*(50), 38-39.

Cartwright, F.F. (1976, March). President's address: Miss Nightingale's dearest friend. *Proceedings of the Royal Society of Medicine, 69*(3), 169-175.

Centenary celebrations [Florence Nightingale] (1954, Nov.). *Nursing Times, 50,* 1213-1214.

Centenary (Editorial). (1960, May). *Nursing Times, 56,* 587.

Charatan, F.B. (1990, Feb.). Florence Nightingale: The most famous nurse in the world. *Today's OR Nurse, 12*(2), 25-30.

Cherescavich, G. (1971, June). *Nursing Clinics of North America, 6,* 217-223.

Choa, G.H. (1971, May). Speech by Dr. the Hon. G.H. Choa at the Florence Nightingale Day Celebration on Wednesday, 12th May, 1971, at City Hall, Hong Kong. *Nursing Journal, 10,* 33-34.

Clayton, R.E. (1974, April). How men may live and not die in India: Florence Nightingale. *Australasian Nurses Journal, 2,* 10-11.

Coakley, M.L. (1989, Winter). Florence Nightingale: A one-woman revolution. *Journal of Christian Nursing, 6,* 20-25.

Collins, W.J. (1945, May 12). Florence Nightingale and district nursing. *Nursing Mirror, 81,* 74.

Cope, Z. (1960, May 13). Florence Nightingale and her nurses. *Nursing Times, 56,* 597.

Coxhead, E. (1973, May 10). Miss Nightingale's country hospital. *Nursing Times, 65,* 615-617.

A criticism of Miss Florence Nightingale. (1907), Feb. 2). *Nursing Times, 3,* 89.

Crowder, E.L. (1978, May). Florence Nightingale. *Texas Nursing, 52*(5), 6-7.

Cruse, P. (1980, Sept.). Florence Nightingale. *Surgery, 88*(3), 394-399.

Davidson, C. (1937, March). Jeanne Mance and Florence Nightingale. *Hospital Progress, 18,* 83-85.

de Guzman, G. (1935, July). [Florence Nightingale]. *Filipino Nurse, 10,* 10-14.

de Tornayay, R. (1976, Nov.-Dec.). Past is prologue: Florence Nightingale, *Pulse, 12*(6), 9-11.

The death of Florence Nightingale. (1910, Sept.). *American Journal of Nursing, 10,* 919-920. (Editorial).

Dennis, K.E., & Prescott, P.A. (1985, Jan.). Florence Nightingale: Yesterday, today, and tomorrow. *Advances in Nursing Science, 7*(2), 66-81.

Draper, J.M. (1907, Jan.). A brief sketch of the life of Florence Nightingale. *Trained Nurse, 38,* 1-4.

Duggan, R. (1981, June). Florence Nightingale memorial service. *Australian Nurses Journal 10*(6), 30.

Dunbar, V.M. (1954, Oct.). Florence Nightingale's influence on nursing education. *International Nursing Review, (ns) 1,* 17-23.

Dwyer, B.A. (1937, Jan.). The mother of our modern nursing system. *Filipino Nurse, 12,* 8-10.

Echos of the past (1907, Nov. 16). *British Journal of Nursing, 39,* 396-397.

Echos of the past (1907, Dec. 21). *British Journal of Nursing, 39,* 497-498.

Ellett, E.C. (1904, May). Florence Nightingale. *Trained Nurse, 32,* 305-310.

Extracts from letters from the Crimea. (1932, May). *American Journal of Nursing, 32,* 537-538.

Fink, L.G. (1934, Dec.). Catholic influences in the life of Florence Nightingale. *Hospital Progress, 15,* 482-489.

Florence Nightingale. (1903, July). *Medical Dial, 5,* 122-124. (Editorial).

Florence Nightingale. (1964, May 15). *Nursing Mirror, 118,* 131. (Editorial).

Florence Nightingale as a leader in the religious and civic thought of her time. (1936, July). *Hospitals, 10,* 78-84.

The Florence Nightingale bibliography (1956, April). *South African Nursing Journal, 22,* 16.

Florence Nightingale bibliography. (1956, Oct.). *Nursing Research, 5,* 87.

Florence Nightingale bibliography is compiled. (1931, May). *Modern Hospital, 36,* 126.

Florence Nightingale: Looking back . . . notes on hospitals. (1979, Sept.). *Lamp, 36,* 39-43.

Florence Nightingale O.M. (1910, Aug. 20). *British Journal of Nursing, 45,* 141-147.

Florence Nightingale: The original geriatric nurse. (1980, May). *Oklahoma Nurse, 25*(4), 6.

Florence Nightingale: Rebel with a cause. (1970, May). *RN, 33,* 39-55.

Florence Nightingale's influence on nursing today. (1969, Jan. 3). *Nursing Times, 65,* 1.

Florence Nightingale's letter. (1932, July 2). *Nursing Times, 28,* 699.

Florence Nightingale's letter of advice to Bellevue. (1911, Feb.). *American Journal of Nursing, 11,* 361-364.

Florence Nightingale's tomb. (1957, June). *Canadian Nurse, 53,* 529.

Florence Nightingale's work for public health. (1914, June). *American Journal of Public Health, 4,* 510-511. (Editorial).

Food for thought. (1958, Aug.) *Nursing Outlook, 6,* 437. (Editorial).

Footnote to a dedicated life. (1958, Aug.). *RN, 21,* 53.

Fraga, M., & Tanenbaum, L. (1980, May). Florence Nightingale: Model for today's nurse. *Florida Nurse, 29*(5), 11.

Frankenstein, L. The lady with a lamp. *Red Cross Courier, 16,* 15-17.

Gordon, J.E. (1972, Oct.). Nurses and nursing in Britain. 21. The work of Florence Nightingale. I. For the health of the army. *Midwife Health Visitor and Community Nurse, 8,* 351-359.

Gordon, J.E. (1972, Nov.). Nurses and nursing in Britain. 22. The work of Florence Nightingale. II. The establishment of nurse training in Britain. *Midwife Health Visitor and Community Nurse, 8,* 391-396.

Gordon, J.E. (1973, Jan.). Nurses and nursing in Britain. 23. The work of Florence Nightingale. III. Her influence throughout the world. *Midwife Health Visitor and Community Nurse, 9,* 17-22.

Gottstein, W.K. (1956, May). Miss Nightingale's personality. *RN, 19,* 58-60, 80, 82.

Gould, M.E. (1970, May 7). A woman of parts. *Nursing Times, 66,* 606.

Graham, S. (1980, Oct. 23). Notes on nursing, 1860-1980: Angels of plain speech. *Nursing Times, 76*(43), 1874.

Greatness in little things (1954, May 8). *Nursing Times, 50,* 508-510.

Grier, B., & Grier, M. (1978, Oct.). Contributions of the passionate statistician (Florence Nightingale). *Research in Nursing and Health, 1*(3), 103-109.

Grier, M.R. (1978, Oct.). Florence Nightingale: Saint or scientist? *Research in Nursing and Health, 1*(3), 91. (Editorial).

Hallowes, R. (1957, Sept. 27). Florence Nightingale. In Distinguished British nurses. *Nursing Mirror, 105,* viii-x.

Hamash Dash, D.M. (1971, June). Florence Nightingale's writings. *Nursing Journal of India, 62,* 179.

Headberry, J. (1966, Feb.). Florence Nightingale and modern nursing. *Australian Nurses Journal, 64,* 32-36.

Headberry, J.E. (1966, Jan.). Florence Nightingale and modern nursing. *Journal of the West Australian Nurses, 32,* 7-16.

Headberry, J.E. (1966, March-April). Florence Nightingale and modern nursing. *UNA Nursing Journal, 64,* 80-87.

Headberry, J.E. (1966, Sept. 2). Florence Nightingale and modern nursing. *Nursing Mirrors, 122,* xiii.

Health as a personal and community asset. (1926, Dec. 13). *Journal of Education, 104,* 566.

Hearn, M.J. (1920, April). Florence Nightingale. *Quarterly Journal of Chinese Nurses, 1,* 12-14.

Her letters [Florence Nightingale]. (1955, June). *Nursing Journal of India, 46,* 210.

Her letters [Florence Nightingale]. (1955, July). *Nursing Journal of India, 46,* 236.

Her letters [Florence Nightingale]. (1955, Aug.). *Nursing Journal of India, 46,* 268.

Her letters [Florence Nightingale]. (1955, Oct.). *Nursing Journal of India, 46,* 326.

Holly, H. (1967, Winter). Wanted: A day's work for a day's pay. *Nevada Nurses Association Newsletter,* 1.

Hurd, H.M. (1920, June). Florence Nightingale: A force in medicine. *Johns Hopkins Nurses Alumnae Magazine, 9,* 68-81.

Ifemesia, C.C. (1976, July-Sept.). Florence Nightingale (1820-1910). *Nigerian Nurse, 8*(3), 26-34.

In her memory. (1957, May). *RN, 20,* 53.

Isler, C. (1970, May). Florence Nightingale, *RN, 33,* 35-55.

Iu, S. (1971, May). President's address at Florence Nightingale Day Celebration 12th May 1971, City Hall Theatre. *Hong Kong Nursing Journal, 10,* 27-32.

Iveson-Iveson, J. (1983, May 11). Nurses in society: A legend in the breaking (Florence Nightingale). *Nursing Mirror, 156*(19), 26-27.

Jake, D.G. (1975, Nov.). Florence Nightingale: Mission impossible. *Arizona Medicine, 32*(11), 894-895.

Jamme, A.C. (1920, May). Florence Nightingale: The great teacher of nurses. *Pacific Coast Journal of Nursing, 16,* 282-285.

Jones, H.W. (1940, Nov.). Some unpublished letters of Florence Nightingale. *Bulletin of the History of Medicine, 8,* 1389-1396.

Jones, O.C. (1972, Aug.). A useful memorial (Florence Nightingale). *Canadian Nurse, 68,* 38-39.

Journey among women: Responsibility at the top. Part II. (1970, June 4). *Nursing Times, 66,* 77.

Kelly, L.Y. (1976, Oct.). Our nursing heritage: Have we renounced it? (Florence Nightingale). *Image* (NY), *8*(3), 43-48.

Kerling, N.J. (1976, July 1). Letters from Florence Nightingale. *Nursing Mirror, 143*(1), 68.

Kiereini, E.M. (1981, June). The way ahead: On the occasion of Florence Nightingale oration at the Perth Concert Hall, Australia, 24th October, 1979. *Kenya Nursing Journal, 10*(1), 5-8.

King, A.G. (1964, June). The changing role of the nurse. *Hospital Topics, 42,* 89.

King, F.A. (1954, Oct. 22). Miss Nightingale and her ladies in the Crimea. *Nursing Mirror, 100,* xi-xii.

King, F.A. (1954, Oct. 29). Miss Nightingale and her ladies in the Crimea. *Nursing Mirror, 100,* viii-ix.

King, F.A. (1954, Nov. 5). Miss Nightingale and her ladies in the Crimea. *Nursing Mirror, 100,* v-vi.

King, F.A. (1954, Nov. 12). Miss Nightingale and her ladies in the Crimea. *Nursing Mirror, 100,* x-xi.

Konderska, Z. (1971, Oct.) [The birthday of nursing, (Florence Nightingale)]. *Pielig Polozna, 8,* 12-13.

Konstatinova, M. (1923, Oct.). In the cradle of nursing. *American Journal of Nursing, 24,* 47-49.

Kopf, E.W. (1978, Oct.). Florence Nightingale as statistician. *Research in Nursing and Health, 1*(3), 93-102.

Kovacs, A.F. (1973, May-June). The personality of Florence Nightingale. *International Nursing Review, 20,* 78-79.

The lady with a lamp. (1929, Feb. 9) *Nursing Times, 25,* 154.

Large, J.T. (1985, May). Florence Nightingale: A multifaceted personality. *Nursing Journal of India, 76*(5), 110, 114.

Lee, C.A. (1987, Feb.). Thrusts of Florence Nightingale in the social context of the 19th century. *Kansas Nurse 62*(2), 3-4.

Lee, C.A. (1987, May). Discussion/life of Florence Nightingale. *Kansas Nurse, 63*(5), 12-13.

Levine, M.E. (1963, April). Florence Nightingale: The legend that lives. *Nursing Forum, 2,* 24.

Literature of Florence Nightingale. (1931, April). *Hospital Progress, 12,* 188.

Loane, S.F. (1911, Feb.). Florence Nightingale and district nursing. *American Journal of Nursing, 11,* 383-384.

McKee, E.S. (1909, Sept.). Florence Nightingale and her followers. *Nashville Journal of Medicine and Surgery, 103,* 385-392.

Mackie, T.T. (1942, Jan.). Florence Nightingale and tropical and military medicine. *American Journal of Tropical Medicine, 22,* 1-8.

Macmillan, K. (1994, April-May). Brilliant mind gave Florence her edge . . . Florence Nightingale. *Registered Nurse, 6*(2), 29-30.

Macrae, J. (1995, Spring). Nightingale's spiritual philosophy and its significance for modern nursing. *Image: Journal of Nursing Scholarship, 27,* 8-10.

Materials for the study of Florence Nightingale. (1931, May). *Trained Nurse and Hospital Review, 86,* 656-657.

The meaning of the lamp. (1956, May). *RN, 19,* 61.

Menon, M. (1980, Aug.). The lamp she lit [Florence Nightingale]. *Nursing Journal of India, 81*(8), 214-215.

Miss Nightingale's book of the Crimea. (1954, May 7). *Nursing Journal of India, 99,* ii-iii.

Monteiro, L. (1972, Nov.-Dec.). Research into things past: Tracking down one of Miss Nightingale's correspondents. *Nursing Research, 21,* 526-529.

Monteiro, L. (1973, Nov. 8). Letters to a friend. *Nursing Times, 69,* 1474-1476.

Monteiro, L.A. (1985, Nov.). Response in anger: Florence Nightingale on the importance of training for nurses. *Journal of Nursing History, 1*(1), 11-18.

The most beautiful old lady. (1951, May 11). *Nursing Journal of India, 93,* 101.

Nagpal, N. (1985, May). Florence Nightingale: A multifaceted personality. *Nursing Journal of India, 76,* 110-114.

Nauright, L. (1984). Politics and power: A new look at Florence Nightingale. *Nursing Forum, 21,* 5-8.

Nelson, J. (1976, May 13). Florence: The legend [Florence Nightingale]. *Nursing Mirror, 142*(2), 40-41.

Newton, M.E. (1951, Sept.). The power of statistics. *Public Health Nursing, 43,* 502-505.

Newton, M.E. (1952, May). Florence Nightingale's concept of clinical teaching. *Nursing World, 126,* 220-221.

Nightingale bibliography. (1957, May). *American Journal of Nursing, 57,* 585.

Nightingale letter to Alice Fisher in Philadelphia (1976, Jan.). *American Nurse, 8*(2), 2.

The Nightingale saga (Vol. 1). (1962, Aug. 13). *Nursing Mirror, 114,* 425.

Ninan, R. (1982, June). The lady with the lamp: A profile. *Nursing Journal of India, 73*(6), 154-155.

No other earth. (1962, Nov.). *Today's Health, 40,* 63.

Noguchi, M. (1969, Oct.). [Nightingale's philosophy and its limitations: My theory on Nightingale]. *Japanese Journal of Nursing Art, 10,* 65-75.

Notting, M.A. (1927, May). Florence Nightingale as a statistician. *Public Health Nursing, 19,* 207-209.

Noyes, C.D. (1931, Jan.). Florence Nightingale: Sanitarian and Hygienist. *Red Cross Courier, 10,* 41-42.

Nuttall, P. (1983, Sept./Oct.). The passionate statistician . . . Florence Nightingale. *Nursing Times, 79*(30), 25-27.

O'Malley, I.B. (1935, May). Florence Nightingale after the Crimean War (1856-1861). *Trained Nurse, 94,* 401-407.

Oman, C. (1950, Nov. 17). Florence Nightingale as seen by two biographers. *Nursing Mirror, 92,* 30-31.

The other side of the coin. (1967, May). *New Zealand Nursing Journal, 60,* 40. (Editorial).

Palmer, I.S. (1976, Sept.-Oct.). Florence Nightingale and the Salisbury incident. *Nursing Research, 25*(5), 370-377.

Palmer, I.S. (1981, June). Florence Nightingale and international origins of modern nursing. *Image, 13,* 28-31.

Palmer, I.S. (1983, July-Aug.). Nightingale revisited. *Nursing Outlook, 31*(4), 229-233.

Palmer, I.S. (1983, Aug. 3). Florence Nightingale: The myth and the reality. *Nursing Times, 79,* 40-42.

Parker, P. (1977, March). Florence Nightingale: First lady of administrative nursing. *Supervisor Nurse, 8,* 24-25.

The passing of Florence Nightingale. (1910, Nov.). *Pacific Coast Journal of Nursing, 6,* 481-519.

A passionate statistician. (1931, May). *American Journal of Nursing, 31,* 566.

Pearce, E.C. (1954, April). The influence of Florence Nightingale on the spirit of nursing. *International Nursing Review, (ns) 1,* 20-22.

Penner, S.J. (1987, May). The remarkable Miss Nightingale. *Kansas Nurse, 62*(5), 11.

Peter, M. (1936, May). A personal interview with Florence Nightingale. *Pacific Coast Journal of Nursing, 32,* 270-271.

Phillips, E.C. (1920, May). Florence Nightingale: A study. *Pacific Coast Journal of Nursing, 16,* 272-274.

Pickering, G. (1974, Dec. 14). Florence Nightingale's illness. *British Medical Journal, 4*(5945), 656. (Letter).

Public health nursing: Florence Nightingale as a consultant. (1920, May). *Pacific Coast Journal of Nursing, 16,* 299-300.

Rains, A.J. (1982, Feb.). Mitchiner memorial lecture: "The Nightingale touch." *Journal of the Royal Army Medical Corps, 128*(1), 4-17.

Rao, G.A. (1971, June). Florence Nightingale's writings. *Nursing Journal of India, 62,* 179.

The real Florence Nightingale. (1912, April 6). *British Journal of Nursing, 48,* 267.

Remembering Florence Nightingale. (1979, Sept.). *Nursing Focus, 1*(1), 34.

The revolting revisionist historian perspective. (1979, Jan.). *Arizona Medicine, 36*(1), 65-66.

Rhynas, M. (1931, May). Intimate sketch of the life of Florence Nightingale. *Canadian Nurse, 27,* 229-233.

Richards, L. (1920, May). Recollections of Florence Nightingale. *American Journal of Nursing, 20,* 649.

Richards, L. (Ed.). (1934). Letters of Florence Nightingale. *Yale Review, 24,* 326-347.

Roberts, M.M. (1937, July). Florence Nightingale as a nurse educator. *American Journal of Nursing, 37,* 773-778.

Rogers, P. (1982, July). Florence Nightingale: The myth and the reality. *Nursing Focus, 3*(11), 10.

The romantic Florence Nightingale. (1968, May). *Canadian Nurse, 64,* 57.

Ross, M. (1954, May). Miss Nightingale's letters. *American Journal of Nursing, 53,* 593-594.

Scovil, E.R. (1911, Feb.). Personal recollections of Florence Nightingale. *American Journal of Nursing, 11,* 365-368.

Scovil, E.R. (1913, Oct.). Florence Nightingale. *American Journal of Nursing, 14,* 28-33.

Scovil, E.R. (1914, Oct.). Florence Nightingale and her nurses. *American Journal of Nursing, 15,* 13-18.

Scovil, E.R. (1916, Dec.). The love story of Florence Nightingale. *American Journal of Nursing, 17,* 209-212.

Scovil, E.R. (1920, May). The later activities of Florence Nightingale. *American Journal of Nursing, 20,* 609-612.

Scovil, E.R. (1927, May). Florence Nightingale's notes on nursing. *American Journal of Nursing, 27,* 355-357.

Seden, F. (1947, July.). Florence Nightingale and Turkish education. *Public Health Nursing, 39,* 349.

Seymer, L.R. (1947, Sept.). Florence Nightingale oration. *International Nursing Bulletin, 3,* 12-17.

Seymer, L.R. (1951, July). Florence Nightingale at Kaiserwerth. *American Journal of Nursing, 51,* 424-426.

Seymer, L.R. (1954, April 2). Florence Nightingale. *Nursing Mirror, 99,* 34-36.

Seymer, L.R. (1960, May). Nightingale Nursing School: 100 years ago. *American Journal of Nursing, 60,* 658.

Seymer, S. (1979, May). The writings of Florence Nightingale. *Nursing Journal of India, 70*(5), 121-128.

Skeet, M. (1980, Oct. 23). Nightingale's notes on nursing, 1860-1980 [interview by Alison Dunn]. *Nursing Times, 76*(43), 1871-1873.

Slater, V.E. (1994, Feb.). The educational and philosophical influences on Florence Nightingale, an enlightened conductor. *Nursing History Review, 2,* 137-152.

Smith, F.T. (1981, May). Florence Nightingale: Early feminist. *American Journal of Nursing, 81,* 1059-1061.

Some letters from Florence Nightingale. (1935, Feb.). *Hospital (London), 31,* 50.

Sotejo, J.V. (1970, April-June). Florence Nightingale: Nurse for all seasons. *ANPHI Papers, 5,* 4.

Sparacino, P.S.A. (1994, March). Clinical practice: Florence Nightingale: A CNS role model. *Clinical Nurse Specialist, 8*(2), 64.

Stewart, I.M. (1939, Dec.). Florence Nightingale: Educator. *Teachers College Record, 41,* 208-223.

Swain, V. (1983, March 16-22). No plaster saint! *Nursing Times, 79*(11), 62-63.

That lamp. (1966, May 13). *Nursing Times, 62,* 631.

Thompson, J.D. (1980, May). The passionate humanist: From Nightingale to the new nurse. *Nursing Outlook, 28*(5), 290-295.

Tinkler, L.F. (1973, Aug. 2). The barracks at Scutari: Start of a nursing legend. *Nursing Times, 69,* 1006-1007.

Tobin, J. (1969, March). Observations on Florence Nightingale. *Tar Heel Nurse, 31,* 52-55.

Tracy, M.A. (1940, July). Florence Nightingale and her influence on hospitals. *Pacific Coast Journal of Nursing, 36,* 406-407.

Trautman, M.J. (1971, April). Nurses as poets. *American Journal of Nursing, 71,* 725-728.

Two unpublished letters. (1937, May). *Public Health Nursing, 29,* 307.

Verney, H. (1980, Spring). The perfect aunt: FN 1820-1910. *News Letter of the Florence Nightingale International Nurses Association, 70,* 13-16.

Walton, P. (1972, Jan.-March). The lady with the lamp: Florence Nightingale. *Philippine Journal of Nursing, 41,* 11-12.

Walton, P. (1986, May). The lady with the lamp (Florence Nightingale). *Nursing Journal of India, 77*(5), 115-116.

Watkin, B. (1976, May 6). Notes on Nightingale. *Nursing Mirror, 142*(19), 42.

Welch, M. (1986, April). Nineteenth-century philosophic influences on Nightingale's concept of the person. *Journal of Nursing History, 1*(2), 3-11.

Westminster Abbey Florence Nightingale Commemorative Service, May 12th, 1970. The 150th anniversary of her birth. (1970, Autumn). *News Letter of the Florence Nightingale International Nurses Association,* pp. 21-24.

White, F.S. (1923, June). At the gate of the temple. *Public Health Nursing, 15,* 279-283.

Whittaker, E., & Olesen, V.L. (1967, Nov.). Why Florence Nightingale? *American Journal of Nursing, 67,* 2338.

The wider education of the nurse. (1951, Sept. 14). *Nursing Journal of India, 93,* 438.

Widerquist, J.G. (1992, Jan.-Feb.). The spirituality of Florence Nightingale. *Nursing Research, 41,* 49-55.

Williams, C.B. (1961, May). Stories from Scutari. *American Journal of Nursing, 61,* 88.

Winchester, J.H. (1967, May). Tough angel of the battlefield. *Today's Health, 45,* 30.

Winslow, C.E.A (1946, July). Florence Nightingale and public health nursing. *Public Health Nursing, 38,* 330-332.

Wolstenholme, G.E. (1980, Dec.). Florence Nightingale: New lamps for old. *Proceedings of the Royal Society of Medicine, 63,* 1282-1288.

Woodham-Smith, Mrs. C. (1947, May 10). Florence Nightingale as a child. *Nursing Mirror, 85,* 91-92.

Woodham-Smith, Mrs. C. (1952, May). Florence Nightingale revealed. *American Journal of Nursing, 52,* 570-572.

Woodham-Smith, Mrs. C. (1954, July 10). The greatest Victorian. *Nursing Times, 50,* 737, 738-741.

The works of mercy window. (1956, May). *American Journal of Nursing, 56,* 574.

Yeates, E.L. (1962, May 11). The prince consort and Florence Nightingale. *Nursing Mirror, 114,* iii-iv.

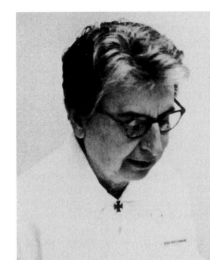

Ernestine Wiedenbach

The Helping Art of Clinical Nursing

Nancy J. McKee, Marguerite Danko, Terrence J. Heidenreiter,
Nancy E. Hunt, Judith E. Marich, Ann Marriner Tomey,
Cynthia A. McCreary, Margery Stuart

CREDENTIALS AND BACKGROUND OF THE THEORIST

Ernestine Wiedenbach's interest in nursing began with her childhood experiences with nurses. She greatly admired the private duty nurse who cared for her ailing grandmother and later enjoyed hearing accounts of nurses' roles in the hospital experiences of

The authors wish to express appreciation to Catherine Martin, Janet Pezelle, and Nancy Preuss for their assistance with data collection and to Ernestine Wiedenbach for critiquing the original chapter.

a young intern her sister was dating. Captivated by the role of the nurse, Wiedenbach enrolled in the Johns Hopkins Hospital School of Nursing after graduating from Wellesley College with a bachelor's degree in liberal arts. After completing her study at Johns Hopkins, she held a variety of positions in hospitals and public health nursing agencies in New York. She also continued her education by attending evening classes at Teachers College, Columbia University, from which she received a master's degree and a Certificate in Public Health Nursing. During this period Hazel Corbin, director of the Maternity

Center Association of New York, persuaded Wiedenbach to enroll in the association's School for Nurse-Midwives. After completing the program, Wiedenbach practiced as a nurse-midwife in the home delivery service of the Maternity Center Association.

In addition to her practice, she also developed her academic career. She taught an evening course in advanced maternity nursing at Teachers College, wrote several articles for professional publications, and remained active in professional nursing organizations. Then in 1952 she moved from New York to Connecticut, where she was subsequently appointed to the faculty of the Yale University School of Nursing. She was the director of graduate programs in maternal-newborn health nursing, which began in 1956.[5] She wrote *Family-Centered Maternity Nursing*, a text on clinical nursing that was published in 1958.

It was out of this vast practical experience and education that she developed her model, and,[9:1] after a long career at Yale, she retired and moved to Florida.

THEORETICAL SOURCES

At Yale, Wiedenbach's theory development benefited from her contact with other faculty members. Ida Orlando Pelletier stimulated Wiedenbach's understanding of the use of self and the effect a nurse's thoughts and feelings has on the outcome of her actions. In addition, Patricia James and William Dickoff, philosophy professors who taught classes for nursing faculty on theory related to research and philosophical concepts, reviewed the manuscript for Wiedenbach's book, *Clinical Nursing: A Helping Art.*[5] In it they identified elements of a prescriptive theory, which Wiedenbach developed more fully in *Meeting the Realities in Clinical Teaching.*[9,10]

USE OF EMPIRICAL EVIDENCE

At present there is no specific research supporting Wiedenbach's work. Her model was developed on the basis of her years of experience in clinical practice and teaching.

MAJOR CONCEPTS & DEFINITIONS

Patient To understand Ernestine Wiedenbach's theory, it is necessary to understand her concepts and how her definitions of common nursing terms may differ from or be similar to the current definitions of those words. She defines a patient as "any individual who is receiving help of some kind, be it care, instruction or advice, from a member of the health professions or from a worker in the field of health."[8:3] Thus, to be a patient, one does not necessarily have to be sick. Someone receiving preventive health care teaching would qualify as a patient.

Need-for-Help Wiedenbach believed every individual experiences needs as a normal part of living. A need is anything the individual may require "to maintain or sustain himself comfortably or capably in his situation."[8:5] An attempt to meet the need is made by the intervention of help, which is "any measure or action that enables the individual to overcome whatever interferes with his ability to function capably in relation to his situation.... To

be meaningful, help must be used by an individual and must succeed in enhancing or extending his capability."[8:5-6] Wiedenbach combines these two definitions into a more critical concept for her theory of a need-for-help.

A need-for-help is "any measure or action required and desired by the individual and which has potential for restoring or extending his ability to cope with the demands implicit in his situation."[8:6] It is crucial to the nursing profession that a need-for-help be based on the individual's perception of his own situation. If one does not perceive a need as a need-for-help, one may not take action to relieve or resolve it.

Nurse "The nurse is a functioning human being. As such she not only acts, but she thinks and feels as well. The thoughts she thinks and the feelings she feels as she goes about her nursing are important; they are intimately involved not only in what she does but also in how she does it. They underlie

Continued

Major Concepts & Definitions—cont'd

every action she takes, be it the form of a spoken word, a written communication, a gesture, or a deed of any kind. For the nurse whose action is directed toward achievement of a specific purpose, thoughts and feelings have a disciplined role to play."[8:8]

Purpose "Purpose—that which the nurse wants to accomplish through what she does—is the overall goal toward which she is striving, and so is constant. It is her reason for being and for doing; it is the *why* of clinical nursing and transcends the immediate intent of her assignment or task by specifically directing her activities towards the 'good' of her patient."[8:13]

Philosophy "Philosophy, an attitude toward life and reality that evolves from each nurse's beliefs and code of conduct, motivates the nurse to act, guides her thinking about what she is to do and influences her decisions. It stems from both her culture and subculture, and is an integral part of her. It is personal in character, unique to each nurse, and expressed in her way of nursing. Philosophy underlines purpose, and her purpose reflects philosophy."[8:13]

Practice "Overt action, directed by disciplined thoughts and feelings toward meeting the patient's need-for-help, constitutes the practice of clinical nursing. . . . [It] is goal-directed, deliberately carried out and patient-centered."[8:23]

Knowledge, judgment, and skills are three aspects necessary for effective practice.[8:25] Identification, ministration, and validation are three components of practice directly related to the patient's care. Coordination of resources is indirectly related to it.[8:31]

Knowledge "Knowledge encompasses all that has been perceived and grasped by the human mind; its scope and range are infinite. Knowledge may be acquired by the nurse, apart from judgment and skills, in a so-called ivory-tower setting. When acquired in this way, it has potentiality for use in directing, teaching, coordinating and planning care

of the patient, but is not sufficient to meet his need-for-help. To be effective in meeting his need, such knowledge must be supplemented by opportunity for the nurse to function in a nurse-patient relationship with responsibility to exercise judgment and to implement skills for the benefit of the patient. Knowledge may be factual, speculative, or practical."[8:25]

Factual knowledge "Factual knowledge is something that may be accepted as existing or as being true."[8:25-26]

Speculative knowledge "Speculative knowledge, on the other hand, encompasses theories, general principles offered to explain phenomena, beliefs or concepts, and the context of such special subject areas as the natural sciences, the social sciences, and the humanities."[8:26]

Practical knowledge "Practical knowledge is knowing how to apply factual or speculative knowledge to the situation at hand."[8:26]

Judgment "Judgment represents the nurse's potentiality for making sound decisions. Judgment grows out of a cognitive process which involves weighing facts—both general and particular—against personal values derived from ideals, principles and convictions. It also involves differentiating facts from assumptions, and relating them to cause and effect. Judgment is personal in character; it will be exercised by the nurse according to how clearly she envisions the purpose to be served, how available relevant knowledge is to her at the time, and how she reacts to prevailing circumstances such as time, setting, and individuals. Decisions resulting from the exercise of judgment will be sound or unsound according to whether or not the nurse has disciplined the functioning of her emotions and of her mind. Uncontrollable emotions can blot out knowledge as well as purpose. Unfounded assumptions can distort facts. Although whatever decision the nurse may make represents her best judgment at the moment of making it, the broader her knowledge and the more

MAJOR CONCEPTS & DEFINITIONS—cont'd

available it is to her, and the greater her clarity of purpose, the firmer will be the foundation on which her decisions rest."[8:27]

Skills "Skills represent the nurse's potentiality for achieving desired results. Skills comprise numerous and varied acts, characterized by harmony of movement, expression and intent, by precision, and by adroit use of self. These acts are always carried out with deliberation to achieve a specific purpose and are not goals in themselves. Deliberation and purpose, therefore, differentiate skills from nurses' actions, which, although they may be carried out with proficiency, are performed with the execution of the act as the end to be attained rather than the means by which it is reached."[8:27]

Skills may be classified as procedural skills or communication skills.

Procedural skills "Procedural skills are potentialities for implementing procedures that the nurse may need to initiate and carry out in order to identify and meet her patient's need-for-help."[8:27-28]

Communication skills "Communication skills are capacities for expression of thoughts and feelings that the nurse desires to convey to her patient and to others associated with his care. Both verbal and nonverbal expression may be used, singly or together, to deliver a message or to elicit a particular response."[8:28]

Identification "Identification involves individualization of the patient, his experiences, and recognition of the patient's perception of his condition."[8:31-32]

"Activities in identification are directed toward ascertaining: (1) whether the patient has a need; (2) whether he recognizes that he has a need; (3) what is interfering with his ability to meet his need; and (4) whether the need represents a need-for-help, in other words, a need that the patient is unable to meet himself."[8:32]

Ministration Ministration is providing the needed help. It requires the identification of the need-for-help, the selection of a helping measure

appropriate to that need, and the acceptability of the help to the patient.[8:32]

Validation Validation is evidence that the patient's functional ability was restored as a result of the help given.[8:32]

Coordination While striving for unity and continuity, the nurse coordinates all services provided to the patient so care will not be fragmented. Reporting, consulting, and conferring are functional elements of coordination.[8:33]

Reporting "Reporting is the act of presenting information in written or oral form and is important in keeping others informed not only about the patient's health and social history, but also about his current condition, reaction, progress, care and plan of care."[8:33-34]

Consulting "Consulting, the act of seeking information or of asking advice, is a means of gaining, from others, an opinion or suggestion that may help the nurse to broaden her understanding before deciding on a course of action."[8:34]

Conferring "Conferring, the act of exchanging and comparing ideas, is most often initiated to review the patient's response to the care he has so far received, and to plan his future care."[8:35]

Art Art is "the application of knowledge and skill to bring about desired results. . . . Art is individualized action. Nursing art, then, is carried out by the nurse in a one-to-one relationship with the patient, and constitutes the nurse's conscious responses to specifics in the patient's immediate situation."[8:36]

The art of clinical nursing is directed toward achievement of four main goals: (1) understanding of the patient and his condition, situation, and need; (2) enhancement of the patient's capability; (3) improvement of his condition or situation within the framework of the medical plan for his care; and (4) prevention of the recurrence of his problem or development of a new one which may cause anxiety, disability or distress."[8:30-31] Nursing art involves three initial operations: stimulus, preconception, and interpretation.[8:38-39] The nurse re-

Continued

MAJOR CONCEPTS *&* DEFINITIONS—cont'd

acts on the basis of those operations. "Her action may be rational, reactionary, or deliberative."[8:40]

Stimulus   The helping process is triggered by a stimulus, which is the patient's presenting behavior.[8:38]

Preconception   Preconception is an expectation of what the patient may be like.

"The preconception is based on knowledge gained from a great variety of sources including the patient's chart, reports from other nurses, doctors or family members, what the nurse has read or heard of patients in similar condition, her own experiences with patients in similar condition, and, finally, her recollection of previous contacts with the patient."[8:38]

Interpretation   Interpretation is comparison of perception with expectation or hope. Perception is an interpretation of the stimulus and may misinterpret the patient's behavior.[8:38]

Rational Action   "Rational action is an overt act taken in response solely or mainly to the doer's immediate perception of another's action—verbal or nonverbal—or situation. In a nurse-patient relationship, the nurse's action would be called rational if she responds in a way guided by only her immediate perception of the patient's behavior—what he says, what he does, or how he appears."[8:40]

Reactionary Action   "Reactionary action, in contrast with rational action, is an overt act taken spontaneously in response to strong feelings the doer experiences when he compares his perception of another's behavior or situation with his expectation or hope about that behavior. In nurse-patient relationship, the nurse's action is reactionary if it is taken solely or mainly in response to her reaction, to the feelings aroused in her by comparing what she perceived as the patient's behavior with what she hoped for or expected."[8:40]

Deliberative Action   "Deliberative action is in contrast with both rational action and reactionary action. A deliberative action is an overt act which, although not failing to take account of the doer's immediate perceptions and feeling-reactions, is,

nonetheless, not based solely on these perceptions or feelings. Rather, deliberative action is interaction, directed toward fulfillment of an explicit purpose and carried out with judgment and understanding of how the other means the behavior which he is manifesting either verbally or nonverbally. In a nurse-patient relationship, the nurse's action is deliberative if her overt action is based on the application—in the fulfillment of her nursing purpose—of principles of helping to gain understanding of how the patient means the behavior he is manifesting."[8:41]

Wiedenbach concluded her consideration of the types of action by saying, "My thesis is that nursing art is not comprised of rational nor reactionary actions but rather of deliberative action."[8:42]

Framework of Nursing   Limits, supports, and research provide a broad framework in which clinical nursing functions. Limits, or boundaries, in a professional service give the individual guidelines to follow in practicing that profession. Professional limits are set by the profession's code; legal limits are those found in state laws and licensing requirements; local limits are set by the hospital, agency, or individual the nurse contracts to work for; and personal limits are self-imposed by the nurse herself.[8:63-73]

Supportive facilities for the practicing nurse are nursing administration, nursing education, and nursing organizations. Although these are rarely found at the patient's bedside or in the one-to-one relationship between the nurse and the patient, they are nevertheless important to the nurse by maintaining standards of quality of nursing care for the profession.[8:73-90]

Wiedenbach recognized that nursing research had not received a great deal of emphasis from the profession in the past, although more nursing research was beginning to occur. She acknowledged that such activity was essential to the growth of nursing and might even "prove to be crucial to the conservation of life and the promotion of health."[8:85]

MAJOR ASSUMPTIONS
Nursing

Nurses ascribe to an explicit philosophy. Basic to this philosophy of nursing are "(1) reverence for the gift of life; (2) respect for the dignity, worth, autonomy, and individuality of each human being; (3) resolution to act dynamically in relation to one's beliefs."[8:16] The rationale for nursing is stated in ". . . the reason she has come into being is that there is a patient who needs her help."[8:3] Wiedenbach identifies five essential attributes of a professional person:

1. Clarity of purpose.
2. Mastery of skill and knowledge essential for fulfilling the purpose.
3. Ability to establish and sustain purposeful working relationships with others, both professional and nonprofessional individuals.
4. Interest in advancing knowledge in the area of interest and in creating new knowledge.
5. Dedication to furthering the goal of mankind rather than to self-aggrandizement.[8:2]

Person

Four explicit assumptions are stated in relation to human nature:

1. Each human being is endowed with unique potential to develop—within himself—resources that enable him to maintain and sustain himself.
2. The human being basically strives toward self-direction and relative independence and desires not only to make best use of his capabilities and potentialities but to fulfill his responsibilities.
3. Self-awareness and self-acceptance are essential to the individual's sense of integrity and self-worth.
4. Whatever the individual does represents his best judgment at the moment of his doing.[8:17]

Earlier Wiedenbach wrote, in relation to the patient's perception of his condition, "An individual should want to be healthy, comfortable, and capable, and . . . when unimpeded, he strives by his own efforts to achieve such states."[8:14]

Health

The concept of health is neither defined nor discussed in Wiedenbach's model. The definitions of nursing, patient, and need-for-help, and the relationships among these concepts, imply health-related concerns in the nurse-patient situation.

Environment

Wiedenbach does not specifically address the concept of environment. She recognized the potential effects of the environment, however. In a statement of purpose for clinical nursing she said, "To facilitate the efforts of the individual to overcome the obstacles which currently interfere with his ability to respond capably to demands made of him by this condition, environment, situation, and time."[8:14-15] So it is implied that the environment may produce obstacles resulting in a need-for-help experienced by the person.

THEORETICAL ASSERTIONS

Identification of the patient's need-for-help involves four steps. First, the nurse uses her powers of observation to look and listen for actual consistencies and inconsistencies in the patient's behavior compared with the nurse's *expectations* for patient behavior. Second, the nurse explores the meaning of the patient's behavior with him. Third, the nurse determines the cause of the patient's discomfort or incapability. Finally, the nurse determines if the patient can resolve his problem or if he has a need-for-help[8:52-57] (Fig. 8-1).

Ministration of help needed involves the nurse making a plan to meet the needs and presenting it to the patient. If the patient concurs with the plan and accepts suggestions for implementing it, the nurse implements it and ministration of help needed occurs. If the patient does not concur with the plan or accept suggestions for implementation, the nurse needs to explore causes of the patient's nonacceptance. If the patient has an interfering problem, the nurse needs to explore the patient's ability to solve the problem. If the patient has a need-for-help, the

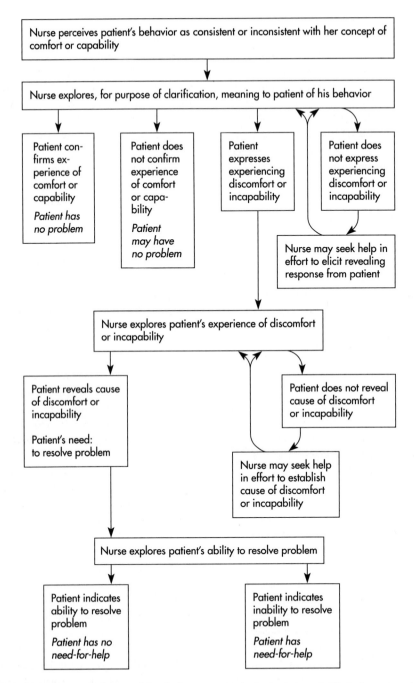

Fig. **8-1** Identification of a need-for-help. *From Wiedenbach, E. (1964).* Clinical nursing: A help-ing art. *New York: Springer, p. 60. Used with permission.*

nurse once again forms a plan to meet the need, presents the plan, and seeks patient concurrence with the plan and acceptance of suggestions for implementation[8:57,61] (Fig. 8-2).

Validation that the need-for-help was met is important. The nurse perceives whether the patient's behavior is consistent with her concept of comfort and seeks clarification from the patient to determine whether he believes his need-for-help was met. Then the nurse needs to take appropriate action on the basis of the feedback[8:57-58,62] (Fig. 8-3).

LOGICAL FORM

Wiedenbach developed this model through induction. The reasoning method in inductive logic begins with observation of specific instances and then combines the specifics into a more generalized whole. The common features of the specific instances allow for grouping the specifics into a larger set of phenomena.[1:61] An analysis of clinical experiences (specific nursing situations) leads to the development and interrelationships of concepts of Wiedenbach's model.[6:79.]

Dickoff, James, and Wiedenbach[2] have identified four levels of theory development in a practice discipline. In order of increasing sophistication these levels are factor-isolating, factor-relating, situation-relating, and situation-producing. Wiedenbach[10] considers her work a situation-producing prescriptive theory.

ACCEPTANCE BY THE NURSING COMMUNITY

Practice

Today, nurses are applying Wiedenbach's concepts to their clinical practice more so than did nurses in the 1950s and 1960s. According to Wiedenbach, the practice of clinical nursing is an "Overt action, directed by disciplined thoughts and feelings toward meeting the patient's need-for-help."[8:23] Drawing from her many years of experience as a nurse-midwife, she published "Childbirth as Mothers Say They Like It." In this article Wiedenbach noted that mothers wanted childbirth to be as natural as possible. In addition, mothers

wanted instruction on childbirth, father participation, full participation in the labor and delivery process, and rooming-in with their infant in the postpartum period.[7:417-421] But not until the 1970s were some or most of these needs-for-help met. In the 1980s the health care industry provided the supposedly unique concept of family-centered care, which Wiedenbach addressed some 20 years ago.

Education

Wiedenbach proposed that nursing education serves the practice of nursing in four major ways:

1. It is responsible for the preparation of future practitioners of nursing.
2. It arranges for nursing students to gain experience in clinical areas of the hospital or in the homes of patients.
3. Its representatives may function in the clinical area and work closely with the staff.
4. It offers educational opportunities to the nurse for special or advanced study.[8:75]

Application of Wiedenbach's model to clinical practice requires the nurse to have a sound knowledge of the normal and pathological states, a thorough understanding of human psychology, competence in clinical skills, and the ability to initiate and maintain therapeutic communication with patient and family. Also, the nurse must develop sound clinical judgment in decision making about patient care and be able to interpret the patient's behavior. These skills require a general education for nurses.

Today, many nursing schools are meeting this need for general education. Students are prepared with 2 years of courses in the humanities, biological science, and the social sciences, followed by 2 years in nursing science. This curriculum prepares a generalist in professional nursing and serves as the basis for graduate study.

Wiedenbach[8:78] saw graduate study as a means for nurses to extend the personal limits of their practice and to realize, to a greater degree than before, their potential for creative and imaginative practice within the area of their responsibility in the total field of health. Today's focus on graduate education is much the same as Wiedenbach's. It is directed toward

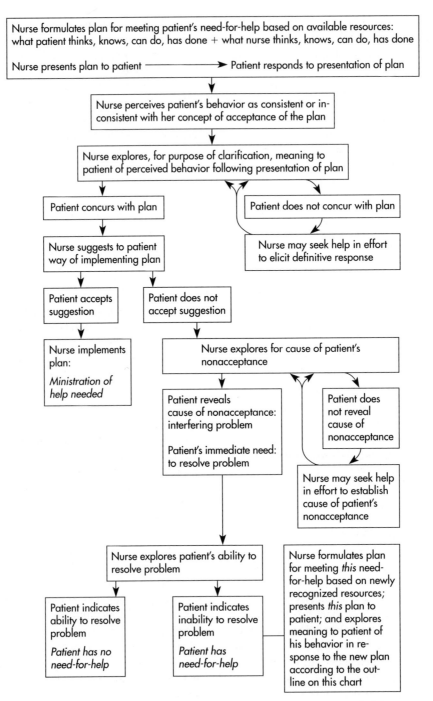

Fig. **8-2** **Ministration of help.** *From Wiedenbach, E. (1964).* Clinical nursing: A helping art. *New York: Springer, p. 61. Used with permission.*

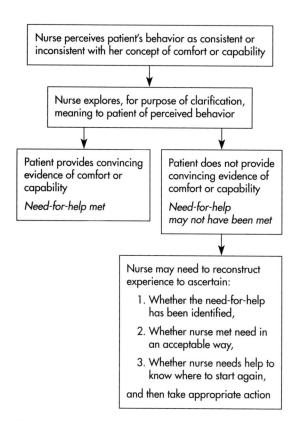

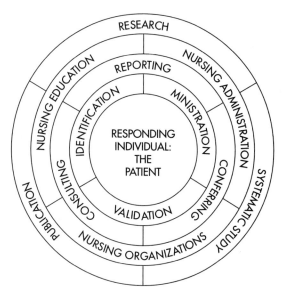

Fig. **8-4** Clinical nursing—the relationship between its focus and its constituents. *From Wiedenbach, E. (1964). Clinical nursing: A helping art. New York: Springer, p. 108. Used with permission.*

Fig. **8-3** Validation that need-for-help was met. *From Wiedenbach, E. (1964). Clinical nursing: A helping art. New York: Springer, p. 62. Used with permission.*

preparing advanced practitioners who are competent, self-directed, and concerned with the exploration of practice, issues, and problems of health care in a selected area of nursing.

Research

Before the development of Wiedenbach's model nursing research focused more on the medical model than on a nursing model. But in Wiedenbach's model the focus of nursing research is to be related to the patient's response to the health care experience. Her model would support research designed to promote family relationships, to control factors responsible for disabling conditions, and to foster sound health care practices. Although not specifically based on

Wiedenbach's model, numerous nursing research studies have been carried out in those areas. The results of those studies have been reported in nursing periodicals such as *Nursing Research*. Because of these nursing studies, nurses are better able to meet the patient's need for help.

Wiedenbach's concept of "need-for-help" was used as a focus for doctoral research completed in 1988. The vocal and bodily behaviors of women in the first stage of labor were videotaped to determine when a "need-for-help" occurred. These tapes were reviewed by the women and the researcher the day after delivery. Findings indicated that care-eliciting behaviors were influenced by a cognitively experienced need-for-help and that these behaviors were observable measures of nonverbalized need-for-help and decreased coping.[4]

Wiedenbach displayed in a graph all the constituent parts of her clinical nursing model at the end of her 1964 treatise[8:108] (Fig. 8-4).

FURTHER DEVELOPMENT

Wiedenbach is a pioneer in the writing of nursing theory. Her model of clinical nursing is one of the early attempts to systematically describe what it is that nurses do and what nursing is all about. It needs to be further developed by more clearly defining the concepts of health and environment. In addition, the component of nursing art needs to be identified in an operational way.

CRITIQUE

Wiedenbach's model evolved out of a desire to describe the practice of professional nursing. Her theory was influenced by Ida Orlando Pelletier and the philosophy of Dickoff and James, her colleagues at Yale University. Hers was one of the earlier nursing theories developed.

Clarity

Wiedenbach's model meets the criterion of clarity in that the concepts and definitions are clear, consistent, and intelligible.

Simplicity

There are too many relational statements for the theory to be classified as a simple theory. The concepts include the need-for-help, nursing practice, and nursing art. All of these concepts are interrelated, equal in importance, and have no meaning aside from their interaction.[6-76] Relationships among the major components can be linked, but it is difficult to diagram some of the concepts in the model. In addition, the concepts describe or explain phenomena but do not predict.

Generality

The scope of the concepts of patient (person), nursing, and need-for-help are very broad and thus possess generality. However, the concept of need-for-help is based on the patient's recognition of his or her need for help. This concept is not applicable to the infant, comatose patient, or many other physio-logically or psychologically incompetent persons. Also, the assumption that all nurses do not share a similar philosophy of nursing lessens the generality of the model.

Empirical Precision

Substantiation of a theory is accomplished through research, and thus the usefulness of the theory is determined. In Wiedenbach's model, the criterion is only partially met. The concepts of nursing practice and need-for-help are operationally defined and measurable. However, the concept of need-for-help is not always applicable. Also, within this theory there is little attempt to operationally define nursing art. Therefore it would be difficult to test this theory.

However, the potential exists for research to be done with this model. J. Fawcett believes three steps must be taken before the model can be tested. "First, the model must be formulated; secondly, a theory must be derived from the model; and third, operational definitions must be given to the concepts, and hypothesis derived."[3:26]

Derivable Consequences

Derivable consequences refer to the overall effect of the theory and its importance to nursing research, practice, and education. Wiedenbach's model fulfills the purpose for which it was developed and that is to describe professional practice. The theory focuses on nurse-patient interactions and regards the patient from a holistic point of view. Wiedenbach's work influenced the work of other early scholars, including Orlando and Peplau.

As one of the early nursing theorists, Wiedenbach made an important contribution to the nursing profession.

CRITICAL THINKING *Activities*

1 Compare Wiedenbach's identification of a need-for-help or no need-for-help to Virginia Henderson's definition of nursing (see Chapter 9).

2 Relate Wiedenbach's model to the nursing process. Determine similarities and differences.

3 Identify communication skills that are necessary to use Wiedenbach's model. Practice these skills with a patient/client, coworker, or friend.

4 Write definitions for health and environment as they are inferred in Wiedenbach's definitions of need-for-help and/or nursing art.

5 Differentiate skills and actions as described in the Wiedenbach model.

6 Compare and contrast deliberative action with rational and reactionary actions.

REFERENCES

1. Chinn, P.L., & Jacobs, M.K. (1983). *Theory and nursing: A systematic approach.* St. Louis: Mosby.
2. Dickoff, J.J., James, P.A., & Wiedenbach, E. (1968, Nov.-Dec.). Theory in a practice discipline. II. Practice-oriented research. *Nursing Research, 17,* 545-554.
3. Fawcett, J. (1984). *Analysis and evaluation of conceptual models of nursing.* Philadelphia: F.A. Davis.
4. Gustafson, D.C. (1988). Signaling behavior in stage I labor to elicit care: A clinical referent for Wiedenbach's need-for-help (Doctoral dissertation, Texas Woman's University, 1988). *Dissertation Abstracts International–B, 49/10,* 4230.
5. Nickel, S., Gesse, T., and MacLaren, A. (1992). Ernestine Wiedenbach: Her professional legacy. *Journal of Nurse-Midwifery, 37,* 161-167.
6. Raleigh, E. (1983). Wiedenbach's model. In J. Fitzpatrick & A. Whall (Eds.), *Conceptual models of nursing: Analysis and application.* Bowie, MD: Robert J. Brady.
7. Wiedenbach, E. (1949, Aug.). Childbirth as mothers say they like it. *Public Health Nursing, 41,* 417-421.
8. Wiedenbach, E. (1964). *Clinical nursing: A helping art.* New York: Springer.
9 Wiedenbach, E. (1969). *Meeting the realities in clinical teaching.* New York: Springer.
10. Wiedenbach, E. (1984, Spring). Written interview.

BIBLIOGRAPHY

Primary sources

Books

Wiedenbach, E. (1958). *Family-centered maternity nursing.* New York: G.P. Putnam's Sons.

Wiedenbach, E. (1964). *Clinical nursing: A helping art.* New York: Springer.
Wiedenbach, E. (1967). *Family-centered maternity nursing* (2nd ed.). New York: G.P. Putnam's Sons.
Wiedenbach, E. (1969). *Meeting the realities in clinical teaching.* New York: Springer.
Wiedenbach, E., & Falls, C.E. (1978). *Communication: Key to effective nursing.* New York: Tiresias.

Book chapter

Wiedenbach, E. (1973). The nursing process in maternity nursing. In J.P. Clausen, et al. (Eds.), *Maternity nursing today.* New York: McGraw-Hill.

Journal articles

Dickoff, J.J., James, P.A., & Wiedenbach, E. (1968, Sept.-Oct.). Theory in a practice discipline I: Practice-oriented theory. *Nursing Research, 14,* 415-435.
Dickoff, J.J., James, P.A., & Wiedenbach, E. (1968, Nov.-Dec.). Theory in a practice discipline II: Practice-oriented theory. *Nursing Research, 17,* 545-554.
Wiedenbach, E. (1940, Jan.). Toward educating 130 million people: A history of the nursing information bureau. *American Journal of Nursing, 40,* 13-18.
Wiedenbach, E. (1949, Aug.). Childbirth as mothers say they like it. *Public Health Nursing, 41,* 417-421.
Wiedenbach, E. (1951). Safeguarding the mother's breasts. *American Journal of Nursing, 51,* 544-548.
Wiedenbach, E. (1960, May). Nurse-midwifery, purpose, practice, and opportunity. *Nursing Outlook, 8,* 256.
Wiedenbach, E. (1963, Nov.). The helping art of nursing. *American Journal of Nursing, 63,* 54-57.
Wiedenbach, E. (1965, Dec.). Family nurse practitioner for maternal and child care. *Nursing Outlook, 13,* 50.
Wiedenbach, E. (1968, May). Genetics and the nurse. *Bulletin of the American College of Nurse Midwifery, 13,* 8-13.
Wiedenbach, E. (1968, June). The nurse's role in family planning: A conceptual base for practice. *Nursing Clinics of North America, 3,* 355-365.
Wiedenbach, E. (1970, May). Nurses' wisdom in nursing theory. *American Journal of Nursing, 70,* 1057-1062.

Secondary sources

Journal articles

Carrington, B.W., Loftman, P.O., Boucher, E., Irish, G., Piniaz, D.K., & Mitchell, J.L. (1994). Modifying a childbirth education curriculum for two specific populations: Inner-city adolescents and substance-using women. *Journal of Nurse-Midwifery, 39,* 312-320.
Dickoff, J., & James, P. (1970). Beliefs and values: Bases for curriculum design. *Nursing Research, 19,* 415-427.
Eisler, J., Wolfer, J.A., & Diers, D. (1972). Relationship between the need for social approval and postoperative recovery welfare. *Nursing Research, 21,* 520-525.

McCabe, P. (1994, Dec./1995, Jan.). Nursing, healing and natural therapies: Testing the waters. *The Lamp,* 35-36.

McKay, S., & Roberts, J. (1990). Obstetrics by ear: Maternal and caregiver perceptions of the meaning of maternal sounds during second stage labor. *Journal of Nurse-Midwifery, 35,* 266-273.

Nelson, M. (1988). Advocacy in nursing: *Nursing Outlook, 36,* 136-141.

Pranulis, M.F. (1986). Re: Toward a theory of nursing: Skills and competency in nurse-patient interaction {Letter to the editor}. *Nursing Research, 35,* 329 & 391.

Rickleman, B.L. (1971). Bio-psycho-social linguistics: A conceptual approach to nurse-patient interaction. *Nursing Research, 20,* 398-403.

Schmidt, J. (1972). Availability: A concept of nursing practice. *American Journal of Nursing, 72,* 1086-1089.

Shields, D. (1978). Nursing care in labor and patient satisfaction: A descriptive study. *Journal of Advanced Nursing, 3,* 535-550.

Thompson, J.B. (1981). Nurse midwives and health promotion during pregnancy. *Birth Defects, 17*(6), 29-57.

Tolley, K.A. (1995). Theory from practice for practice: Is this a reality? *Journal of Advanced Nursing, 21,* 184-190.

Wallace, C.L., & Appleton, C. (1995). Nursing as the promotion of well-being: The client's experience. *Journal of Advanced Nursing, 22,* 285-289.

Wolfer, J. (1993). Aspects of "reality" and ways of knowing in nursing: In search of an integrating paradigm. *Image, 25,*(2), 141-146.

Wolfer, J., & Visintainer, M. (1975). Pediatric surgical patients' and parents' stress responses and adjustment. *Nursing Research, 24,* 244-255.

Wooden, H.E., & Engel, E.L. (1965). Infection control in family-centered maternity care. *Obstetrics and Gynecology, 25,* 232-234.

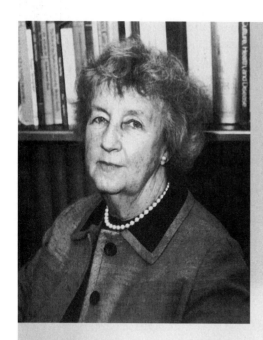

$\mathcal{V}$irginia Henderson

Definition of Nursing

Sr. Judith E. Alexander, Deborah Wertman DeMeester, Tamara Lauer,
Ann Marriner Tomey, Susan E. Neal, Sandy Williams

CREDENTIALS AND BACKGROUND OF THE THEORIST

Virginia Henderson was born in 1897, the fifth of eight children in her family. A native of Kansas City, Missouri, Henderson spent her developmental years in Virginia because her father practiced law in Washington, D.C.

During World War I Henderson developed an interest in nursing. So in 1918 she entered the Army School of Nursing in Washington, D.C. Henderson graduated in 1921 and accepted a position as a staff nurse with the Henry Street Visiting Nurse Service in New York. In 1922 Henderson began teaching nursing in Norfolk Protestant Hospital in Virginia. Five years later she entered Teachers College at Columbia University, where she subsequently earned her B.S. and M.A. degrees in nursing education. In 1929 Henderson served as a teaching supervisor in the clinics of Strong Memorial Hospital in Rochester, New York. She returned to Teachers College in 1930 as a faculty member, teaching courses in the nursing analytical process and clinical practice until 1948.[*]

The authors wish to express appreciation to Virginia Henderson for critiquing the original chapter.

[*]References 3:49; 27:87; 28:116-117.

Henderson enjoyed a long career as an author and researcher. While on the Teachers College faculty she rewrote the fourth edition of Bertha Harmer's *Textbook of the Principles and Practice of Nursing*, published in 1939. The fifth edition of the textbook was published in 1955 and contained Henderson's own definition of nursing. Henderson was associated with Yale University from the early 1950s and did much to further nursing research through this association. From 1959 to 1971 Henderson directed the Nursing Studies Index Project sponsored by Yale. The *Nursing Studies Index* was developed into a four-volume annotated index to nursing's biographical, analytical, and historical literature from 1900 to 1959. Concurrently, Henderson authored or coauthored several other important works. Her pamphlet, *Basic Principles of Nursing Care*, was published for the International Council of Nurses in 1960 and translated into more than 20 languages. Henderson's 5-year collaboration with Leo Simmons produced a national survey of nursing research that was published in 1964. Her book, *The Nature of Nursing*, was published in 1966 and described her concept of nursing's primary, unique function. It was reprinted by the National League for Nursing in 1991. The sixth edition of *The Principles and Practice of Nursing*, published in 1978, was coauthored by Henderson and Gladys Nite and edited by Henderson. This textbook has been widely used in the curriculums of various nursing schools. Her classic textbooks have been translated into more than 25 languages. Through the 1980s, Henderson remained active as a research associate emeritus at Yale. Henderson's achievements and influence in the nursing profession have brought her more than nine honorary doctoral degrees and the first Christiane Reimann Award. Henderson was given the Mary Adelaide Nutting Award from the U.S. National League for Nursing, honorary Fellowship in the American Academy of Nursing, honorary membership in the Association of Integrated and Degree Courses in Nursing, London, and an honorary Fellowship in the Royal College of Nursing in England. In 1983, she received Sigma Theta Tau International's Mary Tolle Wright Founders Award for Leadership, one of the honor society's highest honors. At the 1988 American Nurses Association (ANA) Conven-

tion, she received a special citation of honor for her lifelong contributions to nursing research, education and professionalism.

Henderson died peacefully in March 1996 at the age of 98. Her definition of nursing is known around the world, and her work continues to influence the practice of nursing, nursing education, and nursing research internationally. Henderson became a legend in her lifetime, and because of this Sigma Theta Tau's International Nursing Library is named in her honor. It was fitting that the announcement of Henderson's death traveled through the nursing community on the Internet. Halloran wrote of her, "Miss Virginia Avenel Henderson was to the 20th century as Florence Nightingale was to the 19th. Both wrote extensive works that have influenced the world" (Internet, March 21, 1996).[5]

THEORETICAL SOURCES

Henderson first published her definition of nursing in the 1955 revision of Harmer and Henderson's *The Principles and Practice of Nursing*. There were three major influences on Henderson's decision to synthesize her own definition of nursing. First, she revised *Textbook of the Principles and Practice of Nursing* in 1939. Henderson identified her work for this text as the source that made her realize "the necessity of being clear about the function of nurses."[28:119]

A second source was her involvement as a committee member in a regional conference of the National Nursing Council in 1946. Her committee work was incorporated into Esther Lucile Brown's 1948 report, *Nursing for the Future*. Henderson[9:62] said this report represented "my point of view modified by the thinking of others in the group." Finally, the ANA's 5-year investigation of the function of the nurse interested Henderson, who was not fully satisfied with the definition adopted by the ANA in 1955.

Henderson labeled her work a definition rather than a theory because theory was not in vogue at that time. She described her interpretation as the "synthesis of many influences, some positive and some negative."[7:64] In *The Nature of Nursing* she identifies the following sources of influence during her early years of nursing.

Annie W. Goodrich

Goodrich was the Dean of the Army School of Nursing, where Henderson achieved her basic nursing education, and served as an inspiration to Henderson. Henderson[10:7] recalled, "Whenever she visited our unit, she lifted our sights above techniques and routine." She also attributed Goodrich with "my early discontent with the regimentalized patient care in which I participated and the concept of nursing as merely ancillary to medicine."[10:7]

Caroline Stackpole

Stackpole was a philosophy professor at Teachers College, Columbia University, when Henderson was a graduate student. She impressed upon Henderson the importance of maintaining physiological balance.[10:10-11]

Jean Broadhurst

Broadhurst was a microbiology professor at Teachers College. The importance of hygiene and asepsis made an impact on Henderson.[10:10-11]

Dr. Edward Thorndike

Thorndike worked in psychology at Teachers College. He conducted investigational studies on the fundamental needs of humans. Henderson[10:11] realized that illness is "more than a state of disease" and that most fundamental needs are not met in hospitals.

Dr. George Deaver

Deaver was a physicist at the Institute for the Crippled and Disabled and, later, at Bellevue Hospital. Henderson observed that the goal of the rehabilitative efforts at the institute was rebuilding the patient's independence.[10:12]

Bertha Harmer

Harmer, a Canadian nurse, was the original author of *Textbook of the Principles and Practice of Nursing*, which Henderson revised. Henderson never met Harmer, but similarities of their respective definitions of nursing are obvious. Harmer's 1922 definition begins, "Nursing is rooted in the needs of the humanity."[3:54]

Ida Orlando

Henderson identified Orlando as an influence on her concept of the nurse-patient relationship. She said, "Ida Orlando (Pelletier) [has] made me realize how easily the nurse can act on misconceptions of the patient's needs if she does not check her interpretation of them with him."[10:14]

USE OF EMPIRICAL EVIDENCE

Henderson incorporated physiological and psychological principles into her personal concept of nursing. Her background in these areas stemmed from her associated with Stackpole and Thorndike during her graduate studies at Teachers College.

Stackpole based her physiology course on Claude Bernard's dictum that health depends on keeping lymph constant around the cell.[10:10] From this, Henderson surmised that "A definition of nursing should imply an appreciation of the principle of physiological balance."[10:11] From Bernard's theory, Henderson also gained an appreciation for psychosomatic medicine and its implications for nursing. She stated her view in the following way: "It was obvious that emotional balance is inseparable from physiological balance once I realized that an emotion is actually our interpretation of cellular response to fluctuations in the chemical composition of the intercellular fluids."[10:11]

Henderson did not identify the precise theories that were supported by Thorndike, only that they involved the fundamental needs of human beings. A correlation with Abraham Maslow's hierarchy of needs is seen in Henderson's 14 components of nursing care, which begin with physical needs and progress to the psychosocial components. Although she does not cite Maslow as an influence, she described his theory of human motivation in the sixth edition of *Principles and Practice of Nursing Care* in 1978.

MAJOR CONCEPTS & DEFINITIONS

Nursing Henderson[10:15] defined nursing in functional terms: "The unique function of the nurse is to assist the individual, sick or well, in the performance of those activities contributing to health or its recovery (or to peaceful death) that he would perform unaided if he had the necessary strength, will or knowledge. And to do this in such a way as to help him gain independence as rapidly as possible."

Health Henderson did not state her own definition of health. But in her writing she equated health with independence. In the sixth edition of *The Principles and Practice of Nursing* she cited several definitions of health from various sources, including the one from the charter of the World Health Organization. She viewed health in terms of the patient's ability to perform unaided the 14 components of nursing care. She said it is "the quality of health rather than life itself, that margin of mental/physical vigor that allows a person to work most effectively and to reach his highest potential level of satisfaction in life."[24:122]

Environment Again, Henderson did not give her own definition of environment. She used *Webster's New Collegiate Dictionary*, 1961, which defined environment as "the aggregate of all the external conditions and influences affecting the life and development of an organism."[24:829]

Person (Patient) Henderson[9:65] viewed the patient as an individual who requires assistance to achieve health and independence or peaceful death.

The mind and body are inseparable. The patient and his family are viewed as a unit.

Needs No specific definition of a need is found, but Henderson identified 14 basic needs of the patient, which comprise the components of nursing care.* These include the following needs:

1. Breathe normally
2. Eat and drink adequately
3. Eliminate body wastes
4. Move and maintain desirable position
5. Sleep and rest
6. Select suitable clothes—dress and undress
7. Maintain body temperature within normal range by adjusting clothing and modifying the environment.
8. Keep the body clean and well groomed and protect the integument
9. Avoid dangers in the environment and avoid injuring others
10. Communicate with others in expressing emotions, needs, fears, or opinions
11. Worship according to one's faith
12. Work in such a way that there is a sense of accomplishment
13. Play or participate in various forms of recreation
14. Learn, discover, or satisfy the curiosity that leads to normal development and health and use the available health facilities.

*Reprinted with the permission of Macmillan Publishing Company, *The Nature of Nursing* by Virginia Henderson. Copyright © 1966 by Virginia Henderson.

Major Assumptions

Virginia Henderson did not directly cite what she felt her underlying assumptions included. The following assumptions have been adapted from Henderson's publications.

Nursing

- The nurse has a unique function to help well or sick individuals.
- The nurse functions as a member of a medical team.
- The nurse functions independently of the physician, but promotes his or her plan, if there is a physician in attendance. [Henderson stressed that the nurse, for example, the nurse-midwife can function independently and *must* if he or she is the best-prepared health worker in the situation. The nurse can and *must* diagnose and treat if the situation demands it. Henderson is especially emphatic on this point in the sixth edition of *Principles and Practice of Nursing.*]
- The nurse is knowledgeable in both biological and social sciences.
- The nurse can assess basic human needs.
- The 14 components of nursing care encompass all possible functions of nursing.[9:63;10:16-17;24]

Person (Patient)

- The person must maintain physiological and emotional balance.
- The mind and body of the person are inseparable.
- The patient requires help toward independence.
- The patient and his family are a unit.
- The patient's needs are encompassed by the 14 components of nursing.[10:11]

Health

- Health is a quality of life.
- Health is basic to human functioning.
- Health requires independence and interdependence.
- Promotion of health is more important than care of the sick.[13:33]
- Individuals will achieve or maintain health if they have the necessary strength, will, or knowledge.[10:15]

Environment

- Healthy individuals may be able to control their environment, but illness may interfere with that ability.
- Nurses should have safety education.
- Nurses should protect patients from mechanical injury.
- Nurses should minimize the chances of injury through recommendations regarding construction of buildings, purchase of equipment, and maintenance.
- Doctors use nurses' observations and judgments upon which to base prescriptions for protective devices.
- Nurses must know about social customs and religious practices to assess dangers.[8:652]

Theoretical Assertions
The Nurse-Patient Relationship

Three levels comprising the nurse-patient relationship can be identified, ranging from a very dependent to a quite independent relationship: (1) the nurse as a *substitute* for the patient; (2) the nurse as a *helper* to the patient; and (3) the nurse as a *partner* with the patient. In times of grave illness, the nurse is seen as a "substitute for what the patient lacks to make him 'complete', 'whole', or 'independent', by the lack of physical strength, will, or knowledge."[9:63] Henderson[8:16] reflected this view in her statement that the nurse "is temporarily the consciousness of the unconscious, the love life for the suicidal, the leg of the amputee, the eyes of the newly blind, a means of locomotion for the infant, knowledge and confidence for the young mother, the 'mouthpiece' for those too weak or withdrawn to speak and so on."

During conditions of convalescence, the nurse helps the patient acquire or regain his independence. Henderson[22:120] stated, "Independence is a relative term. None of us is independent of others, but we strive for a healthy interdependence, not a sick dependence."

As partners, the nurse and patient together formulate the care plan. Basic needs exist regardless of diagnosis but are modified by pathology and other conditions such as age, temperament, emotional state, social or cultural status, and physical and intellectual capacities.[8:415]

The nurse must be able to assess not only the patient's needs but also those conditions and pathological states that alter them. Henderson[9:63] said the nurse must "get 'inside the skin' of each of her patients in order to know what he needs." The needs must then be validated with the patient.

The nurse can alter the environment where she deems necessary. Henderson[24:831] believed, "In every situation nurses who know physiologic and psychologic reactions to temperature and humidity, light and color, gas pressures, odors, noise, chemical impurities, and microorganisms can organize and make the best use of the facilities available."

The nurse and the patient are always working toward a goal, whether it be independence or peaceful death. One goal of the nurse must be to keep the patient's day as "normal as possible."[9:67] Promotion of health is another important goal of the nurse. Henderson[13:33] stated, "There is more to be gained by helping every man learn how to be healthy than by preparing the most skilled therapists for service to those in crises."

The Nurse-Physician Relationship

Henderson insisted the nurse has a unique function, distinct from that of physicians. The care plan, formulated by the nurse and patient together, must be implemented in such a way as to promote the physician's prescribed therapeutic plan. Henderson[13:34] stressed that nurses do *not* follow doctor's orders, for she "questions a philosophy that allows a physician to give orders to patients or other health workers." She extended this to emphasize that the nurse helps patients with health management when physicians are unavailable.[24:121] She also indicated that many nurse and physician functions overlap.[20]

The Nurse as a Member of the Health Care Team

The nurse works in interdependence with other health care professionals. The nurse and other team members help each other carry out the total program of care, but they should not do each others' jobs. Henderson[9:63] reminded us that "No one of the team should make such heavy demands on another member that anyone of them is unable to perform his or her unique function."

Henderson compared the entire medical team, including the patient and his family, to wedges on a pie graph (Fig. 9-1). The size of each member's section depends on the patient's current needs and therefore changes as the patient progresses toward independence. In some situations, certain team members are not included in the pie at all. The goal is for the patient to have the largest wedge possible or to take the whole pie.

Just as the patient's needs change, so may the definition of nursing. Henderson[28:121] admitted, "This does not say that it is a definition that will stand for all time. I believe nursing is modified by the era in which it is practiced, and depends to a great extent on what other health workers do."

Henderson believed her sixth edition of *Principles and Practice of Nursing,* coauthored with Gladys Nite, expanded her definition to include nurse practitioners. She said, "Nursing must not exist in a vacuum. Nursing must grow and learn to meet the new health needs of the public as we encounter them."[19]

LOGICAL FORM

Henderson appeared to have the deductive form of logical reasoning to develop her definition of nursing. She deduced her definition of nursing and 14 needs from physiological and psychological principles. One must study the assumptions of Henderson's definition to assess logical adequacy. Many of the assumptions have validity because of their high level of agreement with the literature and research conclusions of scientists in other fields. For example, her 14 basic needs correspond closely to Maslow's widely accepted human needs hierarchy, even though her basic needs were listed before she read Maslow's work.

In her book, *To Be a Nurse,* Evelyn Adam analyzes Henderson's work using a framework she learned from Dorothy Johnson. Adam[1] identifies Henderson's assumptions, values, the goal of nursing, the

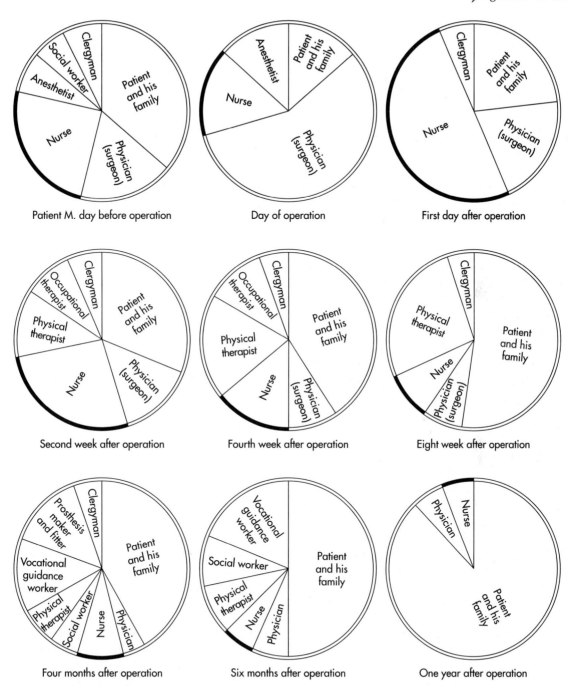

Patient M. day before operation

Day of operation

First day after operation

Second week after operation

Fourth week after operation

Eight week after operation

Four months after operation

Six months after operation

One year after operation

Fig. **9-1** Demonstration of how the nurse's role diminishes as rehabilitation progresses, with the case of the young man having his leg amputated used as an example. *Reprinted with permission of Macmillan Company from* The Nature of Nursing *by V. Henderson. Copyright 1966 by Virginia Henderson.*

client, the role of the nurse, the source of difficulty, the intervention, and the desired consequences.

ACCEPTANCE BY THE NURSING COMMUNITY

Practice

Henderson's definition of nursing as it relates to nursing practice points out that the nurse who sees her primary function as the direct caregiver to the patient will find an immediate reward in the patient's progress from dependence to independence. The nurse must make every effort to understand the patient when he lacks will, knowledge, or strength. As Henderson[10:24] stated, the nurse will "get inside his skin." The nurse can help the patient move to an independent state by assessing, planning, implementing and evaluating each of the 14 components of basic nursing care.

Henderson's approach to patient care was deliberative and involved decision making. Although she did not specifically mention the steps in the nursing process, one can see how the concepts are interrelated. Henderson[18:18,20] believed the nursing process is the problem-solving process and is not peculiar to nursing.

In the assessment phase, the nurse would assess the patient in all 14 components of basic nursing care. After the first component was completely assessed, the nurse would move on to the next component until all 14 areas were assessed. In gathering data, the nurses uses observation, smell, feeling, and hearing. To complete the assessment phase, the nurse must analyze the data she has collected. This requires knowledge of what is normal in health and disease.

Henderson stated, "As long as nursing is the only service available on a 24-hour, 7-day-a-week basis, the ability of nurses to differentiate the normal from the abnormal in patient health, . . . the assessment function of nurses is indisputable."[22]

According to Henderson,[24:416] the planning phase involves making the plan fit the individual's needs, updating the plan as necessary on the basis of the changes, using the plan as a record, and ensuring that it fits with the physician's prescribed plan. A good

plan, in her opinion, integrates the work of all those on the health team.[19]

In the implementation phase, the nurse helps the patient perform activities to maintain health, to recover from illness, or to aid in peaceful death. Interventions are individualized, depending on physiological principles, age, cultural background, emotional balance, and physical and intellectual capacities. Henderson[10:24-31;14] would evaluate the patient according to the degree to which he performs independently. However, the infant cannot be independent, nor can the unconscious. In some phases of illness, we should accept the patient's desire to depend on others.

Education

Henderson[10:69] stated, "In order for a nurse to practice as an expert in her own right and to use the scientific approach to the improvement of practice, the nurse needs the kind of education available only in colleges and universities." The nurse's education demands universal understanding of diverse human beings. The statement supports the position taken in 1965 by the ANA.

In addition, Henderson believed "the value of education comes not only with the added knowledge that is gained but also from the added confidence the individual develops in the institute of higher education environment." She said, "Nursing is a universal occupation and higher education allows you to do it better."[26]

In her book, *The Nature of Nursing: A Definition and Its Implications for Practice, Research, and Education*, Henderson has designed three phases of curriculum development students should progress through in their learning. The focus in all three phases remains the same—assisting the patient when he needs strength, will, or knowledge in performing his daily activities or in carrying out prescribed therapy with the ultimate goal of independence.

In the first phase, emphasis is placed on the fundamental needs of the patient, planning nursing care, and the unique function of the nurse in helping the patient carry out his activities of daily living. In this phase the curriculum plan does not emphasize pathological states or specific illnesses, but takes into account conditions always present that affect basic needs.[10:51] In the second phase, emphasis is placed on helping patients meet their needs during marked body disturbances or pathological states that demand modifications in the nurse's plan of care. The patient presents the student with problems of greater complexity. More medical science is involved, and the student begins to understand the rationale of symptomatic treatment.[10:51] In the third phase, instruction is patient and family centered. The student becomes involved in the complete study of the patient and all his needs.[10:55]

Henderson[17] has stressed the importance of having nursing students develop a habit of inquiry; take courses in biological, physical, and social sciences and in the humanities; study with students in other fields; observe effective care; and give effective care in a variety of settings.

The textbook in which Henderson's definition of nursing is found, *The Principles and Practice of Nursing*, is an excellent source that can be used by nursing students and by practicing nurses. It provides depth usually lacking in such texts. Kelly states, "If only one nursing book can be saved when the bomb falls, *PPN* is that book. In it are the breadth and depth of nursing, framed within the accumulated wisdom of law, medicine, and religion, documented from the world literature, fascinatingly footnoted—and eminently practical."[25:59]

Research

Henderson recommended library research and did a vast amount of it herself. She surveyed library resources and nursing research.[7] She supported developing nurses at the baccalaureate level and believed research was needed to evaluate and improve practice.[6]

"Nurses need to acquire the habit of looking for research upon which to base their practice," Henderson stated.[26] She recommended that nurses make greater use of library resources and hoped nurses would conduct research to improve practice rather than merely for academic respectability.[11;12;15;16;164]

In a survey and assessment of nursing research reported by Henderson and Leo W. Simmons in 1964,

several reasons for lack of research in clinical nursing were identified, including the following reasons:

1. Major energies of the profession have gone into improving the preparation for nursing.
2. Learning how to recruit and to hold sufficient numbers of nurses to meet the growing demand has taken considerable energy.
3. The need for administrators and educators has almost exhausted the supply of degree nurses.
4. A lack of support from administrators, nursing service administrators, and physicians has discouraged researchers.[10:34]

Research questions arise from each of the 14 components for basic nursing care, and it is the nurse's function to assume responsibility for identifying problems, for continually validating her function, for improving the methods she uses, and for reassuring the effectiveness of nursing care.

Henderson[10:39] concluded, "No profession, occupation, or industry in this age can evaluate adequately or improve its practice without research." Research is the most reliable type of analysis.

She believed that until practicing nurses learn how to use library resources, such as indexes from the National Library of Medicine, "nurses will not have taken the most elementary step to becoming part of a research-based profession—a claim nurses now like to make."[20]

FURTHER DEVELOPMENT

Henderson's last revision of her definition of nursing was in 1966.[19] She continued to write and to reflect on the practice of nursing throughout her life. In 1991 she stated that caring for patients was the "essential element of nurses's service."[23:58] Henderson (1982, 1991)[18,23] raised questions regarding nursing practice and the use of the nursing process. She stressed continued assessment of the patient's needs as his condition and goals change. Henderson[17] encouraged nurses to identify new needs beyond the 14 she enumerated. Henderson believed that research in nursing is essential for nursing practice in the age of technological advances.

Halloran (1995) has compiled the writings of Henderson in "*A Virginia Henderson Reader: Excellence in*

Nursing."[4] Nurses unfamiliar with Henderson are introduced to this world-renowned nurse in her own words. The writings and reflections are excerpts from her most important publications, presented and organized so that the reader can appreciate Henderson's work in light of contemporary nursing issues.

CRITIQUE

Before one attempts to evaluate Virginia Henderson's theory of nursing with respect to the generally accepted criteria of simplicity, generality, empirical precision, and derivable consequences, one must understand that she did not intend to develop a definitive nursing *theory*. Instead, she developed a personal concept or definition in an attempt to clarify what she considered to be the unique function of nursing. She stated, "My interpretation of the nurse's function is the synthesis of many influences, some positive and some negative. . . . I should first make clear that I do not expect everyone to agree with me. Rather, I would urge every nurse to develop her own concept."[9:64]

Henderson's definition can be considered a grand theory or philosophy within the preparadigm stage of theory development in nursing. Her concept is descriptive and easy to read. It is defined in common language terms. Her definitions of nursing and enumeration of the 14 basic nursing functions presents a perspective aimed at explaining a totality of nursing behavior. Because she had no intention of developing a theory, Henderson did not develop the interrelated theoretical statements or operational definitions necessary to provide the theory testability. However, that can be done.

Simplicity

Henderson's concept of nursing is complex rather than simplistic. It contains many variables and several different descriptive and explanatory relationships. It is not associated with structural organizations within a framework or model form to enhance simplicity, although some work has been done in this area. Diagrams of Henderson's and Orem's concepts of nursing from the Nursing Developmental Conference Group's book, *Concepts Formation in Nursing*, have been reproduced in Henderson and Nite's book.[24:23] In addition, the 14 basic needs appear simple as stated, but they become complex when an alteration of a need occurs and all the parameters relating to that need are considered. The sixth edition of *The Principles and Practice of Nursing* is extremely comprehensive and well illustrated to add clarity.

Generality

Generality is present in Henderson's definition since it is broad in scope. It attempts to include the function of all nurses and all patients in their various interrelationships and interdependencies.

Derivable Consequences

Henderson's perspective has been useful in promoting new ideas and in furthering conceptual development of emerging theorists. In her many published works she has discussed the importance of nursing's independence from, and interdependence with, other branches of the health care field. She has also influenced curriculum development and made a great contribution in promoting the importance of research in the clinical practice of nursing. She has made extensive use of other theorists' research in her work. Evans[2] states that *The Principles and Practice of Nursing* has made "a revolutionary change in one's thinking about nursing research." He states that the revolutionary thesis of the book is:

> The habits of mind which inform the everyday tasks of a nurse are exactly the same as those which undergird the very finest published research; in this way, every nurse ought not just to *do* simple research tasks as part of her work, but she ought also *always* to *be* a researcher, whether or not she writes or speaks a word in print or public.[2:338-339]

Since Henderson's definition of the unique function of nursing has been widely read, it has functioned as a major stepping stone in the emergence of nursing as a professional scientific discipline.

She continues to be cited in current nursing literature and publications in all areas of nursing practice from holistic nursing to the nursing process.

CRITICAL THINKING *Activities*

1 Can you identify the philosophical beliefs that guided Henderson's definition of nursing?

2 Apply Henderson's definition of nursing to your nursing practice. How does the definition reflect your current nursing practice.

3 As you reread Henderson's definition of nursing, what nursing functions and actions are applicable today?

REFERENCES

1. Adam, E. (1980). *To Be a Nurse.* New York: W.B. Saunders.
2. Evans, D.L. (1980). Every nurse as a researcher: An argumentative critique of *Principles and Practice of Nursing. Nursing Forum, xix*, 335-349.
3. Furukawa, C.Y., & Howe, J.K. (1995). Virginia Henderson. In Nursing Theories Practice Group, J.B. George, Chairperson, *Nursing theories: The base for professional nursing practice.* Englewood Cliffs, NJ: Prentice Hall.
4. Halloran, E.J. (Ed.). (1995). *A Virginia Henderson reader: Excellence in nursing.* New York: Springer.
5. Halloran, E.J. (1996). Internet communication, March 21, 1996.
6. Henderson, V. (1956, Feb.). Research in nursing practice—When? *Nursing Research, 4,* 99.
7. Henderson, V. (1957, Oct.). An overview of nursing research. *Nursing Research, 6,* 61-71.
8. Henderson, V. (1958, May 9). The basic principles of nursing care. *Nursing Mirror, 107,* 337-338, 415-416, 497-498, 583-584, 651-652, 733-734, 803-804.
9. Henderson, V. (1964, Aug.). The nature of nursing. *American Journal of Nursing, 64,* 62-68.
10. Henderson, V. (1966). *The nature of nursing: A definition and its implications for practice, research, and education.* New York: Macmillan.
11. Henderson, V. (1968). Library resources in nursing: Their development and use. *International Nursing Review, 15,* 164-174, 236-246.
12. Henderson, V. (1971, Jan.). Implications for nursing in the library activities of the regional medical programs. *Bulletin of the Medical Library Association, 59,* 53-64.
13. Henderson, V. (1971, March). Health is everybody's business. *Canadian Nurse, 67,* 31-34.
14. Henderson, V. (1973, June). On nursing care plans and their history. *Nursing Outlook, 21,* 378-379.
15. Henderson, V. (1977). Awareness of library resources: A characteristic of professional workers; an essential in research and continuing education. In *Reference resources for research and continuing education in nursing.* Kansas City, MO: American Nurses Association.
16. Henderson, V. (1977, May-June). We've "come a long way," but what of the direction? *Nursing Research, 26,* 163-164.
17. Henderson, V. (1978, March). The concepts of nursing. *Journal of Advanced Nursing, 3,* 13-30.
18. Henderson, V. (1982, March). The nursing process: Is the title right? *Journal of Advanced Nursing, 7,* 103-109.
19. Henderson, V. (1984-1985). Telephone interviews.
20. Henderson, V. (1985, Summer). The essence of nursing in high technology. *Nursing Administration Quarterly, 9*(4), 1-9.
21. Henderson, V. (1985). Personal correspondence.
22. Henderson, V. (1987, May). Nursing process: a critique. *Holistic Nursing Practice, 1*(3), 7-18.
23. Henderson, V. (1991). *The nature of nursing—Reflections after 25 years.* New York: National League for Nursing.
24. Henderson, V., & Nite, G.A. (1978). *The principles and practice of nursing.* New York: Macmillan.
25. Henderson, V., & Watt, S. (1983). 70 plus and going strong: Virginia Henderson, a nurse for all ages. *Geriatric Nursing, 4,* 58-59.
26. Holmes, P. (1985, Aug.). Who's afraid of Virginia Henderson? *Nursing Times, 81*(32), 16-17.
27. Runk, J.A., & Muth Quillin, S.I. (1983). Henderson's definition of nursing. In J.J. Fitzpatrick & A.L. Whall (Eds.), *Conceptual models of nursing: An analysis and application.* Bowie, MD: Robert J. Brady.
28. Safier, G. (1977). Virginia Henderson: Practitioner. In G. Safier (Ed.), *Contemporary American leaders in nursing: An oral history.* New York: McGraw-Hill.

BIBLIOGRAPHY

Primary sources

Books

Harmer, B., & Henderson, V. (1939). *Textbook of the principles and practice of nursing* (4th ed.). New York: Macmillan.

Harmer, B., & Henderson, V. (1955). *Textbook of the principles and practice of nursing* (5th ed.). New York: Macmillan.

Henderson, V. (1966). *The nature of nursing: A definition and its implications for practice, research, and education.* New York: Macmillan.

Henderson, V. (1969). *ICN Basic principles of nursing care.* Geneva: International Council of Nursing.

Henderson, V. (1970). *Basic principles of nursing care.* Basel, Karger. (Pamphlet prepared for International Council of Nurses.)

Henderson, V. (1991). *The nature of nursing: Reflections after 25 years.* New York: National League for Nursing.

Henderson, V., & Nite, G. (1978). *The principles and practice of nursing.* (6th ed.). New York: Macmillan.

Henderson, V., & Simons, L.W. (1957). *The yearbook of modern nursing: 1956.* New York: G.P. Putnam's Sons.

Simmons, L.W., & Henderson, V. (1964). *Nursing research: A survey and assessment.* New York: Appleton-Century-Crofts.

Yale University School of Nursing Index Staff under the direction of Virginia Henderson. (1963-1972). *Nursing Studies Index* (4 vols.). Philadelphia: J.B. Lippincott.

Book chapters

Henderson, V. (1974). On nursing care plans and their history. In *American Journal of Nursing, The nursing process in practice*. Kansas City, MO: American Nurses Association.

Henderson, V. (1977). Annie Warburton Goodrich. In *Dictionary of American Biography: Supplement Five, 1951-1955*. New York: Charles Scribner's Sons.

Henderson, V. (1977). Awareness of library resources: A characteristic of professional workers. In American Nurses Association, *Reference resources for research and continuing education*. Kansas City, MO: American Nurses Association.

Journal articles

Henderson, V. (1937, Jan.). Paper and other substitutes for woven fabric. *American Journal of Nursing, 37*, 23-32.

Henderson, V. (1955, Dec.). Annie Warburton Goodrich. *American Journal of Nursing, 38*, 1203-1216.

Henderson, V. (1956, Feb.). Research in nursing practice—When? *Nursing Research, 4*, 99.

Henderson, V. (1957, Oct.). An overview of nursing research. *Nursing Research, 6, 61-71.*

Henderson, V. (1958, May 2). The basic principles of nursing care. *Nursing Mirror, 107*, 337-338.

Henderson, V. (1958, May 9). The basic principles of nursing care. *Nursing Mirror, 107*, 415-416.

Henderson, V. (1958, May 16). The basic principles of nursing care. *Nursing Mirror, 107*, 497-498.

Henderson, V. (1958, May 23). The basic principles of nursing care. *Nursing Mirror, 107*, 583-584.

Henderson, V. (1958, May 30). The basic principles of nursing care. *Nursing Mirror, 107*, 651-652.

Henderson, V. (1958, June 6). The basic principles of nursing care. *Nursing Mirror, 107*, 733-734.

Henderson, V. (1958, June 13). The basic principles of nursing care. *Nursing Mirror, 107*, 803-804.

Henderson, V. (1964, Aug.). The nature of nursing. *American Journal of Nursing, 64*, 63-68.

Henderson, V. (1965, Jan.-Feb.). The nature of nursing. *International Nursing Review, 12*(1), 23-30.

Henderson, V. (1968, Spring). Some comments for nurses today. *The Alumnae Magazine* (Columbia University-Presbyterian Hospital School of Nursing Alumnae Association), pp. 5-15.

Henderson, V. (1968, April). Library resources in nursing: Their development and use (Part I). *International Nursing Review, 15*(2), 164-182.

Henderson, V. (1968, July). Library resources in nursing: Their development and use (Part II). *International Nursing Review, 15*(3), 236-247.

Henderson, V. (1969, Oct.). Excellence in nursing. *American Journal of Nursing, 69*, 2133, 2137.

Henderson, V. (1968, Oct.). Is the role of the nurse changing? *Weather Vane*, pp.12-43.

Henderson, V. (1968, Oct). Library resources in nursing: Their development and use (Part III). *International Nursing Review, 15*(4), 348-358.

Henderson, V. (1971, Jan.). Implications for nursing in the library activities in regional medical programs. *Bulletin of the Medical Library Association, 59*(1), 53-61.

Henderson, V. (1971, March). Health is everybody's business. *Canadian Nurse, 67*, 31-34.

Henderson, V. (1973, June). On nursing care plans and their history. *Nursing Outlook, 21*, 378-379.

Henderson, V. (1977). The essence of nursing. *Virginia Nurse.*

Henderson, V. (1977, Jan.-Feb.). We've "come a long way," but what of the direction? (Guest editorial). *Nursing Research 26*, 163-164.

Henderson, V. (1978). The concept of nursing. *Journal of Advanced Nursing, 3*, 113-130.

Henderson, V. (1978, May 1). Professional writing. *Nursing Mirror and Midwives Journal*, pp. 5-18.

Henderson, V. (1979, Nov. 22-23). Preserving the essence of nursing in a technological age. *Nursing Times, 75*, 2012.

Henderson, V. (1980, May). Preserving the essence of nursing in a technological age. *Journal of Advanced Nursing, 5*, 245-260.

Henderson, V. (1980, May 22). Nursing—yesterday and tomorrow. *Nursing times, 76*, 905-907.

Henderson, V. (1982, Spring). Is the study of history rewarding for nurses? *Society for Nursing History Gazette, 2*(1), 1-2.

Henderson, V. (1982, March). The nursing process—Is the title right? *Journal of Advanced Nursing , 7*, 103-109.

Henderson, V. (1985, Summer). The essence of nursing in high technology. *Nursing Administration Quarterly, 9*, 1-9.

Henderson, V. (1986, Jan.). Some observations on health care by health services or health industries. *Journal of Advanced Nursing, 11*(1), 1-2.

Henderson, V. (1987, Nov.). The nursing process in perspective [editorial]. *Journal of Advanced Nursing, 12*(6), 657-658.

Henderson, V. (1989). Countdown to 2000: A major international conference for the primary health care team. *Journal of Advanced Nursing, 14*, 81-85.

Henderson, V. (1989, Nov.-Dec.). Nursing information sources [letter comment]. *Nursing Outlet, 37*(6), 256.

Henderson, V. (1990, Apr.). Excellence in nursing 1969 [classic article]. *American Journal of Nursing, 90*, 76-77.

Henderson, V., et al. (1938, Nov.). Oxygen therapy: A study of some aspects of the operation of an oxygen tent. *American Journal of Nursing, 38*, 1203-1216.

Book reviews

Henderson, V. (1969, Jan.). Review of *Edith Cavell: Pioneer and patriot* by A.E. Clark-Kennedy, *Journal of the History of Medicine and Allied Sciences, 24*(1), 100-101.

Henderson, V. (1973). Review of *Mary Adelaide Nutting, Pioneer of modern nursing* by Helen F. Marshall. *Journal of the History of Medicine and Allied Sciences.*

Henderson, V. (1976, Aug.). Review of *Equity in health services: Empirical analysis in social policy* by Ronald Anderson et al. *American Journal of Nursing, 76*(1), 1339-1340.

Henderson, V. (1979, Aug.). Review of *The advance of American nursing* by Philip A. Kalish & Beatrice J. Kalish. *Nursing Outlook, 27*(8), 554.

Henderson, V. (1969, March-April). Review of *A bibliography of nursing literature: 1859-1960* edited by Alice M.C. Thompson. *Nursing Research 18*(2), 174-176.

Thesis

Henderson, V. (1935, June). *Medical and surgical asepsis: The development of asepsis and a study of current practice with recommendations in relation to certain aseptic nursing methods in hospitals.* Department of Nursing Education, Teachers College, Columbia University.

Correspondence

Henderson, V. (1984-1985). Telephone interviews.
Henderson, V. (1985). Personal correspondence.

Interviews

Community Health Nursing Revisited: A conversation with Virginia Henderson. By S.L. Shamansky. *Public Health Nursing, 1*(4).

Henderson, V. (1987, Oct.). A model for nursing (interviewed by Charlotte Alderman). *Nursing Times, 83*(41), 17-18.

Henderson, V. (1988, May 8). Song to today's and tomorrow's nurse (interview by Mette-Marie Davidson). *Sygeplejersken, 88*(20), 5-8.

Henderson, V. (1988, Nov. 26). An interview of Virginia Henderson (interview by Trevor Clay). *Nursing Standard, 3*(9): 18-9.

70 plus and going strong: Virginia Henderson, a nurse for all ages. (1983). *Geriatric Nursing, 4,* 58-59.

Virginia Henderson: A nursing's treasure. (1984). *Focus on Critical Care, 11*(3), 60-61.

Who's afraid of Virginia Henderson? (1977, May 11). By C. Darby. *Nursing Mirror and Midwives Journal, 146,* 15-18.

Videotapes

A conversation with Virginia Henderson. (1989). New York: National League for Nursing. [Videotape]. (Available from the author, 10 Columbus Circle, New York, NY 10019.)

A distinguished leader in nursing: Virginia Henderson. (1979). Capitol Heights, Md: The National Advisory Center. [Videotapes]. (Available from National Institutes of Health, National Library of Medicine, and Sigma Theta Tau International, 1200 Waterway Blvd., Indianapolis, IN: 46202).

Nursing theory: A circle of knowledge. (1987). New York: National League for Nursing. [Videotape]. (Available from the author, 10 Columbus Circle, New York, NY 10019).

The nurse theorists: Portraits of excellence: Virginia Henderson. (1988). Oakland: Studio III. [Videotape]. (Available from Fuld Video Project, 370 Hawthorne Avenue, Oakland, CA 94609.)

Secondary sources
Books

Adam, E. (1980). *To be a nurse.* New York: W.B. Saunders.

Chinn, P.L., & Jacobs, M.K. (1983). *Theory and nursing: A systematic approach.* St. Louis: Mosby.

Walker, L.O., & Avant, K.C. (1983). *Strategies for theory construction in nursing.* Norwalk, CT: Appleton-Century-Crofts.

Book chapters

Furukawa, C.Y., & Howe, J.K. (1980 and 1990). Virginia Henderson. In Nursing Theories Practice Group, J.B. George, Chairperson, *Nursing theories: The base for professional nursing practice.* Englewood Cliffs, NJ: Prentice Hall.

Furukawa, C.Y., & Howe, J.K. (1995). Virginia Henderson. In J.B. George (Ed.). *Nursing theories: The base for professional nursing practice.* (4th ed.), pp. 67-86. Norwalk, CT: Appleton & Lange.

Runk, J.A., & Muth Quillin, S.I. (1983 and 1989). Henderson's definition of nursing. In J.J. Fitzpatrick & A.L. Whall (Eds.), *Conceptual models of nursing: Analysis and application.* Bowie, MD: Robert J. Brady.

Safier, G. (1977). Virginia Henderson: Practitioner. In G. Safier, *Contemporary American leaders in nursing: An oral history.* New York: McGraw-Hill.

Journal articles

Ellis, R. (1968, May-June). Characteristics of significant theories. *Nursing Research 17,* 217-222.

Futton, J.S. (1987, Oct.). Virginia Henderson: Theorist, prophet, poet (biography). *Advances in Nursing Science, 10*(1), 1-9.

Gibbons, B.J. (1994). Venture into nursing cyberspace with the Virginia Henderson International Nursing Library. *Reflections, 20*(2), 14.

Halamandaris, V.J. (1993). Virginia Henderson: First lady of nursing. *Caring People,* 44-54.

Hardy, M.E. (1978). Perspectives on nursing theory. *Advances in Nursing Science, 1,* 37-48.

McBride, A.B. (1996). In celebration of Virginia Avenel Henderson. *Reflections, 22*(1), 22-23.

McCarty, P. (1987). How can nurses prepare for the year 2000? [A response from Virginia Henderson]. *The American Nurse, 19*(1), 3, 6.

Schmieding, N.J. (1990). An integrative theoretical framework. *Journal of Advanced Nursing, 15*(4), 463-467.

Sigma Theta Tau International. (1992). Virginia Henderson, RN: Humanitarian and scholar. *Reflections, 18*(1), 4-5.

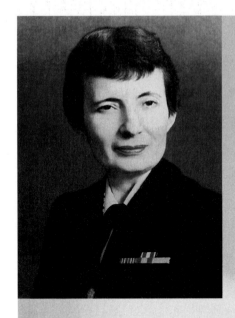

$\mathcal{F}$aye Glenn Abdellah

Twenty-One Nursing Problems

Tamara D. Halterman, Dorothy Kay Dycus, Elizabeth A. McClure,
Donna N. Schmeiser, Flossie M. Taggart, Roseanne Yancey

CREDENTIALS AND BACKGROUND OF THE THEORIST

Faye Glenn Abdellah was born in New York City. A 1942 Magna Cum Laude graduate of Fitkin Memorial Hospital School of Nursing (now Ann May School of Nursing), Abdellah received her B.S., M.A., and Ed.D. from Teachers College at Columbia University. She completed her doctoral work in 1955.

The authors wish to express their appreciation to Dr. Faye G. Abdellah for critiquing the original chapter.

Recognized as "one of the country's leading and best known researchers in health and public policy" as well as an "international expert of health problems,"[8:ix] Abdellah has practiced in many settings. She has been a staff nurse, a head nurse, a faculty member at Yale University and at Columbia University, a public health nurse, a researcher, and an author of more than 147 articles and books. Since 1949, Abdellah has held various positions in the U.S. Public Health Service (USPHS), including nurse consultant to the states, chief of the nurse education branch, senior consultant of nursing research, principal investigator in the progressive patient care project, chief of the research grants branch, director of nursing home affairs, and director of long-term care.

Abdellah was appointed Chief Nurse Officer of the USPHS in 1970, and served in that position for 17 years. Concurrently, in 1982 she was selected as Deputy Surgeon General, the first nurse and first woman to hold the post until her retirement in 1989. In this position, she was the focal point for nursing and a chief advisor on long-term care policy within the Office of the Surgeon General. Abdellah represented the interests of health professionals in all categories in the USPHS. She was advisor on matters related to nursing, long-term care policy, mental retardation, the developmentally disabled, home health services, aging, hospice, and acquired immunodeficiency syndrome (AIDS). Because her efforts were directed toward improvement of the quality of health care for all Americans, she supervised the activities in both health and nonhealth agencies. She is the recipient of more than 72 academic honors and professional awards. These include selection as a charter fellow of the American Academy of Nursing; 11 honorary degrees, including an honorary doctor of laws degree from Case Western Reserve University for pioneering nursing research and being responsible for the advent of the nurse-scientist scholar; an honorary degree from the University of Bridgeport for devoting her career to advancing the quality of health care through research and being an innovative and inspirational leader for nursing professionals; the Federal Nursing Service Award for the advancement of professional nursing; and the Distinguished Service Honor Award of the U.S. Department of Health, Education, and Welfare for exceptional leadership and professional commitment; and the first presidential award of Sigma Theta Tau International. In 1989, she received the prestigious Allied-Signal Achievement Award for research in aging, and in 1992 she received the Gustav O. Lienhard Award, given by the Institute of Medicine, National Academy of Science, in recognition of her contributions to the betterment of the health of all Americans.

In 1988 and 1989, Abdellah received the Surgeon General's Medallion, which was presented by former Surgeon General Koop in recognition of contributions as Chief Nurse Officer, USPHS, and for exemplary service to the Surgeon General.[10]

Abdellah's international involvement is extensive and includes consultation to the Portuguese government in the development of programs for the care of the elderly and disabled. While in the People's Republic of China, she studied the care of the elderly and mentally retarded. She was assigned direct responsibility for developing a resolution to organize the World Assembly on the Elderly in 1982.

Abdellah was instrumental in the implementation of exchange programs for United States/Soviet Union and United States/France with U.S. scientists and health professionals and their counterparts in the then–Soviet Union and France, as well as exchange programs for nurses in developing countries. Her leadership assistance in Yugoslavia resulted in the enactment of a law requiring the establishment of training programs for hospital managers. Her expertise and consultation led to the establishment of nursing research programs at Tel Aviv University in Israel and the development of a prescreening examination used for foreign nurses. She served as consultant to the Japanese Nursing Associations in setting up graduate programs in nursing education and research. Abdellah also participated in a seminar series for nursing home leaders in Australia and nursing education and research meetings in New Zealand. She currently is the dean of the first Uniformed Services Graduate School of Nursing at the Uniformed Services University of the Health Sciences.[10]

Abdellah realized that for nursing to gain full professional status and autonomy, a strong knowledge base was imperative. Nursing also needed to move away from the control of medicine and toward a philosophy of comprehensive patient-centered care. Abdellah and her colleagues conceptualized 21 nursing problems to teach and evaluate students. The typology of 21 nursing problems first appeared in the 1960 edition of *Patient-Centered Approaches to Nursing* and had a far-reaching impact on the profession and on the development of nursing theories (Box 10-1).*

THEORETICAL SOURCES

A critique of Abdellah's work cannot be isolated from the background in which her typology of nursing problems was developed.

Nursing practice and education in the 1950s were facing major problems resulting from technological advancement and social change. Old methods of educational preparation and practice based on functions and medical services were inadequate to meet the demands of the rapid change. The definition of nursing was becoming clouded. In Abdellah's opinion, one of the greatest barriers keeping nursing from a professional status was the lack of a scientific body of knowledge unique to nursing. The educational system was not providing students and practitioners with a means to cope with changing technology. Evaluation of students' clinical experiences based on a services approach provided no measure of the quality of that experience. The delivery of care to patients was organized around

*References 1, 9, 15, 16, 18, 22.

Box 10-1

Abdellah's typology of 21 nursing problems

1. To maintain good hygiene and physical comfort.
2. To promote optimal activity: exercise, rest, sleep.
3. To promote safety through prevention of accident, injury, or other trauma and through the prevention of the spread of infection.
4. To maintain good body mechanics and prevent and correct deformity.
5. To facilitate the maintenance of a supply of oxygen to all body cells.
6. To facilitate the maintenance of nutrition of all body cells.
7. To facilitate the maintenance of elimination.
8. To facilitate the maintenance of fluid and electrolyte balance.
9. To recognize the physiological responses of the body to disease conditions—pathological, physiological, and compensatory.
10. To facilitate the maintenance of regulatory mechanisms and functions.
11. To facilitate the maintenance of sensory function.
12. To identify and accept positive and negative expressions, feelings, and reactions.
13. To identify and accept interrelatedness of emotions and organic illness.
14. To facilitate the maintenance of effective verbal and nonverbal communication.
15. To promote the development of productive interpersonal relationships.
16. To facilitate progress toward achievement and personal spiritual goals.
17. To create and/or maintain a therapeutic environment.
18. To facilitate awareness of self as an individual with varying physical, emotional, and developmental needs.
19. To accept the optimum possible goals in the light of limitations, physical and emotional.
20. To use community resources as an aid in resolving problems arising from illness.
21. To understand the role of social problems as influencing factors in the cause of illness.

MAJOR CONCEPTS & DEFINITIONS

Nursing In writing the typology of 21 nursing problems, which served as a basis of her nursing theory,[6] Abdellah was also creating a guide for nurses to use in identifying and solving patient problems. The concept of nursing was therefore a primary component of her writing. Abdellah[12:24] defined nursing as:

> Service to individuals and families; therefore, to society. It is based upon art and science which mold the attitudes, intellectual competencies, and technical skills of the individual nurse into the desire and ability to help people sick or well cope with their health needs, and may be carried out under general or specific medical direction.

Abdellah was clearly promoting the image of the nurse who was not only kind and caring, but also intelligent, competent, and technically well prepared to provide service to the patient.

Nursing Problem A second major concept in Abdellah's work was the nursing problem. The "nursing problem presented by the patient is a condition faced by the patient or family which the nurse can assist him or them to meet through the performance of her professional functions."[12:7] The problem can be either an overt or covert nursing problem.

Abdellah states that her present perception would be to change nursing problem to patient/client problem. An "overt nursing problem is an apparent condition faced by the patient or family which the nurse can assist him or them to meet through the performance of her professional functions."[2:4] The "covert nursing problem is a concealed or hidden condition faced by the patient or family which the nurse can assist him or them to meet through the performance of her professional functions."[2:4] Both types of nursing or patient problems can now be documented and measured by use of outcome measures based on clinical practice guidelines.[11]

Although Abdellah spoke of the patient-centered approaches, she wrote of nurses identifying and solving specific problems. This identification and classification of problems was called the typology of 21 nursing problems (see Box 10-1). Abdellah's typology[12:11] was divided into three areas: (1) the physical, sociological, and emotional needs of the patient; (2) the types of interpersonal relationships between the nurse and the patient; and (3) the common elements of patient care. Abdellah and her colleagues thought the typology would provide a method to evaluate a student's experiences and also a method to evaluate a nurse's competency based on outcome measures.

Problem Solving "The process of identifying overt and covert nursing problems and interpreting, analyzing, and selecting appropriate courses of action to solve these problems" is problem solving, the final building block of Abdellah's writing.[12:36] Abdellah wrote that the nurse must be able to solve problems to give the best professional nursing care. This process, which closely resembles the steps of the nursing process, involves identifying the problem; selecting data; and formulating, testing and revising hypotheses. According to Abdellah, the patient will not receive quality nursing care if the steps to problem solving are done incorrectly.

Abdellah identifies nursing diagnosis as a subconcept of the problem-solving process. It is defined as the "determination of the nature and extent of nursing problems presented by individual patients or families receiving care."[12:9] meeting the needs of the institution rather than those of the patient.

The problem-solving method is the basis for Abdellah's model. It was formulated as a remedy to the problems facing nursing. The typology of 21 nursing problems and skills was developed to constitute the unique body of knowledge that is nursing.

Abdellah states that "nursing is both an art and a science that mold the attitude, intellectual competencies, and technical skills of the individual nurse into the desire and ability to help people, whether ill or not, cope with their health needs."[17]

Abdellah states that she was influenced by Virginia Henderson and identifies her as a mentor.[7] "Her work is related to Henderson's 14 principles and to her own research studies to establish the classification of nursing problems."[6] Knowledge of the problem-solving approach to nursing problems would provide a method of change with advancing technology. A qualitative assessment of student experiences could be made on the basis of the nursing problems encountered and alleviated while providing patients with patient-centered nursing care. Abdellah, as many other theorists from Columbia University, was of the need school of thought, "based on Maslow's hierarchy of needs and influenced by Erickson's stages of development."[24:252]

USE OF EMPIRICAL EVIDENCE

The typology was developed from several studies conducted during the 1950s. In the study *Appraising the Clinical Resources in Small Hospitals*, Abdellah and Levine[14] classified medical diagnoses of more than 1700 patients into 58 categories thought to represent common nursing problems. The nursing problems presented were identified by diagnostic groups. A similar analytical approach was followed in the development of the problem-oriented medical record more than a decade later and in the development of diagnostic related groups (DRGs) in 1983.

Abdellah's dissertation, *Methods of Determining Covert Aspects of Nursing Problems as a Basis for Improved Clinical Teaching*, reported findings from her study designed to identify what interview technique provided the most complete list of patients' problems.

The study revealed that a free-answer method was the most productive for identifying nursing problems. When used with patients, this method elicited many more covert (emotional-social) problems than did a pictorial interview technique or direct questioning approach.[2] Also in 1955, the National League for Nursing (NLN) Committee on Records formed a subcommittee to develop a meaningful clinical evaluation tool. The subcommittee members, with the assistance of faculties from 40 NLN-accredited collegiate schools of nursing, compressed the 58 patient categories into 21 common nursing problems and reported their development and use in *Patient-Centered Approaches to Nursing* in 1960.

MAJOR ASSUMPTIONS
Nursing

Nursing is a helping profession. In Abdellah's model, nursing care is doing something to or for the person or providing information to the person with the goal of meeting needs, increasing or restoring self-help ability, or alleviating an impairment.

Determination of nursing care strategies to be administered is based on the problem-solving approach. The nursing process is viewed as problem solving and the correct identification of nursing problems is a paramount concern. Direct observation of overt needs may be possible, but determination of covert needs requires mastery of communication skills and patient interaction. Deciding how patient needs can best be met is considered the responsibility of hospital and public health personnel.

"As long as self-help ability is developed and maintained at a level at which need satisfaction can take place without assistance, nursing care will not be required."[12:56] The role of the nurse in health promotion is limited to circumstances of anticipated impairment. In 1960 Abdellah[12:23] stated that physicians need more knowledge about prevention and rehabilitation than nurses do. But in correspondence with the authors in 1984, Abdellah indicated it is important that nurses also know about prevention and rehabilitation.

Also in 1984 she stated, "It is hoped that preoccupation with illness-oriented assessment methods will not diminish concern with the promotion of wellness."[23:111] No consideration is given to achievement of a higher level of wellness than is present when personal needs are met or when actual and anticipated impairments are absent.

Person

Abdellah describes people as having physical, emotional, and sociological needs. These needs may be overt, consisting of largely physical needs, or covert, such as emotional and social needs. The typology of nursing problems is said to evolve from the recognition of a need for patient-centered approaches to nursing. The patient is described as the only justification for the existence of nursing. But as previously discussed, the patient is not the central focus of Abdellah's work.

People are helped by the identification and alleviation of problems they are experiencing. The model implies that by resolving each problem, the person returns to a healthy state or one with which he can cope; therefore the ideal of holism is absent in this model. The whole, which is the patient, is not greater than the sum of its parts, which are his problems.

In Abdellah's model all persons have self-help ability and the capacity to learn, both of which vary from one individual to another. Because identifying these qualities in a comatose patient or an infant without family resources may be difficult, omissions could result when organizing such patients' care with this model.

In 1991 Abdellah[8:24] addressed the importance of self-help, stating:

> There is increased recognition that self-help groups can perform unique and valuable health services. Such groups should become a part of the mainstream health care delivery system. Eventually, self-help will be the other health care delivery system in this country, and it will accept the burden of disease prevention and health promotion.

Health

Health, as Abdellah discussed in *Patient-Centered Approaches to Nursing,* is a state mutually exclusive of

illness. Health is defined implicitly as a state when the individual has no unmet needs and no anticipated or actual impairments. Much of nursing practice in the 1950s focused on remedial or illness care, so it is not surprising that health was not clearly defined. But more than 30 years have passed since the book was published and Abdellah[4] now says she "would certainly place greater emphasis today on health status as an important part of the wellness-sickness continuum." She also fully supports the holistic approach to patient-centered care and the need for greater attention on environmental factors.

Environment

The environment is the least-discussed concept in Abdellah's model. Nursing problem number 17, from the typology, is "to create and/or maintain a therapeutic environment."[12:17] Abdellah also states that if the nurse's reaction to the patient is hostile or negative, the atmosphere in the room may be hostile or negative. This suggests that patients interact with and respond to their environment and that the nurse is part of that environment.

The environment is also the home and community from which the patient comes. Although fleetingly discussed, Abdellah urges that nurses not limit the identification of nursing problems to those existing only in the hospital. She predicts a future community center that will extend beyond the four walls of the hospital into the community.

Abdellah states that in 1988 she would "give greater emphasis to environment and health promotion."[6]

THEORETICAL ASSERTIONS

Several assertions were repeatedly stated by Abdellah although they were not labeled as such:

1. "The nursing problem and nursing treatment typlogies are the principles of nursing practice and constitute the unique body of knowledge that is nursing."[12:12]
2. "Correct identification of the nursing problem influences the nurse's judgment in selecting steps in solving the patient's problem."[18:492]

3. The core of nursing is the patient/client problems that focus on the patient and his/her problems.[6:68]

According to Reynolds[25:68] statements of assertion can be either existence or relational statements. Assertions 1 and 3 are of the existence type, whereas assertion 2 is relational.

Neither the major components of the nursing paradigm nor the central concepts are clearly linked with relational statements. Such structure cannot be diagrammed without imposing the critic's conclusions regarding the existence of relationships. Because the components of person, health, and environment were only implicitly defined, no attempt will be made to propose relationships between them. The major concepts that are more clearly defined by Abdellah are thought to be associated in this manner. Nursing, through the identification of nursing problems and usage of the problem-solving process, helps the client meet his needs. As late as 1972 Abdellah[3:234] stated, "The patient, his needs, and the nurse meeting his needs through nursing service is the only raison d'être for the nursing profession." Abdellah's statement exemplifies her major concerns and implied relationships.

LOGICAL FORM

The logical form can best be described as an inductive approach that generalizes from particulars. Abdellah used her multiple observations from the studies mentioned previously as the basis for her typology. Thus the typology developed inductively from research toward theory.

ACCEPTANCE BY THE NURSING COMMUNITY

In discussing the acceptance by the nursing community, one must be aware of two distinct times within the history of nursing—the mid-1950s through early 1960s and the present. When *Patient-Centered Approaches to Nursing* was published in 1960, the profession of nursing was striving to clarify its practice area and to identify rationale for its actions on the basis of scientific knowledge. The introduction of the

21 nursing problems had profound effects on the areas of practice, education, and research. Now they are associated with nursing diagnosis. Abdellah's studies in research, practice, and education continue to be extensively cited by nursing scholars.

Practice

Abdellah's typology of 21 nursing problems helps nurses practice in an organized, systematic way. The use of this scientific base enabled the nurse to understand the reasons for her actions. The clinical practitioner, using the 21 nursing problems, could assess the patient, make a nursing diagnosis, and plan interventions. Through the problem-solving process the nurse attempted to make the patient, rather than his medical condition, the central figure. By using the typology and the problem-solving process in the clinical setting, nurses gave their practice a scientific basis.

When asked to contrast the 21 nursing problems with the nursing diagnoses being promoted today, Dr. Abdellah says that it would have been heresy to use the term *diagnosis* in relation to nursing 30 years ago. Today she would describe them as being problems presented by patients or clients rather than nursing problems. But, she adds, there is a lot of similarity between the 21 nursing problems and the recently established DRGs. Both involve classification systems. The former could be used to provide the basis for determining acuity of illness, nursing outcomes, and costs of nursing services. This is particularly important as DRGs move into home care and ambulatory settings.[5:32]

Education

"Historically, Abdellah probably had more impact on nursing curriculum development than any other nurse theorist."[20:288] Abdellah's 21 nursing problems had their most dramatic effect on the educational system within nursing. Nursing educators were aware that changes were needed if nurses were to become autonomous. They recognized that the greatest weakness in the profession was the lack of a scientific body of knowledge unique to nursing. The typology provided such a body of knowledge and an opportunity to move away from the medical model of educating nurses. The typology of 21 problems was widely accepted in the nursing community in all types of programs—2-, 3-, and 4-year.

Research

Because the typology of 21 nursing problems was created through research, it is not surprising that more research followed its introduction. Was this typology really necessary from an administrative point of view? Had not hospitals been doing well without it? The amount of time the nurse spent with the patient was examined in the form of function studies. How could the patient receive comprehensive patient care in 18 minutes per 8-hour shift? Does the hospital administration serve the patient or does it serve someone else? To answer these questions Abdellah and Strachan[19] extended the research and used the typology as the basis for developing the nursing care model used for planning staffing patterns in clinical settings. These staffing patterns were based on patients' identified needs and, as Abdellah envisioned, consisted of intensive care, intermediate care, long-term care, self-care, and home-care units. By grouping patients with similar needs instead of diagnoses, nursing service could provide best staffing patterns to meet patients' needs.

In 1991, Abdellah[8:39] stated, "As nurse researchers, we need to be expedient and make a greater effort to let society know about the benefits of our research. This means translating research findings into practice that the patient/client can understand and see as a benefit."

Members of Sigma Theta Tau have been specifically targeted by Abdellah to assist in meeting the goals and challenges of research in health and public policy as clearly outlined in her scholarly publication, *Nursing's Role in the Future: A Case for Health Policy Decision Making*. She continues to author articles on research and has co-authored *Preparing for Nursing Research in the 21st Century*.[17]

FURTHER DEVELOPMENT

According to the categories of Dickoff and James,[21] Abdellah's typology may be recognized as a level one theory—categories or classifications. Currently, the nursing community's use of the 21 nursing problems has moved into a second generation of development, which includes patient problems and patient outcomes rather than nursing problems and nursing outcomes.

Abdellah[4] is pleased with the shift of emphasis from nursing problems to patient outcomes. She believes that 30 years ago the concept of nursing problems was used to identify a strong nursing role in patient care. If the initial emphasis had been on patient problems instead, the concept would *not* have been accepted and the medical model would have been perpetuated.

The concepts of problem-solving and nursing diagnosis continue to be used in the settings of practice, education, and research. Critical thinking and validating of theory in the practice area is needed within the profession. More sophisticated research tools might be designed to thoroughly study problem solving and how nurses apply this concept. The nursing diagnosis classification system may be considered an outgrowth of the typology. Currently, nursing diagnosis is a classification system describing patient signs and symptoms. Expanding this system to explain outcomes may be possible through additional research.

Dr. Abdellah served as Sigma Theta Tau's Distinguished Research Fellow (1990-1991), and she spoke with its members at all seven regional assemblies. There, and in her monograph, published in 1991, she addressed the relevance of nursing's role for policy decision making.

In *Nursing's Role in the Future; a Case for Health Policy Decision Making*, Abdellah "has proposed health policy as a means for influencing legislation at local, state, and national levels for the purpose of making health care accessible to the 37 million persons who do not have it. She has clearly identified nursing's role in policy issues, identified criteria to evaluate health policy decision making and outcomes, and has strongly made the case that more research of these issues by nurses is needed."[8:ix] In addition, Abdellah encourages nurses to read the *Federal Register*, which she calls the "most influential document" in Washington, D.C.[7]

CRITIQUE

Simplicity

The typology is very simple and it is descriptive of nursing problems thought to be common among patients. The concepts of nursing, nursing problems, and the problem-solving process, which are central to this work, are defined explicitly. The concepts of person, health, and environment, which are associated with the nursing paradigm today, are implied. There are no stated relationships between Abdellah's major concepts or those of the nursing paradigm in her writing. This model has a limited number of concepts, and its only structure is a list. A somewhat mixed approach to concept definition is present in this work. Nursing and nursing problems are connotatively defined, whereas the problem-solving process is defined denotatively. These approaches to definitions do not seem to detract from the clarity of definitions. The typology does not yet constitute a theory because it lacks sufficient relationship statements.

Generality

The 21 nursing problems are general and linked to neither time nor environment. "She acknowledges that her list is neither exhaustive nor listed according to priorities."[5:32] With the assumption that persons experience similar needs, the nursing goals stated in the list of 21 problems could be used by nurses in any time frame to meet patients' needs. However, according to this model, some persons do not need nursing.

Other service professions could use the typology of 21 nursing problems to focus on psychosocial and emotional needs presented by patients. The goals of this model vary in generality. The broadest goal is to positively affect nursing education, whereas subgoals are to provide a scientific basis on which to practice and to provide a method of qualitative evaluation of educational experiences for students. The goals are appropriate for nursing.

Empirical Precision

The concepts are very specific with empirical referents that are easily identifiable. The concepts are within the domain of nursing. Ready linkage of the concepts and the typology to reality is secondary to an inductive approach to theory development. Validation of the typology was done by the faculty of 40 collegiate schools of nursing. Chapters 4, 5, and 6 of *Patient-Centered Approaches to Nursing* describe different approaches to implementation and use of the typology in three programs of nursing.

Derivable Consequences

The typology provided a general framework in which to act, but continued neither specific nursing actions nor patient-centered outcomes, despite the title of the book. However, two subsequent publications did address outcome measure (effect variables) and suggested models for organizing curricula to emphasize patient-centered outcomes.[13,14] Except for stating the importance of nursing the whole patient, today's idea of holism is not apparent in this work. The skills list includes skills thought necessary for nurses to meet patients' needs but is not prescriptive. Abdellah suggests nursing research as a method for validating treatments toward resolution of patients' needs.

The emphasis on problem-solving is not limited by time or space and therefore provides a means for continued growth and change in the provision of nursing care. The problem-solving process and the typology of 21 nursing problems can be respectively considered precursors of the nursing care process, classification of nursing diagnoses, and outcome measures in evidence today.

In *Patient-Centered Approaches to Nursing Care*, Abdellah addressed nursing education problems linked to the use of the medical model. Her typology provided a new way to qualitatively evaluate experiences and emphasized a practice based on sound rationales rather than rote.

She proposes that nurses could take a leadership role in making the public aware that quality nursing health care is available. Quality is defined as the care that the patient needs. Need is determined by a classification system that identifies the medical treatment and nursing care essential for that individual.

Abdellah has made significant contributions to patient care, education, and research in nursing and health care in this country and throughout the world.[5:33]

CRITICAL THINKING *Activities*

1 Compare and contrast the 21 nursing problems with NANDA nursing diagnoses.

2 Select a client in your practice setting. Use Abdellah's typology of 21 nursing problems to assess the patient, make a nursing diagnosis, and plan appropriate interventions.

3 You are working on a cardiopulmonary unit and are assigned to two thoracotomy patients. It is the first postoperative day for both patients. What nursing problems do you anticipate? Is it correct to assume that both patients will exhibit the same problems and needs?

REFERENCES

1. Abdellah, F.G. (1955). *Methods of determining covert aspects of nursing problems as basis for improved clinical teaching.* Doctoral dissertation, New York Teachers College, Columbia University.
2. Abdellah, F.G. (1957, June). Methods of identifying covert aspects of nursing problems. *Nursing Research, 6,* 4.
3. Abdellah, F.G. (1972). Evolution of nursing as a profession: Perspective on manpower development. *International Nursing Review, 19,* 3.
4. Abdellah, F.G. (1984, March 7). Personal correspondence.
5. Abdellah, F.G. (1986, Oct.). Faye G. Abdellah—Working to enrich the profession (interview). *Focus on Critical Care, 13*(5), 32-33.
6. Abdellah, F.G. (1988, April 28). Personal correspondence.
7. Abdellah, F.G. (Speaker, Keynote Panel). (1989, Nov. 13). [Audiocassette]. Plenary Session I: Scientific Session, Sigma Theta Tau Biennial National Conference, Indianapolis, IN.
8. Abdellah, F.G. (1991). Nursing's role in the future; a case for health policy decision making. *Monograph Series No. 91.* Indianapolis: Sigma Theta Tau International, Inc.
9. Abdellah, F.G. (1992, April). Telephone interview.
10. Abdellah, F.G. (1996, April). Vitae.
11. Abdellah, F.G. (1996, July). Telephone interview.
12. Abdellah, F.G., Beland, I.L., Martin, A., & Matheny, R. (1960). *Patient-centered approaches to nursing.* New York: Macmillan.
13. Abdellah, F.G., Beland, I.L, Martin, A., & Matheny, R. (1973). *New directions in patient-centered nursing: Guidelines for systems of service, education, and research.* New York: Macmillan.
14. Abdellah, F.G., & Levine, E. (1954). *Appraising the clinical resources in small hospitals.* (U.S. Public Health Service. Pub. No. 389). Washington, D.C.: U.S. Government Printing Office.
15. Abdellah, F., & Levine, E. (1958). Effect of nurse staffing on satisfactions with nursing care. In *Hospital Monograph Series No. 4.* Chicago: American Hospital Association.
16. Abdellah, F.G., & Levine. (1965). *Better patient care through nursing research.* New York: Macmillan.
17. Abdellah, F.G., Levine, E. (1996). *Preparing for nursing research in the 21st century: Evolution, methodologies, challenges.* New York: Springer.
18. Abdellah, F.G., Levine, E., & Levine, B.S. (1986). *Better patient care through nursing research* (3rd ed.). New York: Macmillan.
19. Abdellah, F.G., & Strachan, E.J. (1959, May). Progressive patient care, *American Journal of Nursing, 59,* 5.
20. Barnum, B.S. (1990). *Nursing theory.* (3rd ed.). Glenview, IL: Scott, Foresman.
21. Dickoff, J., & James, P. (1968, March). A theory of theories: A position paper. *Nursing Research 17,* 3.
22. Falco, S.M. (1980). Faye G. Abdellah. In Nursing Theories Conference Group & J.B. George, Chairperson. *Nursing theories: The base for professional practice.* Englewood Cliffs, NJ: Prentice Hall.
23. Levine, E., & Abdellah, F.G. (1984, Summer). DRGs: Nursing has been using them for a long time. *Inquiry.*
24. Meleis, A.J. (1991). *Theoretical nursing: Development and progress* (2nd ed.). Philadelphia: J.B. Lippincott.
25. Reynolds, P.D. (1971). *A primer in theory construction.* Indianapolis: Bobbs-Merrill.

BIBLIOGRAPHY
Primary sources
Books and monographs

Abdellah, F.G. (1954). *For better nursing in Michigan: A survey.* Detroit: Cunningham Drug Company Foundation.
Abdellah, F.G. (1954, April). *Job guide for medical occupations.* Washington, D.C.: U.S. Department of Labor.
Abdellah, F.G. (1962, Sept.). *The elements of progressive patient care* (U.S. Public Health Service Publication No. 930-C-1). Washington, D.C.: U.S. Government Printing Office.
Abdellah, F.G. (1968). *An overview of nurse-scientist programs in the country.* National League for Nursing, No. 15-1342.
Abdellah, F.G. (1969). *Research in nursing: 1955-1968.* (U.S. Public Health Service Publication No. 1356). Washington, D.C.: U.S. Government Printing Office.
Abdellah, F.G. (1971, Nov.). *Extending the scope of nursing practice: A report of the secretary's committee to study extended roles for nurses,* Washington, D.C.: U.S. Department of Health, Education, and Welfare.

Abdellah, F.G. (1972). *A career in nursing.* (B'nai B'rith Career and Counseling Services Occupational Brief Series). Washington, D.C.: B'nai B'rith.

Abdellah, F.G. (1972). *Extending the scope of nursing practice.* National League for Nursing Pub. No. 16-1473.

Abdellah, F.G. (1975). Models for health care systems. In *Models for health care delivery: Now and for the future*, pp. 3-19. Publication Code G-1192M5/75. (Papers presented at the annual meeting of the American Academy of Nursing held on January 20-21, 1975). Kansas City: American Nurses Association.

Abdellah, F.G. (1976). *How to select a nursing home.* (No. 017-022-00502-6 DHEW [OS] 76-50045). Washington, D.C.: U.S. Government Printing Office.

Abdellah, F.G. (1976, March). Assessing health care needs in skilled nursing facilities: Health professional perspectives. *Long term care facility improvement monograph No. 1.* (DHEW Publication No. [OS] 76-50049). Washington, D.C.: U.S. Government Printing Office.

Abdellah, F.G. (1976, June). Physicians' drug prescribing patterns in skilled nursing facilities. Monograph No. 2 (DHEW Publication No. [OS] 76-50050). Washington, D.C.: U.S. Government Printing Office.

Abdellah, F.G. (1991). *Nursing's role in the future: The case for health policy decision making. Monograph Series No. 91.* Indianapolis: Sigma Theta Tau International, Inc.

Abdellah, F.G., Beland, I.L., Martin, A., & Matheney, R.V. (1960). *Patient-centered approaches to nursing.* New York: Macmillan.

Abdellah, F.G., Beland, I.L, Martin, A., & Matheney, R.V. (1968). *Patient-centered approaches to nursing.* (2nd ed.). New York: Macmillan.

Abdellah, F.G., Beland, I.L, Martin, A., & Matheney, R.V. (1973). *New directions in patient-centered nursing.* New York: Macmillan.

Abdellah, F.G., Beland, I.L., Martin, A., & Matheney, R.V. (1982, Nov.). *Report on hospice care in the United States.* Washington, D.C.: U.S. Department of Health and Human Services. (Publication No. HCFA-82-02152).

Abdellah, F.G., & Harper, B. (1981). Fact sheet on Hospice Care in the U.S. In *Information for Health Professionals.* Washington, D.C.: U.S. Public Health Service/Department of Health and Human Service.

Abdellah, F.G., & Levine, E. (1954). *Appraising the clinical resources in small hospitals.* (U.S. Public Health Service Pub. No. 389). Washington, D.C.: U.S. Government Printing Office.

Abdellah, F.G., & Levine, E. (1957). *Patients and personnel speak: A method of studying patient care in hospitals.* (U.S. Public Health Service Publication No. 527). Washington, D.C.: U.S. Government Printing Office.

Abdellah, F.G., & Levine, E. (1958). *Effect of nurse staffing on satisfactions with nursing care: A study of how omissions in nursing services, as perceived by patients and personnel, are influenced by the number of nursing hours available.* Chicago: American Hospital Association.

Abdellah, F.G., & Levine, E. (1965). *Better patient care through nursing research.* New York: Macmillan.

Abdellah, F.G., & Levine, E. (1979). *Better patient care through nursing research.* (2nd ed.). New York: Macmillan.

Abdellah, F.G., & Levine, E. (1994). *Preparing for nursing research in the 21st century: Evolution, methodologies, challenges.* New York: Springer.

Abdellah, F.G., Levine, E., & Levine, B.S. (1986). *Better patient care through nursing research.* (3rd ed.). New York: Macmillan.

Abdellah, F.G., Meltzer, L.E., & Kitchell, J.R. (Eds.). (1969). *Concepts and practices of intensive care for nursing specialists.* Philadelphia: Charles Press.

Abdellah, F.G., Meltzer, L.E., & Kitchell, J.R. (Eds.). (1976). *Concepts and practices of intensive care for nursing specialists.* (2nd ed.). Bowie, MD: Charles Press.

Abdellah, F.G., & Moore, S.R. (1988). *Surgeon General's workshop on health promotion and aging.* Proceedings. Washington, DC: Department of Health and Human Services, U.S. Public Health Service.

Abdellah, F.G., Moore, S., Moritsugu, K., & Wickizer, S. (1994). *Public Health Service flag officer's manual.* Washington, DC: Office of the Surgeon General, U.S. Public Health Service.

Abdellah, F.G., Schwartz, D.R., & Smoyak, S.A. (1975). *Models for health care delivery: Now and for the future.* (American Nurses Association No. G119). American Academy of Nursing.

Abdellah, F.G., Walsh, M.E., & Brown, E.L. (1979). *Health care in the 1980's: Who provides? Who plans? Who pays?* (Publication No. 52-1755). National League for Nursing.

Meltzer, L., Abdellah, F.G., & Kitchell, J.R. (Eds.). (1973). *Intensive care een handleiding voor intensive verpleging.* Amsterdam: Excerpta Medica.

Dissertation

Abdellah, F.G. (1955). *Methods of determining covert aspects of nursing problems as basis for improved clinical teaching.* New York Teachers College, Columbia University.

Book chapters

Abdellah, F.G., (1959). Improving the teaching of nursing through research in patient care. In *The improvement of nursing through research* (pp. 74-91). Washington, DC: The Catholic University Press.

Abdellah, F.G. (1968). An overview of nurse-scientist programs in the country. In *Extending the boundaries of nursing education: The preparation and role of the nurse scientist* (pp. 11-24). New York: National League for Nursing.

Abdellah, F.G. (1972). The nursing role in coronary care system. In L.E. Meltzer & A.J. Dunning (Eds.), *Textbook of coronary care* (pp. 35-51). Amsterdam: Excerpta Medica.

Abdellah, F.G. (1974). Overview of emerging health services delivery projects. In M. Leininger (Ed.), *Health care dimensions* (pp. 125-139). Health Care Issues Series. Philadelphia: F.A. Davis.

Abdellah, F.G. (1977). Criterion measures for research in nursing. In P.J. Verhonick (Ed.), *Nursing research II*. Boston: Little, Brown.

Abdellah, F.G. (1981). The National Health Service Corps: Providing settings for nursing practice. In L.H. Aiken (Ed.), *Health policy and nursing practice*. American Academy of Nursing. New York: McGraw-Hill.

Abdellah, F.G. (1981). New directions in the care of the elderly. In L.A. Copp (Ed.), *Recent advances in nursing 2: Care of the aging*. New York: Churchill Livingstone.

Abdellah, F.G. (1985). Public health aspects of rehabilitation of the aged. In S.J. Brody (Ed.), *Aging and rehabilitation*. New York: Springer.

Abdellah, F.G. (1985). The aging woman and the future of health care delivery. In M.R. Haug, A.B. Ford, & M. Scheafor (Eds.), *The physical and mental health of aged women*. New York: Springer.

Abdellah, F.G. (1986). The nature of nursing science. In L.H. Nicoll (Ed.), *Perspectives on nursing theory*. Boston: Little, Brown.

Abdellah, F.G. (1986). Nurses as primary health care providers in the USA. In *The accountability of nurses in changing society*. International Nurses' Foundation of Japan .

Abdellah, F.G. (1988). Future directions: Refining, implementing, testing, and evaluating the nursing minimum data set. In H.H. Werley & N.M. Lang (Eds.), *Identification of the nursing minimum set*. New York: Springer.

Abdellah, F.G. (1988, Jan.). Welcome and opening remarks from the Public Health Service. In *Evaluating the environmental health work force*. (Publication No. HRP 0907160). Washington, DC: Department of Health and Human Services/ U.S. Public Health Service.

Abdellah, F.G. (1991). Public policy impacting on nursing care of older adults. In E.M. Baines (Ed.), *Perspectives on gerontological nursing*. Newbury, CA: Sage Publications.

Abdellah, F.G. (1991). Nursing research in the 21st century: An unfinished revolution. In S.R. Moore (Ed.), *The C. Everett Koop Honorary Lectures 1991-1996* (pp. 13-31). Rockville, MD: Anchor & Caduceus Society, Inc.

McCormick, K.A., & Abdellah, F.G. (1984). Respiratory failure: Technological care in the home and hospital. In S.J. Reiser & M. Anbar (Eds.), *The machine at the bedside*. Cambridge, MA: Harvard University Press.

Journal articles

Abdellah, F.G. (1952, June). State nursing surveys and community action. *Public Health Reports, 67*, 554-560.

Abdellah, F.G. (1953, July). Some trends in nursing education. *American Journal of Nursing 53*, 841-843.

Abdellah, F.G. (1954, May). Surveys stimulate community action. *Nursing Outlook, 2*, 268-270.

Abdellah, F.G. (1955). Let the patients tell us where we fail. *Modern Hospital, 85*(2), 71-74.

Abdellah, F.G. (1955, March). Data from patients, nurses, and doctors on the needs for nursing service. *Military Medicine 16*, 205-208.

Abdellah, F.G. (1955, June). Area of responsibility: Supervisor, head nurse, staff nurse—levels at which they perform. *Ohio Nurses' Review*.

Abdellah, F.G. (1957, June). Methods of identifying covert aspects of nursing problems. *Nursing Research, 6*, 4.

Abdellah, F.G. (1959, Jan. 16). Symposium on progressive patient care. *Hospitals, 33*, 42-46.

Abdellah, F.G. (1959, May). How we look at ourselves. *Nursing Outlook, 7*, 273.

Abdellah, F.G. (1960, Jan.). The five elements of progressive patient care. *Bulletin, Texas Graduate Nurses' Association*.

Abdellah, F.G. (1960, Jan. 19). Progressive patient care. *Research in Patient Care*, New York, National Health Council.

Abdellah, F.G. (1960, March). Progressive patient care, some questions and challenges. *Bulletin, Texas Graduate Nurses' Association*.

Abdellah, F.G. (1960, June). Progressive patient care: A challenge for nursing. Hospital Management, 89, 102-106, 135-137.

Abdellah, F.G. (1960, Aug.). Nursing patterns vary in progressive care. *Modern Hospital, 95*, 85.

Abdellah, F.G. (1961, April). The decision is yours. *Nursing Outlook, 9*, 223.

Abdellah, F.G. (1961, Winter). Criterion measures in nursing. *Nursing Research, 10*, 21.

Abdellah, F.G. (1965, Oct.). Search or research? An experiment to stimulate research. *Nursing Outlook, 13*, 65-67.

Abdellah, F.G. (1966). Doctoral preparation for nurses. *Nursing Forum, 5*(3), 44-53.

Abdellah, F.G. (1966). Frontiers in nursing research. *Nursing Forum, 5*, 28-38.

Abdellah, F.G. (1967, Fall). Approaches to protecting the rights of human subjects. *Nursing Research, 16*, 315-320.

Abdellah, F.G. (1969, Sept.-Oct.). The nature of nursing science. *Nursing Research, 18*, 390-393.

Abdellah, F.G. (1969, Dec.). Nursing research in the health services. [Editorial], *Nursing Research Reports, 4*, 2.

Abdellah, F.G. (1970, Jan.-Feb.). Overview of nursing research: 1955-1968 (Part I). *Nursing Research, 19*, 6-17.

Abdellah, F.G. (1970, March-April). Overview of nursing research: 1955-1968 (Part II). *Nursing Research, 19*, 151-162.

Abdellah, F.G. (1970, May). Training and development of the health care team. *AORN Journal, 11*, 86-91.

Abdellah, F.G. (1970, May-June). Overview of nursing research: 1955-1968 (Part III). *Nursing Research, 19*, 239-252.

Abdellah, F.G. (1970, Summer). Conference on the nature of science in nursing. The nature of nursing science. *Japanese Journal of Nursing Research, 3*, 248-252.

Abdellah, F.G. (1971, May). Problems, issues, challenges of nursing research. *Canadian Nurse, 67*, 44-46.

Abdellah, F.G. (1972). Evolution of nursing as a profession: Perspective on manpower development. *International Nursing Review, 19*, 219-238.

Abdellah, F.G. (1972, Sept). The physician-nurse team approach to coronary care. In Symposium on Concepts in Cardiac Nursing. *Nursing Clinics of North America, 7*(3), 423-430.

Abdellah, F.G. (1972, Oct.). No legal bars to expanded nursing practice. *Stat, 41,* 4.

Abdellah, F.G. (1973, Jan.-Feb.). Criterios de avaliac as em enfermagen. *Revista Brasileira de Enfermagem, 26,* 17-32. (Portugal).

Abdellah, F.G. (1973, May). Research on career development in the health professions: Nursing. *Occupational Health Nursing 21,* 12-16.

Abdellah, F.G. (1973, June). School nurse practitioner: An expanded role for nurses. *Journal of the American College Health Association, 21,* 423-432.

Abdellah, F.G. (1973, Dec.). Nursing and health care in the USSR. *American Journal of Nursing , 73,* 2096-2099.

Abdellah, F.G. (1974). A national health strategy for the delivery of long-term health care: Implications for nursing. *Journal of New York State Nurses' Association 5*(4), 7-13.

Abdellah, F.G. (1974, Spring). Long-term care: A top health priority. (Guest editorial). *Journal of Long-Term Care Administration, 2*(2), 1-3.

Abdellah, F.G. (1974, Fall). Health care issues: Overview of emerging health services delivery projects. *Health Care Dimensions,* pp, 125-139.

Abdellah, F.G. (1975). Campaign for improvement for long-term care [editorial]. *Public Health Reports, 90*(6).

Abdellah, F.G. (1975). A national health strategy for the delivery of long-term health care: Implication for nursing. *Nursing Digest 4*(5), 15-17.

Abdellah, F.G. (1975). Nursing home infection control held 'essential.' *Hospital Infection Control, 2*(8), 103-104.

Abdellah, F.G. (1975, Jan.-Feb.). National Library of Medicine is official nursing archives. [letter]. *Nursing Research, 24*(1), 64.

Abdellah, F.G. (1975, Sept.-Oct.). The nursing archives at the National Library of Medicine [letter]. *Nursing Research, 24*(5), 389.

Abdellah, F.G. (1975, Nov.). Three views. Patient assessment: Its potential and use (Part I). *American Health Care Association Journal, 1,* 69.

Abdellah, F.G. (1976). HEW task force examines ways to upgrade and expand home health care programs. (Viewpoint). *Geriatrics, 12,* 31-43, 46.

Abdellah, F.G. (1976, March). Nurse practitioners and nursing practice. [editorial]. *American Journal of Public Health, 66*(3), 245-246.

Abdellah, F.G. (1976-Aug.). Nursing's role in future health care. *AORN Journal, 24*(2), 236-240.

Abdellah, F.G. (1977, Jan.-Feb.). A nationwide study to evaluate the care of patients in nursing homes. *Public Health Reports, 92*(1), 30-32.

Abdellah, F.G. (1977, July-Aug.). U.S. Public Health Service's contribution to nursing research: Past, present, future. *Nursing Research, 27*(4), 244-249.

Abdellah, F.G. (1978). The future of long-term care. *Bulletin of the New York Academy of Medicine, 54*(3), 261-270.

Abdellah, F.G. (1978, July). Long-term care policy issues: Alternatives to institutional care. *American Academy of Political and Social Science Annals, 438,* 28-29.

Abdellah, F.G. (1979). Cross-cultural comparison: Care of the elderly in China and U.S.S.R. *The Journal of Intercare, 1*(2), 1, 3, 8, 12-14.

Abdellah, F.G. (1981). Thirty-second world health assembly: Actions and implications for nursing. *The Journal of Intercare, 1,* 1,3,6,7,10-13.

Abdellah, F.G. (1981, Nov.). Nursing care of the aged in the United States of America. *Journal of Gerontological Nursing, 7*(11), 657-663.

Abdellah, F.G. (1982, Summer). The nurse practitioner 17 years later: Present and emerging issues. *Inquiry, 19*(2), 105-116.

Abdellah, F.G. (1982, Dec.). Keynote address, 75th anniversary of the West Virginia State Nurses' Association. *Weather Vane, 51*(6), 10-13,15.

Abdellah, F.G. (1983, Feb.-March). Future directions: Impact of the NSNA 1982 and 2012. *Imprint, 30*(1), 66-74.

Abdellah, F.G. (1983, March-April 6-7). 1983-2008: Nursing Practice. *Arizona Nurse, 36*(2), 6-7.

Abdellah, F.G. (1983, April-May). Future directions: Impact of the NSNA 1982 and 2012. *Imprint, 30*(2), 91-97.

Abdellah, F.G. (1984, Feb.). New roles in the Federal Nursing Services. *Today's OR Nurse, 6*(2), 6.

Abdellah, F.G. (1984, July). Nursing in the world: 35 years of development after World War II. Changes affecting nursing in the United States 1949-1984. *Kango Tenbo, 36*(3), 2-10. (Japanese Journal of Nursing Science).

Abdellah, F.G. (1984, Aug.). Changes affecting nursing in the United States 1949-1984. *Kango.* International Nursing Index ISSN 022-8362, pp. 2-10.

Abdellah, F.G. (1985, June 5-11). Standards of care: Hospitals mean business. *Nursing Times, 81*(23), 36-37.

Abdellah, F.G. (1987, Feb.). Practice mode of nursing the "Health for All." *Kango Tenbo 12*(2), 164-169. (Japanese Journal of Nursing Science).

Abdellah, F.G. (1987, Sept.-Oct.). The federal role in nursing education. *Nursing Outlook, 35*(5), 224-225.

Abdellah, F.G. (1988). Incontinence: Implications for health care policy. *Nursing Clinics of North America, 23*1, 1, 291-297.

Abdellah, F.G. (1990). Agency for health care policy and research: A challenge for nurse researchers. *Journal for Professional Nursing, 6*(6), 325.

Abdellah, F.G. (1990). Management of clinical trials. *Journal of Professional Nursing, 6,* 4, 189.

Abdellah, F.G. (1990). The National Library of Medicine: A treasure trove for nurse researchers [editorial]. *Journal of Professional Nursing, 6,* 3, 134.

Abdellah, F.G. (1990). Peer review: The only answer to high-quality research? *Journal of Professional Nursing, 6,* 2, 70.

Abdellah, F.G. (1990). Reflections of a recurring theme: Historical perspective of nursing shortage. *Nursing Clinics of North America, 25,* 509-516.

Abdellah, F.G. (1990). Scientific misconduct: Myth or reality? *Journal of Professional Nursing, 6,* 1, 6, 63.

Abdellah, F.G. (1990). Self-help groups offer prime areas for nurse researchers. *Journal of Professional Nursing, 6*(5), 257.

Abdellah, F.G. (1991). The funding crisis in biomedical research: Addressing the issue (Part 1). *Journal of Professional Nursing, 7*(1), 7.

Abdellah, F.G. (1991). The funding crisis in biomedical research: Options for action. (Part 2). *Journal of Professional Nursing, 7*(2), 75.

Abdellah, F.G. (1991). The human genome initiative: Implications for nurse researchers. *Journal of Professional Nursing, 7*(6), 332.

Abdellah, F.G. (1992). The politics of health and policy formation. *Reflections, 18*(1), 23.

Abdellah, F.G. (1993). Doctoral preparation and research productivity. *Journal of Professional Nursing, 9*(2), 71.

Abdellah, F.G. (1995). Management perspectives: "I'm the aspiring vice president of nursing at a university hospital, and I'm wondering how to avoid hitting the 'glass ceiling.'" *Nursing Spectrum of Washington D.C., 5*(9), 7.

Abdellah, F.G., Burke, C., & Chall, C.L. (1956). A time study of nursing activities in psychiatric hospital. *Nursing Research, 5*(1), 27-35.

Abdellah, F.G., Chamberlain, J.G., & Levine, I.S. (1986, Sept.-Oct.). Role of nurses in meeting needs of the homeless: Summary of a workshop for providers, researchers, and educators. *Public Health Reports, 101*(5), 494-498.

Abdellah, F.G., & Chow, R.K. (1976, Nov.-Dec.). The long-term care facility improvement campaign: The PACE project. *Association of Rehabilitation Nurses' Journal, 1*(7), 3-4.

Abdellah, F.G., & Chow, R.K. (1976, Winter). Long-term care facility improvement: A nationwide research effort. *Journal of Long-Term Care Administration, 4*(1), 5-19.

Abdellah, F.G., Foerst, H.V., & Chow, R.K. (1979, June). PACE: An approach to improving the care of the elderly. *American Journal of Nursing 79*(6), 1109-1110.

Abdellah, F.G., & Haldeman, J.C. (1959, May 16). The concept of progressive patient care. *Hospitals,* (Part 1, Part 2).

Abdellah, F.G., & Levine, E. (1952, January). Survey shows only 19 percent of West Virginia workers covered by in-plant nursing services. *Occupational Health, 12*(1), 4-6. Federal Security Agency, U.S. Public Health Service.

Abdellah, F.G., & Levine, E. (1954, June). Why nurses leave home. *Hospitals, 28,* 80-81.

Abdellah, F.G., & Levine, E. (1954, June). Work sampling applied to the study of nursing personnel. *Nursing Research, 3*(1), 11-16.

Abdellah, F.G., & Levine, E. (1957, Feb.). Developing a measure of patient and personnel satisfaction with nursing care. *Nursing Research, 5,* 100.

Abdellah, F.G., & Levine, E. (1957, Nov. 1). Polling patients and personnel: What patients say about their nursing care (Part 1). *Hospitals, 31,* 44-48.

Abdellah, F.G., & Levine, E. (1957, Nov. 16). What factors affect patients' opinions of their nursing care? (Part 2). *Hospitals, 31,* 61-64.

Abdellah, F.G., & Levine, E. (1957, Dec. 1). What personnel say about nursing care (Part 3). *Hospitals, 3,* 53-57.

Abdellah, F.G., & Levine, E. (1957, Dec. 16). What hospitals have done to improve patient care (Part 4). *Hospitals, 31,* 43-44.

Abdellah, F.G., & Levine, E. (1965, April). Better patient care through nursing research. *International Journal of Nursing Studies, 2,* 1.

Abdellah, F.G., Levine, E. (1965, Winter). The aims of nursing research. *Nursing Research, 14,* 27-32.

Abdellah, F.G., & Levine, E. (1966, Jan.). Future directions of research in nursing. *American Journal of Nursing, 66,* 112-116.

Abdellah, F.G., Levine, E. (1968, Summer). The aims of nursing research. *Comprehensive Nursing Monthly, 3,* 12-31. (Japan).

Abdellah, F.G., & Levine, E. (1982, Aug.). Better patient care through nursing research (Part 1). *Kango Tenbo, 7*(8), 714-719. (Japanese Journal of Nursing Science).

Abdellah, F.G., & Strachan, E.J. (1959, May). Progressive patient care. *American Journal of Nursing, 59,* 649.

Fuller, E.O., Hasselmeyer, E.G., Hunter, J.C., Abdellah, F.G., & Hinshaw, A.S. (1991). Summary statements of the NIH nursing research grant applications. *Nursing Research, 40*(6), 346-351.

Levine, E., & Abdellah, F.G. (1984, Summer). DRGs: A recent refinement to an old method. *Inquiry, 21*(2), 105-112.

Matarazzo, J.D., & Abdellah, F.G. (1971, Sept.-Oct.). Doctoral education for nurses in the U.S. *Nursing Research, 20,* 404-414.

Muller, J.E., Abdellah, F.G. , Billings, F.T., Hess, A.E., Petit, D., & Egeberg, R.D. (1972, March). The Soviet health system: Aspects of relevance for medicine in the U.S. *New England Journal of Medicine, 286,* 693-702.

Conferences

Abdellah, F.G. (1959, Feb. 24-Mar. 7). Criterion measures in nursing for experimental research. *Report on Nursing Research Conference.* Walter Reed Army Medical Center, Washington, DC.

Abdellah, F.G. (1972, May 31). An effective health care delivery system: Can it be achieved? (Commencement Address at the Cornell University Medical College and Cornell University-New York Hospital School of Nursing, New York City), 26 p.

Abdellah, F.G. (1975, July 27-31). Long term care facility improvement: A nationwide research effort. *Proceedings of the First North American Symposium on Long Term Care Administration* (pp. 3-22). Toronto, Ontario, Canada: American College of Nursing Home Administrators.

Abdellah, F.G. (1976, June 4). A nursing issue: Administration of medications by unlicensed personnel. In *A Look to the Future* (pp. 17-18). Conference sponsored by American Nurses' Association, Council of State Boards of Nursing, Shelburne Hotel, Atlantic City, NJ.

Abdellah, F.G. New nurse practitioners and care of the aging. In *Care of the Aging* (pp. 37-55). Conference report of Josiah Macy, Jr. Foundation. Feb. 1978.

Abdellah, F.G. (1986, Nov. 6-8). Elder abuse. In A.Z. Reed & J.C. Sullivan (Eds.), *Violence in America* (pp. 23-25). Proceedings of the Southern Regional Research Conference. Family Advocacy Program of USAF and LBJ School of Public Affairs, University of Texas, Austin.

Abdellah, F.G. (1987, Sept. 20-22). Department of Health and Human Services/U.S. Public Health Service. *Report of the Surgeon General's Workshop on Self-Help and Public Health.* Proceedings. Los Angeles, CA.

Abdellah, F.G., & Moore, S.R. (Eds.). (1988, March 20-23). *Surgeon General's Workshop on Health Promotion and Aging.* Background Papers. Department of Health and Human Services/U.S. Public Health Service, Washington, DC.

Chow, R.K., & Abdellah, F.G. (1974, Sept.). Intensive nursing care of the patient in myocardial failure: A videotaped case study. *Abstracts, World Congress of Cardiology.* Buenos Aires, Argentina. No. 399.

Hogness, J.R., Atkinson, H., Abdellah, F.G., Foster, J., Haley, R.W., & Patterson, R.A. (1984, March 29-30). International Conference on the Reuse of Disposable Medical Devices in the 1980's. Final Report of the Conference Panel, Washington, DC: Institute for Health Policy Analysis, Georgetown University Medical Center. (Conference proceedings also published by the Institute for Health Policy Analysis.)

Forewords

Abdellah, F.G. (1971) Foreword in *Theoretical Issues in Professional Nursing*, edited by J.F. Murphy, 196 p. New York: Meredith.

Department of Health, Education, and Welfare. (1975). Foreword by F.G. Abdellah in *Long Term Care Facility Improvement Study: Introductory Report.* 137 p. Washington, DC: U.S. Government Printing Office.

Correspondence

Abdellah, F.G. (1984, March 7). Personal letter.
Abdellah, F.G. (1988, April 28). Personal letter.
Abdellah, F.G. (1992, March). Vitae.
Abdellah, F.G. (1992, April 4). Telephone interview.

Secondary sources

Book reviews

Abdellah, F.G. (1972). Review of the book *The Physician's Assistant: Today and Tomorrow.*
The New England Journal of Medicine, 287(24), 1257-1258.

Abdellah, F.G., Beland, I.L., Martin, A., & Matheney, R.V. (1963). [Review of the book, *Patient-centered approaches to nursing*].
Hospital Administration, 8, 48, Spring, 1963.

Abdellah, F.G., Beland, I.L, Martin, A., & Matheny, R.V. (1973). [Review of the book, *New directions in patient-centered nursing*].
American Journal of Nursing, 73, 1439, Aug. 1973.
Nursing Outlook, 22, 555, Sept. 1974.

Abdellah, F.G., & Levine, E. (1957). [Review of the book, *Patients and personnel speak: A method of studying patient care in hospitals*].
American Journal of Nursing, 59, 634-635, May 1959.

Abdellah, F.G., & Levine, E. (1965). [Review of the book, *Better patient care through nursing research*].
Hospitals, 39, 115, Nov. 1965.
Nursing Outlook, 13, 18, Dec. 1965.
Catholic Nurse, 14, 63, March 1966.
American Journal of Nursing, 66, 828, April 1966.
Nursing Research, 15, 217, Summer 1966.
Nursing Research Reports, 2, 6, June 1967.

Abdellah, F.G., & Levine, E. (1979). [Review of the book, *Better patient care through nursing research* (2nd ed.)].
American Journal of Nursing, 80, 67-68, Jan. 1980.

Abdellah, F.G., & Levine, E. (1986). [Review of the book, *Better patient care through nursing research* (3rd ed.)].
Journal of Advanced Nursing, 12(3), 400, 1987.

Interviews

Abdellah, F.G. (1984, Jan.). Interview with Faye Abdellah (interview by Judith Rodin). *American Psychologist, 39*(1), 67-70.

Abdellah, F.G. (1986, May). An interview with Faye G. Abdellah (interview by S. Senno). *Kango Tenbo, 11*(6), 592-593. *(Japanese Journal of Nursing Science).*

News releases

Appointments (1971, Jan.). H.S.M.H.A. *Health Report, 36,* 27-38.

Department of Health, Education, and Welfare (1971, Jan.-Feb.). Faye G. Abdellah: A New Appointment. *Journal of Continuing Education in Nursing, 2,* 9.

Public Health Service Now Has Two Lady Admirals: Jessie Scott and Faye Abdellah. (1970, Nov.). *American Journal of Nursing, 70,* 2281.

Two Named to Top Nurse Rank in P.H.S. (1970, Nov.). *Nursing Outlook, 18,* 10.

Biographical sources

Directory of Nurses with Doctoral Degrees. (1980, Aug.). American Nurses Association.(ANA Publication No. G-143).

Faye Abdellah Sees Bright Future for Nurses. (1980, Sept.). *American Journal of Nursing, 80,* 1671-1672.

The National Nursing Directory, (1982). Rockville, MD: Aspen Systems.

Who's Who in America: 1981-1983 (42nd ed.). (1982). Chicago: Marquis.

Books

Dolan, J.A., Fitzpatrick, M.L., & Hermann, E.K. (1983). *Nursing in society: A historic perspective* (15th ed.). Philadelphia: W.B. Saunders.

Griffin, J.G., & Griffin, J.K. (1973). *History and trends of professional nursing.* St. Louis: Mosby.

Nursing Theories Conference Group, J.B. George, Chairperson. (1980). *Nursing theories: The base for professional practice.* Englewood Cliffs, NJ: Prentice Hall.

Orem, D.E. (Ed.). (1979). *Concept formalization in nursing, process and product.* Boston: Little, Brown.

Book chapter

Falco, S.M. (1980). Faye Abdellah. In Nursing Theories Conference Group, J.B. George, Chairperson. *Nursing theories: The base for professional nursing practice.* Englewood Cliffs, NJ: Prentice Hall.

Journal articles

Abraham, I.L., Chalifoux, Z.L., Evers, G.C.M., & DeGeest, S. (1995). Conditions, interventions, and outcomes in nursing research: A comparative analysis of North American and European International journals. (1981-1990). *International Journal of Nursing Studies, 32*(2), 173-187.

Adebo, E.O, (1974). Identifying problems for nursing research. *International Nursing Review, 21*(2), 53.

Alward, R.R. (1983). Patient classification system. The ideal vs. reality. *Journal of Nursing Administration, 13*(2), 14-19.

Armiger, B. (1977). Ethics of nursing research: Profile, principles perspective. *Nursing Research, 26*(5), 330-336.

Auger, J.A., & Dee, V. (1983). A patient classification system based on the behavioral system model of nursing. *Journal of Nursing Administration, 13*(4), 38-43.

Auster, D. (1978). Occupational values of male and female nursing students. *Sociology of Work and Occupations, 5*(2), 209-233.

Avis, M. (1995). Valid arguments? A consideration of the concept of validity in establishing the credibility of research findings. *Journal of Advanced Nursing, 22*(6), 1203-1209.

Ballard, K.A., Gray, R.F., Knauf, R.A., & Uppal, P. (1993). Measuring variations in nursing care per DRG. *Nursing Management, 24*(4), 40-41.

Ballard, S. , & McNamara, R. (1983). Qualifying nursing needs in home health care. *Nursing Research, 32*(4), 236-241.

Becker, G., & Kaufman, S. (1988). Old age, rehabilitation and research: A review of the issues. *Gerontologist, 28*(4), 459-468.

Bergman, R., Stocker, R.A., Shavit, N., Sharon, R., Feinberg, O., & Danon, A. (1981). Role, selection and preparation of unit head nurses (Part 1). *International Journal of Nursing Studies, 18*(2), 123-152.

Bergman, R., Stocker, R.A., Shavit, N., Sharon, R., Feinberg, O., & Danon, A. (1981). Role, selection and preparation of unit head nurses (Part 2). *International Journal of Nursing Studies, 18*(3), 191-211.

Bergman, R., Stocker, R.A., Shavit, N. Sharon, R., Feinberg, O., & Danon, A. (1981). Role, selection and preparation of unit head nurses (Part 3). *International Journal of Nursing Studies, 18*(4), 237-250.

Bernal, H., Church, O.M., Arevian, M., & Schensul, S.L. (1995). Community health nursing in a former Soviet Union Republic: A case study of change in Armenia. *Nursing Outlook, 43*(2), 78-83.

Bircumshaw, D., & Chapman, C.M. (1988). A study to compare the practice style of graduate and non-graduate nurses and midwives: The pilot study. *Journal of Advanced Nursing, 13*(5), 605-614.

Blancett, S.S. (1991). The ethics of writing and publishing. *The Journal of Nursing Administration, 21*(5), 31-36.

Boschma, G. (1994). The meaning of holism in nursing: Historical shifts in holistic nursing ideas. *Public Health Nursing, 11*(5), 324-330.

Brickhill, C.E. (1995). ICU for the '90s: The "intensive customer unit." *Nursing Management, 26*(1), 44-48.

Brown, G.D. (1995). Understanding barriers to basing nursing practice upon research: A communication model approach. *Journal of Advanced Nursing, 21*(1), 154-157.

Buttriss, G., Kuiper, R., & Newbold, B. (1995). The use of a homeless shelter as a clinical rotation for nursing students. *Journal of Nursing Education, 38*(8), 375-377.

Carnegie, M.E. (1975). Financial assistance for nursing research: Past and present. *Nursing Research, 24*(3), 163.

Carter, M.D. (1973). Identification of behaviors displayed by children experiencing prolonged hospitalization. *International Journal of Nursing Studies, 10*(2), 125-135.

Cateriniccho, R.P., & Davis, R.H. (1983). Developing a client focused allocation statistic of inpatient nursing resource use: An alternative to the patient day. *Social Science and Medicine, 17*(5), 259-272.

Chamorro, I.L., Davis, M.L., Green, D., & Kramer, M. (1973). Development of an instrument to measure premature infant behavior and caretaker activities: Time-sampling methodology. *Nursing Research, 22*(4), 300-309.

Chamorro, T. (1981). The role of a nurse clinician in joint practice with a gynecologic oncologist. *Cancer, 48*(2), 622-631.

Chandler, M.C., & Mason, W.H. (1995). Solution-focused therapy: An alternative approach to addictions in nursing. *Perspectives in Psychiatric Care, 31*(1), 8-13.

Chow, R.K. (1974). Significant research and future needs for improving patient care. *Military Medicine, 139*(4), 302-306.

Clay, T. (1986). Unity for change? *Journal of Advanced Nursing, 11*(1), 21-33.

Colaizzi, J. (1975). Proper object of nursing science. *International Journal of Nursing Studies, 12*(4), 197-200.

Conine, T.A., & Hopper, D.L. (1978). Work sampling: Tool in management. *American Journal of Occupational Therapy, 32*(5), 301-304.

Connelly, C.E. (1986). Replication research in nursing. *International Journal of Nursing Studies, 23*(1), 71-77.

Copp, L.A. (1973). Professional change: Which trends do nurses endorse? *International Journal of Nursing Studies, 10*(1), 55-63.

Copp, L.A. (1974). Critical concerns and commitments of a new department of nursing. *International Journal of Nursing Studies, 11*(4), 203-210.

Cornell, S.A. (1974). (1974). Development of an instrument for measuring quality of nursing care. *Nursing Research, 23*(1), 103-117.

Corner, J. (1991). In search of more complete answers to research questions. Quantitative versus qualitative methods: Is there a way forward? *Journal of Advanced Nursing, 16*(16), 718-727.

Craig, S.L. (1980). Theory development and its relevance for nursing. *Journal of Advanced Nursing, 5*(4), 349-355.

Cronenwett, L.R. (1983). Helping and nursing models. *Nursing Research, 6*(6), 342-346.

Crow, R.A. (1981). Research and the standards of nursing care: What is the relationship? *Journal of Advanced Nursing, 6*(6), 491-496.

Daeffler, R.J. (1977). Outcomes of primary nursing for the patient. *Military Medicine, 142*,(3), 204-208.

DeGroot, H.A. (1989). Patient classification system evaluation. Part I: Essential system elements. *The Journal of Nursing Administration, 19*(6), 30-35.

Delacuestra, C. (1983). The nursing process: From development to implementation. *Journal of Advanced Nursing, 8*(5), 365-371.

DeLeon, P.H., Kjervik, D.K., Kraut, A.G., & VandenBos, G.R. (1985). Psychology and nursing: A natural alliance. *American Psychologist, 40*(11), 1153-1164.

Denton, J.A., & Wisenbaker, V.B. (1977). Death experience and death anxiety among nurses and nursing students. *Nursing Research, 26*(1), 61-64.

Dickoff, J., James, P., & Semradek, J. (1975). Designing nursing research: Eight points to encounter. *Nursing Research, 24*(3), 164-176.

Dickoff, J., James, P., & Semradek, J. (1975). Stance for nursing research: Tenacity or inquiry? *Nursing Research, 24*(2), 84-88.

Dickson, W.M. (1978). Measuring pharmacist time use: Note on use of fixed interval work sampling. *American Journal of Hospital Pharmacy, 35*(10), 1241-1243.

DiMarco, N., Castels, M.R., Carter, J.H. & Corrigan, M.K. (1976). Nursing resources on nursing unit and quality of patient care. *International Journal of Nursing Studies, 13*(3), 139-152.

Doerr, B.C., & Jones, J.W. (1979). Effect of family preparation on the state anxiety level of the C.C.U. patient. *Nursing Research, 28*(5), 315-316.

Doessel, D.P., & Marshall, J.V. (1985). A rehabilitation of health outcome in quality assessment. *Social Science and Medicine, 21*(12), 1319-1328.

Duhart, J., & Chartonb, J. (1973). Hospital reform and health care in medical ordinance. *Revue Francaise De Sociologie, 14*, 77-101.

Dungy, C.I., & Mullins, R.G. (1981). School nurse practitioner: Analysis of questionnaire and time-motion data. *Journal of School Health, 51*(7), 475-478.

Dunning, T. (1995). Development of nursing care manual to improve the knowledge of nurses caring for hospitalized patients with diabetes. *Journal of Continuing Education in Nursing, 26*(6), 261-266.

Edwardson, S. R. (1988). Outcomes of coronary care in the acute care setting. *Research in Nursing and Health, 11*, 215-222.

Edwardson, S.R., & Giovannetti, P.B. (1994). Nursing workload measurement systems. *Annual Review of Nursing Research, 12*, 95-123.

Ellis, R. (1977). Fallibilities, fragments, and frames: Contemplation on 25 years of research in medical-surgical nursing. *Nursing Research, 26*(3), 177-182.

Elms, R.R. (1972). Recovery room behavior and postoperative convalescence. *Nursing Research, 21*(5), 390-397.

Eriksen, L.R. (1987, July). Patient satisfaction: An indicator of nursing care quality? *Nursing Management, 18*(7), 31-35.

Falcone, A.R. (1983). Comprehensive functional assessment as an administrative tool. *Journal of the American Geriatrics Society, 31*(11), 642-650.

Fiedler, J.L. (1981). A review of the literature on access and utilization of medical care with special emphasis on rural primary care, social science and medical (Part c). *Medical Economics, 15*(3c), 129-142.

Flook, E. (1973). Health services research and R and D in perspective. *American Journal of Public Health and the Nations Health, 63*(8), 681-686.

Fortinsky, R.H., Granger, C.F., & Seltzer, G.B. (1981). The use of functional assessment in understanding home care needs. *Medical Care, 19*(5), 489-497.

Foster, S.B. (1974). Adrenal measure for evaluating nursing effectiveness. *Nursing Research, 23*(2), 118-124.

Fowler, S.B. (1995). Hope: Implications for neuroscience nursing. *Journal of Neuroscience Nursing, 27*(5), 298-304.

Fox, R.N., & Ventura, M.R. (1983). Small scale administration of instruments procedures. *Nursing Research, 32*(2), 122-125.

Frelick, R.W., & Frelick, J.H. (1976). Coming to grips with main issues. *American Journal of Public Health, 66*(8), 795.

French, K. (1981). Methodological considerations in hospital patient opinion surveys. *International Journal of Nursing Studies, 18*(1), 7-32.

Fuhrer, M.J. (1983). Commentary: Communicating and utilizing research in medical rehabilitation. *Archives of Physical Medicine and Rehabilitation, 64*(12), 608-610.

Glover, T.L. (1995). Preliminary exploration of variables related to operating room staffing methods. *Surgical Services Management, 1*(4), 37-41.

Golden, A.S. (19175). Task analysis in health manpower development and utilization. *Medical Care, 13*(8), 704-710.

Goodwin, J.D., & Edwards, B.S. (1975). Developing a computer program to assist nursing process: Phase 1: From systems analysis to an expandable program. *Nursing Research, 24*(4), 299-305.

Gordon, M. (1980). Determining study topics. *Nursing Research, 2*, 83-87.

Gordon, M., Sweeney, M.A., & McKeehan, K. (1980). Development of nursing diagnoses. *American Journal of Nursing, 4*, 669.

Gortner, S.R., & Nahm, H. (1977). Overview of nursing research in the United States. *Nursing Research, 26*(1), 10-33.

Greaves, F. (1980). Objectively toward curriculum improvement in nursing: Education in England and Wales. *Journal of Advanced Nursing, 5*(6), 591-599.

Grier, M.R., & Schnitzler, C.P. (1979). Nurses' propensity to risk. *Nursing Research, 28*(3), 186-191.

Grobe, S.J. (1990). Nursing intervention lexicon and taxonomy study: Language and classification methods. *Advances in Nursing Science, 13*(2), 22-35.

Gunter, L.M., & Miller, J.C. (1977). Toward a nurse gerontology. *Nursing Research, 26*(3), 209-221.

Hagell, E.I. (1989). Nursing knowledge: Women's knowledge—a sociological perspective. *Journal of Advanced Nursing, 14*(3), 226-233.

Hall, J.A., & Dornan, M.C. (1988). What patients like about their medical care and how often they are asked: A meta-analysis of the satisfaction literature. *Social Science and Medicine, 27*(9), 935-939.

Halloran, E.J. (1985). Nursing workload, medical diagnosis related groups and nursing diagnosis. *Research in Nursing and Health, 8*(4), 421-433.

Halloran, E.J., & Kiley, M. (1985). The nurses' role and length of stay. [letter]. *Medical Care, 23*(9), 1122-1124.

Handa, A. (1995). Sex education for adolescents. *Nursing Journal of India, 86*(8), 173-177.

Hanucharurnkul, S. (1989). Comparative analysis of Orem's and King's theories. *Journal of Advanced Nursing, 14*(5), 365-372.

Hardy, L.K. (1982). Nursing models and nursing: A restrictive view. *Journal of Advanced Nursing, 7*(5), 447-451.

Harrington, A. (1995). Spiritual care: What does it mean to RNs? *Australian Journal of Advanced Nursing, 12*(4), 5-14.

Hawthorne, P.J. (1984). Measuring change in nursing practice. *Journal of Advanced Nursing, 9*(3), 239-247.

Hayesbautista, D.E. (1976). Classification of practitioners by urban Chicano patients: Aspects of sociology of lay knowledge. *American Journal of Optometry and Physiological Optics, 53*(3), 156-163.

Heagarty, M.C., Boehringer, J.R., Lavinge, P.A., Brooks, E.G., & Evans, M.E. (1973). Evaluation of activities of nurses and pediatricians in a university outpatient department. *Journal of Pediatrics, 83*(5), 875-879.

Hendrickson, G., Doddato, T.M., & Kovner, C.T. (1990). How do nurses use their time? *Journal of Nursing Administration, 20*(3), 31-38.

Hodgman, E.L. (1979). Closing the gap between research and practice: Changing the answer to the who, the where and the how of nursing research. *International Journal of Nursing Studies, 16*(1), 105-110.

Holmes, S. (1989). Use of a modified symptom distress scale in assessment of the cancer patient. *International Journal of Nursing Studies, 26*(1), 69-79.

Holmes, S. (1991). Preliminary investigations of symptom distress in two cancer patient populations: Evaluation of a measurement instrument. *Journal of Advanced Nursing, 16*(4), 439-446.

Holmes, S., & Eburn, E. (1989). Patients' and nurses' perceptions of symptom distress in cancer. *Journal of Advanced Nursing, 14*(10), 840-846.

Hooker, B.B. (1977). Diploma school of nursing: Option in post secondary education. *Journal of Nursing Education, 16*(3), 36-42.

Horn, S.D., & Horn, R.A. (1986). Reliability and validity of the Severity of Illness Index. *Medical Care, 24*(2), 159-168.

Hubbard, S.M. & Donehower, M.G. (1980). The nurse in a cancer research setting. *Seminars in Oncology, 1*, 9-17.

Huckabay, L.M., & Roberts, S.L. (1984). Effect of verbal mediators on cognitive learning, transfer of learning, and effective behaviors of student nurses as they apply to the care of patients with myocardial infarctions. *Heart and Lung, 13*(3), 280-286.

Jackson, B.S., & Kinney, M.R. (1978). Energy-expenditure, heart rate, rhythm and blood pressure in normal female subjects engaged in common hospitalized patient positions and modes of patient transfer. *International Journal of Nursing Studies, 15*(3), 115-128.

Jacobsen, B.S., & Meininger, J.C. (1985). The designs and methods of published nursing research: 1956-1983. *Nursing Research, 34*(5), 306-312.

Jennings, B.M. (1988). Merging nursing research and practice: A case of multiple identities. *Journal of Advanced Nursing, 13*(6), 752-758.

Jennings, C.P., & Jennings, T.F. (1977). Containing costs through perspective reimbursement. *American Journal of Nursing, 77*(7), 1155-1159.

Ketefian, S. (1975). Application of selected nursing research findings into nursing practice. Pilot study. *Nursing Research, 24*(2), 89-92.

Ketefien, S. (1976). Curriculum change in nursing education: Sources of knowledge utilized. *International Nursing Review, 23*(4), 107-115.

Krueger, J.C. (1980). Establishing priorities for evaluation and evaluation research: Nursing perspective. *Nursing Research, 2*, 115-118.

Kuhn, B.G. (1980). Prediction of nursing requirements from patient characteristics. *International Journal of Nursing Studies, 1*, 5-15.

Lanara, V.A. (1976). Philosophy of nursing and current nursing problems. *International Nursing Review, 23*(2), 48-54.

Levow, J.L. (1974). Consumer assessments of quality of medical care. *Medical Care, 12*(4), 328-337.

Leininger, M. (1976). Doctoral trends for nurses: Trends, questions, and projected plans. Part I: Trends, questions and issues on doctoral programs. *Nursing Research, 25*(3), 201-210.

Levine, E., & Abdellah, F.G. (1984). DRGs: A recent refinement to an old method. *Inquiry, 21*(2), 105-112.

Lewandowski, L.A., & Kositsky, A.M. (1983). Research priorities for critical care nursing: A study by the American Association of Critical Care Nurses. *Heart and Lung, 12*(1), 35-44.

Leyden, D.R. (1983). Measuring patients attitudes in a comprehensive health care setting. *Computers in Biology and Medicine, 13*(2), 99-124.

Lindeman, C.A. (1975). Delphi survey of priorities in clinical nursing research. *Nursing Research, 24*(6), 434-441.

Lindquist, R.D., Tracy, M.F., Treat-Jacobson, D. (1995). Peer review of nursing research proposals. *American Journal of Critical Care, 4*(1), 59-65.

Linn, L.S., Brook, R.H., Clark, V.A., Davies, A.R., Fink, A., & Kosecoff, J. (1985). Physician and patient satisfaction as factors related to the organization of internal medicine group practices. *Medical Care, 23*(10), 1171-1178.

Loomis, M.E. (1985). Emerging content in nursing: An analysis of dissertation abstracts and titles: 1976-1982. *Nursing Research, 34*(2), 113-118.

Lynaugh, J. (1990). Moments in nursing history: Four hundred postcards. *Nursing Research, 39*(4), 254-256.

MacGuire, J.M. (1990). Putting nursing research findings into practice: Research utilization as an aspect of the management of change. *Journal of Advanced Nursing, 15*(5), 614-620.

Maddox, M.A., & Fishbein, E.G. (1994). Survey results: Academic courses of women's health across the lifespan. *Journal of Gerontological Nursing, 20*(6), 43-47.

Majesky, S.J., Brester, M.H., & Nishio, K.T. (1978). Development of a research tool: Patient indications of nursing care. *Nursing Research, 27*(6), 365-371.

Martin, K. (1988). Research in home care. *Nursing Clinics of North America, 23*(2), 363-385.

McGee, D.C. (1995). The perinatal nurse practitioner: An innovative model of advanced practice. *Journal of Obstetric Gynecologic and Neonatal Nursing, 24*(7), 602-606.

McGilloway, F.A. (1980). The nursing process: A problem-solving approach to patient care. *International Journal of Nursing Studies, 2,* 79-90.

McKinnon, E.L. (1978). Circulation research: Exploring its potential in clinical nursing. *Nursing Research, 21*(6), 494-498.

McLane, A.M. (1978). Core competencies of masters-prepared nurses. *Nursing Research, 27*(1), 48-53.

McMillan, S.C. (1985). A comparison of professional performance examination scores of graduating associate and baccalaureate degree nursing students. *Research in Nursing and Health, 8*(2), 167-172.

Meleis, A.I. (1979). Development of a conceptually based nursing curriculum: International experiment. *Journal of Advanced Nursing, 6,* 659-671.

Mickely, B.B. (1974). Physiologic and psychologic responses of elective surgical patients: Early definite or late indefinite scheduling of surgical procedures. *Nursing Research, 23*(5), 392-401.

Miller, A. (1984). Nurse/patient dependency: A review of different approaches with particular reference to studies of the dependency of elderly patients. *Journal of Advanced Nursing, 9*(5), 479-486.

Minnick, A., Young, W.B., & Roberts, M.J. (1995). 2,000 patients relate their hospital experiences. *Nursing Management, 26*(12), 29-31.

Mitchell, D., & Hicks, M. (1995). Components of Life Model in practice. *Accident and Emergency Nursing, 3*(4), 190-200.

Molde, S., & Diers, D. (1985). Nurse practitioner research: Selected literature review and research agenda. *Nursing Research, 34*(6), 362-367.

Molzahn, A.E. (1993). An evaluation of the nephrology nursing research literature: 1979-1989 . . . including commentary by Abbink C. with author response. *ANNA Journal, 20*(4), 395-428.

Moores, B., & Thompson, A.G.H. (1986). What 1357 hospital inpatients think about aspects of their stay in British acute hospitals. *Journal of Advanced Nursing, 11*(1), 87-102.

Munro, C.L., & Pickler, R.H. (1994). The technology and use of blastomere analysis. *Journal of Obstetric Gynecologic and Neonatal Nursing, 23*(3), 229-234.

Newman, B. (1995). Enhancing patient care: Case management and critical pathways. *Australian Journal of Advanced Nursing, 13*(1), 16-24.

Newman, S.J. (1985). Housing and long-term care: The suitability of the elderly's housing to the provision of in-home services. *Gerontologist, 25*(1), 35-40.

Nunnally, D.M. (1974). Patients' evaluation of other prenatal and delivery care. *Nursing Research, 23*(6), 469-474.

Orr, J.A. (1979). Nursing and the process of scientific inquiry. *Journal of Advanced Nursing, 6,* 603-610.

Paradis, L.F., & Cummings, S.B. (1986). The evolution of hospice in America toward organizational homogeneity. *Journal of Health and Social Behavior, 27*(4), 370-386.

Penchansky, R., & Thomas, J.W. (1981). The concept of access: Definitions and relationship to consumer satisfaction. *Medical Care, 19*(2), 127-140.

Peters, D.A. (1988). Development of a Community Health Intensity Rating Scale. *Nursing Research, 37*(4), 202-207.

Proudfoot, L.M., Farmer, E.S., & McIntosh, J.B. (1994). Testing incontinence pads using single-case research designs. *British Journal of Nursing, 3*(7), 316.

Rankin, M.A. (1974). Pienschke's theoretical framework for guardedness or openness on the cancer unit. [letter]. *Nursing Research, 23*(5), 434.

Razquin, M.I.S., Solis, M.H.N., Sastre, R.S., Izco, M.S., & Garchitorena, E.C. (1995). Health problems identified in patients in a cardiovascular surgery department [Spanish]. *Enfermeria Clinica, 5*(4), 150-156.

Risser, N.L. (1975). Development of an instrument to measure patient satisfaction with nurses and nursing care in primary care settings. *Nursing Research, 24*(1), 45-52.

Roberts, K.L (1985). Theory of nursing as curriculum content. *Journal of Advanced Nursing, 10*(3), 209-215.

Rodgers, M.W. (1986). Implementing faculty practice: A question of human and financial resources. *Journal of Advanced Nursing, 11*(6), 687-696.

Santus, G., Ranzenigo, A., Caregnato, R., & Inzoli, M.R. (1990). Social and family integration of hemiplegic elderly patients 1 year after stroke. *Stroke, 21*(7), 1019-1022.

Sarnecky, M.T. (1990). Historiography: A legitimate research methodology for nursing. *Advances in Nursing Science, 12*(4), 1-10.

Schlotfeldt, R.M. (1975). Research in nursing and research training for nurses: Retrospect and prospect. *Nursing Research, 24*(3), 177-183.

Schuster, C. (1995). Have we forgotten the older adults? An argument in support of more health promotion programs for and research directed toward people 65 years and older. *Journal of Health Education, 26*(6), 338-344.

Seither, F.G. (1974). Predictive validity study of screening measures used to select practical nursing students. *Nursing Research, 23*(1), 60-63.

Sheahan, J. (1980). Some aspects of the teaching and learning of nursing. *Journal of Advanced Nursing, 5*(5), 491-511.

Shopa, M.A. (1975). Historical materials in nursing. *Nursing Research, 24*(4), 308.

Shukla, R.K., & Turner, W.E. III (1984). Patients perception of care under primary and team nursing. *Research in Nursing and Health, 7*(2), 93-99.

Simms, L.M., Pfoutz, S.K., & Price, S.C. (1986) Caring for older people: A challenge for nurse administrators. *Nursing Outlook 34*(3), 145-148.

Smoyak, S.A. (1976). Is practice responding to research? *American Journal of Nursing, 76*(7), 1146-1150.

Spiegel, A.D, Hyman, H.H., & Gary, L.R. (1980). Issues and opportunities in the regulation of home health care. *Health Policy and Education, 1*(3), 237-253.

Stevenson, J.S. (1987). Forging a research discipline. *Nursing Research, 36*(1), 60-64.

Stolte, K., Myers, S.T., & Owen, W.L. (1994). Changes in maternity care and the impact on nurses and nursing practice. *Journal of Obstetric Gynecologic and Neonatal Nursing, 23*(7), 603-608.

Stratton, T.D., Dunkin, J.W., & Juhl, N. (1995). Redefining the nursing shortage: A rural perspective. *Nursing Outlook, 43*(2), 71-77.

Sutcliffe, J., & Holmes, S. (1991). Quality of life: Verification and use of a self-assessment scale in two patient populations. *Journal of Advanced Nursing, 16*(4), 490-498.

Taylor, S.D. (1974). Development of a classification system for current nursing research. *Nursing Research, 23*(1), 63-68.

Taylor, S.D. (1975). Bibliography on nursing research: 1950-1974. *Milbank, 24*(3), 207-225.

Temkingreener, H. (1983). Interprofessional perspectives on teamwork in health care: A case study. *Milback Memorial Fund Quarterly: Health and Society, 61*(4), 641-658.

Thompson, D.R., & Sutton, T.W. (1985). Nursing decision making in a coronary care unit. *International Journal of Nursing Studies, 22*(3), 259-266.

Thurston, N. (1995). Hospital research comes of age. *Canadian Nurse, 91*(4), 34-38.

Tiesinga, L.J., Halfens, R.J.G., Algera-Osinga, J.T., & Hasman, A. (1994). The application of a factor evaluation system for community nursing in the Netherlands. *Journal of Nursing Management, 2*(4), 175-179.

Tornary, R.D. (1977). Nursing research: Road ahead. *Nursing Research, 26*(6), 404-407.

Trivedi, V.M., & Hancock, W.J. (1975). Measurement of nursing workload using head nurses' perceptions. *Nursing Research, 24*(5), 371-376.

Trivedi, V.M., & Warner, D.M. (1976). Branch and bound algorithm for optimum allocation of float nurses. *Management Science, 22*(9), 972-981.

Turnbull, E.M. (1978). Effect of basic preventive health practices and mass-media on practice of breast self-examination. *Nursing Research, 27*(2), 98-102.

Ventura, M.R., & Waligoraserofur, B. (1981). Study priorities identified by nurses in mental health setting. *International Journal of Nursing Studies, 19*(1), 41-46.

Vredevoe, D.L. (1972). Nursing research involving physiological mechanisms: Definitions of variables. *Nursing Research, 21*(1), 68-72.

Wade, G.H. (1995). Is research in the patient setting feasible? *Journal of Continuing Education in Nursing, 26*(6), 253-256.

Wade, S. (1995). Partnership in care: A critical review. *Nursing Standard, 9*(48), 29-32.

Wagner, V.D., Kee, C.C., & Gray, D.P. (1995). A historical decline of educational perioperative clinical experiences. *AORN Journal, 62*(5), 771-772.

Ware, J.E., & Berwick, D.M. (1990). Conclusions and recommendations (of a Pilot-study: patient judgements of hospital quality). *Medical Care, 28*(9), S39-S44.

Warner, D.M. (1976). Nurse staffing, scheduling, reallocation in hospital. *Hospital and Health Services Administration, 21*(3), 77-90.

Webber, P.B. (1994). National response to the nursing shortage: Implications for nursing education. *Journal of Nursing Education, 33*(3), 107-111.

White, M.B. (1972). Importance of selected nursing activities. *Nursing Research, 21*(1), 4-14.

Wolfer, J.A. (1973). Definition and assessment of surgical patients' welfare and recovery. *Nursing Research, 22*(5), 394-401.

Wright, D. (1984). An introduction to the evaluation of nursing care: A review of the literature. *Journal of Advanced Nursing, 9*(5), 457-467.

Yurick, A., Burgio, L., & Paton, S.M. (1995). Assessing disruptive behaviors of nursing home residents: Use of microcomputer technology to promote objectivity in planning nursing interventions. *Journal of Gerontological Nursing, 21*(4), 29-34.

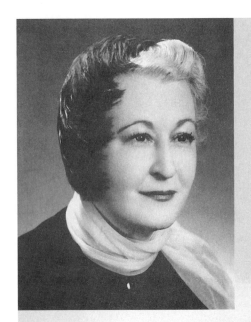

Lydia E. Hall

Core, Care, and Cure Model

Carolyn H. Fakouri, Marcy Grandstaff, S. Brook Gumm,
Ann Marriner Tomey, Kim Tippey Peskoe

CREDENTIALS AND BACKGROUND OF THE THEORIST

Lydia Hall began her prestigious career in nursing as a graduate of the York Hospital School of Nursing in York, Pennsylvania. She then earned her B.S. and M.A. degrees from Teachers College, Columbia University, in New York, like many other contemporary nursing theorists.

Hall had faculty positions at the York Hospital School of Nursing and the Fordham Hospital School of Nursing and was a consultant in nursing educa-

tion to the nursing faculty at State University of New York, Upstate Medical Center. She also was an instructor of nursing education at Teachers College.

Hall's career interests revolved around public health nursing, cardiovascular nursing, pediatric cardiology, and nursing of long-term illnesses. She authored 21 publications, with the bulk of articles and addresses regarding her nursing theories published in the early to middle 1960s. In 1967 she received the Award for Distinguished Achievement in Nursing Practice from Columbia University.

Perhaps Hall's greatest achievement in nursing was her design and development of the Loeb Center for Nursing at Montefiore Hospital in New York City. Established to apply her theory to nursing practice, the center opened in January 1963. Hall designed the 80-bed Loeb Center for persons aged 16 years or older who were no longer having acute biological disturbances. Candidates for the Loeb Center were recommended by their physician and had favorable potential for recovery and return to their community. Within the nondirective setting, patients demonstrated success and provided empirical evidence to support the major concepts in Hall's theory. Hall served as administrative director of the Loeb Center for Nursing from its opening until her death in February 1969.

The Loeb Center remains a vital part of Montefiore Medical Center. The skilled nursing facility provides a team approach to assist hospital patients who are recovering from an acute illness or surgical procedure. Consistent with Hall's original model, nurses and the interdisciplinary rehabilitation staff work together with the patient and family to assist the patient to make the transition from hospital to home.

THEORETICAL SOURCES

Hall drew extensively from the schools of psychiatry and psychology in theorizing about the nurse-patient relationship. She was a proponent of Carl Rogers' philosophy of "client-centered therapy." This method of therapy entails establishing a relationship of warmth and safety, conveying a sensitive empathy with the client's feelings and communications as expressed.[14:34] A major premise Hall borrowed from Rogers[14:280] is that patients achieve their maximal potential through a learning process. Rogers[14:47] states that psychotherapy facilitates significant learning by (1) pointing out and labeling unsatisfying behaviors, (2) exploring objectively with the client the reasons for the behaviors, and (3) establishing through reeducation more effective problem-solving habits. In client-centered therapy, changes occur when:

1. The person accepts himself and his feelings more fully

2. He becomes more self-confident and self-directing

3. He changes maladaptive behaviors, even chronic ones

4. He becomes more open to evidence of what is going on both inside and outside of himself[14:280-281]

Extensive documentation indicates the result of this treatment is that physiological and psychological tensions are reduced and that the change lasts.[14:65]

The major therapeutic approach advocated by Hall is also Rogerian. This approach is the use of reflection, a nondirective method of helping the patient clarify, explore, and validate what he says. Rogers[14:43] states, "The therapist procedure which [clients] had found most helpful was that the therapist clarified and openly stated feelings which the client had been approaching hazily and hesitantly."[14:73]

Hall derived her postulates regarding the nature of feeling-based behavior from Rogers, who repeatedly speaks to the interaction of known feelings and feelings out-of-awareness. Rogers[14:36] hypothesizes that in a client-centered relationship the patient:

> Will re-organize himself at both the conscious and deeper levels of his personality in such a manner as to cope with life more constructively. . . . He shows . . . more of the characteristics of the healthy, well-functioning person. . . . He is less frustrated by stress, and recovers from stress more quickly.

Hall also adopted Rogers's theory on motivation for change. In this theory Rogers asserts that, although the therapist does not motivate the client, neither is the motivation supplied by the client. Alternatively, motivation for change "springs from the self-actualizing tendency of life itself."[14:285] In the proper psychological climate, this tendency is released.

In addition to utilizing Rogers's theories, Hall also integrated educational and interpersonal theories into her theory. Hall developed her ideas regarding interpersonal behavior from Harry Stack Sullivan and also utilized teaching and learning ideas integrated from John Dewey. Hall did not utilize ideas of the contemporary nursing theorists. The influence of Dewey can be seen in Hall's emphasis on the teaching-learning process with the nurse's primary responsibility as one of teacher. Sullivan's influence was evidenced in the role of the nurse as nurturer for the patient within the "Core" circle.[15:11-12]

USE OF EMPIRICAL EVIDENCE

Rogers's theories have received wide acclaim in the fields of psychiatry, psychology, and social work. His methods of therapy have been used in caring for clients and in the area of education, where a nondirective approach is less than common. In *On Becoming a Person*, one of Rogers's students, Samuel Tenen-

baum, discussed learning through a nondirective approach and then teaching that way.[14:285]

The application of client-centered therapy in play therapy for children is addressed by Elaine Dorfman in Rogers's book, *Client-Centered Therapy*. In this specialized area, the therapist must work at the child's level of communication. Even with small children, reflection and clarification techniques are instrumental in helping children examine their feelings[13] in leadership and administration situations. Thomas Gordon has addressed Rogers's concepts as they relate to group dynamics and group-centered leadership.[14] Gordon believes a leader can strive to

MAJOR CONCEPTS & DEFINITIONS

Behavior Hall broadly defines behavior as everything that is said or done. Behavior is dictated by feelings, both conscious and unconscious.

Reflection Reflection is a Rogerian method of communication in which selected verbalizations of patients are repeated back to them with different phraseology, to invite them to explore feelings further.[4:88]

Self-Awareness Self-awareness refers to the state of being that nurses endeavor to help their patients achieve. The more self-awareness persons have of their feelings, the more control they have over their behavior.

Phases of Medical Care Hall divides medical care into two phases: biologically critical and evaluative follow-up. Biologically critical medicine lasts a few days to a week or more and is the period when physicians devise treatment plans that help the patient reach the second phase. During the first phase, the patient receives intensive medical care and multiple diagnostic tests.[4:84]

Second-Stage Illness The patient enters the second phase of medical care once the doctors begin giving only follow-up care. Hall defines second-stage illness as the nonacute recovery phase of illness. This stage is conducive to learning and rehabilitation.[4:84] The need for medical care is minimal

although the need for nurturing and learning is great. Therefore this is the ideal time for wholly professional nursing care.

Wholly Professional Nursing Wholly professional nursing implies nursing care given exclusively by professional registered nurses educated in the behavioral sciences who take the responsibility and opportunity to coordinate and deliver the total care of their patients.[4:91] This concept includes the roles of nurturing, teaching, and advocacy in the fostering of healing.

Nursing circles of Care, Core, and Cure are the central concepts of Hall's theory (Fig. 11-1). Care alludes to the "hands-on," intimate bodily care of the patient and implies a comforting, nurturing relationship.[4:85] While intimate physical care is provided, the nurse and patient develop a close relationship representing the teaching-learning aspect of nursing. Core involves the therapeutic use of self in communicating with the patient. The nurse, through the use of reflective technique, helps the patient clarify motives and goals, facilitating the process of increasing the patient's self-awareness. Cure is the aspect of nursing involved with administration of medications and treatments. The nurse functions in this role as an investigator and potential "painer."[3:152] create a nonthreatening psychological climate by conveying warmth and acceptance; clarification statements can be used to link chains of thought.

The multiplicity of applications of Rogerian theory in everyday life is almost endless. Rogers deserves his venerable title of the "founder of nondirective client-centered therapy."[6] His writings would have constituted the most current literature on this topic in the 1960s, when Hall was building her theory of nursing.

Although Hall did not actually research her theory, Blue Cross Insurance studies indicated that patients at Loeb recovered in half the time, at less than half the cost, and with fewer readmissions than patients who stayed in Montefiore Hospital. Twenty-two home-care programs in the New York area had a readmission rate five times higher than Loeb's.[5:91-92] On a follow-up questionnaire, 40 physicians indicated the hospital stay of patients at the Loeb Center ranged from 3 to 43 days shorter than at other hospitals, with the usual difference of 1 to 3 weeks. Patients and physicians were both pleased with the care.[5:82]

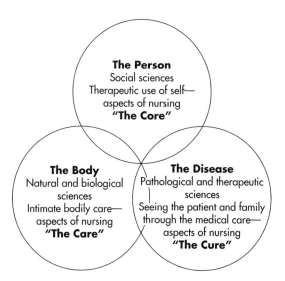

Fig. **11-1** Core, Care, and Cure Model. *From Hall, L. (1964, Feb.). Nursing: What is it? The Canadian Nurse, 60 (2), 151. Reproduced with permission from The Canadian Nurse.*

Not only did studies conducted at Loeb show increased patient satisfaction and decreased length of stay, but increased nurse satisfaction was also found. A study done in 1968 recorded perceptions of baccalaureate graduates hired at Loeb Center and compared nurses at similar educational levels working in a hospital setting. The researchers found that the philosophy at Loeb and the support of administration created a greater amount of satisfaction for nurses at Loeb compared with their hospital cohorts.[15:12]

MAJOR ASSUMPTIONS

The following assumptions are basic to Hall's theory of nursing. They are explicit and for the most part are adequately defined in her writings.

Nursing

Nursing can and should be professional.[4:81] Hall stipulated patients should be cared for only by professional registered nurses who can take total responsibility for the care and teaching of their patients. The following interesting afternote appears in one of her articles on the Loeb Center[4:95]:

> We hire from 3-year schools, community colleges, baccalaureate, and even master's degree programmes. . . . Although all learn to master satisfactorily, those from the 2 and 3-year programmes reach a plateau. The baccalaureate graduates keep on learning and being and don't seem to stop growing in their ability to gain skills in the nurturing process.

The professional nurse functions most therapeutically when patients have entered the second stage of their hospital stay.[4:84] The second stage is the recuperating, or nonacute, phase of illness. The first stage of illness is a time of biological crisis, with nursing being ancillary to medicine. After the crisis period the patient is more able to benefit and learn from the teaching that nurses can offer.

Nursing is all complex.[4:84] The patient is certainly complex. Not only is he/she a human being, bringing with him/her the influences of his/her culture and environment, but he/she may be suffering from an illness that medicine is still struggling to understand and treat. The nurse giving the care is also a unique human being, interacting with the patient in a complex process of teaching and learning.

Nursing expertise centers around the body.[4:85] This statement refers to Hall's theoretical model because she viewed the patient as composed of Body, Pathology, and Personality. The uniqueness of nursing lies not only in knowing bodily care but also in knowing how to modify these processes in line with the pathologic process and treatment, and amend them in line with the personality of the patient.

Person

Patients achieve their maximal potential through a learning process; therefore the chief therapy they need is teaching.[4:82] Rehabilitation is a process of learning to live within limitations. Physical and mental skills must be learned, but a prerequisite to these is learning about oneself as a person, becoming aware of feelings and behaviors, and clarifying motivations. Hall believed the teaching-learning process could best be facilitated by the professional nurse educated in communication skills.

People strive for their own goals, not goals others set for them.[4:82] Hall declared that in the usual medical setting the doctor defines the goals for the patient, but too often these goals do not coincide with the patient's goals for himself/herself. In this situation, effective teaching and learning cannot occur.

A patient is composed of three aspects: Body, Pathology, and Person.[4:84] (These elements are discussed later.) This particular assumption is crucial to Hall's theory of nursing.

People behave on the basis of their feelings, not on the basis of knowledge.[4:89] The evidence that learning has occurred is a resultant change in some behavior. Changes in behavior do not usually happen strictly as a result of knowing information. Actions occur in conjunction with feelings, and feelings are not influenced by rationality.

There are two types of feelings: known feelings and feelings-out-of-awareness.[4:90] When people act on the basis of known feelings, they are *free* and in control of their behavior. When they act on feelings-out-of-awareness, they have no choice as to their behavior and the feelings make them act.

Health

Becoming ill is behavior,[4:90] according to Hall's definition of behavior. Illness is directed by one's feelings-out-of-awareness, which are the root of adjustment difficulties.

Healing may be hastened by helping people move in the direction of self-awareness.[4:90] Once people are brought to grips with their true feelings and motivations, they become free to release their own powers of healing.

Through the process of reflection, "the patient has a chance to move from the unlabeled threat of anxiety . . . through a mislabeled threat of 'phobia' or 'disease' . . . to a properly labeled threat (fear) with which he can deal constructively."[4:91]

Environment

Hospital nursing services are organized to accomplish tasks efficiently.[4:83] Hall viewed these organizations as being an end unto themselves. She did not believe they had patient care and teaching as their goal, but rather that their goal was helping physicians and administrators get their work done.

Hall was not pleased with the concept of team nursing. She said, "Any career that is defined around the work that has to be done, and how it is divided to get it done, is a trade."[4:83] She vehemently opposed the ideas of anyone other than educated, professional nurses taking direct care of patients and decried the fact that nursing has trained nonprofessionals to function as practical nurses so that professional nurses can function as practical doctors.

There are two phases of medical care practiced in medical centers: biological crisis and evaluative medicine.[4:84] The biological crisis phase involves intensive medical and diagnostic treatment of the patient. The evaluative medicine phase follows and generally is the time when the patient is observed to appraise whether he/she is meeting the doctor's goals.

Theoretical Assertions

Hall's theory consists of three major tenets. The first is that nursing functions differently in the three interlocking circles that constitute aspects of the patient.[4:81] These three circles are interrelated and are influenced by each other. The three circles are the patient's Body, the Disease affecting the body, and the Person of the patient, which is being affected by both of the other circles. Nursing operates in all three circles, but shares them with other professions to different degrees. Because pathological conditions are treated with medical care (Cure), nursing shares this circle with physicians. The Person aspect (Core) is cared for by therapeutic use of the self. Therefore this arena is shared with psychiatry, psychology, social work, and religious ministry. The body of the patient is cared for exclusively by nursing (Care). The care circle includes all intimate bodily care such as feeding, bathing, and toileting the patient. The Care component is the exclusive domain of nursing.

Hall's second assertion[2:806] is the Core postulate of her theory. As the patient needs less medical care, he/she needs more professional nursing care and teaching. This inversely proportional relationship alters the ratio of nursing care in the three circles. Patients in the second stage of illness (nonacute phase) are primarily in need of rehabilitation through learning; thus, the Care and Core circles predominate the Cure circle. The Loeb Center was designed for the care of nonacute patients in need of teaching and rehabilitation; the fact that it is staffed and run by nurses with physicians functioning as ancillaries is no surprise.

The third assertion of this theory is that wholly professional nursing care will hasten recovery. Hall decried the concept of team nursing, which gives the care of less complicated cases to caregivers with less training. Nurses are complex people using a complex process of teaching and learning in caring for complex patients with complex diseases. Only professional nurses are inherently qualified to provide the teaching, counseling, and nurturing needed in the second stage of illness.[3:150;4:83-84] At the Loeb Center, secretaries and messenger-attendants were employed for the indirect patient care. But they were not permitted to do anything directly related to the patient.

The professional nurse is the coordinator for all her patients' therapies, and all disciplines act in a consulting capacity to nursing.[4:82]

Logical Form

Hall's theory is formulated using inductive logic, moving from specific observations to a generalized concept. For example:

- Nursing care shortens patient recovery time.
- Nursing care facilitates patient recovery.
- Professional nursing improves patient care.
- Therefore "wholly professional nursing will hasten recovery."[5:82]

Acceptance by the Nursing Community

Practice

Hall's theory closely resembles the modern nursing model of primary care. Her emphasis on the professional nurse as the primary caregiver parallels primary care nursing to the extent that continuity and coordination of patient care are provided. In addition, Hall's concepts of nurses being accountable and responsible for their own practice are ideas that are pertinent and applicable today. Concern for these concepts demonstrates support for her theory.

Education

Hall's theory delineates definite ideas regarding nursing care being provided for by a professional nursing staff. The acceptance of this philosophy can be seen in the shift toward professional staffing in some health care facilities, and in the growing trend toward the BSN degree as the minimum entry level requirement for professional practice. Hall[2:806] also emphasized the concept of nurses practicing nursing while completing their educational programs, instead of practicing as practical doctors. Today's issues of narrowing the divide between nursing education and service, and of using nursing diagnoses as a guide for patient care instead of medical diagnoses, support Hall's concepts from her theory.

Research

Until the late 1980s, research testing Hall's theory had been conducted only at Loeb Center. Now two different facilities in Europe are utilizing the ideas of Hall to develop nursing care units. Pearson, Durand, and Punton (1988) compared patients in an acute care hospital with patients receiving care at a nursing unit. All patients were more than 65 years old and had fractures of the femoral neck. The researchers compared length of acute stay, quality of nursing care, and life satisfaction 6 months after discharge. Those patients who received care on the nursing unit spent less time in acute care, received more consistent quality of nursing care, and reported improvements in level of life satisfaction after 6 months.[11]

Pearson, Durand, and Punton again conducted a larger scale study similar to the 1988 study. They found the same results of increased satisfaction for patients who received care on a nursing unit. Hall's theory is also being implemented in Oxford, United Kingdom.[12] No specific research studies were done, but McMahon (1989) wrote two articles detailing the use and success of the Oxford Nursing Development Unit.[7,8] Implementation of Hall's theory in nursing units within the United States was not found outside the Loeb Center.

Given the changes in health care in the United States, it may be difficult to further test Hall's assertion that wholly professional nursing care will hasten recovery in a skilled nursing center. Even at the Loeb Center in the 1990s the staffing patterns have changed. In addition to a geriatric nurse-practitioner and professional rehabilitation nurses, nurse-attendants now assist with patient care. Tasks such as hair and nail care are performed by nursing attendants.

FURTHER DEVELOPMENT

Much research and testing of Hall's theory is needed before it can be applicable and useful to areas of nursing other than long-term illnesses and rehabilitative nursing. In particular, the theory needs to be adapted to health care facilities that differ from the Loeb Center for Nursing before its true impact and contribution to nursing can be judged. This step would require flexibility and change in several of Hall's main concepts and relationships, particularly those relating to the age and illness orientation of the client. It would be interesting to further develop in a variety of settings the concept of increased nursing care as a means to hasten patient recovery. This tenet has been highly successful at the Loeb Center in reducing both patient days and health care costs.

Home health care is one domain of nursing in which testing could be done to see if utilizing Hall's ideas could decrease readmissions to the hospital. With the installation of diagnostic related groups, patients leave the hospital as soon as the acute phase of illness is resolved. Home health nurses could utilize Hall's ideas of teaching-learning by using reflection to increase self-awareness. Because the patient was ill while hospitalized, the patient would not have learned all needed information for proper care at home. Home health nurses can intervene to ensure the patient learns all needed information for proper care.

CRITIQUE
Simplicity

Hall's theory is simple and easily understood. The major concepts and relationships are limited and clear. The three aspects of professional nursing are identified both individually and as they relate to each other in the total process of patient care. Hall designed basic models to represent the major concepts and relationships of her theory, using individual and interlocking circles to define the three aspects of the patient and their relationships to the three aspects of nursing. The language used to define and describe the theory is easily understood and is indigenous to nursing.

Generality

Perhaps the most serious flaw in Hall's theory of nursing is its limited generality. Hall's primary target[5:80] in nursing theory is the adult patient who has passed the acute phase of his/her illness and has a relatively good chance at rehabilitation. This concept severely limits application of the theory to a small population of patients of specific age and stage of illness. Although the ideas of Core, Care, and Cure can possibly be applied to patients in the acute phase of their illness, the theory would be most difficult to apply to infants, small children, and comatose patients. In addition, Hall[5:80,82] devotes her theory to adult individuals who are ill. The function of the nurse in preventive health care and health maintenance is not addressed, nor is the nurse's role in community health, although the model could be adapted.

Hall viewed the role of the nurse as heavily involved in the Care and Core aspects of patient care. Unfortunately, this concept provides for little interaction between the nurse and the family, because her theory delineates the family aspect of patient care only in the Cure circle.[3:151;4:87]

The use of therapeutic communication to help patients look at and explore their feelings regarding their illnesses and the potential changes the illnesses might cause is discussed in the Core aspect of nursing care. Therapeutic communication is also thought to motivate patients by making them aware of their true feelings. However, the only communication technique Hall[4:91] described in her theory as a means to assist the patient toward self-awareness was reflection. This is a very limited approach to therapeutic communication because not all nurses can effectively use the technique of reflection, and it is not always the most effective and successful communication tool in dealing with patients.[1:47]

Empirical Precision

Hall's concept of professional nursing hastening patient recovery with increased care as the patient improves has been subjected to a great amount of testing at the Loeb Center for Nursing.[5:80] The fact that the theory is identified with empirical reality cannot be disputed. Evidence obtained through research at the Loeb Center demonstrates that Hall's theory[4:92] does in fact obtain its goal of shortening patient recovery time through concentrated, professional nursing efforts. Currently, the available literature supports the results obtained at the Loeb Center in testing the theory. Although research support has been demonstrated by the success of the Center, a wider range of

testing in various settings is necessary to allow for increased empirical precision of the theory.

Hall's theory has been tested at two other facilities and has been found to be successful. These two facilities still only care for adults, mainly those more than 65 years old. Therefore empirical precision of Hall's theory continues to be limited and further testing in facilities not caring for adults will still be needed.

Derivable Consequences

The theory provides a general framework for nursing, and the concepts are within the domain of nursing, although the aspects of Cure and Core are shared with other health professionals and family members. Although the theory does not provide for the resolution of specific issues and problems, it does address itself to the pertinent and contemporary issues of accountability, responsibility, and professionalism. Application of the theory in practice has produced valued outcomes in all three areas. In addition, the theory demonstrates a great impact on the educational preparation of nursing students. Hall[2:806] stated, "With early field experience in a center where nursing rather than medicine is emphasized, the student may emerge a nurse first." Hall believed that in nursing centers the student would benefit from experiencing nursing as it is taught to them in the classroom.

Despite the shortcomings of Hall's theory of nursing, her contribution to nursing practice is tremendous. Her insight into the problems of nursing in the 1960s has provided a base for professional practice in the multidimensional modern domain of nursing.

CRITICAL THINKING *Activities*

1 Given the demands in nursing practice to meet the physical aspects of Care, some nurses question whether a nurse can develop a genuine caring relationship with all patients as advocated by Hall.[9:63-65] Which patients require a close nurse-patient relationship?

2 Advanced practice nurses (nurse-practitioners, clinical nurse specialists, nurse-midwives, and nurse-anesthetists) include advocacy as an integral part of the nurse-patient relationship. Some nurse theorists refer to advocacy as an extension of the Care concept.[10:103-115] How can advanced practice nurses use Hall's Core, Care, Cure Model in their clinical practice?

3 In the 1960s Hall described the Cure concept in her model as helping the patient and family through the medical, surgical, and rehabilitation phases of a pathological process. The Cure concept was directed by the physician and shared with other members of the health team. Given nursing's knowledge of stress-related illness, for example, could Hall's Cure Model be expanded within current advanced practice nursing roles? Under which situations can a nurse cure an illness?

REFERENCES

 1. Hale, K., & George, J. (1980). Lydia E. Hall. In Nursing Theories Conference Group, J.B. George, Chairperson, *Nursing theories: The base for professional practice.* Englewood Cliffs, NJ: Prentice Hall.
 2. Hall, L.E. (1963, Nov). Center for nursing. *Nursing Outlook, 11,* 805-806.
 3. Hall, L.E. (1964, Feb.). Nursing: What is it? *Canadian Nurse, 60;* 150-154.
 4. Hall, L.E. (1969). The Loeb Center for Nursing and Rehabilitation. *International Journal of Nursing Studies, 6;* 81-95.
 5. Henderson, C. (1964, June). Can nursing care hasten recovery? *American Journal of Nursing, 64;* 80-83.
 6. Knech, D. (1976). *Psychology: A basic course.* New York: Alfred A. Knopf.
 7. McMahon, R. (1989). Partners in care. *Nursing Times, 85* (8), Feb. 22, 34-37.
 8. McMahon, R. (1989). Primary nursing: One to one. *Nursing Times, 85* (2), Jan. 11, 39-40.
 9. Muxlow, J. (1995, Oct.). The relationship between nurse and patient. *Professional Nurse, 11* (1), 63-65.
10. Nelson, M.L. (1995). Client advocacy. In M. Snyder & M.P. Mirr (Eds.), *Advanced practice nursing: A guide to professional development.* New York: Springer.
11. Pearson, A., Durand, I., & Punton, S. (1988). The feasibility and effectiveness of nursing beds. *Nursing Times, 84* (47), Nov. 23, 48-50.
12. Pearson, A., Durand, I., & Punton, S. (1989). Determining quality in a unit where nursing is the primary intervention. *Journal of Advanced Nursing, 14,* 269-273.
13. Rogers, C. (1951). *Client-centered therapy.* Boston: Houghton Mifflin.
14. Rogers, C. (1961). *On becoming a person.* Boston: Houghton Mifflin.
15. Wiggins, L.R. (1980). Lydia Hall's place in the development of theory in nursing. *Image, 12* (1), 10-12.

BIBLIOGRAPHY

Primary sources

Book chapters

Hall, L. (1965). Nursing: What is it? In H. Baumgarten, Jr., *Concepts of nursing home administration.* New York: Macmillan.
Hall, L. (1966). Another view of nursing care and quality. In M.K. Straub, *Continuity of patient care: The role of nursing.* Washington, DC: Catholic University of America Press.

Journal articles

Hall, L. (1955, June). Quality of nursing care. *Public Health News, 36* (6); 212-215. (New Jersey State Department of Health.)
Hall, L. (1963, Nov.). Center for nursing. *Nursing Outlook, 11,* 805-806.
Hall, L. (1964, Feb.). Nursing: What is it? *Canadian Nurse, 60,* 150-154.
Hall, L. (1969). The Loeb Center for nursing and rehabilitation. *International Journal of Nursing Studies, 6,* 81-95.
Hall, L., Hauck, M., & Rosenson, L. (1949, March). The cardiac child in school and community. *New York Heart Association Publication.*

Pamphlets

Hall, L. (1951). *What the classroom teacher should know and do about children with heart disease.* American Heart Association.
Loeb Center: A specialized nursing facility at Montefiore. New York: Montefiore Medical Center: Office of Publication.

Reports

Hall, L. (1960). *Report of a work conference on nursing in long-term chronic disease and aging.* (National League for Nursing as a League Exchange #50) New York: National League for Nursing.
Hall, L. (1963, June). *Report of Loeb Center for nursing and rehabilitation project report.* Congressional Record hearings before the Special Subcommittee on Intermediate Care of the Committee on Veterans' Affairs. Washington, DC, pp. 1515-1562.

Secondary sources

Book chapters

Alfano, G.J. (1987). The Loeb Center for Nursing and Rehabilitation: A model for extended care. In B.C. Vladeck & G.J. Alfano (Eds.), *Medicare and extended care: Issues, problems and prospects.* Owings Mills, MD: Rynd Communications.

Chinn, P.L., & Jacobs, M.K. (1987). Theory in nursing: A current overview. In P.L. Chinn & M. K. Jacobs, *Theory and nursing.* St. Louis: Mosby.

George, J.B. (1995). Lydia E. Hall. In J.B. George (Ed.), *Nursing theories: The base for professional nursing practice.* Norwalk, CT: Appleton & Lange.

Griffith, J. (1982). Other frameworks and models. In J. Griffith & P. Christenson, *Nursing process: Application of theories, frameworks, and models.* St. Louis: Mosby.

Hale, K., & George, J. (1980). Lydia E. Hall. In Nursing Theories Group Conference, J.B. George, Chairperson, *Nursing theories: The base for professional practice.* Englewood Cliffs, NJ: Prentice Hall.

Journal articles

Alfano, G.J. (1988, Jan.-Feb.). A different kind of nursing. *Nursing Outlook, 36,* 34-37.

Alfano, G. (1964, June). Administration means working with nurses. *American Journal of Nursing, 64,* 83-85.

Beasley, T., Gerbis, P., & Lyon, J. (1995, Feb.). Workplace advocacy: New roles for nurses. *Nevada-RNformation, 4* (1), 1-2.

Bernardin, E. (1964, June). Loeb Center: As the staff nurse sees it. *American Journal of Nursing, 64,* 85-86.

Bowar-Ferres, S. (1975, May). Loeb Center and its philosophy of nursing. *American Journal of Nursing, 65,* 810.

Bryan, C. (1995, Jan.). Practice nursing: A study of the role. *Nursing Standard, 9,* 25-29.

Glasgow, G.M. (1990). Quality of care in occupational health through nursing diagnosis. *AAOHN Journal, 38* (3), 105-109.

Henderson, C. (1964, June). Can nursing care hasten recovery? *American Journal of Nursing, 64,* 80-83.

Isler, C. (1964, June). New concepts in nursing therapy: More care as the patient improves. *RN, 27,* 58-70.

Kitson, A.L. (1987). Raising standards of clinical practice: The fundamental issue of effective nursing practice. *Journal of Advanced Nursing, 12,* 321-329.

McMahon, R. (1989). Primary nursing: One to one. *Nursing Times, 85* (2), Jan. 11, 39-40.

McMahon, R. (1989, Feb. 22). Partners in care. *Nursing Times, 85* (8), 34-37.

Pearson, A., Durand, I., & Punton, S. (1988, Nov. 23). The feasibility and effectiveness of nursing beds. *Nursing Times, 84* (47), 48-50.

Pearson, A., Durand, I., & Punton, S. (1989). Determining quality in a unit where nursing is the primary intervention. *Journal of Advanced Nursing, 14,* 269-273.

Tabak, N., & Ben-Or, T. (1994). The nurse's challenge in coping with ethical dilemmas in occupational health. *Nursing Ethics, 1* (4), 208-215.

Wiggins, L.R. (1980). Lydia Hall's place in the development of theory in nursing. *Image, 12* (1), 10-12.

Wilkinson, R.A. (1994, July). A more autonomous and independent role: Primary nursing versus patient allocation. *Professional Nurse, 9,* (10), 680-684.

Correspondence

Alfano, G.J. (1984, Jan. 26). Personal correspondence.

Alfano, G.J. (1984, Feb. 15). Personal correspondence.

Oodal, D. (1996, July 12). (Secretary of the Loeb Center) Telephone interview.

Wender, B. (1984, Jan. 25). (Secretary of the Loeb Center) Telephone interview.

Other sources

Chinn, P.L., & Jacobs, M.K. (1983). *Theory and nursing.* St. Louis: Mosby.

Rogers, C. (1951). *Client-centered therapy.* Boston: Houghton Mifflin.

Rogers, C. (1961). *On becoming a person.* Boston: Houghton Mifflin.

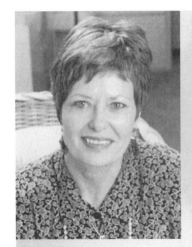

Jean Watson

Philosophy and Science of Caring

Tracey J.F. Patton, Deborah A. Barnhart, Patricia M. Bennett,
Beverly D. Porter, Rebecca S. Sloan

CREDENTIALS AND BACKGROUND OF THE THEORIST

Margaret Jean Harman Watson was born in southern West Virginia and grew up during the 1940s and 1950s in the small town of Welch, West Virginia, in the Appalachian Mountains. As the youngest of eight children, she was surrounded by an extended family-community environment.

After graduating from high school in West Virginia, she attended the Lewis-Gale School of Nursing in Roanoke, Virginia, graduating in 1961. After

The authors wish to express appreciation to Dr. Jean Watson for critiquing the chapter. A special thanks to Jean for her assistance in the revision of the introductory section of this chapter.

graduation she married her husband, Douglas, and moved west to his native state of Colorado. They have two grown daughters, Jennifer (1963) and Julie (1967). Watson and her husband have continued to live in Boulder, Colorado, since 1962.

After moving to Colorado, Watson continued her nursing education and graduate studies at the University of Colorado. She earned a B.S. in Nursing in 1964 at the Boulder campus; an M.S. in Psychiatric-Mental Health Nursing in 1966 at the Health Sciences campus; and a Ph.D. in Educational Psychology and Counseling in 1973 at the Graduate School, Boulder campus.

After Watson completed her Ph.D. degree, she joined the School of Nursing faculty of the University of Colorado Health Sciences Center in Denver, where she has served in both faculty and administrative positions. She has been Chair and Assistant Dean of the undergraduate program and she was involved in early planning and implementation of the nursing Ph.D. program in Colorado, which was initiated in 1978. She was Coordinator and Director of the Ph.D. program between 1978 and 1981. In 1981 and 1982 she pursued sabbatical studies and upon her return was Dean of the University of Colorado School of Nursing and Associate Director, Nursing Practice, University Hospital from 1983 to 1990. Currently she is Professor of Nursing and Director of the Center for Human Caring at the University of Colorado Health Sciences Center in Denver.

During her deanship she was instrumental in the development of a post-baccalaureate nursing curriculum in human caring, health, and healing, which leads to a career professional clinical doctoral degree (ND). This pilot ND program has been selected and funded as a national demonstration program by the Helene Fuld Health Trust in New York and Colorado clinical agencies. The program was implemented in 1990 as a partnership between nursing education and practice, whereby clinical and academic agencies in Colorado work jointly to simultaneously restructure nursing education and nursing practice for the future.

Dr. Watson has also helped to establish the Center for Human Caring at the University of Colorado, which is the nation's first interdisciplinary center with an overall commitment to develop and use knowledge of human caring and healing as the moral and scientific basis of clinical practice and nursing scholarship and as the foundation for efforts to transform the current health care system. The center develops and sponsors numerous clinical, educational, and community scholarship activities and projects in human caring, including national and international scholars in residence.

During her career, Watson has been active in community programs, having served as one of the early founders, clinical consultants, and members of the Board of Boulder County Hospice. The recipient of several research and advanced education federal grants and awards, Watson also has received numerous university and private grants and extramural funding for her faculty and administrative projects and scholarships in human caring.

Other honors include four honorary doctoral degrees from Assumption College, Worcester, Massachusetts (1985), the University of Akron (1987), the University of West Virginia (1996), and Göteborg University in Sweden (1996). Watson also received the high honor of Distinguished Professor of Nursing at the University of Colorado in 1992. Between 1993 and 1996, Watson served as a member of the executive committee, governing board and officer for the National League for Nursing (NLN). She served as the president of the NLN from 1995 to 1996.[34]

Dr. Watson's national and international work includes distinguished lectureships throughout the United States and in other countries at universities, including Boston College, Catholic University, Adelphi University, Columbia University-Teachers College, State University of New York, and the University of Montreal in Canada.

Her international activities include an International Kellogg Fellowship in Australia (1982), a Fulbright Research and Lecture Award to Sweden and other parts of Scandinavia (1991), and a lecture tour in the United Kingdom. She has also been involved in international projects and invitations in New Zealand, India, Thailand, Taiwan, Israel, and Japan.

Watson is also featured in several national videos on nursing theory. These include "Circles of Knowledge" and "Conversations on Caring with Jean Watson and Janet Quinn" from the NLN, "Portraits of Excellence: Nursing Theorists and their Work" from the Helene Fuld Health Trust, and "Theory in Practice" from the NLN, which features the Denver Nursing Project in Human Caring, a nurse-directed Caring Center for persons with acquired immunodeficiency syndrome (AIDS). The Denver Nursing Project in Human Caring is a clinical (caring-theory based) demonstration project of the University of Colorado Center for Human Caring/School of Nursing.[32]

Dr. Watson's publications reflect the evolution of her theory of caring. Her writings have been geared toward educating nursing students and providing them the ontological and epistomological basis for their praxis and research directions. Much of her current work began with the 1979 publication, *Nursing: The Philosophy and Science of Caring*, which she says began as class notes for a course she was developing. Although Watson refers to this book as a treatise on nursing, the nursing community considers this book a theory for nursing.

Her second major work, *Nursing: Human Science and Human Care, A Theory of Nursing*, was published in 1985 (rereleased in 1988). The purpose of this book was to address some of the conceptual and philosophical problems that still existed in nursing. She hoped that others would join her as she seeks to "elucidate the human care process in nursing, preserve the concept of the person in our science, and better our contribution to society."[31:ix]

The discrepancy in nursing between theory and practice is well known. To reduce this dichotomy, Watson proposed a philosophy and science of caring. She refers to caring as the essence of nursing practice.[9:xii]

Caring is a moral ideal rather than a task-oriented behavior and includes such elusive aspects of the actual caring occasion as the transpersonal caring relationship between the nurse and the client. The goal is the preservation of human dignity and humanity in the health care system. Watson[27:40] believes professional nursing care is developed through a combined study of the sciences and the humanities and culminates in a human care process between nurse and client that transcends time and space and has spiritual dimensions.

According to Watson, the goal of nursing is to facilitate the individual's gaining "a higher degree of harmony within the mind, body, and soul which generates self-knowledge, self-reverence, self-healing, and self-care processes while allowing increasing diversity."[31:49] Watson states that the goal is attained through the human-to-human caring process and caring transactions.

One way Watson has attempted to bridge the gap between theory and practice is through the development of the Center for Human Caring and the ND program at the University of Colorado Health Sciences Center. Both the center and the ND program provide opportunities to "integrate the arts, humanities, and social and behavioral sciences into human care and the healing process."[23:1]

THEORETICAL SOURCES

In addition to traditional nursing knowledge and the works of Nightingale, Henderson, Krueter, and Hall, Watson acknowledges the work of Leininger and Gadow[27:10] as background for her work. In her more recent work, Watson refers to the works of others such as Maslow, Heidegger, Erikson, Seyle, and Lazarus. To develop her framework, Watson drew heavily on the sciences and the humanities, providing a phenomenological, existential, and spiritual orientation.

Watson attributes her emphasis on the interpersonal and transpersonal qualities of congruence, empathy, and warmth to the views of Carl Rogers and recent transpersonal psychology writers. Rogers describes several incidents leading to the formulation of his thoughts on human behavior. One such episode involves his learning "that it is the client who knows what hurts and that the facilitator should allow the direction of the therapeutic process to come from the client."[17:11-12] Rogers[17:18-19] believed that through understanding the client would come to accept himself, an initial step toward a positive outcome. The therapist helps by clarifying and stating feelings about which the client has been unclear. To accomplish this goal, the therapist must be able to understand the meaning, feeling, and attitudes of the client. A warm interest facilitates understanding. Rogers presents an unpublished thesis by R.D. Quinn who studied recorded therapists' statements both in and out of context. Degree of understanding was judged to be high in both contexts, and Quinn[17:44] concluded that understanding is primarily a desire to understand.

Another concept of Rogerian theory is that the therapist-client relationship is more important to the outcome than adherence to traditional methods. Rogers[17:33] states:

> In my early professional years I was asking the question, How can I treat, or cure, or change this person? Now I phrase the question in this way: How can I provide a relationship which this person may use for his own personal growth?

To support his concept, Rogers notes a study by Betz and Whitehorn[1] describing the differences in degree of improvement for schizophrenic patients treated by two methods. Those patients treated by physicians who endeavored to understand the personal meaning of their patients' behavior fared better than patients of doctors who saw their clients as symptomatic of a specific diagnosis.[1:89-117,25] Additionally, Seeman's study[19] describes the effectiveness of psychotherapy when this approach is characterized by mutual affection and respect between the therapist and client.

Watson believes a strong liberal arts background is also essential to the process of holistic care for clients. She believes the study of the humanities expands the mind and increases thinking skills and personal growth. Watson[25,35] compares the current status of nursing to the mythological Danaides, who attempted to fill a broken jar with water, only to see water flow through the cracks. Until nursing merges theory and practice through combined study of the sciences and the humanities, she believes similar cracks will be evident in the scientific basis of nursing knowledge.

Yalom's 11 curative factors stimulated Watson's thinking[24:xvi] about the psychodynamic and human components that could apply to nursing and caring and, consequently, to her 10 carative factors in nursing.

Watson's work has been called a treatise, a conceptual model, a framework, and a theory. This chapter uses the terms *theory* and *framework* interchangeably.

USE OF EMPIRICAL EVIDENCE

Watson and her colleagues have attempted to study the concept of caring by collecting data to use in classifying caring behaviors, to describe the similarities and differences between what nurses consider care and what clients consider care, and to generate testable hypotheses around the concept of nursing care. They studied responses from registered nurses, student nurses, and clients to the same open-ended questionnaire covering a variety of aspects of "(1) taking care of and (2) caring about" patients. Their findings revealed a discrepancy in the values considered most important by clients, student nurses, and registered nurses. They stressed the need for further study to clarify what behaviors and values are important from each viewpoint. The study also raised a question about differences in values for persons in various situations, as well as the question of meeting minimum care needs before the quality of care can be evaluated.[25]

Watson's research into caring incorporates empiricism but emphasizes methodologies that begin with nursing phenomena rather than the natural sciences.[9:344] She used a human science, empirical phenomenology, and transcendent phenomenology in her latest work. More recently she has been investigating new language, such as metaphor and poetry, to communicate, convey, and elucidate human caring and healing.[29]

MAJOR CONCEPTS & DEFINITIONS

Watson[24:9-10] bases her theory for nursing practice on the following 10 carative factors. Each has a dynamic phenomenological component that is relative to the individuals involved in the relationship as encompassed by nursing. The first three interdependent factors serve as the "philosophical foundation for the science of caring."[24:9-10]

1. Formation of a humanistic-altruistic system of values. Humanistic and altruistic values are learned early in life but can be greatly influenced by nurse-educators. This factor can be defined as satisfaction through giving and extension of the sense of self.[24:10-12]

2. Instillation of faith-hope. This factor, incorporating humanistic and altruistic values, facilitates the promotion of holistic nursing care and positive health within the client population. It also describes the nurse's role in developing effective nurse-client interrelationships and in promoting wellness by helping the client adopt health-seeking behaviors.[24:12-16]

3. Cultivation of sensitivity to one's self and to others. The recognition of feelings leads to self-actualization through self-acceptance for both the nurse and the client. As nurses acknowledge their sensitivity and feelings, they

Continued

become more genuine, authentic, and sensitive to others.[24:16-19]

4. Development of a helping-trust relationship. The development of a helping-trust relationship between the nurse and client is crucial for transpersonal caring. A trusting relationship promotes and accepts the expression of both positive and negative feelings. It involves congruence, empathy, nonpossessive warmth, and effective communication.[24:23-41] Congruence involves being real, honest, genuine, and authentic.[24:26-28] Empathy is the ability to experience and thereby understand the other person's perceptions and feelings and to communicate those understandings.[24:28-30] Nonpossessive warmth is demonstrated by a moderate speaking volume; a relaxed, open posture; and facial expressions that are congruent with other communications.[24:30-34] Effective communication has cognitive, affective, and behavior response components.[24:24-41]

5. Promotion and acceptance of the expression of positive and negative feelings. The sharing of feelings is a risk-taking experience for both nurse and client. The nurse must be prepared for either positive or negative feelings. The nurse must recognize that intellectual and emotional understandings of a situation differ.[24:41-48]

6. Systematic use of the scientific problem-solving method for decision making. Use of the nursing process brings a scientific problem-solving approach to nursing care, dispelling the traditional image of nurses as the "doctor's handmaiden." The nursing process is similar to the research process in that it is systematic and organized.[24:51-66]

7. Promotion of interpersonal teaching-learning. This factor is an important concept for nursing in that it separates *caring* from *curing*. It allows the client to be informed and thus shifts the responsibility for one's wellness and health to the client. The nurse facilitates this process with teaching-learning techniques that are designed to enable clients to provide self-care, determine personal needs, and provide opportunities for their personal growth.[24:69-79]

8. Provision for supportive, protective, and/or corrective mental, physical, sociocultural, and spiritual environment. Nurses must recognize the infuence that internal and external environments have on the health and illness of individuals. Concepts relevant to the internal environment include the mental and spiritual well-being and sociocultural beliefs of an individual. In addition to epidemiological variables, other external variables include comfort, privacy, safety, and clean, aesthetic surroundings.[24:81-101]

9. Assistance with gratification of human needs. The nurse recognizes the biophysical, psychophysical, psychosocial, and intrapersonal needs of self and client. Clients must satisfy lower-order needs before attempting to attain higher-order ones. Food, elimination, and ventilation are examples of lower-order biophysical needs, whereas activity/inactivity and sexuality are considered lower-order psychophysical needs. Achievement and affiliation are higher-order psychosocial needs. Self-actualization is a higher order intrapersonal-interpersonal need.[24:105-203]

10. Allowance for existential-phenomenological forces. Phenomenology describes data of the immediate situation that help people understand the phenomena in question.[24:208] Existential psychology is a science of human existence that uses phenomenological analysis.[24:209] Watson considers this factor to be difficult to understand. It is included to provide a thought-provoking experience leading to a better understanding of ourselves and others.[24:205-215]

Watson believes that nurses have the responsibility to go beyond the 10 carative factors and to facilitate clients' development in the area of health promotion through preventive health actions. This goal is accomplished by teaching clients personal changes to promote health, providing situational support, teaching problem-solving methods, and recognizing coping skills and adaptation to loss.[24]

MAJOR ASSUMPTIONS

In her first book, *Nursing: The Philosophy and Science of Caring*, Watson[24:8-9] states the major assumptions of the science of caring in nursing:

1. Caring can only be effectively demonstrated and practiced interpersonally.
2. Caring consists of carative factors that result in the satisfaction of certain human needs.
3. Effective caring promotes health and individual or family growth.
4. Caring responses accept a person not only as he/she is now but for what he/she may become.
5. A caring environment offers the development of potential while allowing the person to choose the best action for himself/herself at a given time.
6. Caring is more "healthogenic" than is curing. The practice of caring integrates biophysical knowledge with knowledge of human behavior to generate or promote health and to provide ministrations to those who are ill. A science of caring therefore is complementary to the science of curing.
7. The practice of caring is central to nursing.

Gaut identified three conditions necessary for caring. These include "(1) an awareness and knowledge about one's need for care; (2) an intention to act, and actions based on knowledge; (3) a positive change as a result of caring, judged solely on the basis of welfare of others."[6:313-324] Watson expanded Gaut's work by adding two additional conditions: "an underlying value and moral commitment to care; and a will to care."[32:33]

In her second book, Watson says that "Nursing education and the health care delivery system must be based on human values and concern for the welfare of others."[32:33] To further define the social and ethical responsibilities of nursing and to explicate the human care concepts in nursing, Watson proposes the following 11 assumptions related to human care values:

1. Care and love comprise the primal and universal psychic energy.
2. Care and love, often overlooked, are the cornerstones of our humanness; nourishment of these needs fulfills our humanity.
3. The ability to sustain the caring ideal and ideology in practice will affect the development of civilization and determine nursing's contribution to society.
4. Caring for ourselves is a prerequisite to caring for others.
5. Historically, nursing has held a human-care and caring stance in regard to people with health-illness concerns.
6. Caring is the central unifying focus of nursing practice—the essence of nursing.
7. Caring, at the human level, has been increasingly deemphasized in the health care system.
8. Nursing's caring foundation has been sublimated by technological advancements and institutional constraints.
9. A significant issue for nursing today and in the future is the preservation and advancement of human care.
10. Only through interpersonal relationships can human care be effectively demonstrated and practiced.
11. Nursing's social, moral, and scientific contributions to humankind and society lie in its commitments to human care ideals in theory, practice, and research.[31:34]

THEORETICAL ASSERTIONS

According to Watson, nursing is interested in understanding health, illness, and the human experience. Within the philosophy and science of caring, she tries to define an outcome of scientific activity with regard to the humanistic aspects of life. She attempts to make nursing an interrelationship of quality of life, including death, and the prolongation of life.[24:xvii]

Watson believes nursing is concerned with health promotion and restoration and illness prevention. *Health*, more than the absence of illness, is an elusive concept because of its subjective nature.[24:219] Health refers to "unity and harmony within the mind, body, and soul"[31:48] and is associated with the "degree of congruence between the self as perceived and the self as experienced."[31:48]

According to Watson, *caring* is a nursing term, representing the factors nurses use to deliver health care to clients.[26] She states that by responding to others as unique individuals, the caring person perceives the feelings of the other and recognizes the uniqueness of the other.[26,30-32]

Using the 10 carative factors, the nurse provides care to various clients. [24:6] Each carative factor describes the caring process of how a client attains, or maintains, health or dies a peaceful death. On the other hand, Watson describes curing as a medical term referring to elimination of disease.[24:7]

In her initial work, *Nursing: The Philosophy and Science of Caring*, Watson[24:8] describes the basic premises of a science for nursing:

1. Caring (and nursing) has existed in every society. Every society has had some people who have cared for others. A caring attitude is transmitted by the culture of the profession as a unique way of coping with its environment. The opportunities for nurses to obtain advanced education and engage in higher level analyses of problems and concerns in their education and practice have allowed nursing to combine its humanistic orientation with the relevant science.
2. There is often a discrepancy between theory and practice or between the scientific and artistic aspects of caring, partly because of the disjunction between scientific values and humanistic values.

Expanding on her previous work, Watson added the following components for the context of human science theory development.[27:16]

1. A philosophy of human freedom, choice, and responsibility
2. A biology and psychology of holism (nonreducible persons interconnected with others and nature)
3. An epistemology that allows not only for empirics but also for advancement of esthetics, ethical values, intuition, and process discovery
4. An ontology of time and space
5. A context of interhuman events, processes, and relationships
6. A scientific world view that is open

As Watson's work evolves, she continued to focus more on the human care process, the transpersonal aspects of caring. The basic premises stated by Watson in *Nursing: Human Science and Human Care* are a reflection of the interpersonal-transpersonal-spiritual aspects of her work.[30,33:50-51] These aspects represent an integration of her beliefs and values about human life and provide the foundation for the further development of her theory.

1. A person's mind and emotions are windows to the soul.
2. A person's body is confined in time and space, but the mind and soul are not confined to the physical universe.
3. Access to a person's body, mind, and soul is possible as long as the person is perceived as and treated as a whole.
4. The spirit, inner self, or soul (giest) of a person exists in and for itself.
5. People need each other in a caring, loving way.
6. To find solutions it is necessary to find meanings.
7. The totality of experience at any given moment constitutes a phenomenal field.

Watson continues to work on various aspects of her theory. Currently, much of her work focuses on developing and defining ontological caring competencies.

LOGICAL FORM

The framework is presented in a logical form. It contains broad ideas and addresses many situations on the health-illness continuum. Watson's definition of *caring* as opposed to *curing* delineates nursing from medicine. This concept is helpful in classifying the body of nursing knowledge as a separate science.

The development of the theory since 1979 has been toward clarifying the person of the nurse and the person of the client. Another emphasis has been on existential-phenomenological and spiritual factors.

Watson's theory has foundational support from theorists in other disciplines, such as Rogers, Erikson, and Maslow. She is adamant in her support for nursing education that incorporates holistic knowledge from many disciplines and integrates the humanities, arts, and sciences. She believes the increasingly complex requirements of the health care system and patient needs require nurses to have a broad, liberal education. The ideals/content/theory of liberal education must be integrated into professional nursing education.[18:43]

Watson has recently incorporated dimensions of a postmodern paradigm shift throughout her theory of transpersonal caring. Modern theoretical underpinnings have been associated with concepts such as steady state maintenance, adaptation, linear interactions, and problem-based nursing practice. The postmodern approach moves beyond this point; the redefining of such a nursing paradigm leads to a more holistic, humanistic, open system wherein harmony, interpretation, and self-transcendence are the emerging directions reflected in this epistemological shift. Watson believes that nursing must be challenged to construct and co-construct ancient and new knowledge toward an ever-evolving humanity of possibilities to further clarify nursing for a new era.[33]

ACCEPTANCE BY THE NURSING COMMUNITY

Practice

Institutions that are seeking a holistic approach to nursing care are integrating many aspects of Watson's theoretical commitment to caring. An example is nursing journals that are concerned with the delivery of nursing care contain increasing numbers of articles that reference Watson and incorporate the importance of caring as an essential domain of nursing.[2:25]

The theory is being clinically validated in a variety of settings and with various populations. The clinical settings have included critical care units,[3,5,15] neonatal intensive care units,[21] and pediatric and gerontological care units.[20]

The populations have included women who have miscarried, women who have had newborns in intensive care units, and women identified as socially at risk[22]; postmyocardial infarction patients[5]; oncology patients[8]; persons with AIDS[13]; and the elderly.[4] The relationship of caring to nursing administration has also been examined.[10,14,16]

The acuity level of hospitalized individuals, the short length of hospital stays, and the increasing complexity of technology have been identified as possibly interfering with implementation of the caring theory.

Education

Watson has been active in curriculum planning at the University of Colorado. Her framework is being taught in numerous baccalaureate nursing curricula, including Bellarmine College in Louisville, Kentucky; Assumption College in Worcester, Massachusetts; Indiana State University in Terre Haute, Indiana; and Florida Atlantic University in Boca Raton, Florida. In addition, these concepts are now widely used in nursing programs in Australia, Sweden, Finland, and the United Kingdom.

Critics of the author's work have concentrated on the use of undefined terms, incomplete treatment of subject matter when describing the 10 carative factors, and a lack of attention to the pathophysiological aspect of nursing. Watson[24:xv] addresses these aspects in the preface of her second book, where she defines her intent to describe the *core* of nursing—those aspects of the nurse-client relationship resulting in a therapeutic outcome—rather than the *trim* of nursing—the procedures, tasks, and techniques used by various practice settings. With this focus, the framework is not limited to any nursing specialty.

Watson hopes her work will help nurses develop a meaningful moral and philosophical base for practice.[27:50-51] A study of Watson's framework leads the reader through a thought-provoking experience by emphasizing communication skills, use of self-transpersonal growth, attention to both nurse and patient, and the human caring process that potentiates human health and healing.

With other national and international scholars and faculty, Dr. Watson's work continues through the University of Colorado Center for Human Caring. The Center has become a focal point nationally and internationally for the continuation and further testing and implementation of caring in education, research, and clinical practice.[32]

Research

Watson and others[7,11,12,28] are attempting to research the caring framework and to arrive at empirical data amenable to research techniques. This abstract framework, however, is difficult to study concretely.

Watson believes there is often a chasm between the essential qualities and subject matter of nursing and the methods used for research. As with her concern for uniting the liberal arts with nursing education, she hopes that nursing research will incorporate and explore esthetic, metaphysical, empirical, and contextual methodologies.[9:343-344;29]

Morse, Solberg, Neander, and Bottorff[11,12] have analyzed the "caring" literature for themes related to conceptual and theoretical development. They conclude that the development of a knowledge base in Watson's caring theory has been limited by the abstractness of the concept and clinical reality in some situations (for example, the brief interactions with clients afforded by outpatient or office visits), whether caring exists in nursing situations that have yet to develop interpersonally, and whether caring is unique to nursing. Patient outcomes in caring transactions need further study.

Research and practice must focus on both subjective and objective patient outcomes in determining whether caring is the "essence of nursing." The development of behaviors and predictors of change is critical to further development of this work.

FURTHER DEVELOPMENT

Nursing research has traditionally followed the *received view* format in which single-factor methodology is compared against rigorous standards of truth, operational definitions, and observational criteria.[19,25] Watson concludes that this methodology does not apply to the multifactorial study of nursing care. She proposes that as nursing advances in its own doctoral programs, the process of scientific development will be used on itself. Nursing research will adopt the received view, reject it, and synthesize new ideas, which will result in a new nursing model for the 1990s and the next century.

Watson has identified several critical issues for future research: conditions that foster the person as an end and not a means in a highly technological society and conditions that promote caring when humanity is threatened.[27;21] This theory lends itself to creative research methodologies that assist nursing in formulating a philosophical base for professional human care concepts.

CRITIQUE
Clarity

Watson's theory is easily read and uses nontechnical language that provides clarity. In *Nursing: Human Science and Human Care*, Watson expands the philosophical nature of her theory. The reader's comprehension of her theory is enhanced by an understanding of philosophy.

Simplicity

Watson draws on a number of disciplines to formulate her theory. The reader must have an understanding of a variety of subject matters to understand the theory as it is presented. It is seen as complex when considering the existential-phenomenological nature of her work, due in part to the limited liberal arts background of many nurses and the limited integration of liberal arts in baccalaureate nursing curricula.

Generality

The theory seeks to provide a moral and philosophical basis for nursing. The scope of the framework encompasses all aspects of the health-illness continuum. In addition, the theory addresses aspects of preventing illness and experiencing a peaceful death, thereby increasing its generality. The carative factors, described by Watson, have provided important guidelines for nurse-client interactions; however, some critics have stated that the generality is limited due to the emphasis placed on the psychosocial aspects rather than on the physiological aspects of caring.

Empirical Precision

Although the framework is difficult to study empirically, Watson draws heavily on widely accepted work from other disciplines. This solid foundation strengthens her views. Watson describes her theory as descriptive. She acknowledges the newness of the theory. She welcomes input by others as she continues to develop her theory.

The theory does not lend itself to research conducted with traditional scientific methodologies. In her second book, Watson addresses the issue of methodology. The methodologies relevant to studying transpersonal caring and developing nursing as a human science and art can be classified as qualitative, naturalistic, or phenomenological. Watson does acknowledge that a combination of qualitative-quantitative inquiry may also be useful.

Derivable Consequences

Although further testing is necessary, Watson's theory continues to provide a useful and important metaphysical orientation for the delivery of nursing care. Watson's theoretical concepts, such as use of self, client-identified needs, the caring process, and the spiritual sense of being human, may help nurses and their clients find meaning and harmony in a period of increasing complexity.

CRITICAL THINKING *Activities*

Critical thinking with Watson's philosophy and science of caring offers a holistic and humanistic approach in the assessment, diagnosis, planning, implementation, and evaluation phases of the nursing process. The basis of ten carative assumptions, Watson's theory provides a framework on which nurses establish a precedence of collaboration to assist the client in gaining control, knowledge, and health. The following exercises demonstrate critical thinking from the perspective of Watson's theory.

1 Examine your own values and beliefs to ascertain how each of Watson's ten carative assumptions would fit with your own personal philosophy of caring in relation to the client, environment, health, and nursing.

2 Jonas has been hospitalized with recurrent chest pain and possible myocardial infarction. He is 47 years old and currently working two jobs as well as volunteering as a Boy Scout guide in his free time. He is married and has four children ranging in age from seven to sixteen years old. At present, he and his family are building an addition to his house, which will include an extra bedroom for his ill mother who will be coming to live with his family. Using Watson's theory as a guide, formulate a care plan that focuses on the priority diagnosis of this client and the interventions that will best meet his needs.

3 You have been chosen to serve on the curriculum revision committee within your institution. The curriculum that you will be revising is from an upper-year transition course that is intended to provide students with advanced theory and practice focused on leadership, problem-solving, and decision-making skills.

a. How will you propose development of a curriculum based on the integration of Watson's ten carative assumptions?

b. How will these factors influence your choice of content, teaching strategies, and evaluation measure for the newly proposed curriculum?

c. How do these differ from the traditional approaches formerly implemented within a behavioristic paradigm of thought?

d. What types of conflict or challenges do you foresee (for faculty and students) in implementing the newly revised curriculum?

REFERENCES

1. Betz, B.J., & Whitehorn, J.C. (1956). The relationship of the therapist to the outcome of therapy in schizophrenia. *Psychiatric Research Reports #5.* Research techniques in schizophrenia. Washington, DC: American Psychiatric Association.
2. Brenner, P., Boyd, C., Thompson, T., Cervantez, M., Buerhaus, P., & Leininger, M. (1986, Jan.). The care symposium: Considerations for nursing administrators. *JONA, 16*(1), 25-26.
3. Byrd, R. (1988). Positive therapeutic effects of intercessory prayer in a coronary care unit population. *Southern Medical Journal, 81*(7), 826-829.

4. Clayton, G. (1989). Research testing Watson's theory. In J. Riehl-Siska (Ed.), *Conceptual models for nursing practice* (pp. 245-252). Norwalk, CT: Appleton & Lange.

5. Cronin, S., & Harrison, B. (1988). Importance of nursing care behaviors as perceived by patient after myocardial infarction. *Heart and Lung, 17*(4), 374-380.

6. Gaut, D. (1983). Development of a theoretically adequate description of caring. *Western Journal of Nursing Research, 5*(4), 313-324.

7. Hester, N.O., & Ray, M.A. (1987). *Assessment of Watson's carative factors: A qualitative research study.* Paper presented at the International Nursing Research Congress, Edinburgh, Scotland.

8. Larson, P. (1987). Comparison of cancer patients' and professional nurses' perceptions of important nurse caring behaviors. *Heart and Lung, 16*(2), 187-193

9. Leininger, M. (1979). Preface. In J. Watson, *Nursing: The philosophy and science of caring.* Boston: Little, Brown.

10. Miller, K. (1987). The human care perspective in nursing administration. *Journal of Nursing Administration, 17*(2), 10-12.

11. Morse, J., Bottorff, J., Neander, W., & Solberg, S. (1991). Comparative analysis of conceptualizations and theories of caring. *Image: Journal of Nursing Scholarship, 23*(2), 119-126.

12. Morse, J., Solberg, S., Neander, W., Bottorff, J., & Johnson, J. (1990). Concepts of caring and caring as a concept. *Advances in Nursing Science, 13*(1), 1-14.

13. Neil, R. (1990). Watson's theory of caring in nursing: The rainbow of and for people living with AIDS. In M.E. Parker (Ed.), *Nursing theories in practice* (pp. 289-301). New York: National League for Nursing.

14. Nyberg, J. (1989). The element of caring in nursing administration. *Nursing Administration Quarterly, 13*(3), 9-16.

15. Ray, M. (1987). Technological caring: A new model in critical care. *Dimensions of Critical Care Nursing, 6*, 166-173.

16. Ray, M. (1989). The theory of bureaucratic caring in nursing practice in the organizational culture. *Nursing Administration Quarterly, 13*(2), 31-42.

17. Rogers, C.R. (1961). *On becoming a person: A therapist's view of psychology.* Boston: Houghton Mifflin.

18. Sakalys, J.A., & Watson, J. (1986). Professional education: Post-baccalaureate education for professional nursing. *Journal of Professional Nursing, 2*(2), 91-97.

19. Seeman, J. (1954). Counselor judgments of therapeutic process and outcome. In C.R. Rogers & R.F. Dymond (Eds.), *Psychotherapy and personality change* (pp. 272-299). Chicago: University of Chicago Press.

20. Sithichoke-Rattan, N. (1989). A clinical application of Watson's theory. *Pediatric Nursing, 15*(5), 458-462.

21. Swanson, K. (1990). Providing care in the NICU: Sometimes an act of love. *Advances in Nursing Science, 13*(1), 60-73.

22. Swanson, K. (1991). Empirical development of a middle range theory of caring. *Nursing Research, 40*(3), 161-166.

23. The dean speaks out: Center for human caring established. (1986, Dec.). *The University of Colorado School of Nursing News*, pp. 1-6.

24. Watson, J. (1979). *Nursing: The philosophy and science of caring.* Boston: Little, Brown.

25. Watson, J. (1981, July). Nursing's scientific quest. *Nursing Outlook, 29*, 413-416.

26. Watson, J. (1984). Telephone interview.

27. Watson, J. (1985). *Nursing: Human science and human care.* Norwalk, CT: Appleton-Century-Crofts.

28. Watson, J. (1985). Reflections on new methodologies for study of human care. In M. Leininger (Ed.), *Qualitative research methods in nursing* (pp. 343-349). Orlando, FL: Grune & Stratton.

29. Watson, J. (1987). Nursing on the caring edge: Metaphorical vignettes. *Advances in Nursing Science, 10*(1), 10-17.

30. Watson, J. (1988). Telephone interview.

31. Watson, J. (1988). *Nursing: Human science and human care—a theory of nursing.* New York: National League for Nursing.

32. Watson, J. (1992). Personal communication, Aug. 3, 1992.

33. Watson, J. (1995). Post modernism and knowledge development in nursing. *Nursing Science Quarterly, 8*(2), 60-64.

34. Watson, J. (1996). Telephone interview.

35. Watson, J., Burckhardt, C., Brown, L., Boock, D., & Hester, N. (1979). *A model of caring: An alternative health care model for nursing practice and research.* American Nurses Association NP-59 3W 8179190, Clinical and Scientific Sessions, Div. of Practice, Kansas City, MO, pp. 32-44.

BIBLIOGRAPHY

Books

Bevis, E.O., & Watson, J. (1989). *Toward a caring curriculum: A new pedagogy for nursing.* New York: National League for Nursing.

Chinn, P., & Watson, J. (Eds.). (1994). *Art and aesthetics of nursing.* New York: National League for Nursing.

Leininger, M., & Watson, J. (Eds.). (1990). *The caring imperative in education.* New York: National League for Nursing.

Taylor, R., & Watson, J. (Eds.). (1989). *They shall not hurt: Human suffering and human caring.* Boulder, CO: University Press of Colorado.

Watson, J. (1979). *Nursing: The philosophy and science of caring.* Boston: Little, Brown. 2nd printing (1985), Boulder, CO: University Press of Colorado.

Watson, J. (1985). *Nursing: Human science and human care.* Norwalk; CT: Appleton-Century-Crofts. 2nd printing (1988). New York: National League for Nursing. Translated into Japanese (1990).

Watson, J. (Ed.). (1994). *Applying the art and science of human caring.* New York: National League for Nursing.

Watson, J., & Ray, M. (Eds.). (1988). *The ethics of care and the ethics of cure: Synthesis in chronicity.* New York: National League for Nursing.

Chapters and monographs

Watson, J. (1980). Self losses. In F. Bower (Ed.), *Nursing and the concept of loss* (pp. 51-84). New York: Wiley.

Watson, J. (1981). Some issues related to a science of caring for nursing practice. In M. Leininger (Ed. & Author), Proceedings from National Caring Conference, Universtiy of Utah, *Caring: An essential human need* (pp. 61-67). Thorofare, NJ: Charles B. Slack.

Watson, J. (1982). The nurse-client relationship. In L. Sonstegard, K. Kowalski, & B. Jennings (Eds.), *Women's health care* (pp. 45-56). New York: Grune & Stratton.

Watson, J. (1983). Delivery and assurance of quality health care: A rights based foundation. In R. Luke, J. Krueger, & R. Madrow (Eds.), *Organization and change in health care quality assurance* (pp. 13-19). Rockville, MD: Aspen Systems.

Watson, J. (1985). Reflection on different methodologies for the future of nursing. In M. Leininger (Ed.), *Qualitative research methods in nursing* (pp. 343-349). Orlando, FL: Grune & Stratton.

Watson, J. (1987). The dream curriculum. In National League for Nursing (Ed.), *Patterns in nursing: Strategic planning for nursing education* (pp. 91-104). New York: Author.

Watson, J. (1988). A case study: Curriculum in transition. In National League for Nursing (Ed.), *Curriculum revolution: Mandate for change* (pp. 1-8). New York: Author.

Watson, J. (1988). Introduction. In J. Watson & M. Ray (Eds.), *The ethics of care and the ethics of cure: Synthesis in chronicity* (pp. 1-3). New York: National League for Nursing.

Watson, J. (1988). The professional doctorate as an entry level into practice. In National League for Nursing (Ed.), *Perspectives* (p. 41-47). New York: Author.

Watson, J. (1989). Human caring and suffering: A subjective model for health sciences. In R. Taylor & J. Watson (Eds.), *They shall not hurt* (pp. 125-135). Boulder, CO: University Press of Colorado.

Watson, J. (1989). Preface and introduction. In M. Krysl, *Midwife and other poems on caring* (p. v, vii-viii). New York: National League for Nursing.

Watson, J. (1989). Watson's philosophy and theory of human caring in nursing. In J. Riehl-Sisca (Ed.), *Conceptual models for nursing practice* (3rd ed.). (pp. 219-236). Norwalk, CT: Appleton & Lang.

Watson, J. (1990). Foreword. In L. Hill & N. Smith (Eds.), *Self care nursing: Promotion of health* (pp. xi-xii). Norwalk, CT: Appleton & Lange.

Watson, J. (1990). Preface. In *Proceedings of the 12th International Caring Conference.* New York: National League for Nursing.

Watson, J. (1990). Human caring: A public agenda. From revolution to renaissance. In J. Stevenson & T. Tripp-Reiner (Eds.), *Knowledge about care and caring: State of the art and future developments* (pp.41-48). Proceedings of a Wingspread Conference, Racine, Wisconsin, Feb. 1-3, 1989. St. Louis: American Academy of Nursing.

Watson, J. (1990). Informed moral passion. In *Proceedings for the 1989 National Forum of Doctoral Education in Nursing,* Indianapolis: Indiana University School of Nursing.

Watson, J. (1990). Preface. In M. Leininger & J. Watson (Eds.), *The caring imperative in education* (pp. xiii-xiv). New York: National League for Nursing.

Watson, J. (1990). Transformation in nursing: Bring care back to health care. In National League for Nursing (Ed.), *Curriculum revolution: Redefining the student-teacher relationship* (pp. 15-20). New York: National League for Nursing.

Watson, J. (1990). Transpersonal caring: A transcendent view of person, health, and healing. In M. Parker (Ed.), *Nursing theories in practice* (pp. 277-288). New York: National League for Nursing.

Watson, J. (1991). Preface: The caring imperative on education. In R. Neil & R. Watts (Eds.), *Caring and nursing: Explorations in feminist perspectives* (pp. ix-x). New York: National League for Nursing.

Watson, J. (1991). Introduction. In M. Leininger, *Theory of transcultural nursing.* New York: National League for Nursing.

Watson, J. (1992). Notes on nursing: Guidelines for caring then and now. In F. Nightingale, *Notes on nursing.* Philadelphia: J.B. Lippincott.

Watson, J. (1992). Prelude. In E. Gee, *The light around the dark.* New York: National League for Nursing.

Watson, J. (1993). Foreword. In N. Diekelman, *Transforming nursing education.* New York: National League for Nursing.

Watson, J. (1994). A frog, a rock, a ritual: An eco-caring cosmology. In E. Schuster & C. Brown (Eds.), *Caring and environmental connection.* New York: National League for Nursing.

Watson, J. (1994). Foreword/chapter. In C. Johns (Ed.), *The Burford NDU model. Caring in practice.* Oxford: Blackwell Scientific.

Watson, J. (1994). Poeticizing as truth through language. In P.L. Chinn & J. Watson (Eds.), *Art and aesthetics in nursing* (pp. 3-17). New York: National League for Nursing.

Watson, J. (1996). Beyond art & science. In D. Marks-Mara (Ed.), *Reconstructing nursing: Beyond art & science.* London: Bailliere Tindall. In press.

Watson, J. (1996). Poeticizing as truth on nursing inquiry. In J. Kikuchi, H. Simmons, & D. Romyn (Eds.), *Truth on nursing inquiry* (pp. 125-139). Thousand Oaks, CA: Sage.

Watson, J., & Bevis, E. (1990). Coming of age for a new age. In N. Chaska (Ed.), *The nursing profession: Turning points* (pp. 100-105). St. Louis: Mosby.

Watson, J., & Chinn, P.L. (1994). Art and aesthetics as passage between centuries. In P.L. Chinn & J. Watson (Eds.), *Art and aesthetics in nursing* (pp. xiii-xviii). New York: National League for Nursing.

Watson, J., & Chinn, P. (1994). Introduction to aesthetics and art of nursing. In P. L. Chinn & J. Watson (Eds.), *Anthology on art and aesthetics in nursing.* New York: National League for Nursing.

Watson, J., Burckhardt, C., Brown, L., Bloch, D., & Hester, N. (1979). A model of caring: An alternative health care model for nursing practice and research. *Clinical and Scientific Sessions* (pp. 32-44). Kansas City, MO: American Nurses Association, Division of Practice.

Watson, J., et al. (1994). *Overview of caring theory.* In Watson, J. (Ed.), *Applying the art and science of human caring.* New York: National League for Nursing.

Journal articles

Carozza, V., Congdon, J.A., & Watson, J. (1978, Nov.). An experimental educationally sponsored pilot internship program. *Journal of Nursing Education, 17,* 14-20.

Krysl, M., & Watson, J. (1988, Jan.). Poetry on caring and addendum on center for human caring. *Advances in Nursing Science, 10*(2), 12-17.

Sakalys, J., & Watson, J. (1985, Sep./Oct.). New directions in higher education. A review of trends. *Journal of Professional Nursing, 1*(5), 293-299.

Sakalys, J., & Watson, J. (1986, Mar./Apr.). Professional education: Post-baccalaureate education for professional nursing. *Journal of Professional Nursing, 2*(2), 91-97.

Watson, J. (1968, Feb.). Death—A necessary concern for nurses. *Nursing Outlook* (47-48). Reprinted in *The dying patient: A nursing perspective.* (Contemporary Nursing Series, 1972, 196-200). New York: American Journal of Nursing Publication Co.

Watson, J. (1973, May). Self examination—A necessary concern for counselors. *Awareness,* a journal of the Colorado Personnel and Guidance Association, Denver, CO.

Watson, J. (1976). Research and literature on children's responses to injections: Some general nursing implications. *Pediatric Nursing, 2*(1), 7-8.

Watson, J. (1976). Research: Question-Answer. Creative approach to researchable questions. *Nursing Research, 25*(6), 439.

Watson, J. (1976, Jan./Feb.). The quasirational element in conflict: A review of selected conflict literature. *Nursing Research, 25,* 19-23.

Watson, J. (1977). Follow-up study of University of Colorado undergraduate nursing program. *Colorado Nurse, 77*(1), 6-19.

Watson, J. (1978). Conceptual systems of undergraduate nursing students compared with college students at large and practicing nurses. *Nursing Research, 27*(3), 151-155.

Watson, J. (1979). Research answer. Content analysis. *Western Journal of Nursing Research, 1*(3), 214-219.

Watson, J. (1980). Response to review of *Nursing: Philosophy and science of caring. Western Journal of Nursing Research, 2*(2), 514-515.

Watson, J. (1980). Review of *Starting point: An introduction to the dialectic of existence. Western Journal of Nursing Research, 2*(3), 637-638.

Watson, J. (1981). Conceptual systems of students and practicing nurses. *Western Journal of Nursing Research, 3*(2), 172-192.

Watson, J. (1981). The lost art of nursing. *Nursing Forum, 20*(3), 244-249 (1983 release).

Watson, J. (1981). Nursing's scientific quest. *Nursing Outlook, 29*(7), 413-416.

Watson, J. (1981). Response to *Conceptual systems, students, practitioner. Western Journal of Nursing Research, 3*(2), 197-198.

Watson, J. (1981, Aug.). Professional identity crisis—Is nursing finally growing up? *American Journal of Nursing, 81,* 1488-1490.

Watson, J. (1982, Aug.). Traditional v. tertiary: Ideological shifts in nursing education. *The Australian Nurses Journal, 12*(2), 44-46.

Watson, J. (1983, Fall). Commentary on instructor directed research model. *Western Journal of Nursing Research, 5*(4), 310-311.

Watson, J. (1987). Academic and clinical collaboration: Advancing the art and science of human caring. *Communicating Nursing Research,* Vol. 20, *Collaboration in Nursing Research: Advancing the Science of Human Care* (pp. 1-16). Western Institute of Nursing. Proceedings of the Western Society for Research in Nursing Conference, Tempe, AZ.

Watson, J. (1987). Review of *Health as expanding consciousness. Journal of Profesional Nursing, 3*(5), 315.

Watson, J. (1987). Review of Myron F. Weiner, MD (Author), *Practical psychotherapy. Journal of Psychosocial Nursing and Mental Health Services, 25*(3), 42.

Watson, J. (1987, Oct.). Nursing on the caring edge: Metaphorical vignettes. *Advances in Nursing Science,* 10-18.

Watson, J. (1988). New dimensions of human caring theory. *Nursing Science Quarterly, 1*(4), 175-181.

Watson, J. (1988). Human caring as moral context for nursing education. *Nursing and Health Care, 9*(8), 422-425.

Watson, J. (1988). Response to *Caring and practice. Construction of the nurses' world. Scholarly Inquiry for Nursing Practice: An International Journal, 2*(3), 217-221.

Watson, J. (1988, July). Of nurses, women, and the devaluation of caring. *Review of Images of Nurses: Perspectives for history, art, and literature. Medical Humanities Review, 2*(2), 60-62.

Watson, J. (1989, Oct.). Keynote address: Caring theory. *Journal of Japan Academy of Nursing Science, 9*(2), 29-37.

Watson, J. (1990). Caring knowledge and informed moral passion. *Advances in Nursing Science, 13*(1), 15-24.

Watson, J. (1990). The moral failure of the patriarchy. *Nursintg Outlook, 28*(2), 62-66.

Watson, J. (1990). Reconceptualizing nursing ethics: A response. *Scholarly Inquiry for Nursing Practice: An International Journal, 4*(3), 219-221.

Watson, J. (1991). From revolution to renaissance. *Revolution: Journal of Nurse Empowerment, 1*(1), 94-100.

Watson, J. (1991). Robb, Dock, and Nutting: I wish I'd been there. In T.A. Kippenbrock, I wish I'd been there: A sense of nursing history. *Nursing & Health Care, 12*(4), 210.

Watson, J. (1992, Summer). Caring, virtue through a foundation for nursing ethics. A response to Pamela Salsberry, *Scholarly Inquiry for Nursing Practice: An International Journal, 6*(2), 169-171.

Watson, J. (1993). Dr. Jean Watson with E. Henderson—An interview. *Alberta Association of Registered Nurses Newsletter, 49,*(6), 10-12.

Watson, J. (1992). Response to *Caring, virtue, theory, and a foundation for nursing ethics. Scholarly Inquiry for Nursing Practice: An International Journal, 6*(2), 169-171.

Watson, J. (1993). Should NPs, CNM, and CNAs, etc., add graduate credentials? *National League for Nursing. Open Mind, 2*(3), 2.

Watson, J. (1994). Have we arrived or are we on our way out? Promises, possibilities, and paradigms. (Invited editorial). *Image: Journal of Nursing Scholarship, 26*(2), 86.

Watson, J. (1994). Guest editorial. *Nursing praxis in New Zealand, 9*(1), 2-5.

Watson, J. (1994). Postmodern crisis in science and method. Proceedings of National Insitutes of Health-Office of Alternative Medicine Conference, Bethesda, MD.

Watson, J. (1995). A Fulbright in Sweden: Runes, academics, archetypal motifs, and other things. *Image: Journal of Nursing Scholarship, 27*(1), 71-75.

Watson, J. (1995). Advanced nursing practice and what might be. *Journal of Nursing & Health Care, 16*(2), 78-83.

Watson, J. (1995). Concerning the spiritual in caring. *British Journal of Nursing.* A publication effort with the Scottish Highlands Center for Human Caring and the University of Colorado School of Nursing Center for Human Caring. In press.

Watson, J. (1995). Postmodernism and knowledge development in nursing. *Nursing Science Quarterly, 8*(2), 60-64.

Watson, J. (1995, July). Nursing's caring-healing model as exemplar for alternative medicine. *Journal of Alternative Therapies in Health and Medicine, 1*(3), 64-69.

Watson, J. (1995, Aug.). A yearning for new debates. *National League for Nursing Update, 1*(3), 6-8.

Watson, J. (1996). Nursing, caring-healing paradigm. In D. Pesat (Ed.), *Capsules of comments in psychiatric nursing.* St. Louis: Mosby.

Watson, J. (1996, May). The wait, the wonder, the watch: Caring in a transplant unit. *Journal of Clinical Nursing, 5*(3), 199-200.

Watson, J., et al. (1995). The wait, the wonder, the watch: caring in a transplant unit. *Journal of Clinical Nursing, 5*(3), 199-200.

Watson, J., & Phillips, S. (1992, Jan.-Feb.). A call for educational reform: Colorado nursing doctorate model as exemplar. *Nursing Outlook, 40*(1), 20-26.

Abstracts and other publications

Bevis, E., & Watson, J. (1989). *Coming of age for a new age (Abstract).* International Council of Nurses, 19th Quadrennial Congress. Seoul, Korea.

Watson, J. (1975, Dec.). Invitational farewell address to graduating class of 1975. *CU School of Nursing Commencement Exercise Bulletin.*

Watson, J. (1977, Feb.). Preparation of faculty for nurse practitioner role. *The Future of Nurse Practitioners,* Proceedings of WICHE Conference. Boulder, CO: WICHE.

Watson, J. (1978, Jan.). Integration of practitioner skills in an undergraduate nursing curriculum. Proceedings of HEW, Division of Nursing Conference, Denver, CO.

Watson, J. (1979, Dec.). Terminal Progress Report, HEW Research Project, Division of Nursing Research, Conceptual Systems, Students, Practitioners, NU-000590.

Watson, J. (1981, April 14). The need to clarify faculty governance. *Silver and Gold Record* (p. 2), University of Colorado publication.

Watson, J. (1982). A hospice home care program. *Kellogg Publication (No. 2).* Centre for Advanced Studies in Health Sciences, W.A.I.T., Western Australia, June 1982. (Based on presentation at International Conference—Care of Dying in Australia and Third World, Perth, Western Australia.)

Watson, J. (1982). Changing demands and perspectives in nursing education. *Kellogg Publication (No. 4).* Centre for Advanced Studies in Health Sciences, W.A.I.T., Western Australia.

Watson, J. (1982). Ethical issues in nursing and health sciences. *Kellogg Publication (No. 6).* Centre for Advanced Studies in Health Sciences, W.A.I.T., Western Australia.

Watson, J. (1982). Final Report. Visiting Kellogg Fellow Centre for Advanced Studies Division of Health Sciences. Western Australian Institute of Technology, Bentley, Western Australia.

Watson, J. (1982). Ideological shifts between traditional hospital training and tertiary nursing education. *Kellogg Publication (No. 7).*Centre for Advanced Studies in Health Sciences, W.A.I.T., Western Australia.

Watson, J. (1982). Issues of interdisciplinary health education and practice. *Kellogg Publication (No. 3).* Centre for Advanced Studies in Health Sciences, W.A.I.T., Western Australia.

Watson, J. (1982). Nursing's "new" art and "new" science. *Kellogg Publication (No. 5).* Centre for Advanced Studies in Health Sciences, W.A.I.T., Western Australia.

Watson, J. (1982). Review of *The misguided cell. Kellogg Publication (No. 8).* Centre for Advanced Studies in Health Sciences. Sunderland, MA: Sinauer Associates.

Watson, J. (1982). Understanding loss and grief. *Kellogg Publication (No. 1).* Centre for Advanced Studies in Health Sciences, W.A.I.T., Western Australia, June, 1982. (Based on presentation at International Conference—Care of Dying in Australia and Third World, Perth, Western Australia.)

Watson, J. (1983-1984). University of Colorado planning directions for year 2000. *University of Colorado School of Nursing Newsletter.*

Watson, J. (1984-1990). The Dean speaks out. *University of Colorado School of Nursing Newsletter* (Dean's column).

Watson, J. (1985, Jan.). Nursing education and current trends—Needs and supply data. Report to Colorado Commission on Higher Education.

Watson, J. (1989). *Humanitarian–human caring paradigm for nursing education (Abstract).* International Council of Nurses, 19th Quadrennial Congress. Seoul, Korea.

Watson, J. (1989, Sep. 11). Colorado shows leadership in solving the nursing crisis (Guest editorial). *Boulder Daily Camera.*

Watson, J. (1993). Poeticizing as truth. Proceedings of 1993 Institute for Philosophical Nursing, University of Alberta, Canada.

Watson, J. (1995). President's message: Challenges and summons from within and without. *Journal of Nursing & Health Care, 16*(6), 340. (Official publication of the National League for Nursing.)

Watson, J. (1995, Sep./Oct.). President's message: Visioning on: Toward action and transformation. *Journal of Nursing & Health Care, 16*(5), 290. (Official publication of the National League for Nursing.)

Watson, J. (1996, March/April). President's message: From discipline specific to "inter" to "multi" to "transdisciplinary" health care education and practice. *Journal of Nursing & Health Care, 17*(2), 0-91. (Official publication of the National League for Nursing.)

Watson, J. (1996, May). Review of the book *Healing nutrition,* Kegan, L. *Journal Alternative Therapies Health & Medicine, 2*(3), 91.

Unpublished manuscript

Watson, J. (1973). The effect of feelings and various forms of feedback upon conflict in a political group problem-solving situation. Unpublished doctoral dissertation, University of Colorado.

Audiovisual or media productions

Watson, J. (1974). Interview of patient with progressive-permanent threat to steady state maintenance—Mr. J. (Audiotape). University of Colorado School of Nursing Learning Resource Laboratory, Denver.

Watson, J. (1981, Fall). A phenomenological approach to person [Videotape]. University of Colorado Health Sciences Center Educational Resources Production, Denver.

Watson, J. (1987, Feb.). The balance between objectivity and caring [Audiotape]. The Value of Many Voices Conference, Rose Medical Center, The Center for Applied Biomedical Ethics, Denver, CO.

Watson, J. (1988). Center for Human Caring Video. University of Colorado Health Sciences Center, School of Nursing.

Watson, J. (1994). *Applying the art and science of human caring.* National League for Nursing in conjunction with the University of Colorado, Center for Human Caring, New York.

Watson, J., Chinn, P., & Schroeder, C. (1992). A dialogue with nursing theorists. University of Colorado Health Sciences Center Production (President's Grant).

Watson, J, Peterson, C., & Walsh, K. (1974, Nov.). Surgical preparation of hospitalized child [Videotape]. University of Colorado Medical Center Educational Resources Production, Denver.

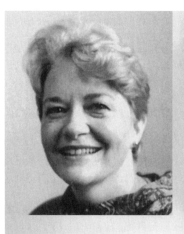

$\mathcal{P}$atricia Benner

From Novice to Expert: Excellence and Power in Clinical Nursing Practice

Jullette C. Mitre, Sr. Judith E. Alexander, Susan L. Keller

CREDENTIALS AND BACKGROUND OF THE THEORIST

Patricia Benner was born in Hampton, Virginia, and spent her childhood in California, where she received her early and professional education. Majoring in nursing, she obtained a bachelor of arts degree from Pasadena College in 1964. In 1970, she earned a master's degree in nursing, with her major emphasis in medical-surgical nursing from the University of California, San Francisco School of Nursing. She worked as a research assistant to Richard Lazarus at the University of California, Berkeley, while working on her

The authors wish to express appreciation to Patricia Benner for critiquing the original chapter.

Ph.D. in stress, coping, and health, which was conferred in 1982.

Benner has a wide range of clinical experience including acute medical-surgical, critical care, and home health care. She has held staff and head nurse positions.

Benner has a rich background in research and began this part of her career in 1970 as a postgraduate nurse researcher in the school of nursing at the University of California, San Francisco. In 1982, Benner achieved the position of associate professor in the Department of Physiological Nursing at the University of California, San Francisco, and in 1989 was tenured to professor, a position she currently holds. She teaches primarily at the doctoral and master's levels and serves on 8 to 10 dissertation committees per year.

Benner acknowledges that her thinking in nursing has been greatly influenced by Virginia Henderson. Henderson[32] writes that Benner's *From Novice to Expert* as clinically focused research might materially affect practice and preparation of nurses for practice. The foreword to Benner's work *The Primacy of Caring: Stress and Coping in Health and Illness*[21] was written by Virginia Henderson.

The most recent book by Benner, Tanner, and Chesla, *Expertise in Nursing Practice: Caring, Clinical Judgment, and Ethics* (1996), is in many ways a continuation and expansion of *From Novice to Expert*. These authors provide several implications for nursing administration, practice, and education. The foreword to this work was written by Barbara Stevens Barnum. She writes, "This work continues to challenge our traditional understanding of what it means to know, to be, and to act skillfully and ethically in nursing practice. Equally important, the book enables the reader to see how we might begin to shape our systems to better accommodate expert caring work. One of the truths of learning made clear by the work is that clinical learning is a dialogue between principles and practice."[3:vii-viii]

Hubert Dreyfus, a philosophy professor at Berkeley, introduced Benner to phenomenology. Stuart Dreyfus, in operations research, and Herbert Dreyfus, in philosophy, developed the Dreyfus Model of Skill Acquisition, which Benner applied in her work *From Novice to Expert*.[6] She credits Jane Rubin's scholarship, teaching, and colleagueship as sources of inspiration and influence, especially in relationship to the works of Heidegger and Kierkegaard. R.S. Lazarus, with whom she worked at Berkeley, has involved her in the field of stress and coping. Judith Wrubel has been a participant and coauthor with Benner for years, collaborating on the ontology of caring and caring practices.

Benner has published extensively and has been the recipient of numerous honors and awards, including the 1984 and 1988 *American Journal of Nursing* Book of the Year awards for *From Novice to Expert* and *The Primacy of Caring*, respectively.

The book *The Crisis of Care: Affirming and Restoring Caring Practice in the Helping Professions*, edited

by Susan S. Phillips and Patricia Benner, was selected for the CHOICE list of Outstanding Academic Books for 1995. Benner's books have been translated into eight languages. Several of her articles have also been translated and read worldwide.

In 1985 Benner was inducted into the American Academy of Nurses; in 1989 she received the National League for Nursing's Linda Richards Award for Leadership in Education. In 1990, she received the Excellence in Nursing Research/Education Award from the Organization of Nurse Executives–California. She also received the Alumnus of the Year Award from Point Loma Nazarene College (formerly Pasadena College) in 1993. In 1994, Benner became an Honorary Fellow in the Royal College of Nursing, United Kingdom. In 1995, she was the faculty member recognized at the University of California, San Francisco, for her contribution to nursing science and research. She was awarded The Helen Nahm Research Lecture Award. She is invited worldwide to lecture and lead workshops on health, stress and coping, skill acquisition, and ethics.

Benner expressed that nursing is a cultural paradox in a highly technical society and that we are slow to value and articulate caring practices. She feels that the value of extreme individualism makes it difficult to perceive the brilliance of caring in expert nursing practice.

THEORETICAL SOURCES

Benner studied clinical nursing practice in an attempt to discover and describe the knowledge embedded in nursing practice, that is, that knowledge that accrues over time in a practice discipline, and to describe the difference between practical and theoretical knowledge[6:1] One of the first theoretical distinctions Benner made was related to theory itself. Benner stated that knowledge development in a practice discipline "consists of extending practical knowledge (know-how) through theory-based scientific investigations and through the charting of the existent 'know-how' developed through clinical experience in the practice of that discipline."[6:3]

She believes that nurses have been delinquent in documenting their clinical learning and "this lack of charting of our practices and clinical observations deprives nursing theory of the uniqueness and richness of the knowledge embedded in expert clinical practice."[5:36] It is the description of the know-how of nursing practice that Benner has contributed.

Scientists have long distinguished interactional causal relationships as "knowing that" from "knowing how." Citing philosophers of science Kuhn and Polanyi, Benner emphasized the difference in "knowing how," a practical knowledge that may elude formulations, and "knowing that," or theoretical explanations.[6:2] "Knowing that" is the way one comes to know by establishing causal relationships between events. "Knowing how" is that skill acquisition that may defy the "knowing that," that is, one may know how before the development of a theoretical explanation. Benner stated that practical knowledge may extend theory or be developed ahead of scientific formulas. Clinical situations are always more varied and complicated than theoretical accounts, and therefore clinical practice is an area of inquiry and knowledge development. Clinical practice embodies the notion of excellence; by studying it we can uncover new knowledge. Nursing must develop the knowledge base of its practice (know-how) and through scientific investigation and observation begin to record and develop the know-how of clinical expertise. In an ideal world, practice and theory set up a dialogue that creates new possibilities. Theory is derived from practice and then practice is altered or extended by theory.

Dreyfus and Dreyfus's (1980, 1986) Model of Skill Acquisition and Skill Development was adapted by Benner to clinical nursing practice. The Dreyfus model was developed by Stuart and Hubert Dreyfus, both professors at the University of California at Berkeley. The model is situational and describes five levels of skill acquisition and development: novice, advanced beginner, competent, proficient, and expert. The model posits that in movement through the levels of skill acquisition, changes in four aspects of performance occur: (1) movement from a reliance on abstract principles and rules to use of past, concrete experience; (2) shift from reliance on analytical, rule-based thinking to intuition; (3) change in the learner's perception of the situation from one in

which it is viewed as a compilation of equally relevant bits to an increasingly complex whole in which certain parts are relevant; and (4) passage from detached observer, standing outside the situation, to one of a position of involvement, fully engaged in the situation.[18:14] The performance level can be determined only by consensual validation of expert judges and the assessment of the outcomes of the situation.[6:293]

In subsequent research further explicating the Dreyfus model, Benner identified two interrelated aspects of practice that also distinguish the levels of practice from advanced beginner to expert. First, clinicians at different levels of practice live in different clinical worlds, recognizing and responding to different guides for action. Second, clinicians develop what Benner terms agency, or the sense of responsibility toward the patient, and evolve into becoming a member of the health care team.[18:14]

Benner attempted to highlight the growing edges of clinical knowledge rather than to describe a typical nurse's day. Benner's explanation of nursing practice goes beyond the rigid application of rules and theories and instead is based on "reasonable behavior that responds to the demands of a given situation."[6:xx] The skills acquired through nursing experience and the perceptual awareness expert nurses develop as decision makers from the "gestalt of the situation" lead them to follow their hunches as they search for evidence to confirm the subtle changes they observe in patients.[6:xviii]

The concept of experience defined as the outcome when preconceived notions are challenged, refined, or refuted in the situation is based on Heidegger and Gadamer.[31:8] As the nurse gains experience, clinical knowledge becomes a blend of practical and theoretical knowledge. Expertise develops as the clinician tests and modifies principle-based expectations in the actual situation. Heidegger's influence is evident in this and in Benner's subsequent writings on the primacy of caring. Benner refutes the dualistic Cartesian descriptions of mind-body person and espouses Heidegger's phenomenological description of person as a self-interpreting being who is defined by concerns, practices, and life experiences. Persons are always situated, that is, engaged meaningfully in the context of where they are. Persons come to situations with an understanding of the self in the world. Heidegger called the kind of knowing that occurs when one is involved in the situation *practical knowledge*. Persons share background meanings, skills, and habits derived from their cultural practices. Benner and Wrubel state: "Skilled activity, which is made possible by our embodied intelligence, has been long regarded as 'lower' than intellectual, reflective activity" but argue that intellectual, reflective capacities are dependent on embodied knowing.[21:43] Embodied knowing and the meaning of being are premises for the capacity to care; things matter to us and "cause us to be involved in and defined by our concerns."[21:42]

While doing her doctoral studies at Berkeley, Benner was a research assistant to Richard S. Lazarus, who is known for his development of stress and coping theory. As part of Lazarus's larger study, Benner conducted a study of midcareer men's meaning of work and coping, which was published as *Stress and Satisfaction on the Job: Work Meanings and Coping of Mid-Career Men*.[22] In this study *coping* is defined as a form of practical knowledge, and it was determined that work meanings influence what is experienced as stress and what coping options are available to the individual.

Lazarus's Theory of Stress and Coping is described as phenomenological, that is, the person is understood to constitute and be constituted by meanings. Stress is described as the disruption of meanings, and coping is what the person does about the disruption. Both doing something and refraining from doing anything about the stressful situation are ways of coping. Coping is bounded by the meanings inherent in what the person counts as stressful. The person must be understood as a "participant self" in a situation that is shaped by reflective and nonreflective meanings and concerns. "The way the person is *in* the situation sets up different possibilities."[21:63] Benner uses this key concept to describe clinical nursing practice in terms of nurses making a positive difference by being in the situation in a caring way.

USE OF EMPIRICAL EVIDENCE

Benner's early work focused on the anticipatory socialization of nurses. Benner and Kramer[16] studied the differences between nurses who worked in special care units and those who worked in regular hospital units. She was a research consultant for a nursing activity study to determine the use and productivity of nursing personnel in 1974 and 1975. Concurrently, she was a consultant on a study of new nurse work-entry. Benner and Benner[15] conducted a systematic evaluation of the competencies, the job-finding, and work-entry problems of new graduate nurses. Benner also studied methods of increasing teacher competencies through the use of a mobile microteaching laboratory.

From 1978 to 1981 she was the author and project director of a federally funded grant, "Achieving Methods of Intraprofessional Consensus, Assessment and Evaluation," known as the AMICAE Project. This research led to the publication of *From Novice to Expert*[6] and numerous articles. Benner and Wrubel have further explained and developed the background to this study in *The Primacy of Caring: Stress and Coping in Health and Illness,* "an interpretive theory of nursing practice as it is concerned with helping patients cope with the stress of illness."[21:7] The primacy of caring is three-pronged "as the producer of both stress and coping in the lived experience of health and illness, . . . as the enabling condition of nursing practice (indeed any practice), and the ways that nursing practice based in such caring can positively affect the outcome of an illness."[21:7]

Benner[11] continues to conduct research focusing on practical knowledge or skilled clinical knowledge developed by practicing nurses and the stress and coping techniques of patients with chronic illness. Currently she is investigating end-of-life decision making and care of the dying in critical care.[14]

Benner directed the AMICAE Project to develop evaluation methods for participating schools of nursing and hospitals in the San Francisco area. It was an interpretive descriptive study that led to the use of Dreyfus's five levels of competency to describe skill acquisition in clinical nursing practice. In describing the interpretive approach, Benner stated that a rich description of nursing practice from observation and narrative accounts of actual nursing practice provide the test for interpretation (hermeneutics). The nurses' descriptions of patient care situations in which they made a positive difference "present the uniqueness of nursing as a discipline and an art."[6:xxvi] Over 1200 nurse participants completed questionnaires and interviews and were observed by trained researchers. Twenty-one paired preceptor-preceptee interviews about patient care situations they had in common were conducted with beginning nurses and nurses who were recognized for their expertise. "The research was aimed at discovering if there were distinguishable, characteristic differences in the novice's and expert's descriptions of the same clinical incident."[6:14] Further interviews and participant observations were conducted with 51 nurse-clinicians and other newly graduated nurses and senior nursing students to "describe characteristics of nurse performance at different stages of skill acquisition."[6:15] The purpose "of the inquiry has been to uncover meanings and knowledge embedded in skilled practice. By bringing these meanings, skills, and knowledge into public discourse new knowledge and understandings are constituted."[6:218]

The Dreyfus Model of Skill Acquisition was developed as a result of studying the performance of pilots in emergency situations and chess players. In applying the model to nursing, Benner noted that skilled nursing requires a sound educational base that allows for a safer and quicker experience-based skill acquisition. Skill and skilled practice, as defined by Benner, means skilled nursing interventions and clinical judgment skills in actual clinical situations. In no case does this refer to context-free psychomotor skills or other demonstrable enabling skills outside the context of nursing practice.

Thirty-one competencies emerged from analysis of the transcripts of interviews with nurses's detailed descriptions of patient care episodes, including their intentions and interpretations of the events. From these competencies identified from actual practice situations, the following seven domains were inductively derived on the basis of similarity of function and intent:

- The helping role
- The teaching-coaching function
- The diagnostic and patient-monitoring function

- Effective management of rapidly changing situations
- Administering and monitoring therapeutic interventions and regimens
- Monitoring and ensuring the quality of health care practices
- Organizational work-role competencies[6:46]

Each of these domains was described with the related competencies from the exemplars describing nursing practice.

Benner extended her research presented in *From Novice to Expert: Excellence and Power in Clinical Nursing Practice* (1984) and presents the work in the book *Expertise in Nursing Practice: Caring, Clinical Judgment, and Ethics* (1996). The book is based on a 6-year study of 130 hospital nurses, primarily critical care nurses, examining the acquisition of clinical expertise and the nature of clinical knowledge, clinical inquiry, clinical judgment, and expert ethical comportment.[19:xiii] The key aims of the study were to:

1. Delineate the practical knowledge embedded in expert practice
2. Describe the nature of skill acquisition in critical care nursing practice
3. Identify institutional impediments and resources for the development of expertise in nursing practice
4. Begin to identify educational strategies that encourage the development of expertise[19:xvi]

Benner states, "In the study we found that examining the nature of the nurse's agency, by which we mean the sense and possibilities for acting in particular clinical situations, gave new insights about how perception and action are both shaped by a practice community."[19:xiii] As a result of the study, there was a clearer understanding of the distinctions between engagement with a problem or situation and the requisite nursing skills of involvement. It appears that the requisite nursing skills of involvement with patients and families are learned over time experientially.[19:xiii] The skill of involvement with patients and families seem central in gaining nursing expertise. And researchers came to see the interlinkage of clinical and ethical decision making—how one's notions of good and poor outcomes and visions of excellence shape clinical judgments and actions.[19:xiv]

Novice In the novice stage of skill acquisition from the Dreyfus model, one has no background experience of the situation in which one is involved. Context-free rules and objective attributes must be given to guide performance. There is difficulty discerning between relevant and irrelevant aspects of a situation. Generally, this level applies to students of nursing, but Benner has suggested that nurses at higher levels of skill in one area of practice could be classified at the novice level if placed in an unfamiliar area or situation.[6:20-21]

Advanced Beginner The advanced beginner stage in the Dreyfus model develops when one can demonstrate marginally acceptable performance, having coped with enough real situations to note, or to have pointed out by a mentor, the recurring meaningful components of the situation. The advanced beginner has enough experience to grasp aspects of the situation.[6:291] Unlike attributes and features, aspects cannot be completely objectified because they require experience based on recognition in the context of the situation.

Nurses functioning at this level are rule guided and task-completion oriented and have difficulty grasping the current patient situation in terms of the larger perspective. However, Dreyfus and Dreyfus state, "Through practical experience in concrete situations with meaningful elements which neither the instructor nor student can define in terms of objective features, the advanced beginner starts intuitively to recognize these elements when they are present. We call these newly recognized elements 'situational' to distinguish them from the objective elements of the skill domain that the beginner can recognize prior to seeing concrete examples."[26:38].

Clinical situations are viewed as a test of the nurses' abilities and the demands it placed on them rather than in terms of the patient needs and responses.[18:17] Advanced beginners feel highly responsible for managing patient care yet still largely rely on the help of those more experienced.[18:19] Benner places most newly graduated nurses at this level.

Competent Through learning from actual practice situations and by following the actions of others, the advanced beginner moves to the competent level.[18:19] The competent stage of the Dreyfus model is typified by considerable conscious and deliberate planning that determines which aspects of the current and future situations are important and which can be ignored.[6:292]

"Consistency, predictability, and time management are important, and gaining a sense of mastery through planning and predictability is the accomplishment."[18:20] There is an increased level of efficiency but "the focus is on time management and the nurse's organization of the task world rather than on timing in relation to the patient's needs."[18:20] The competent nurse may display hyperresponsibility for the patient, often more than is realistic, and exhibit an ever-present and critical view of the self.[18:23]

The competent stage is most pivotal in clinical learning because it is at this stage that the learner must begin to recognize patterns and determine which elements of the situation warrant attention and which can be ignored. The competent nurse devises new rules and reasoning procedures for a plan while, at the same time, applying already learned rules for action on the basis of the relevant facts of that situation. To become proficient, the competent performer must allow the situation to guide responses.[26:39-40] Study points to the importance of active teaching and learning in the competent stage to coach nurses making the transition from competency to proficiency.

Proficient At the proficient stage of the Dreyfus model, the performer perceives the situation as a whole (the total picture) rather than in terms of aspects, and the performance is guided by maxims. The proficient level is a qualitative leap beyond the competent. Now the performer recognizes the most salient aspects and has an intuitive grasp of the situation based on background understanding.[6:297]

Nurses at this level demonstrate a new ability to see changing relevance in a situation including the recognition and the implementation of skilled responses to the situation as it evolves. They no

Major Concepts & Definitions—cont'd

longer rely on preset goals to organize and they demonstrate an increased confidence in their own knowledge and abilities.[18:23-24] At the proficient stage, there is much more involvement with the patient and family. The proficient stage is a transition into expertise.[19:141]

Expert The fifth stage of the Dreyfus model is achieved when "the expert performer no longer relies on analytical principle (rule, guideline, maxim) to connect her or his understanding of the situation to an appropriate action."[6:31] Benner described the expert nurse as having an intuitive grasp of the situation and as being able to identify the region of the problem without wasting consideration on a range of alternative diagnoses and solutions. There is a qualitative change as the expert performer "knows the patient," meaning knowing typical patterns of responses and knowing the patient as a person. Key aspects of the expert nurse's practice are: (1) a clinical grasp and resource-based practice, (2) embodied know-how, (3) seeing the big picture, and (4) seeing the unexpected.[19:145]

The expert nurse has this ability of pattern recognition on the basis of deep experiential background. For the expert nurse, meeting the patient's actual concerns and needs is of utmost importance, even if it means planning and negotiating for a change in the plan of care. There is almost a transparent view of the self.[18:27]

Aspects of a Situation The characteristics of the situation recognized and understood in context because of prior experience.

Attribute of a Situation Measurable properties of a situation that can be explained without previous experience in the situation.

Competency Competency is "an interpretively defined area of skilled performance identified and described by its intent, functions, and meanings."[6:292] This term is unrelated to the competent stage of the Dreyfus model.

Domain An area of practice having a number of competencies with similar intents, functions, and meanings.

Exemplar An example of a clinical situation that conveys one or more intents, meanings, functions, or outcomes easily translated to other clinical situations.[6:293]

Experience Not a mere passage of time but an active process of refining and changing preconceived theories, notions, and ideas when confronted with actual situations; implies there is a dialogue between what is found in practice and what is expected.[20:11]

Maxim A cryptic description of skilled performance that requires a certain level of experience to recognize the implications of the instructions.[6:294]

Paradigm Case A clinical experience that stands out and alters the way one perceives and understands future clinical situations.[6:296] Paradigm cases create new clinical understanding and open new clinical perspectives and alternatives.

Salience A perceptual stance of embodied knowledge whereby aspects of a situation stand out as more or less important.

Major Assumptions

Benner incorporated assumptions from the Dreyfus model, "that with experience and mastery the skill is transformed."[6:38] "This model assumes that all practical situations are far more complex than can be described by formal models, theories and textbook descriptions."[6:178]

In her subsequent writing Benner explicated the themes of nursing, person, situation, and health.

Nursing

Nursing is described as a caring relationship, an "enabling condition of connection and concern."[21:4]

"Caring is primary because caring sets up the possibility of giving help and receiving help."[21:4] "Nursing is viewed as a caring practice whose science is guided by the moral art and ethics of care and responsibility."[21:xi] Benner understands nursing practice as the care and study of the lived experience of health, illness, and disease and the relationships among these three.[21:8]

Person

Benner has used Heidegger's phenomenological description of person: "A person is a self-interpreting being, that is, the person does not come into the world predefined but gets defined in the course of living a life. A person also has . . . an effortless and nonreflective understanding of the self in the world."[21:41] "The person is viewed as a participant in common meanings."[21:23]

Finally, the person is embodied. Benner and Wrubel[21] have conceptualized the major aspects of understanding the person must deal with as the role of the situation, the role of the body, the role of personal concerns, and the role of temporality. Together these aspects of the person make up the person in the world. This view of the person is based on the works of Heidegger,[31] Merleau-Ponty,[34] and Dreyfus.[25] Their goal is to overcome Cartesian dualism, namely, the view that the mind and body are distinct, separate entities.[38] Benner and Wrubel[21] give a central place to embodiment in their theory and defined *embodiment* as the capacity of the body to respond to meaningful situations. On the basis of the work of Merleau-Ponty[34] and Dreyfus (1979), they outline five dimensions of the body: (1) the unborn complex, the unacculturated body of the fetus and newborn baby; (2) the habitual skilled body, the social learned postures, gestures, customs, and skills evident in bodily skills such as seeing and "body language" that are "learned over time through identification, imitation, and trial and error"[21:71]; (3) the projective body, the way the body is set (predisposed) to act in specific situations, for example, opening a door or walking; (4) the actual projected body, one's current bodily orientation or projection in a situation that is flexible and varied to fit the situation, such as when one is skillful in using a keyboard; and (5) the phenomenal body, the body aware of itself, that ability to imagine and describe kinesthetic sensations. Benner and Wrubel point out that nurses attend to the body and the role of embodiment in health, illness, and recovery.

Health

On the basis of the work of Heidegger and Merleau-Ponty, Benner "focuses on the lived experience of being healthy and being ill."[21:7] *Health* is defined as what can be assessed, whereas well-being is the human experience of health or wholeness. Well-being and being ill are understood as distinct ways of being in the world. Health is described as not just the absence of disease and illness. Also a person may have a disease and not experience himself as ill because illness is the human experience of loss or dysfunction, whereas disease is what can be assessed at the physical level.[21:8]

Situation

Benner uses the term *situation* rather than *environment* because *situation* conveys a people environment with social definition and meaningfulness.[21:80] She uses the phenomenological terms of being *situated* and *situated meaning,* which are defined by the person's engaged interaction, interpretation, and understanding of the situation. "To be situated implies that one has a past, present, and future and that all of these aspects . . . influence the current situation."[21:80] Persons "enter into situations with their own sets of meanings, habits, and perspectives."[21:23] "Personal interpretation of the situation is bounded by the way the individual is *in* it."[21:84]

THEORETICAL ASSERTIONS

Benner stated that theory is crucial to form the right questions to ask in a clinical situation; theory directs the practitioner in looking for problems and anticipating care needs. There is always more to any situation than theory predicts.[6:178] The skilled practice of nursing exceeds the bounds of formal theory. Concrete experience provides the learning about the exceptions and shades of meaning in a situation. The knowledge embedded in practice discovers and interprets theory, precedes and extends theory, and synthesizes and adapts theory in caring nursing practice. Some of the relationship statements included in Benner's work follow:

Discovering assumptions, expectations, and sets can uncover an unexamined area of practical knowledge that can then be systematically studied and extended or refuted.[6:8]

The clinician's knowledge is embedded in perceptions rather than precepts.[6:43]

Perceptual awareness is central to good nursing judgment and . . . begins with vague hunches and global assessments that initially bypass critical analysis; conceptual clarity follows more often than it precedes.[6:xviii]

Formal rules are limited and discretionary judgment is used in actual clinical situations.[6:xix]

Knowledge . . . accrues over time in the practice of an applied discipline.[6:1]

Expertise develops when the clinician tests and refines propositions, hypotheses, and principle-based expectations in actual practice situations.[6:3]

LOGICAL FORM

Through qualitative descriptive research, Benner applied the Dreyfus model of skill acquisition to clinical nursing practice. By following the logical sequence developed by Dreyfus, Benner was able to identify the performance characteristics and teaching-learning needs inherent at each level of skill. From her research, Benner identified 31 competencies of expert practice, which she classified inductively into seven domains of nursing practice. In reporting her research, Benner used exemplars taken directly from interviews and observation of expert practice to help the reader form a clear picture of such practice. Benner accomplished the goal of her research, which she stated to be "to uncover meanings and knowledge embedded in skilled practice . . .

by bringing these meanings, skills, and knowledge into public discourse, new knowledge and understanding are constituted."[6:218]

ACCEPTANCE BY THE NURSING COMMUNITY
Practice

Benner has described clinical nursing practice by using an interpretive approach. Included in *From Novice to Expert* are several examples of application of her work in practice settings. The model has been used to aid in the development of clinical ladders of promotion, new graduate orientation programs, and clinical knowledge development seminars. Symposiums focusing on excellence in nursing practice have been held for staff development, recognition, and reward and as a way of demonstrating clinical knowledge development in practice.[24]

Fenton[29] reported the use of Benner's approach in an ethnographic study of the performance of clinical nurse-specialists. She found that the nurses were functioning at an advanced level of preparation but that "we have not yet developed accurate written and verbal descriptions of that advanced practice."[28:37] Balasco and Black[1] and Silver[36;37:32] used Benner's model as a basis for differentiating clinical knowledge development and career progression in nursing.

Neverveld[35] used Benner's rationale and format in her development of basic and advanced preceptor workshops.

Crissman and Jelsma applied Benner's findings in developing a cross-training program to aid in staffing imbalances. "Cross-training delineates specific performance objectives for the nurse in her novice role and provides a preceptor in the setting for the clinical area unfamiliar to her. There, as a novice, she aims to become an advanced beginner able to function independently with an experienced nurse available as a resource."[23:64D]

Benner has been cited extensively in nursing literature regarding nursing practice concerns and the role of caring in such practice. She continues to publish applications of the model to clinical situations.[7-9,17]

Benner's current research project, funded by the Helene Fuld Foundation, is to develop an approach to teaching clinical judgment.[14]

Education

Benner[4] has critiqued the concept of competency-based testing by contrasting it with the complexity of the proficiency and expert stages described in the Dreyfus Model of Skill Acquisition and the 31 competencies. In summary, she stated, "competency-based testing seems limited to the less situational, less interactional areas of patient care where the behavior can be well defined and patient and nurse variations do not alter the performance criteria."[4:309]

Fenton[28,29] described the application of the domains of expert practice as the basis for studying the skilled performance of master's-prepared nurses. The analysis verified the performance skills of expert nurses reported in the AMICAE project and identified new areas of skilled performance and five preliminary categories relevant for curriculum evaluation in the graduate program.

According to Barnum, surprisingly it is not Benner's development of the seven domains of nursing practice that has had the greatest impact on nursing education but rather the "appreciation of the utility of the Dreyfus model in describing learning and thinking in our discipline." Nursing educators have realized that learning needs at the early stages of clinical knowledge development are different from those required at later stages. These differences must be acknowledged and valued when educators develop teaching curriculums.[2:170]

Benner, Tanner, and Chesla, in *Expertise in Nursing Practice: Caring, Clinical Judgment, and Ethics* emphasize the importance of learning the skill of involvement and caring through practical experience, the articulation of knowledge with practice, and the use of narratives in undergraduate education.[19:307-309]

Research

The preceding example by Fenton[28,29] presented an application of educational research. Lock and Gordon,[33] medical anthropologists who had been re-search assistants on the AMICAE project, extended the inquiry to study the formal models used in nursing practice and medicine. They concluded that formal models may serve as maps directing care and can substitute for knowledge and result in conformity. Gordon[30] cautions that a misuse of formal models occurs when nurses apply models without using judgment, use them to exert control, and use language from them that can cover up meanings, or not really know what they mean. Finally, "formal models should be used with discretion" as tools and so as not to eclipse the relational, holistic, intuitive aspects of nursing.[6:242]

FURTHER DEVELOPMENT

Benner and Wrubel have extended the basis and interpretation of the study of clinical nursing practice in *The Primacy of Caring: Stress and Coping in Health and Illness.*[21] This work explores the philosophies affecting our thinking and practice. Benner and Wrubel suggest that the adoption of a phenomenological view of person with shared meanings in the situation gives the potential for an understanding of caring and expert nursing practice and stress and coping. "Theory must be informed by real-world experience and experiments, which are in turn subject to theoretical interpretation. . . . A theory is needed that describes, interprets, and explains not an imagined ideal of nursing, but actual expert nursing as it is practiced day by day."[21:5]

Benner's application of the Dreyfus model in clinical nursing practice has provided rich descriptions of nursing as it is practiced. In the interpretation of the five levels of practice, Benner provided suggestions for matching competency to nursing practice and for the development of each stage on the basis of experience. It is better to place a new graduate with a competent nurse preceptor who can explain nursing practice in ways that the beginner comprehends. The intuitive knowledge of the expert will elude beginners who do not have the experienced know-how to grasp the situation.

To date, the model provides concept definitions and in-depth descriptions of each from nursing practice. From these situated descriptions, 31 competencies in seven domains have been derived from actual nursing practice. By maintaining the context of these situated performances, the descriptions are holistic or synthetic, rather than procedural and elemental.[6:45] "The competencies within each domain [are] in no way intended as an exhaustive list."[6:45] A situation-based interpretive approach to describing nursing practice overcomes some of the problems of reductionism . . . and overcomes the problem of global and overly general descriptions based on nursing process categories."[6:46]

In recent research, Benner examined the role of narrative accounts in understanding the notion of good or ethical caring in expert clinical nursing practice. "The narrative memory of the actual concrete event is taken up in embodied know-how and comportment, complete with emotional responses to situations. The narrative memory can evoke perceptual or sensory memories that enhance pattern recognition."[12:16]

Dunlop[27] explored the nursing literature related to the science of caring. She draws a distinction between a science for caring and a science of caring. "A science of caring implies that caring can be operationalized in some way as a set of behaviors which can be observed, counted or measured."[27:666] Benner has taken a hermeneutical form to uncover the knowledge embedded in clinical nursing practice. "As she does this, she is also uncovering the nursing-caring with which it is deeply intertwined."[27:668] Dunlop noted that, although useful, "it does not provide us with any universal truths about caring in general or about nursing-caring in particular—indeed it does not make any such pretension."[27:668]

CRITIQUE
Simplicity

Benner has developed an interpretive descriptive account of clinical nursing practice. The concepts are the levels of skilled practice from the Dreyfus model, including novice, advanced beginner, competent, proficient, and expert. She uses the five concepts to describe nursing practice from interviews, observations, and the analysis of transcripts of exemplars provided by the nurses. From these descriptions, 31 competencies were identified, and these were grouped into seven domains of nursing practice on the basis of common intentions and meanings. The model is relatively simple with regard to the five stages of skill acquisition and provides a comparative guide for identifying levels of nursing practice from individual nurse descriptions and observations of actual nursing practice. The interpretations are validated by consensus. A degree of complexity is encountered in the subconcepts for differentiation among the levels of competency and the need to identify meanings and intentions. This interpretive approach is designed to overcome the constraints of the rational-technical approach to the study and description of practice. Although providing a decontextualized (i.e., object) description of the novice level of performance is possible, the limits of objectification are encountered as soon as an understanding of the situation is required for expert performance. Clinical knowledge is relational and contextual and often deals with local, specific, historical issues. To capture the contextual and relational aspects of practice, Benner uses narrative accounts of actual clinical situations and maintains that the exemplar enables the reader to recognize similar intents and meanings, although the "objective" circumstances may be quite different.

Generality

The descriptive model of nursing practice has the potential for universal application as a framework, but the descriptions are limited by dependence on the actual clinical nursing situations from which they must be derived. Its use depends on the understanding of the five levels of competency and the ability to identify the characteristic intentions and meanings inherent at each level of practice. The model has universal characteristics in that it is not restricted by age, illness, health, or location of nursing practice. The characteristics of theoretical universality, however, imply properties of operationalization for prediction that are not a part of this perspective. Indeed, this phenomenological perspective critiques the limits of "universality" in studies of human practices.

Empirical Precision

The model was empirically tested using qualitative methodologies, and 31 competencies and seven domains of nursing practice were derived inductively. Subsequent research suggests that the framework is applicable and useful in providing knowledge of the description of nursing practice. Benner stated that "if we choose only scientific, technical and organizational strategies for legitimizing expert nursing care, we will miss the primacy of caring and the central ethic of care and responsibility embedded in expert nursing practice."[10] It is precisely the use of alternative models of discovering nursing knowledge that makes it difficult to address the work of *From Novice to Expert* within a rational-empirical framework for critique. Utilizing the scientific approach, one would look for lawlike relational statements to predict practice. Nevertheless, using the qualitative methods in an interpretive approach, Benner describes expert nursing practice in many exemplars. Positivistic science takes an alternative approach by seeking formulas and models to apply. Her work seems to be hypothesis generating rather than hypothesis testing. Benner provides no universal "how to" for nursing practice but rather provides a methodology for uncovering and entering into the situated meaning of expert nursing care. The interpretation of the meaning and level of nursing practice will no doubt frustrate "objective" researchers who seek precision and control. The strength of the Benner model is that it is data-based research that contributes to the science of nursing.

Derivable Consequences

Benner's *From Novice to Expert*[6] model provides a general framework for identifying, defining, and describing clinical nursing practice. Benner uses a phenomenological approach to describe persons and derives meaning and abilities from interactions in life situations. The significance of Benner's research findings lies in her conclusion that "a nurse's clinical knowledge is relevant to the extent to which its manifestation in nursing skills makes a difference in patient care and patient outcomes."[20:11]

Nursing is the involved interaction with persons in a caring mode. *The Primacy of Caring*[21] further develops these themes. Benner described her work as a description of the knowledge embedded in actual nursing practice. The five levels of competencies are descriptions of the practical nursing knowledge of each level in the context of the situations described. The approach to generalization is through common meanings, skills, practices, and embodied capacities rather than through general ahistorical laws. The knowledge embedded in clinical nursing practice should no longer be ignored but brought forth as public knowledge so that a greater understanding of nursing practice can occur. Benner[6] believes the scope and complexity of nursing practice are too extensive simply to rely on idealized, decontextualized views of practice or experiments. "The platonic quest to get to the general so that we can get beyond the vagaries of experience was a misguided turn. . . . We can redeem the turn if we subject our theories to our unedited, concrete, moral experience and acknowledge that skillful ethical comportment calls us not to be beyond experience but tempered and taught by it."[12:19]

The generalizations are depicted through exemplars that demonstrate relational and contextually relevant intents and aspects of clinical knowledge. This approach takes issue with the common approaches used for universality or generalization in physics and the natural sciences and claims that the basis for generalization in clinical knowledge cannot be structural or mechanistic but rather must be based on common meanings and practices. The strategies for generalization are not based on abstraction through removing the situation or context (objectification) but rather by showing how the skilled knowledge, the intent, content, and notion of good in clinical knowledge must be depicted by exemplars that illustrate the role of the situation. Benner claims that this is not a privativistic or subjectivistic approach but rather an attempt to overcome the limits of subject-object descriptions. Benner's call is to "increase public storytelling"[12:19] to validate nursing as an ethical caring practice and "to extend, alter, and preserve ethical distinctions and concerns."[12:20] Benner states that, "We have overlooked practitioner stories that demonstrate that compassion can be wise and, in the long run, less costly than 'defensive' adversarial commodified technocures."[13:35-36] Benner's work is useful in that it has framed nursing practice from the context of what nursing actually is and does rather than from idealized theoretical descriptors that are context-free.

CRITICAL THINKING *Activities*

The three patients described below are admitted to a nursing unit at the same time. Explain, describe, and provide a rationale for how a nurse at each of the stages of skills acquisition (novice, advanced beginner, competent, proficient, and expert) would do the following:

- Prioritize or categorize each patient
- Assess each patient
- Intervene with each patient

1 A 69-year-old male with a history of chronic obstructive pulmonary disease has an acute exacerbation of respiratory distress. His respirations are 38 per minute, shallow, and labored, and he is using the accessory muscles to assist in breathing. He is diaphoretic and pale and has decreased breath sounds bilaterally. His arterial blood gas values are pH 7.27, Po_2 59, Pco_2 57, HCO_3^- 21.

2 A 2-year-old female is diagnosed with bilateral otitis media, and she has a rectal temperature of 105.2° F. Her skin color is flushed, and she has a dry cough and rhinorrhea and a pulse oximetry of 89% on room air.

3 A 35-year-old woman complains of acute onset of right lower quadrant abdominal pain and nausea, and she has vomited three times. Her color is ashen, her oral temperature is 99.2° F, her pulse 118 beats per minute, her respiration 24 per minute, and her blood pressure 90/50 mm Hg. She is diagnosed with a ruptured right ovarian cyst.

REFERENCES

1. Balasco, E.M., Black, A.S. (1988). Advancing nursing practice: Description, recognition, and reward. *Nursing Administration Quarterly, 12*(2), 52-62.
2. Barnum, B.J. (1990). *Nursing theory: Analysis, application, evaluation.* Glenview, IL: Scott, Foresman.
3. Barnum, B. (1996). Foreword. In P. Benner, C. Tanner, & C. Chelsa, *Expertise in nursing practice: Caring, clinical judgment, and ethics.* New York: Springer.
4. Benner, P. (1982), May). Issues in competency-based training. *Nursing Outlook, 20*(5), 303-309.
5. Benner, P. (1983). Uncovering the knowledge embedded in clinical practice. *Image: The Journal of Nursing Scholarship, 15*(2), 36-41.
6. Benner, P. (1984). *From novice to expert: Excellence and power in clinical nursing practice.* Menlo Park, CA: Addison-Wesley.
7. Benner, P. (1985, Feb.). The oncology clinical nurse specialist: An expert coach. *Oncology Nursing Forum, 12*(2), 40-44.
8. Benner, P. (1985, Oct.). Quality of life: A phenomenological perspective on explanation, prediction, and understanding in nursing science. *Advances in Nursing Science, 8*(1), 1-14.
9. Benner, P. (1987, Sept.). A dialogue with excellence. *American Journal of Nursing, 87*(9), 1170-1172.
10. Benner, P. (1988). Personal correspondence.
11. Benner, P. (1992). Personal correspondence.
12. Benner, P. (1992). The role of narrative experience and community in ethical comportment. *Advances in Nursing Science, 14*(2), 1-21.
13. Benner, P. (1996). Embodiment, caring and ethics: A nursing perspective: The 1995 Helen Nahm Lecture. *The Science of Caring, 8*(2), 30-36.
14. Benner, P. (1996). Personal correspondence.
15. Benner, P., & Benner, R.V. (1979). *The new nurses' work entry: A troubled sponsorship.* New York: Tiresias.
16. Benner, P., & Kramer, M. (1972, Jan.). Role conceptions and integrative role behavior of nurses in special care and regular hospital nursing units. *Nursing Research, 21*(1), 20-29.
17. Benner, P., & Tanner, C. (1987, Jan.). Clinical judgment: How expert nurses use intuition. *American Journal of Nursing, 87*(1), 23-31.
18. Benner, P., Tanner, C., & Chesla, C. (1992). From beginner to expert: Gaining a differentiated clinical world in critical care nursing. *Advances in Nursing Science, 14*(3), 13-28.
19. Benner, P., Tanner, C., & Chesla, C. (1996). *Expertise in nursing practice: Caring, clinical judgment, and ethics.* New York: Springer.
20. Benner, P., & Wrubel, J. (1982). Skilled clinical knowledge: The value of perceptual awareness. *Nurse Educator, 7*(3), 11-17.

21. Benner, P., & Wrubel, J. (1989). *The primacy of caring: Stress and coping in health and illness.* Menlo Park, CA: Addison-Wesley.

22. Benner, P.E. (1984). *Stress and satisfaction on the job: Work meanings and coping of mid-career men.* New York: Praeger.

23. Crissman, S., & Jelsma, N. (1990). Cross-training: Practicing effectively on two levels. *Nursing Management, 21*(3), 64a-64h.

24. Dolan, K. (1984). Building bridges between education and practice. In P. Benner (Ed.), *From novice to expert.* Menlo Park, CA: Addison-Wesley.

25. Dreyfus, H.L. (1991). *Being-in-the-world: A commentary on being and time dimension I.* Cambridge, MA: M.I.T. Press.

26. Dreyfus, H.L, & Dreyfus, S.E. (1996). The relationship of theory and practice in the acquisition of skill. In P. Benner, C. Tanner, & C. Chesla, *Expertise in nursing practice: Caring, clinical judgment, and ethics* (pp. 29-47). New York: Springer.

27. Dunlop, M.J. (1986). Is a science of caring possible? *Journal of Advanced Nursing, 11,* 661-670.

28. Fenton, M.V. (1984). Identification of the skilled performance of master's prepared nurses as a method of curriculum planning and evaluation. In P. Benner, *From novice to expert* (pp. 262-274). Menlo Park, CA: Addison-Wesley.

29. Fenton, M.V. (1985). Identifying competencies of clinical nurse specialists. *Journal of Nursing Administration, 15*(12), 31-37.

30. Gordon, D.R. (1984). Research application: Identifying the use and misuse of formal nursing models in nursing practice. In P. Benner, *From novice to expert,* (pp. 225-243). Menlo Park, CA: Addison-Wesley.

31. Heidegger, M. (1962). *Being and time.* (MacQuarrie, J., & Robinson, E., Trans.) New York: Harper & Row.

32. Henderson, V. (1989). Foreword. In P. Benner & J. Wrubel, *The primacy of caring: Stress and coping in health and illness.* Menlo Park, CA: Addison-Wesley.

33. Lock, M., & Gordon, D.R. (Eds.). (1989). *Biomedicine examined.* Boston, MA: Kluwer Academic.

34. Merleau-Ponty, M. (1962). *Phenomenology of perception..* (C. Smith, Trans.) London: Routledge and Kegan Paul.

35. Neverveld, M.E. (1990, July, Aug.). Preceptorship: One step beyond. *Journal of Nursing Staff Development,* 186-189.

36. Silver, M. (1986). A program for career structure: A vision becomes a reality. *The Australian Nurse, 16*(2), 44-47.

37. Silver, M. (1986). A program for career structure: From neophyte to expert. *The Australian Nurse, 16*(2), 38-41.

38. Visintainer, M. (1988). Review of the book *The primacy of caring: Stress and coping in health and illness. Image: Journal of Nursing Scholarship, 20*(2), 113-114.

BIBLIOGRAPHY

Primary sources

Books

Benner, P. (1984). *From novice to expert: Excellence and power in clinical nursing practice.* Menlo Park, CA: Addison-Wesley.

Benner, P.E. (1984). *Stress and job satisfaction on the job: Work meanings and coping of mid-career men.* New York: Praeger.

Benner, P. (1987). *Practica progresiva en enfermeria: Manual de comportamiento profesiona* (Spanish translation). Barcelona: Ediciones Grijalbo.

Benner, P. (1994). *Interpretive phenomenology: Embodiment, caring and ethics in health and illness.* Thousand Oaks, CA: Sage.

Benner, P. , & Benner, R.V. (1979). *The new nurses' work entry: A troubled sponsorship.* New York: Tiresias Press.

Benner, P., Tanner, C., & Chesla, C. (1996). *Expertise in nursing practice: Caring, clinical judgment, and ethics.* New York: Springer.

Benner, P., & Wrubel, J. (1989). *The primacy of caring: Stress and coping in health and illness.* Menlo Park, CA: Addison-Wesley.

Phillips, S., & Benner, P. (Eds.). (1994). *The crisis of care: Affirming and restoring caring practices in the helping professions.* Washington, DC: Georgetown University Press.

Book chapters

Allen, D., Benner, P., & Diekelmann, N. (1986). Three paradigms for nursing research-methodology implications. In P.L. Chinn (Ed.), *Nursing research methodology.* Rockville, MD: Aspen.

Benner, P. (1974). Reality testing a "Reality Shock" program. In M. Kramer (Ed.), *Reality shock: Why nurses leave nursing* (pp. 191-215). St. Louis: Mosby.

Benner, P. (1975). Nurses in the intensive care unit. In M. Davis, M. Kramer, & A. Straus (Eds.), *Nurses in practice: A perspective on work environment* (pp. 106-128). St. Louis: Mosby.

Benner, P. (1975). Process and persistence of value transmission. In M. Davis, M. Kramer, & A. Straus (Eds.), *Nurses in practice: A perspective on work environment* (pp. 166-176). St. Louis: Mosby.

Benner, P. (1990). The moral dimensions of caring. In J.S. Stevenson & T. Tripp-Reimer (Eds.), *Knowledge about care and caring: State of the art and future developments.* Kansas City, MO: American Academy of Nursing.

Benner, P. (1990). Performance expectations of new graduates. In *Critical care in the nursing curriculum: Linking education and practice.* Newport Beach, CA: American Association of Critical Care Nurses.

Benner, P. (1991). Coping with cancer. In S. Baird, R. McCorkle, & M. Grant (Eds.), *Cancer nursing: A comprehensive textbook.* Philadelphia: W.B. Saunders.

Benner, P. (1991). Response to hermeneutical inquiry by Janice Thompson. In L.E. Moody (Ed.). *Advancing theory for nursing science through research,* Vol. 2. Newbury Park, CA: Sage.

Benner, P. (1994). Caring as a way of knowing and not knowing. In S. Phillips & P. Benner (Eds.), *The crisis of care: Affirming and restoring caring practices in the helping professions* (pp. 42-62). Washington, DC: Georgetown University Press.

Benner, P. (1994). Discovering challenges to ethical theory in experience-based narratives of nurses' everyday ethical comportment. In J.F. Monagle & D.C. Thomasina (Eds.), *Health care ethics: Critical issues* (pp. 401-411). Gaithersburg, MD: Aspen.

Benner, P. (1994). The role of articulation in understanding practice and experience as sources of knowledge. In J. Tully & D.M. Weinstock (Eds.), *Philosophy in a time of pluralism: Perspectives on the philosophy of Charles Taylor* (pp. 136-155). Cambridge: Cambridge University Press.

Benner, P., & Kramer, M. (1977). Work shoes speak. In M. Kramer & C. Schmallenberg (Eds.), *Path to biculturalism* (pp. 204-232). Wakefield, MA: Contemporary Publishers.

Benner, P., Roskies, E., & Lazarus, R. (1980). Stress and coping under extreme conditions. In J.E. Dimsdale (Ed.), *Survivors, victims and perpetrators: Essays on the Nazi holocaust* (pp. 219-258). New York: Hemisphere.

Wrubel, J., Benner, P., & Lazarus, R.S. (1981). Social competence from the perspective of stress and coping. In J.D. Wine & M.D. Smye (Eds.), *Social competence* (pp. 61-99). New York: Guilford Press.

Journal articles

Benner, P. (1981, Aug.). Retaining experienced nursing is key to quality care. *The American Nurse, 13*(8), 4, 15.

Benner, P. (1982, March). From novice to expert. *American Journal of Nursing, 82*(3), 402-407.

Benner, P. (1982, May). Issues in competency-based testing. *Nursing Outlook, 30*(5), 303-309.

Benner, P. (1983, Spring). Uncovering the knowledge embedded in clinical practice. *Image, Journal of Nursing Scholarship, 15*(2), 36-41.

Benner, P. (1985). General systems theory and nursing. *Japanese Journal of Nursing Research, 18*(1), 61-71.

Benner, P. (1985). Why does nursing need a theory? *Japanese Journal of Nursing Research, 18*(1), 3-30.

Benner, P. (1985, March/April). The oncology clinical nurse specialist: An expert coach. *Oncology Nursing Forum, 12*(2), 40-44.

Benner, P. (1985, Aug.). Preserving caring in an era of cost-containment and high technology (pp. 12-20). *Yale Nurse.*

Benner, P. (1985, Oct.). Quality of life: A phenomenological perspective on explanation, prediction, and understanding in nursing science. *Advances in Nursing Science, 8*(1), 1-14.

Benner, P. (1986, Oct.). Advice for new graduate nurses on their first job. *The American Nurse* (invited column).

Benner, P. (1987, Sept.). A dialogue with excellence. *American Journal of Nursing, 87*(9), 1170-1172.

Benner, P. (1989, Dec.). *Nursing as a caring profession.* Working paper presented at the meeting of the American Academy of Nursing, Kansas City, MO.

Benner, P. (1990, Spring). Phenomenology as theory and method. *Japanese Journal of Nursing Research,* 25-34.

Benner, P. (1992). Patricia Benner: Uncovering the wonders of skilled practice by listening to nurses' stories (interview by Michael Villaire). *Critical Care Nurse, 12*(6), 82-89.

Benner, P. (1992). The role of narrative experience and community in ethical comportment. *Advances in Nursing Science, 14*(2), 1-21.

Benner, P. (1992, March). The power of our practice: A source for a national care agenda (editorial). *Nursing Health Care, 13*(3), 115-116.

Benner, P. (1993). The phenomenology of knowing the patient. *Image: The Journal of Nursing Scholarship, 25*(4), 273-280.

Benner, P. (1996). Embodiment, caring and ethics: A nursing perspective. The 1995 Helen Nahm Lecture. *Science of Caring, 8*(2), 30-36.

Benner, P., & Kramer, M. (1972, Jan./Feb.). Role conceptions and integrative role behavior of nurses in special care and regular hospital nursing units. *Nursing Research, 21*(1), 20-29.

Benner, P., & Tanner, C. (1987, Jan.). Clinical judgment: How expert nurses use intuition. *American Journal of Nursing, 87*(1), 23-31.

Benner, P., Tanner, C., & Chesla, C. (1990). The nature of clinical expertise in intensive care units. *Anthropology of Work Review, 11*(3), 16-19.

Benner, P., Tanner, C., & Chesla, C. (1992). From beginner to expert: Gaining a differentiated clinical world in critical care nursing. *Advances in Nursing Science, 14*(3), 13-28.

Benner, P., & Wrubel, J. (1982, May). Skilled clinical knowledge: The value of perceptual awareness, Part 1. *Journal of Nursing Administration, 12*(5), 11-14.

Benner, P., & Wrubel, J. (1982, May/June). Skilled clinical knowledge: The value of perceptual awareness. *Nurse Educator, 7*(3), 11-17.

Benner, P., & Wrubel, J. (1982, June). Skilled clinical knowledge: The value of perceptual awareness, Part 2. *Journal of Nursing Administration, 12*(6), 28-33.

Benner, P., & Wrubel, J. (1988). Caring comes first. *American Journal of Nursing, 88*(8), 1072-1075.

Benner, R., & Benner, P. (1991, July/Aug.) Stories from the front line. *Health Care Forum Journal, 34,* 69-74.

Benner, R.V., & Benner, P. (1979, Sept./Oct.). Follow-through evaluation: A resource for curriculum planning and development. *Nurse Educator, 4*(5), 16-21.

Brandt, S., & Benner, P. (1980, March). Infection control in hospitals: What are the challenges? *American Journal of Nursing, 80*(3), 432-434.

Diekelmann, N., & Benner, P. (1985). Three paradigms for research in nursing education. *Progressions Education Research Notes, A Publication of Division 1: Education in the Progressions of American Educational Research Association, 7*(1), 6-10.

Eaton, S., & Benner, P. (1977). Discussion stoppers in teaching. *Nursing Outlook, 25*(9), 578-583.

Marculescu, G.L., & Benner, P. (1987, Dec.). A dialogue with excellence: Early warning (commentary). *American Journal of Nursing, 87*(12), 1556-1558.

Meleis, A.L., & Benner, P. (1975, May). Process vs. product evaluation? *Nursing Outlook, 23*(5), 303-307.

Videotape

Nursing theory: A circle of knowledge (1987). New York: National League for Nursing.

Other sources

Dreyfus, H.L. (1979). *What computers can't do.* New York: Harper & Row.

Dreyfus, H.L., & Dreyfus, S.E. (1986). *Mind over machine.* New York: The Free Press.

Dreyfus, H.L., & Rabinow, P. (1982). *Michel Foucault.* Chicago: University of Chicago Press.

Dreyfus, S.E., & Dreyfus, H.L. (1980, Feb.). *A five-stage model of the mental activities involved in directed skill acquisition.* Unpublished report supported by the Air Force Office of Scientific Research (AFSC), USAF (Contract F49620-79-c-0063), University of California at Berkeley.

Good, B.J., & Good, M.J. DelVecchio. (1982). The meaning of symptoms: A cultural hermeneutic model for clinical practice. In L. Eisenberg & A. Kleinman (Eds.), *The relevance of social sciences for medicine.* Boston: D. Reidel.

Lazarus, R.S. (1985). The trivialization of distress. In J.C. Rosen & L.J. Solomon (Eds.), *Preventing health risk behaviors and promoting coping with illness* (Vol. 8). Vermont Conference on the Primary Prevention of Psychopathology (pp. 279-298). Hanover, NH: University Press of New England.

Lazarus, R.S., & Folkman, S. (1984). *Stress appraisals and coping.* New York: Springer.

Palmer, R.E. (1969). *Hermeneutics.* Evanston, IL: Northwestern University Press.

Polanyi, M. (1958). *Personal knowledge.* Chicago: University of Chicago Press.

Taylor, C. (1971, Sept.). Interpretation and the sciences of man. *Review of Metaphysics, 25*(1), 3-34, 45-51.

Publications in press

Benner, P., & Gordon, S. (1996). The knowledge and skill embedded in caregiving. In S. Gordon, P. Benner, & N. Noddings (Eds.), *The care voice and beyond.* Philadelphia: University of Pennsylvania Press.

Unpublished manuscripts

Benner, P., Hooper, P., & Stannard, D. (1995). *Nursing therapeutics in critical care: Caring practices linked to treatment.* Unpublished manuscript, University of California, San Francisco.

Benner, P., Wrubel, J., Phillips, S., Chesla, C., & Tanner, C. (1995). *Critical caring: The knowledge and skill embedded in helping.* Unpublished manuscript, University of California, San Francisco.

UNIT

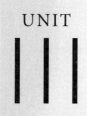

Conceptual Models: Grand Theories

- Nursing conceptual models are concepts, definitions, and propositions that specify their interrelationship to form an organized perspective for viewing phenomena specific to the discipline.

- Grand theories are conceptual structures that are nearly as abstract as the nursing models from which they are derived but propose outcomes based on utilization and application of the model in nursing practice.

- Conceptual models provide different ways of thinking about nursing and address the broad metaparadigm concepts that are central to its meaning.

- This unit has been expanded to include a work that is a nursing model that has been used over the last three decades in Scotland in addition to the seven nursing models commonly recognized in the United States.

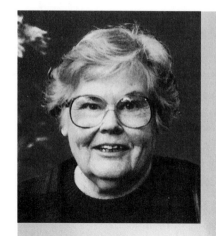

CHAPTER

14

$\mathcal{D}$orothea E. Orem

Self-Care Deficit Theory of Nursing

Susan G. Taylor, Angela Compton, Jeanne Donohue Eben,
Sarah Emerson, Nergess N. Gashti, Ann Marriner Tomey,
Margaret J. Nation, Sherry B. Nordmeyer

CREDENTIALS AND BACKGROUND OF THE THEORIST

Dorothea Elizabeth Orem, one of America's foremost nursing theorists, was born in Baltimore, Maryland. Her father was a construction worker who liked fishing, and her mother was a homemaker who liked reading. The younger of two daughters, Orem began her nursing career at Providence Hospital School of Nursing in Washington, D.C., where she received a diploma of nursing in the early 1930s. Orem continued her education and received a B.S.N. from The Catholic University of America in 1939

The authors wish to express appreciation to Dorothea E. Orem for critiquing the first edition.

and an M.S. in nursing education in 1945 from the same university.

Her nursing experience included private duty nursing, hospital staff nursing, and teaching. Orem held directorship of both the nursing school and the department of nursing at Providence Hospital, Detroit, from 1940 to 1949. After leaving Detroit, Orem spent 7 years (1949-1957) in Indiana working in the Division of Hospital and Institutional Services of the Indiana State Board of Health. While there her goal was to upgrade the quality of nursing in general hospitals throughout the state. During this time, Orem developed her definition of nursing practice.

In 1957 Orem moved to Washington, D.C., where she was employed by the Office of Education, U.S.

Department of Health, Education, and Welfare, (HEW) as a curriculum consultant from 1958 to 1960. While at HEW she worked on a project to upgrade practical nursing training that stimulated a need to address the question, What is the subject matter of nursing? As a result, *Guidelines for Developing Curricula for the Education of Practical Nurses* was published in 1959.[91]

In 1959, Orem became an assistant professor of Nursing Education at The Catholic University of America. She subsequently served as acting dean of the School of Nursing and as associate professor of nursing education. She continued to develop her concept of nursing and self-care while at The Catholic University. While there, she wrote "The Hope of Nursing" (1962), which was published in the *Journal of Nursing Education.* In 1970 Orem left The Catholic University and began her own consulting firm of Orem and Shields, Inc., of Chevy Chase, Maryland. Orem's first book, published in 1971, was *Nursing: Concepts of Practice.*[92] This was followed by *Concept Formalization in Nursing: Process and Product* (1972).[93] Georgetown University conferred Orem with the honorary degree of Doctor of Science in 1976. "Levels of Nursing Education and Practice" was published in the alumnae magazine of Johns Hopkins School of Nursing in 1979. She received the Catholic University of America Alumni Association Award for Nursing Theory in 1980. Other honors received include honorary Doctor of Science, Incarnate Word College, 1980; Doctor of Humane Letters, Illinois Wesleyan University, 1988; Linda Richards Award, National League for Nursing, 1991; and honorary Fellow of the American Academy of Nursing, 1992.

Subsequent editions of *Nursing: Concepts of Practice* were published in 1980, 1985, 1991, and 1995.[94-96] Orem retired in 1984 and resides in Savannah, Georgia, where she enjoys reading, traveling, consulting, and attending nursing conferences to discuss her theory. Orem has been working alone and with colleagues on the continued conceptual development of Self-Care Deficit Nursing Theory (SCDNT). She participates in conferences and prepares papers about various conceptual elements of the theory. She continues to contribute to the work of her colleagues through discussions about the structure of the theory and its use in nursing.

THEORETICAL SOURCES

While Orem cites Eugenia K. Spaulding as a great friend and teacher, she indicates that no particular nursing leader was a direct influence on her work. She believes association with many nurses over the years provided many learning experiences, and she views her work with graduate students and collaborative works with colleagues as valuable endeavors. While crediting no one as a major influence, she does cite many other nurses' works in terms of their contributions to nursing including, but not limited to, Abdellah, Henderson, Johnson, King, Levine, Nightingale, Orlando, Peplau, Riehl, Rogers, Roy, Travelbee, and Wiedenbach. She also cites numerous authors in other disciplines including, but not limited to, Gordon Allport, Chester Barnard, René Dubos, Erich Fromm, Gartly Jaco, Robert Katz, Kurt Lewin, Ernest Nagel, Talcott Parsons, Hans Selye, Magda Arnold, Bernard Lonergan,[96:463-465] and Ludwig von Bertalanffy.

Orem has identified her philosophical view as that of "moderate realism."[130] Action theory, from the perspective of the person as deliberate actor or agent, forms the basis for the theory. Concepts of speculative and practical science are also foundational.[95]

USE OF EMPIRICAL EVIDENCE

Orem formulated her concept of nursing in relation to self-care as part of a study on the organization and administration of hospitals done while she was at the Indiana State Department of Health.[90] She became aware of the need for such a description while writing her report. Orem experienced a spontaneous insight about why individuals required and could be helped through nursing. This knowledge enabled her to formulate and express her concept of nursing. Her knowledge of the features of nursing practice situations was acquired over many years. Since the SCDNT was first published, there has been extensive empirical evidence. This has been incorporated into the continuing development of the theory; however, the basics of the theory remain unchanged.

Orem labels her self-care deficit theory of nursing as a general theory composed of three related theories: (1) the theory of self-care (describes why and how people care for themselves), (2) the theory of self-care deficit (describes and explains why people can be helped through nursing), and (3) the theory of nursing systems (describes and explains relationships that must be brought about and maintained for nursing to be produced). The major concepts of these theories are identified here and discussed more fully in Orem's book *Nursing: Concepts of Practice*[96:166-177] (Fig. 14-1).

Self-Care The practice of activities that maturing and mature persons initiate and perform, within time frames, on their own behalf in the interests of maintaining life, healthful functioning, continuing personal development, and well-being.[96:461]

Self-Care Requisites A formulated and expressed insight about actions to be performed that are known or hypothesized to be necessary in the regulation of an aspect(s) of human functioning and development continuously or under specified conditions and circumstances. A formulated self-care requisite names (1) the factor to be controlled or managed to keep an aspect(s) of human functioning and development within norms compatible with life and health and personal well-being and (2) the nature of the required action. Formulated and expressed self-care requisite constitutes the formalized purposes of self-care. They are the reasons for which self-care is undertaken; they express the intended or desired results—the goals of self-care.[96:461]

Universal Self-Care Requisites Universally required goals to be met through self-care or dependent-care have their origins in what is known and what is validated or in process of validation about human structural and functional integrity at various stages of the life cycle. Six self-care requisites common to men, women, and children are suggested:

1. The maintenance of a sufficient intake of air, water, and food.
2. The provision of care associated with elimination processes and excrements.

3. The maintenance of balance between activity and rest
4. The maintenance of balance between solitude and social interaction.
5. The prevention of hazards to human life, human functioning, and human well-being.
6. The promotion of human functioning and development within social groups in accord with human potential, known human limitations, and the human desire to be normal. *Normalcy* is used in the sense of that which is essentially human and that which is in accord with the genetic and constitutional characteristics and talents of individuals.[96:191]

Developmental Self-Care Requisites Developmental self-care requisites were separated from universal self-care requisites in the second edition of *Nursing: Concepts of Practice*. They promote processes for life and maturation and prevent conditions deleterious to maturation or mitigate those effects.[96:96]

Health Deviation Self-Care Requisites These self-care requisites exist for persons who are ill or injured, who have specific forms of pathologic conditions or disorders, including defects and disabilities, and who are undergoing medical diagnosis and treatment. The characteristics of health deviation as conditions extending over time determine the kinds of care demands that individuals experience as they live with the effects of pathologic conditions and live through their duration.

Disease or injury affects not only specific structures and physiologic or psychological mechanisms but also integrated human functioning. When integrated functioning is seriously affected (severe mental retardation, comatose states, autism), the individual's developing or developed powers of agency are seriously impaired either permanently or temporarily. In abnormal states of health, self-care requisites arise from both the disease state and the measures used in its diagnosis or treatment. There are six categories of health-deviation self-care requisites.

Continued

Care measures to meet existent health-deviation self-care requisites must be made action components of individuals' systems of self-care or dependent-care. The complexity of self-care or dependent-care systems is increased by the number of kinds of health-deviation requisites that must be met in specific time frames.[96:200-202]

Therapeutic Self-Care Demand The summation of care measures necessary at specific times or over a duration of time for meeting all of an individual's known self-care requisites particularized for existent conditions and circumstances using methods appropriate for (1) controlling or managing factors identified in the requisites the values of which are regulatory of human functioning, for example, sufficiency of air, water, food; and (2) fulfilling the activity element of the requisite, for example, maintenance, promotion, prevention, and provision.

Therapeutic self-care demand at any point in time (1) describes factors in the patient or the environment that (for the sake of the patient's life, health, or well-being) must be held steady within a range of values or brought within and held within such a range and (2) has a known degree of instrumental effectiveness derived from the choice of technologies and specific techniques for using a changing, or in some way controlling, patient or environmental factors.[96:462,189]

Self-Care Agency The complex acquired ability of mature and maturing persons to know and meet their continuing requirements for deliberate, purposive action to regulate their own human functioning and development.[96:461]

Agent The person who engages in a course of action or who has the power to do so.[96:456]

Dependent-Care Agent Maturing adolescents or adults who accept and fulfill the responsibility to know and meet the therapeutic self-care demand of relevant others who are socially dependent on them or to regulate the development or exercise of these persons' self-care agency.[96:457]

Self-Care Deficit A relation between the human properties therapeutic self-care demand and self-care agency in which constituent developed self-care capabilities within self-care agency are not op-erable or not adequate for knowing and meeting some or all components of the existent or projected therapeutic self-care demand.[96:461]

Nursing Agency The developed capabilities of persons educated as nurses that empower them to represent themselves as nurses and within the frame of a legitimate interpersonal relationship to act, know, and help persons in such relationships to meet their therapeutic self-care demands and to regulate the development or exercise of their self-care agency.[96:458]

Nursing Design A professional function performed both before and after nursing diagnosis and prescription through which nurses, on the basis of reflective practical judgments about existent conditions, synthesize concrete situational elements into orderly relations to structure operational units. The purpose of nursing design is to provide guides for achieving needed and foreseen results in the production of nursing toward the achievement of nursing goals; the units taken together constitute the pattern to guide the production of nursing.[96:458]

Nursing Systems Series and sequences of deliberate practical actions of nurses performed at times in coordination with actions of their patients to know and meet components of their patients' therapeutic self-care demands and to protect and regulate the exercise or development of patients' self-care agency.[96:303,459]

Helping Methods A helping method from a nursing perspective is a sequential series of actions, which, if performed, will overcome or compensate for the health-associated limitations of persons to engage in actions to regulate their own functioning and development or that of their dependents. Nurses use all the methods, selecting and combining them in relation to the action demands on persons under nursing care and their health-associated action limitations[96:14-15]:

1. Acting for or doing for another
2. Guiding and directing
3. Providing physical or psychological support
4. Providing and maintaining an environment that supports personal development
5. Teaching

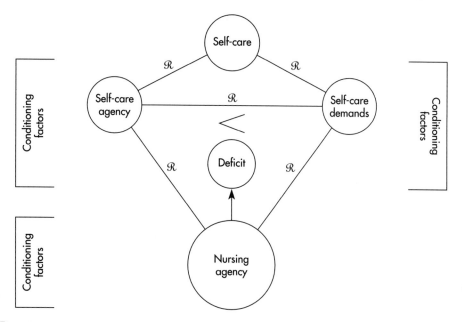

Fig. **14-1** A conceptual framework for nursing. *R*, Relationship; <, deficit relationship, current or projected. *From Orem, D.E. (1995).* Nursing: Concepts of practice. *St. Louis: Mosby, p. 435. Used with permission.*

MAJOR ASSUMPTIONS

Assumptions basic to the general theory were formalized in the early 1970s and were first presented at Marquette University School of Nursing in 1973. Orem identifies the five premises underlying the general theory of nursing:

1. Human beings require continuous deliberate inputs to themselves and their environments to remain alive and function in accord with natural human endowments.
2. Human agency, the power to act deliberately, is exercised in the form of care of self and others in identifying needs for and in making needed inputs.
3. Mature human beings experience privations in the form of limitations for action in care of self and others involving and making of life-sustaining and function-regulating inputs.
4. Human agency is exercised in discovering, developing, and transmitting to others ways and means to identify needs for and make inputs to self and others.
5. Groups of human beings with structured relationships cluster tasks and allocate responsibilities for providing care to group members who experience privations for making required deliberate input to self and others.[96:169]

Orem lists presuppositions for the theory of self-care, the theory of self-care deficit, and the theory of nursing systems in *Nursing: Concepts of Practice.*[96:171-172]

THEORETICAL ASSERTIONS

The model shows that when an individual's self-care capabilities are inadequate or inappropriate to meet the therapeutic self-care demand, the nurse may design and produce a nursing system that compensates for the limitations expressed as self-care or dependent-care deficit. The relational structure is discussed in Orem's book, *Nursing: Concepts of Practice,* as presuppositions, central ideas, and propositions of the three related theories of self-care, self-care deficit, and nursing system. Propositions are defined as statements that serve as principles and guides for further development of the theories.[96:179] The three theories are elaborated and described, including descriptions of processes, in other chapters. In the most recent edition, Orem expressed the theory in three sets of sentences that include: (I) facts, occurrences, and circumstances observed or observable in society in concrete situations of human living for which the theory was devised; (II) the central idea of the theory (the expressed model); and (III) a summary of the materials and models on which the central idea is based.[96:10]

It is important to note that the three constituent theories taken together in relationship constitute the SCDNT. The Theory of Nursing Systems is the most general and includes all the essential terms. It establishes the structure and content of nursing practice. The Theory of Nursing Systems subsumes the Theory of Self-Care Deficit and with it the Theory of Self-Care. The Theory of Self-Care Deficit develops the reason a person may benefit from nursing. The Theory of Self-Care is foundational.[96:167-178]

Theory of Nursing Systems

The Theory of Nursing Systems proposes that nursing is human action; nursing systems are action systems formed (designed and produced) by nurses through the exercise of their nursing agency for persons with health-derived or health-associated limitations in self-care or dependent-care. Nursing agency includes concepts of deliberate action, including intentionality and operations of diagnosis, prescription, and regulation. Fig. 14-2 shows the basic nursing systems categorized according to the relationship between patient action and nurse action. Nursing systems may be produced for individuals, for persons who constitute a dependent-care unit, for groups whose members have therapeutic self-care demands with similar components or who have similar limitations for engagement in self-care or dependent-care, or for families or other multiperson units.[96:176]

Theory of Self-Care Deficit

The central idea of the Theory of Self-Care Deficit is that requirements of persons for nursing are as-

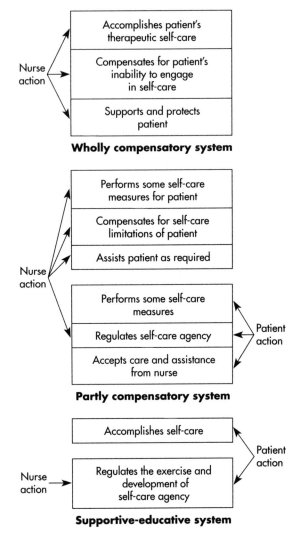

Fig. **14-2** Basic nursing systems. *From Orem, D.E. (1995). Nursing: Concepts of practice. St. Louis: Mosby, p. 307. Used with permission.*

sociated with the subjectivity of mature and maturing persons to health-related or health-care-related action limitations that render them completely or partially unable to know existent and emerging requisites for regulatory care for themselves or their dependents and to engage in the continuing performance of care measures to control or in some way manage factors that are regulatory of their own or their dependents' functioning and development[96:175]

Self-care deficit is a term that expresses the relationship between the action capabilities of individuals and their demands for care. Self-care deficit is an abstract concept that, when expressed in terms of action limitations, provides guides for selection of methods of helping and understanding patient roles in self-care.[96:175]

Theory of Self-Care

Self-care is a human regulatory function that individuals must, with deliberation, perform for themselves or have performed for them to maintain life, health, development, and well-being. Self-care is an action system. The elaboration of the concepts of self-care, self-care demand, and self-care agency provide the foundation for understanding the action requirements and action limitations of persons who may benefit from nursing.[96:171-174] Self-care as a human regulatory function stands in distinction to other types of regulation of human functioning and development such as neuroendocrine regulation. Self-care must be *learned* and it must be *deliberately performed continuously* in time and in conformity with the regulatory requirements of individuals associated, for example, with their stages of growth and development, states of health, specific features of health or developmental states, environmental factors, and levels of energy expenditure.[96:172]

LOGICAL FORM

Orem's insight led to her initial formalization and subsequent expression of a general concept of nursing. That generalization then made possible inductive and deductive thinking about nursing.

Susan Taylor and Thomas Taylor from the University of Missouri at Columbia have worked with Orem's general theory of nursing using a mathematical logic approach to explicate its syntactical structure or internal logic as a step toward identifying rules and modes of inquiry. By 1993, development of the theoretical constructs was reaching the stage that allowed transformation to computerized nursing information systems.[5,6,82]

ACCEPTANCE BY THE NURSING COMMUNITY

Orem's Self-Care Deficit Nursing Theory has achieved a significant level of acceptance by the nursing community as evidenced by the magnitude of published material. Over 600 references can be found through computerized search. A review of 225 of the most recent (since 1990) forms the basis for the content in this section.

In reviewing articles referenced as self-care, the searcher is cautioned that not all references to self-care are references to Orem's Theory of Nursing. The reader is also cautioned that not all uses of Orem's theory accurately reflect the most current state of theory development as expressed in the fifth edition of *Nursing: Concepts of Practice* (1995).[96] Much of the published literature uses Orem's Theory of Self-Care and Self-Care Deficit or other components of the theory as a way to explain practice. Orem cautions that the appropriate use of the SCDNT entails use of *all three* theories: self-care, self-care deficits, and nursing systems.

Practice

The first documented use of Orem's theory as the basis for structuring practice can be found in descriptions of nurse-managed clinics at Johns Hopkins Hospital in 1973.[1,2] Since that time there have been descriptions of the use of Orem's theory in a variety of clinical populations and age groups, from neonates to the elderly. The literature also includes the use of SCDNT in a number of ethnically and culturally diverse populations.

Multiple research articles have been published on teaching self-care to individuals with diabetes mellitus.[38-40,68,79] Likewise, there is a large section of research on end-stage renal failure, hemodialysis and peritoneal dialysis, and renal transplant,* all of which use the core concepts of SCDNT. Pain assessment

*References 12, 56, 58, 71, 100, 111.

and control is another highly researched area that makes use of Orem's theory.[21,42,67,128,129] This research not only assesses pain but teaches individuals to prevent, control, and alleviate pain. SCDNT is used frequently in cardiac research.[9,35,36,62,124-126] Cardiology nurses researched everything from self-care after a stroke to body image resulting from cardiac-related illnesses. Oncology has used SCDNT in a vast amount of research.* Oncology focuses a great deal on educating individuals either through cancer prevention or on how to maintain self-care after being diagnosed with malignancies. Dodd has done extensive work on self-care and patients with cancer.[23-29] Psychiatry and mental health is another research area that often uses Orem's theory.† This research primarily focuses on assessment and intervention of psychiatric disorders.

Multiple ethnic and cultural populations have been researched with the use of the SCDNT.‡ Wellness promotion in underprivileged ethnic groups and perceptions of self-care are two of the recently researched areas. Another highly researched area using Orem's theory is the elderly population.§ The elderly have many chronic illnesses and provide a variety of research topics. Many researchers are currently focusing on health promotion, self-care for the independent elderly, and family caregiver stress.[20,22,79,85]

In addition to the use of the theory for these clinical populations, the theory has been used in a variety of settings.[1,120] The Vancouver Health Department has done major work in designing community population-based care using Orem's conceptualizations.[31] Newark Beth Israel was one of the first acute-care hospitals to structure the delivery of nursing and the documentation system from Orem's theory.[86] Some in occupational health nursing are basing their practice on SCDNT. There are many health hazards and job-related risk factors of which nurses must be

aware. The ability to identify health problems, interpret findings, and draw correct conclusions is critical in occupational nursing.[70] Binghamton General Hospital is using Orem's theory as part of the orientation process for their new graduate nurses. For new graduates the first work experience is often the most difficult. There is some conflict with school teachings and real-world work values. SCDNT helps assist these nurses in combining their school teachings with the real nursing work that occurs after graduation.[34] Other future uses of the SCDNT will be on user-friendly intuitive computerized information systems that support nursing practices in a variety of settings.[5-6,81]

Orem's theory has been used to define and describe various roles for nurses within multiple settings. The clinical nurse-specialist role,[87] the case management role,[59,61,87,123] and the administrative role[17,80] have all been documented as having gained meaning through the application of the theory. A relatively new area explored is in teaching SCDNT to multiskilled workers and nurses' aides to assist them in becoming more aware of their roles and the patients' roles in the care given.[72]

There are several reports of the use of Orem's SCDNT in the development of clinical measurement approaches. The first major work done in this area was the study by Horn and Swain.[60] They developed criteria measures of nursing care focused around the universal self-care requisites and health-deviation self-care requisites. Since then a number of other clinical instruments have been developed. In 1989, Moore and Gaffney[84] developed the Dependent Care Agent (DCA) questionnaire to measure mothers' performance of self-care activities for children. Individual requisites for self-care are evidenced in the DCA. Hayward et al.[56] utilized Orem's theory when creating the Kidney Transplant Recipient Stress Scale (KTRSS), which was developed to identify stressors in renal transplant recipients. Graff and coworkers[43] developed a postoperative self-assessment form with Orem's concept of the nurse assisting the client in self-care. The Appraisal of Self-Care Agency (ASA) scale was developed to measure a core-concept of Orem's SCDNT.[32]

---

*References 14, 15, 44-47, 57, 65, 75, 82, 88, 99, 101-103, 107, 108, 127, 134.
†References 13, 18, 30, 37, 48, 74, 97, 105, 110, 133, 137.
‡References 11, 16, 19, 30, 54, 55, 69, 73, 106, 135.
§References 4, 8, 10, 33, 35, 48, 49, 50, 63, 64, 66, 98, 109, 112, 131, 132, 136.

Orem's theory has been translated into Italian, French, Spanish, Dutch, and Japanese; currently, there are translations of some or all of her recent work going on in Germany, Thailand, and Norway, among others. Her work is known to be used throughout the world. Practitioners of nursing in Great Britain, Taiwan, Thailand, Japan, Korea, Canada, Australia, New Zealand, South Africa, Israel, Germany, Spain, Italy, France, Belgium, the Netherlands, Bolivia, Colombia, and Mexico report their use of Orem's theory.[98]

There has been little work on the theory of nursing systems. No studies were found that directly refer to nursing systems as they are designed and implemented for individuals or populations.[115]

Education

While Orem's original insights about self-care and the reasons why persons need nursing occurred in a research-on-practice setting, the second stage of development of the theory was done in the context of education. Much of the initial work was done with the Nursing Models Committee at The Catholic University of America. The first publication relating the theory and education was the *Guidelines for Developing Curricula for the Education of Practical Nurses* (1959). In each of Orem's subsequent publications, there are sections on education.

There are a number of reports in the literature describing the use of SCDNT as the basis for the curriculum.[3,52,53] At least 45 schools of nursing are known to use SCDNT as the basis for their curriculums (data from the International Orem Society). Taylor (1985) described the use of the theory in preservice nursing education and in teaching[113,114] The Sinclair School of Nursing, University of Missouri at Columbia, has used SCDNT as the framework for curriculum and teaching since 1978. The theory is used at all levels of the curriculum and in continuing education. Oakland University, College of St. Benedict, and Anderson College are three schools with curricula designed within SCDNT. Samples of their courses may be accessed through the Internet by searching for Self-Care Deficit Nursing Theory.

Research

The research related to or derived from Orem's theory can be classified as that relating to (1) the development of research instruments for measuring the conceptual elements of the theory and (2) studies that test elements of the theory in specific populations. There is also a large body of research literature in which the use of SCDNT or components is merely tangential; these are not reviewed here.

A number of instruments for research have been developed. The first instrument to measure the exercise of self-care agency was published in 1979. Since then there have been others developed and critiqued.[7] The SCDNT was the conceptual groundwork for Kearney and Fleisher's Exercise of Self-Care Agency in 1979,[67] Denyes' Self-Care Agency in 1981,[20] and Hanson and Bickel's Perception of Self-Care Agency in 1981.[77,78] The SCDNT was a pivotal construct in the design of the Self-As-Carer Inventory (SCI). This inventory permits individuals to express their perceived capacity to care for their self.[41] McBride[78] did a comparative analysis of three instruments designed to measure self-care agency: Denyes' Self-Care Agency Instrument (DSCAI), Kearney and Fleisher's Exercise of Self-Care Agency (ESCA), and Hanson and Bickel's Perception of Self-Care Agency. To identify latent traits and their relationships, a common factor analysis and canonical correlation was done. The results supported the multidimensionality of Orem's concept of self-care agency. McBride also points out that the use of only one instrument does not adequately reflect this multidimensionality. McBride also examined the reliability and construct validity of the ESCA. To test for construct validity the Self-Directed Learning Readiness Scale (SDLRS) was used. Findings showed that the ESCA was significantly correlated with all eight factors of the SDLRS for the student group and with only three factors for the patient group, with need for further study of the construct validity.[77] Geden and Taylor[41] tested the construct and empirical validity of the SCI and found that the SCI seemed to possess strong theoretical validity but that further validity testing should also be done. Currently, validity of nursing theory for use within computerized nursing information systems (CNIS) is occurring. Bliss-Holtz, McLaughlin, and Taylor have performed some research within this area.[5]

The research instruments most frequently used include the Denyes Self-Care Agency Instrument (DSCAI),[39,40] Denyes Self-Care Practice Instrument (DSCPI),[39,40] ASA,[32] and SCI.[41] Others include Maieutic Dimensions of Self-Care Agency Scale (MDSCAS)[89] and Moore and Gaffney's DCA questionnaire.[84]

Some examples of these tools utilized are as follows. The MDSCAS is a sensitive outcome measure for use in educative-supportive nursing systems where the outcome of interest is enhancement. Moore[77] utilized the Child and Adolescent Self-Care Practice Questionnaire, the DSCAI, and the ESCA when she measured the self-care practices of children and adolescents.

McCaleb and Edgil[79] used the DCSPI to measure self-concept and self-care practices of health adolescents. To assess and teach self-care to youths with diabetes mellitus, Frey and Fox used the DSCPI and Denyes Health Status Instrument along with the Diabetes Self-Care Practice Instrument.[40]

For evaluation of a hemodialysis patient program and support program, the ESCA was used.[71] Whetstone and Reid[136] also used the ESCA to measure health promotion in older adults and perceived barriers. Research with the elderly tends to utilize the ASA and the ESCA often to assess their self-care agencies and abilities.* Folden used the ESCA to measure the effect of a supportive-educative nursing intervention on older adults' perceptions of self-care after a stroke.[35] When measuring perceptions of self-care in Sweden, Whetstone and Hansson[135] used the ESCA and the Self-Concept Inventory. Research with pregnant women often uses the ESCA and the ASA to assess basic conditioning factors and self-care abilities related to their health and that of their infants.[51,76,104]

FURTHER DEVELOPMENT

From the publication of the first edition of *Nursing: Concepts of Practice*[92] in 1971, to the present, Orem

has been engaged in continual development of her conceptualizations. She has done this work by herself and with colleagues. The fifth edition was completed and published in 1995.[96] Orem is presently working with a group of scholars, known as the Orem Study Group, to further develop the various conceptualizations and to structure nursing knowledge using the elements of the theory. The development of SCDNT has been done by a number of researchers and scholars throughout the years.[117-119,122]

The fifth edition is organized in two parts: nursing as a unique field of knowledge and nursing as practical science. It includes an expansion of content on nursing practice and the theory of nursing systems. Design units, first described in the fourth edition, have been amplified. The caring dimensions of nursing are explored. There is new work done on the interpersonal features of nursing. The fifth edition also includes a new chapter on nursing in multiperson situations, family, and community, written by Taylor and Renpenning.[121]

There is further development of Orem's conceptualization of nursing administration that is being done by Allison, Renpenning, and others. Work in progress includes the development of a theory of dependent care, the relationship or use of the theory in primary care, and further exploration of the theoretical foundations of the work. Ongoing research by many nursing scholars will clarify certain conceptualizations and will demonstrate the relationship of theory and practice. Orem, in collaboration with Vardiman, has developed a concept of positive mental health.[97]

The International Orem Society for Nursing Science and Nursing Scholarship (IOS) was established in 1993. Incorporated as a not-for-profit organization, the purpose of the IOS is to advance nursing science and scholarship through the use of Dorothea E. Orem's nursing conceptualizations in nursing education, practice, and research. The IOS semiannually publishes a newsletter. This can be accessed through the Internet, Self-Care Deficit Theory home page, maintained by the University of Missouri at Columbia, Sinclair School of Nursing.

*References 57, 58, 63, 64, 101, 109.

CRITIQUE

Clarity

The terms used by Orem are precisely defined. The language of the theory is consistent with the language used in action theory and philosophy. There are no created words. The terminology of the theory is congruent throughout. The term *self-care* has multiple meanings across disciplines; Orem has defined the term and elaborated the substantive structure of the concept in a way that is unique but also congruent with other interpretations. There have been references to the difficulty of Orem's language; the limitation generally resides in the reader's lack of familiarity with the field of action science.

Simplicity

Orem's general theory (SCDNT) comprises three constituent theories, that of self-care, self-care deficits, and nursing systems. The self-care deficit theory of nursing is a "synthesis of knowledge about the theoretical entities self-care (and dependent-care), self-care agency (and dependent-care agency), therapeutic self-care demand, the relational entity self-care deficit and nursing agency."[96:170]

The entity nursing system is also included. The development of the theory using these six entities is parsimonious. The relationship between and among these entities can be presented in a simple diagram. The substantive structure of the theory is found in the development of these entities.

Generality

Orem herself has commented on the generality or universality of the theory:

> The self-care deficit theory of nursing is not an explanation of the individuality of a particular concrete nursing practice situation, but rather the expression of a singular combination of conceptualized properties or features common to all instances of nursing. As a general theory, it serves nurses engaged in nursing practice, in development and validation of nursing knowledge, and in teaching and learning nursing.[96:167]

A review of the research and other literature attests to the generality of the theory.

Empirical Precision

Orem's theory has been used for research using both qualitative and quantitative methodologies. The theoretical entities are well defined and lend themselves to being measurable; however, instruments have not been developed for all of the entities, for example, nursing agency.

Furthermore, the values of the theoretical entities are not constant across populations. For example, the Theory of Self-Care Deficit is a function of the self-care requisites and basic conditioning factors. This necessitates the development of multiple instruments to measure the Theory of Self-Care Deficit. The most appropriate methods of inquiry for this theory, as well as for all nursing theories, are yet to be determined. The beauty of Orem's theory lies in the scope, complexity, and clinical usefulness; it is useful for generating hypotheses and adding to the body of knowledge that is nursing.

Derivable Consequences

The SCDNT differentiates the focus of nursing from other disciplines. While other disciplines find the theory of self-care helpful and contribute to its development, the theory of nursing systems provides the unique focus for nursing. There is ample evidence in the literature that the theory is useful in developing and guiding practice and research.[116,117] It gives direction to nursing-specific outcomes related to knowing and meeting the therapeutic self-care demands, regulating the development and exercise of self-care agency, establishing self-care and self-management systems, and others.

The theory is also useful in the design of curriculums[3,53,113,114] for preservice, graduate, and continuing nursing education. The theory also gives direction to nursing administration. The development of theory-based computer systems, assessment forms, and the overall structuring of the delivery of care attests to the usefulness of the theory.[86]

The significance of Orem's work extends far beyond the development of the SCDNT. In her works she has provided us with the expression of the form of nursing science as practical science, with a structure for ongoing development of nursing knowledge in the stages of development of theory. She has presented a visionary view of contemporary nursing practice, education, and knowledge development expressed through the general theory.

CRITICAL THINKING *Activities*

1 Not all of Orem's writings are expositions of the Self-Care Deficit Nursing Theory. Review some of her writings and identify that which is theory and that which is application or related ideas about nursing.

2 Review the definitions provided in the glossary, *Nursing: Concepts of Practice*, fifth edition. Classify them as conceptual or operational, denotative or connotative. Explain your thinking.

3 Select a research article that purports to use SCDNT as the conceptual framework. Is the research question derived from the theory? What contribution does it make to further understanding of the theory?

4 Make a list of the definitions of nursing used by the theorists. Which ones are specific to nursing? Evaluate Orem's description of the proper object of nursing. How does that relate to others?

REFERENCES

1. Allison, S.E. (1973). A framework for nursing action in a nurse-conducted diabetic managed clinic. *Journal of Nursing Administration, 3*(4), 53-60.
2. Backsheider, J. (1974). Self-care requirements, self-care capabilities and nursing systems in the diabetic nurse managed clinic. *American Journal of Public Health, 64*(12), 1138-1146
3. Berbiglia, V.A. (1991). A case study: Perspectives on a self-care deficit nursing theory–based curriculum. *Journal of Advanced Nursing, 16*(10), 1158-63.
4. Biggs, A.J. (1990). Family caregiver versus nursing assessments of elderly self-care abilities. *Journal of Gerontological Nursing, 16*(8), 11-16.
5. Bliss-Holtz, J., McLaughlin, K., Taylor, S.G. (1990). Validating nursing theory for use within a computerized nursing information system. *Advances in Nursing Science, 13*(2), 46-52.
6. Bliss-Holtz, J., Taylor, S.G., & McLaughlin, K. (1992). Nursing theory as a base for a computerized nursing information system. *Nursing Science Quarterly, 5*(3), 124-128.
7. Bottorff, J.L. (1988). Assessing an instrument in a pilot project: The self-care agency questionnaire. *Canadian Journal of Nursing Research, 20*(1), 7-16.
8. Bracher, E. (1989). A model approach. *Nursing Times, 85*(43), 42-43.
9. Brundage, D.J. (1993). Self-care instruction for patients with COPD. *Rehabilitation Nursing, 18*(5), 321-325.
10. Buntings, S.M. (1989). Stress on caregivers of the elderly. *Advanced Nursing Science, 11*(2), 63-73.
11. Butler, F.R. (1987). Minority wellness promotion: A behavioral self-management approach. *Journal of Gerontological Nursing, 31*(8), 23-28.
12. Collins, B. (1995). End-stage renal failure: The challenge to the nurse. *Nursing Times, 8*(91), 27-29.
13. Compton, P. (1989). Drug abuse: A self-care deficit. *Journal of Psychosocial Nursing, 27*(3), 22-27.
14. Coward, D.D. (1988). Hypercalcemia knowledge assessment in patients at risk of developing cancer-induced hypercalcemia. *Oncology Nursing Forum, 15*(4), 471-476.
15. Cretain, G.K. (1989). Motivational factors in breast self-examination: Implications for nurses. *Cancer Nursing, 12*(4), 250-256.
16. Dashiff, C.J. (1992). Self-care capabilities in black girls in anticipation of menarche. *Health Care for Women International, 13*, 67-76
17. Davidhizar, R. (1993). Self-care and mentors to reduce stress and enhance administrative ability. *Geriatric Nursing, 14*, 146-149.
18. Davidhizar, R., & Cosgray, R. (1990). The use of Orem's model in psychiatric rehabilitation assessment. *Rehabilitation Nursing, 15*(1), 39-41.
19. Dennis, L.I. (1989). Soviet hospital nursing: A model for self-care. *Journal of Nursing Education, 28*(2), 76-77.
20. Denyes, M.J. (1988). Orem's model used for health promotion: Directions from research. *Advances in Nursing, 11*(1), 13-21.
21. Denyes, M.J., Neuman, B.M., & Villarruel, A.M. (1991). Nursing actions to prevent and alleviate pain in hospitalized children. *Issues in Comprehensive Pediatric Nursing, 14*, 31-48.
22. Denyes, M.J., O'Connor, N.A., Oakley, D., & Ferguson, S. (1989). Integrating nursing theory, practice, and research through collaborative research. *Journal of Advanced Nursing, 14*(2), 141-145.
23. Dodd, M.J. (1982). Assessing patient self-care for side effects of cancer chemotherapy. *Cancer Nursing, 5*(6), 447-451.

24. Dodd, M.J. (1982). Chemotherapy knowledge in patients with cancer: Assessment and informational interventions. *Oncology Nursing Forum,* (3), 39-44.

25. Dodd, M.J. (1983). Self-care for side effects of cancer chemotherapy: An assessment of nursing interventions. *Cancer Nursing,* 6(1), 63-67.

26. Dodd, M.J. (1988). Efficacy of proactive information on self-care in chemotherapy patients. *Patient Education and Counseling,* 11, 215-225.

27. Dodd, M.J. (1988). Patterns of self-care in patients with breast cancer. *Western Journal of Nursing Research,* 10(1), 7-14.

28. Dodd, M.J. (1991). *Managing side effects of chemotherapy and radiation therapy for cancer: A guide for patients and families* (2nd ed.). Englewood Cliffs, NJ: Prentice-Hall.

29. Dodd, M.J., Thomas, M.L., & Dibble, S.L. (1991). Self-care for patients experiencing cancer chemotherapy side effects: A concern for home care nurses. *Home Healthcare,* 9(6), 21-26.

30. Duffey, J. (1993). Psychiatric home care: A framework for assessment and intervention. *Home Healthcare Nurse,* 11(2), 22-28.

31. Duncan, S., & Murphy, F. (1988). Embracing a conceptual model. *Canadian Nurse,* 84(4), 24-26.

32. Evers, G.C.M., Isenberg, M.A., Philipsen, H., Senten, M., & Brouns, G. (1993). Validity testing of the Dutch translation of the appraisal of the self-care agency A.S.A. scale. *International Journal of Nursing Studies,* 30(4), 331-342.

33. Fawcett, J., Ellis, V., Underwood, P., Naqvi, A., & Wilson, D. (1990). The effect of Orem's self-care model on nursing care in a nursing home setting. *Journal of Advanced Nursing,* 15, 659-666.

34. Feldsine, F.T. (1982). Options for transition into practice: Nursing process orientation program. *Journal, N.Y.S.N.A.,* 13(1), 11-16.

35. Folden, S.L. (1993). Effect of a supportive-educative nursing intervention on older adults' perceptions of self-care after a stroke. *Rehabilitation Nursing,* 18(3), 162-167.

36. Frances, Sr. (1989). Self-care in pregnancy-induced hypertension. *Nursing Journal of India,* 7, 188-189.

37. Frederick, J., & Cotanch, P. (1994). Self-help techniques for auditory hallucinations in schizophrenia. *Issues in Mental Health Nursing,* 16, 213-224.

38. Frey, G.M. (1990). Stressors in renal transplant recipients at six weeks after transplant. *ANNA Journal,* 17(6), 443-446.

39. Frey, M.A., & Denyes, M.J. (1989). Health and illness self-care in adolescents with IDDM: A test of Orem's theory. *Advanced Nursing Science,* 12(1), 67-75.

40. Frey, M.A., & Fox, M.A. (1990). Assessing and teaching self-care to youths with diabetes mellitus. *Pediatric Nursing,* 16(6), 597-599.

41. Geden, E., & Taylor, S. (1991). Construct and empirical validity of the self-as-carer inventory. *Nursing Research,* 40(1), 47-50.

42. Good, M. (1995). A comparison of the effects of jaw relaxation and music on postoperative pain. *Nursing Research,* 44(1), 52-57.

43. Graff, B.M., Thomas, J.S., Hollingsworth, A.O., Cohen, S.M., Rubin, M.M. (1992). Development of a postoperative self-assessment form. *Clinical Nurse Specialist,* 6(1), 47-50.

44. Graling, P.R., & Grant, J.M. (1995). Demographics and patient treatment choice in stage I breast cancer. *AORN Journal,* 62(3), 376-384.

45. Grant, M. (1990). The effect of nursing consultation on anxiety, side effects, and self-care of patients receiving radiation therapy. *Oncology Nursing Forum,* 17(3), 31-36.

46. Hagoplan, G.A. (1991). The effects of a weekly radiation therapy newsletter on patients. *Oncology Nursing Forum,* 18(7), 1199-1203.

47. Hanucharurnkul, S. (1988). Predictors of self-care in cancer patients receiving radiotherapy. *Cancer Nursing,* 12(1), 21-27.

48. Harris, J. (1990). Self-care actions of chronic schizophrenics associated with meeting solitude and social interaction requisites. *Archives of Psychiatric Nursing,* 4(5), 298-307.

49. Harris, J.L., & Williams, L.K. (1991). Universal self-care requisites as identified by homeless elderly men. *Journal of Gerontological Nursing,* 17(6), 39-43.

50. Harris, M.D., Rhinehart, J.M., & Gertsman, J. (1993). Animal-assisted therapy for the homebound elderly. *Holistic Nurse Practitioner,* 8(1), 27-37.

51. Hart, M.A. (1995). Orem's self-care deficit theory: Research with pregnant women. *Nursing Science Quarterly,* 8(3), 120-126.

52. Hartweg, D.L. (1986). Self-care attitude changes of nursing students enrolled in self-care curriculum—A longitudinal study. *Research in Nursing & Health,* 9(4), 347-353.

53. Hartweg, D.L. (1995). Curricular decisions: Using Orem's conceptualizations to guide curriculum and student clinical practice. *International Orem Society Newsletter,* 3(1), 8-9.

54. Hartweg, D.L. (1996). Determining the adequacy of a health promotion self-care interview guide with healthy, middle-aged, Mexican American women: A pilot study. *Health Care for Women International,* 17(1), 57-68.

55. Hautman, M.A. (1987). Self-care responses to respiratory illnesses among Vietnamese. *Western Journal of Nursing Research,* 9(2), 223-243.

56. Hayward, M.B., Kish, J.P., Frey, G.M., Kirchner, J.M., Carr, L.S., & Wolfe, C.M. (1989). An instrument to identify stressors in renal transplant recipients. *ANNA Journal,* 16(2), 81-84.

57. Hiromoto, B.M., & Dungan, J. (1991). Contract learning for self-care activities: A protocol study among chemotherapy outpatients. *Cancer Nursing,* 14(3), 148-154.

58. Hoffart, N. (1982). Self-care decision making by renal transplant recipients. *AANNT Journal, 9*(3), 43-47.

59. Holzemer, W.L. (1992). Linking primary health care and self-care through case management. *International Nursing Review, 39*(3), 83-89.

60. Horn, B.J., & Swain, M.A. (1977). Development of criterion measures of nursing care (Vols. 1 and 2). *University of Michigan and National Center for Health Services Research.* U.S. Department of Commerce (NTIS Publication No. 267-004 and 267-005.)

61. Issel, M. (1995). Evaluating case management programs. *MCN, 20,* 67-74.

62. Jaarsma, T., Kastermans, M., Dassen, T., & Philipsen, H. (1995). Problems of cardiac patients in early recovery. *Journal of Advanced Nursing, 21,* 21-27.

63. Jirovec, M.M., & Kasno, J. (1990). Self-care agency as a function of patient-environmental factors among nursing home residents. *Research in Nursing & Health, 13,* 303-309.

64. Jirovec, M.M., & Kasno, J. (1993). Predictors of self-care abilities among the institutionalized elderly. *Western Journal of Nursing Research, 15*(3), 314-326.

65. Jones, A. (1988). A level of independence. *Nursing Times, 84*(15), 54-57.

66. Jopp, M., Carroll, M.C., & Waters, L. (1993). Using self-care theory to guide nursing management of the older adult after hospitalization. *Rehabilitation Nursing, 18*(2), 91-94.

67. Kearney, B., & Fleischer, B.J. (1972). Development of an instrument to measure exercise of self-care agency. *Research in Nursing Health, 2,* 25-34.

68. Keohane, N.S., & Lacey, L.A. (1991). Preparing the woman with gestational diabetes for self-care: Use of a structured teaching plan by nursing staff. *JOGNN, 20*(3), 189-193.

69. Kerkstra, A., Castelein, E., & Philipsen, H. (1991). Preventive home visits to elderly people by community nurses in the Netherlands. *Journal of Advanced Nursing, 16,* 631-637.

70. Komulainen, P. (1991). Occupational health nursing based on self-care theory. *AAOHN Journal, 39*(7), 333-335.

71. Korniewicz, DM., & O'Brien, M.E. (1994). Evaluation of a hemodialysis patient education and support program. *ANNA Journal, 21*(1), 33-38.

72. Kostovich, C.T., Mahneke, S.M., Meyer, P.A., & Healy, C. (1994). The clinician technician as a member of the patient-focused healthcare delivery team. *JONA, 24*(12), 32-38.

73. Lile, J.L., & Hoffman, R. (1991). Medication-taking by the frail elderly in two ethnic groups. *Nursing Forum, 26*(4), 19-24.

74. MacDonald, G. (1991). Plans for a better future. *Nursing Times, 87*(31), 42-43.

75. Mack, C.H. (1992). Assessment of the autologous bone marrow transplant patient according to Orem's self-care model. *Cancer Nursing, 15*(6), 429-436.

76. Mapanga, K.G., & Andrews, C.M. (1995). The influence of family and friends' basic conditioning factors and self-care agency on unmarried teenage primiparas' engagement in contraceptive practice. *Journal of Community Health, 12*(2), 89-100.

77. McBride, S. (1987). Validation of an instrument to measure exercise of self-care agency. *Research in Nursing & Health, 10,* 311-316.

78. McBride, S. (1991). Comparative analysis of three instruments designed to measure self-care agency. *Nursing Research, 40*(1), 12-16.

79. McCaleb, A.M., & Edgil, A. (1994). Self-concept and self-care practices of healthy adolescents. *Journal of Pediatric Nursing, 9*(4), 233-238.

80. McCoy, S. (1989). Teaching self-care in a market-oriented world. *Nursing Management, 20*(5), 22-26.

81. McLaughlin, K., Taylor, S., Bliss-Holtz, J., Sayers, P., & Nickle, L. (1990). Shaping the future; The marriage of nursing theory and informatics. *Computers in Nursing, 8*(4), 174-179.

82. Meriney, D.K. (1990). Application of Orem's conceptual framework to patients with hypercalcemia related to breast cancer. *Cancer Nursing, 13*(5), 316-323.

83. Moore, J.B. (1995). Measuring the self-care practice of children and adolescents: Instrument development. *Maternal-Child Nursing Journal, 23*(3), 101-108.

84. Moore, J.B., & Gaffney, K.F. (1989). Development of an instrument to measure mothers' performance of self-care activities for children. *Advanced Nursing Science, 12*(1), 76-84.

85. Mulkeen, H. (1989). Diabetes: Teaching the teaching of self-care. *Nursing Times, 85*(3), 63-5.

86. National League for Nursing Editorial Review Board News. (1987, Dec.). Newark Beth Israel Medical Center adopts Orem's Self-Care Model. *Nursing and Health Care, 8*(10), 593-594.

87. Norris, M.K.G., & Hill, C. (1991). The clinical nurse specialist: Developing the case manager role. *Dimensions of Critical Care Nursing, 10*(6), 346-353.

88. Oberst, M.T., Chang, A.S., & McCubbin, M.A. (1991). Self-care burden, stress appraisal, and mood among persons receiving radiotherapy. *Cancer Nursing, 14*(2), 71-78.

89. O'Connor, N.A. (1995). Maieutic dimensions of self-care agency: Instrument development. *Dissertation Abstracts International, 56-05,* 2563.

90. Orem, D.E. (1956). Nursing service: An analysis. Report to the Division of Hospital and Institutional Services of the Indiana State Board of Health.

91. Orem, D.E. (1959). *Guidelines for developing curricula for the education of practical nurses.* Washington, DC: U.S. Government Printing Office.

92. Orem, D.E. (1971). *Nursing: Concepts of practice.* New York: McGraw-Hill.

93. Orem, D.E. (1979). *Concept formalization in nursing: Process and product* (2nd ed.). Boston: Little, Brown.

94. Orem, D.E. (1985). *Nursing: Concepts of practice* (3rd ed.). New York: McGraw-Hill.

95. Orem, D.E. (1988, May). The form on nursing science. *Nursing Science Quarterly, 1*(2), 75-79.

96. Orem, D.E. (1995). *Nursing: Concepts of practice* (5th ed.). St Louis: Mosby.

97. Orem, D.E., & Vardiman, E.M. (1995). Orem's nursing theory and positive mental health: Practical considerations. *Nursing Science Quarterly, 8*(4), 165-173.

98. Padula, C.A. (1992). Self-care and the elderly: Review and implications. *Public Health Nursing, 9*(1), 22-28.

99. Palmer, P., & Meyers, F.J. (1990). An outpatient approach to the delivery of intensive consolidation chemotherapy to adults with acute lymphoblastic leukemia. *Oncology Nursing Forum, 17*(4), 553-558.

100. Perras, S.T., & Zappacosta, A.R. (1982). The application of Orem's theory in promoting self-care in a peritoneal dialysis facility. *AANNT Journal, 9*(3), 37-9, 55.

101. Rhodes, V. (1990). Nausea, vomiting, and retching. *Nursing Clinics of North America, 25*(4), 855-900.

102. Rhodes, V.A., Watson, P.M., & Hanson, B.M. (1988). Patients' descriptions of the influence of tiredness and weakness on self-care abilities. *Cancer Nursing, 11*(3), 186-194.

103. Richardson, A. (1992). Studies exploring self-care for the person coping with cancer treatment: A review. *International Journal of Nursing Studies, 29*(2), 191-204.

104. Riesch, S.K. (1988). Changes in the exercise of self-care agency. *Western Journal of Nursing Research, 10*(3), 257-273.

105. Roper, J.M., Shapira, J., & Chang, B.L. (1991). Agitation in the demented patient: A framework for management. *Journal of Gerontological Nursing, 17*(3), 17-21.

106. Roy, O., & Collin, M.E.F. (1994). La personne agee atteinte de demence. *L'Infirmiere Canadienne, 90*(1), 39-43.

107. Smith, M.C., Holcombe, J.K., & Stullenbarger, E. (1994). A meta-analysis of intervention effectiveness for symptom management in oncology nursing research. *Oncology Nursing Forum, 21*(7), 1201-1209.

108. Smith, M.K. (1995). Implementing annual cancer screenings for elderly women. *Journal of Gerontological Nursing, 21*(7), 12-17.

109. Smits, M.W. (1992). Correlates of self-care among the independent elderly: Self-concept affects well-being. *Journal of Gerontological Nursing, 18*(9), 13-18.

110. Steele, S., Russell, F., Hansen, B., & Mills, B. (1989). Home management of URI in children with Down syndrome. *Pediatric Nursing, 15*(5), 484-488.

111. Summerton, H. (1995). End-stage renal failure: The challenge to the nurse. *Nursing Times, 91*(6), 27-29.

112. Taira, F. (1991). Teaching independently living older adults about managing their medications. *Rehabilitation Nursing, 16*(6), 322-326.

113. Taylor, S.G. (1985). Curriculum development for preservice programs using Orem's theory of nursing. In J. Riehl-Sisca (Ed.), *The science and art of self-care* (pp. 25-32). Norwalk CT: Appleton-Century-Crofts.

114. Taylor, S.G. (1985). Teaching self-care deficit theory to generic students. In J. Riehl-Sisca (Ed.), *The art and science of self-care.* New York: Appleton-Century-Crofts.

115. Taylor, S.G. (1986). *Defining clinical populations from self-care deficit theory (SCDT) perspective.* In S.G. Taylor (Ed.). Papers presented at the Fifth Annual Self-Care Deficit Theory Conference presented by the School of Nursing, University of Missouri–Columbia (pp.29-35), St. Louis.

116. Taylor, S.G. (1987). *Clinical decision-making from the perspective of self-care deficit theory (SCDT).* In S.G. Taylor (Ed.), Paper presented at the Sixth Annual Self-Care Deficit Theory Conference presented by the School of Nursing, University of Missouri–Columbia (pp.78-90), St. Louis.

117. Taylor, S.G. (1988). Nursing theory and nursing process. *Nursing Science Quarterly, 1*(3), 111-119.

118. Taylor, S.G. (1989). The interpretation of family from the perspective of self-care deficit nursing theory. *Nursing Science Quarterly, 2*(3), 131-137.

119. Taylor, S.G. (1991). The structure of nursing diagnosis from Orem's theory. *Nursing Science Quarterly, 4*(1), 24-32.

120. Taylor, S.G., & McLaughlin, K. (1991, Winter). Orem's theory and community. *Nursing Science Quarterly, 4*(4), 153-160.

121. Taylor, S.G., & Renpenning, D. (1995). The practice of nursing in multiperson situations: Family and community. In D.E. Orem, *Nursing: Concepts of practice* (5th ed) (pp. 348-380). St. Louis: Mosby.

122. Taylor, S.G., & Robinson-Purdy, A.V. (1989). *Assessing self-management and dependent care capabilities of hospitalized adults and care givers in preparation for discharge.* Paper presented at the First International Self-Care Deficit Nursing Theory Conference presented by the School of Nursing, University of Missouri–Columbia (pp. 4-16), Kansas City, MO.

123. Togno-Armanasco, V.T., Olivas, G.S., & Harter, S. (1989). Developing an integrated nursing case management model. *Nursing Management, 29*(10), 26-29.

124. Toyama, A.K., Edlefsen, P., Krozek, K.S., Ballantyne, S., Hostrup, M., & Wuertzer, P.R. (1988). Assisting long-term patient recovery through a nonmonitored maintenance component in a cardiac rehabilitation program. *Journal of Cardiovascular Nursing, 2*(3), 13-22.

125. Utz, S.W., Hammer, J., Whitmire, V.M., & Grass, S. (1990). Perceptions of body image and health status in persons with mitral valve prolapse. *IMAGE: Journal of Nursing Scholarship, 22*(1), 18-22.

126. Utz, S.W., & Ramos, M.C. (1993). Mitral valve prolapse and its effects: A programme of inquiry within Orem's self-care deficit theory of nursing. *Journal of Advanced Nursing, 18*, 742-751.

127. Utz, S.W., Shuster, G.F., Merwin, E., & Williams, B. (1994). A community-based smoking cessation program: Self-care behaviors and success. *Public Health Nursing, 11*(5), 291-299.

128. Vesely, C. (1995). Pediatric patient-controlled analgesia: Enhancing the self-care construct. *Pediatric Nursing, 21*(2), 124-128.

129. Villarruel, A.M., & Denyes, M.J. (1991). Pain assessment in children: Theoretical and empirical validity. *Advanced Nursing Science, 14*(2), 32-41.

130. Wallace, W.A. (1979). *From a realist point of view: Essays on the philosophy of science.* Washington, DC: Universal Press of America.

131. Wanich, C.K., Sullivan-Max, E.M., Gottlieb, G.L., & Johnson, J.C. (1992). Functional status outcomes of a nursing intervention in hospitalized elderly. *IMAGE: Journal of Nursing Scholarship, 24*(3), 201-207.

132. Ward-Griffen, C., & Bramwell, L. (1990). The congruence of elderly client and nurse perceptions of the clients' self-care agency. *Journal of Advanced Nursing, 15,* 1070-1077.

133. Whall, A.L. (1994). What is the nursing treatment for depression? *Journal of Gerontological Nursing,* 42,45.

134. Whenery-Tedder, M. (1991). Teaching acceptance. *Nursing Times, 87*(12), 36-39.

135. Whetstone, W.R., & Hansson, A.O. (1989). Perceptions of self-care in Sweden: A cross-cultural replication. *Journal of Advanced Nursing, 14,* 962-969.

136. Whetstone, W.R., & Reid, J. (1991). Health promotion of older adults: Perceived barriers. *Journal of Advanced Nursing, 16,* 1343-1349.

137. Youssef, F.A. (1987). Discharge planning for psychiatric patients: The effects of a family-patient teaching programme. *Journal of Advanced Nursing, 12,* 611-616.

BIBLIOGRAPHY

Primary sources

Books

Orem, D.E. (Ed.). (1959). *Guides for developing curricula for the education of practical nurses.* Vocational Division #274. Trade and Industrial Education #68, Washington, DC: U.S. Department of Health Education, and Welfare.

Orem, D.E. (1971). *Nursing: Concepts of practice.* Scarborough, Ontario: McGraw-Hill.

Orem, D.E. (Ed.). (1973). *Concepts formalization in nursing: Process and product.* Boston: Little, Brown.

Orem, D.E. (Ed.). (1979). *Concept formalization in nursing: Process and product* (2nd ed.). Boston: Little, Brown.

Orem, D.E. (1980). *Nursing: Concepts of practice.* (2nd ed.). New York: McGraw-Hill.

Orem, D.E. (1985). *Nursing: Concepts of practice.* (3rd ed.). New York: McGraw-Hill.

Orem, D.E. (1991). *Nursing: Concepts of practice.* (4th ed.). St. Louis: Mosby.

Orem, D.E. (1995). *Nursing: Concepts of practice.* (5th ed.). St. Louis: Mosby.

Orem, D.E., & Parker K.S. (Eds.)(1963). *Nurse practice education workshop proceedings.* Washington, DC: The Catholic University of America.

Orem, D.E., & Parker, K.S. (Eds). (1964). *Nursing content in preservice nursing curriculum.* Washington, DC: The Catholic University of America Press.

Book chapters

Orem, D.E. (1966). Discussion of paper—Another view of nursing care and quality. In K.M. Straub & K.S. Parker (Eds.), *Continuity of patient care: The role of nursing.* Washington, DC: The Catholic University of America Press.

Orem, D.E. (1969). Inservice education and nursing practice forces effecting nursing practice. In D.K. Petrowski & K.M. Staub (Eds.), *School of nursing education.* Washington, DC: The Catholic University of America Press.

Orem, D.E. (1981). Nursing: A triad of action systems. In G.E. Lasker (Ed.), *Applied systems and cybernetics* (Vol. IV). *Systems research in health care, biocybernetics and ecology.* New York: Pergamon Press.

Orem, D.E. (1982). Nursing: A dilemma for higher education. In Sister A. Power (Ed.), *Words commemorated: Essays celebrating the centennial of Incarnate Word College.* San Antonio, TX: Incarnate Word College.

Orem, D.E. (1983). The self-care deficit theory of nursing: A general theory. In I. Clements & F. Roberts (Eds), *Family health: A theoretical approach to nursing care.* New York: Wiley Medical Publications.

Orem, D.E. (1984). Orem's conceptual model and community health nursing. In M.K. Asay & C.C. Ossler, *Proceedings of the Eighth Annual Community Health Nursing Conference: Conceptual models of nursing applications in community health nursing.* Chapel Hill: University of North Carolina, Department of Public Health Nursing, School of Public Health.

Orem, D.E., & Taylor, S. (1986). Orem's general theory of nursing. In P. Winstead-Fry (Ed.), *Case studies in nursing theory* (pp. 37-71). Pub. No. 15-2152. New York: National League for Nursing.

Orem, D.E. (1988). Nursing administration: A theoretical approach. In B. Henry, C. Arndt, M. DiVincenti, & A. Marriner-Tomey (Eds.), *Dimensions of nursing administration.* Boston: Blackwell Scientific.

Orem, D.E. (1990). A nursing practice theory in three parts, 1956-1989. In M.E. Parker (Ed.), *Nursing theories in practice.* New York: National League for Nursing.

Journal articles

Orem, D.E. (1962, Jan.). The hope of nursing. *Journal of Nursing Education, 1,* 5.

Orem, D.E. (1979, March). Levels of nursing education and practice. *Alumnae Magazine, The Johns Hopkins School of Nursing, 68,* 2-6.

Orem, D.E. (1985, May-June). Concepts of self-care for the rehabilitation client. *Rehabilitation Nursing, 10*(3), 33-36.

Orem, D.E. (1988, May). The forum of nursing science. *Nursing Science Quarterly, 1*(2), 75-79.

Orem, D.E., & O'Malley, M. (1952, Aug.). Diagnosis of hospital nursing problems. *Hospitals, 26*, 63.

Orem, D.E., & Vardiman, E. (1995, Winter). Orem's nursing theory and positive mental health: practical considerations. *Nursing Science Quarterly, 8*(4), 165-173.

Reports

Orem, D.E. (1955). *Indiana hospitals: A report.* Author of three sections of 10-year report of status and problems of Indiana hospitals. Indiana State Board of Health.

Orem, D.E. (1956). *Hospital nursing service: An analysis and report of a study of administrative positions in one hospital nursing service.* Indiana State Board of Health.

Orem, D.E., Dear, M., & Greenbaum, J. (1976). *Organization of nursing faculty responsibilities.* (Project Report, Public Health Service Grant No. 03D-005-3666.) Washington, DC: Georgetown University School of Nursing.

Audiotape

Orem, D.E. (1978, Dec.). Paper presented at the Second Annual Nurse Educator Conference, New York. (Audiotape available from Teach 'em, Inc., 160 E. Illinois Street, Chicago, IL 60611.)

Videocassettes

National League for Nurses. (1987). *Nursing theory: A circle of knowledge.* (Available from the author, 10 Columbus Circle, New York, NY 10019.)

The Nurse Theorists. Portraits of excellence: Dorothea Orem. (1988). *Excellence in Action: Dorothea Orem* (1992). Oakland: Studio III. (Available from Fuld Video Project, Studio III, 370 Hawthorne Avenue, Oakland, CA 94609.)

Secondary sources

Book reviews

Orem, D.E. (1971). *Nursing: Concepts of practice.*
Canadian Nurse, 67, 47, Dec. 1971.
Supervisor Nurse, 3, 45-46, Jan. 1972.
American Journal of Nursing, 72, 1330, July 1972.

Orem, D.E. (1980). *Nursing: Concepts of practice* (2nd ed.).
Registered Nurse Association of British Columbia, 12, 25, Nov. 1980.
AORN Journal, 24, 776, Oct. 1981.
Nursing Times, 78, 1671, Oct. 6-12, 1982.
Journal of Advanced Nursing, 8(1), 89, Jan. 1983.

Dissertations

Aish, A.E. (1993). *An investigation of a nursing system to support nutritional self-care in post myocardial infarction patients.* Unpublished doctoral dissertation, Wayne State University.

Alberto, J.E. (1990). *A test of a model of the relationship between time orientation, perception of threat, hope, and self-care behavior of persons with chronic obstructive pulmonary disease.* Unpublished doctoral dissertation, Indiana University School of Nursing.

Alfred, N. (1990). *Effect of a health promotion program on self-care agency of children.* Unpublished doctoral dissertation, University of Alabama at Birmingham.

Baas, L.S. (1992). *The relationship among self-care knowledge, self-care resources, activity level and life satisfaction in persons three to six months after a myocardial infarction.* Unpublished doctoral dissertation, The University of Texas at Austin.

Baker, C.J. (1993). *The development of the self-care ability to detect early signs of relapse among individuals who have schizophrenia.* Unpublished doctoral dissertation, The University of Texas at Austin.

Baker, L.K. (1991). *Predictors of self-care in adolescents with cystic fibrosis: A test and explication of Orem's theories of self-care and self-care deficit.* Unpublished doctoral dissertation, Wayne State University.

Baker, S.P. (1993). *The relationship of self-care agency and self-care actions to caregivers' strain as perceived by female family caregivers of elderly parents.* Unpublished doctoral dissertation, New York University.

Beatty, E.R. (1991). *Locus-of-control, self-actualization and self-care agency among registered nurses.* Unpublished doctoral dissertation, Columbia University Teachers College.

Beecroft, P.C. (1990) *The effects of cognitive restructuring and assertation skills training on the self-efficacy and self-care agency of adolescents undergoing hemodialysis.* Unpublished doctoral dissertation, The University of Texas at Austin.

Bess, C.J. (1995). *Abilities and limitation of adult type II diabetic patients with integrating of self-care practices into their daily lives.* Unpublished doctoral dissertation, University of Alabama at Birmingham.

Blecke, J. (1991). *Children's perceived self-care health behavior within differing family contexts.* Unpublished doctoral dissertation, Michigan State University.

Campbell, H.L. (1993). *Factors that predict self-care behaviors of non-insulin-dependent African Americans.* Unpublished doctoral dissertation, Northern Illinois University.

Chaiphibalsarisdi, P. (1990). *Self-care responses of rural Thai perimenopausal women.* Unpublished doctoral dissertation, University of Illinois at Chicago, Health Sciences Center.

Cull, V.V. (1995). *Exposure to violence and self-care practices of adolescents.* Unpublished doctoral dissertation, University of Alabama at Birmingham.

Daniels, R.D. (1994). *Exploring the self-care variables that explain a wellness lifestyle in spinal cord injured wheelchair basketball athletes.* Unpublished doctoral dissertation, The University of Texas at Austin.

Daniels, R.D. (1994). *Beyond job satisfaction: The phenomenon of joy in work.* Unpublished doctoral dissertation, Georgia State University.

Engberg, S.J.H. (1993). *Urinary incontinence: The relationship between common sense perceptions and self-care behaviors in rural community-dwelling older women.* Unpublished doctoral dissertation, University of Pittsburgh.

Folden, S.L. (1990). *The effect of supportive-educative nursing interventions on poststroke older adults' self-care perceptions.* Unpublished doctoral dissertation, University of Miami.

Freeman, E.M. (1992). *Self-care agency in gay men with HIV infection.* Unpublished doctoral dissertation, University of California, San Francisco.

Fuller, F.J. (1992). *Health of elderly male dependent-care agents for a spouse with Alzheimer's disease.* Unpublished doctoral dissertation, University of Alabama at Birmingham.

Hart, M.A. (1993). *Self-care agency and prenatal care actions: Relationships to pregnancy outcomes.* Unpublished doctoral dissertation, Case Western Reserve University.

Hartweg, D.L. (1991). *Health promotion self-care actions of healthy, middle-aged women.* Unpublished doctoral dissertation, Wayne State University.

Horsburgh, M.E. (1994). *The contribution of personality to adult well-being: A test and explication of Orem's theory of self-care.* Unpublished doctoral dissertation, Wayne State University.

Huddleston, D.S.T. (1991). *Determinants of self-care response patterns of perimenopausal women.* Unpublished doctoral dissertation, University of Illinois at Chicago, Health Sciences Center.

Hurst, J.D. (1991). *The relationship among self-care agency, risk-taking, and health risks in adolescents.* Unpublished doctoral dissertation, University of Alabama at Birmingham.

James, K.S. (1991). *Factors related to self-care agency and self-care practices of obese adolescents.* Unpublished doctoral dissertation, University of San Diego.

Jesek-Hale, S.R. (1994). *Self-care agency and self-care pregnant adolescents: A test of Orem's theory.* Unpublished doctoral dissertation, Rush University, College of Nursing.

Keith, C.C. (1991). *Caring for the older parent: Transformation of the family into a parentcare system.* Unpublished doctoral dissertation, The University of Wisconsin-Milwaukee.

Kellegrew, D.H. (1994). *The impact of daily routines and opportunities on the self-care skill performance of young children with disabilities.* Unpublished doctoral dissertation, University of California, Santa Barbara.

Koster, M.K. (1995). *A comparison of the relationship among self-care agency, self-determinism, and absenteeism in two groups of school-age children.* Unpublished doctoral dissertation, The University of Texas at Austin.

Kreulen, G.J. (1994). *Self-care, utilization, cost, quality and health status outcomes of a psychobehavioral nursing intervention: Women experiencing treatment for breast cancer.* Unpublished doctoral dissertation, The University of Arizona.

Lutz, R.D. (1993). *Self-efficacy and self-care in the hypertensive female patient.* Unpublished doctoral dissertation, Loma Linda University.

Mapanga, K.G. (1994). *The influence of family and friends' basic conditioning factors, and self-care agency on unmarried teenage primiparas' engagement in contraceptive practice.* Unpublished doctoral dissertation, Case Western Reserve University.

Mccaleb, K.A. (1991). *Self-concept and self-care practices of health adolescents.* Unpublished doctoral dissertation, University of Alabama at Birmingham.

Mcquiston, C.M. (1993). *Basic conditioning factors and self-care agency of unmarried women at risk for sexually transmitted disease.* Unpublished doctoral dissertation, Wayne State University.

O'Connor, N.A. (1995). *Maieutic dimensions of self-care agency: Instrument development.* Unpublished doctoral dissertation, Wayne State University.

Ortiz-Martinez, M.A. (1994). *The self-care model for nursing in Puerto Rico: A cross-cultural study of the implementation of change.* Unpublished doctoral dissertation, Walden University.

Patterson, D.L.F. (1992). *Self-care of menstrual health in collegiate athletes.* Unpublished doctoral dissertation, University of Pennsylvania.

Pettine, A. (1995). *Development of self-care: A problem for elementary-age children?* Unpublished doctoral dissertation, Colorado State University.

Rios Iturrion, H. (1992). *Hispanic diabetic elders: Self-care behaviors and explanatory models.* Unpublished doctoral dissertation, The University of Iowa.

Robinson, M.K. (1995). *Determinants of functional status in chronically ill adults.* Unpublished doctoral dissertation, University of Alabama at Birmingham.

Rosenow, D.J. (1992). *Multidimensional scaling analysis of self-care actions for reintegrating holistic health after a myocardial infarction: Implications for nursing.* Unpublished doctoral dissertation, The University of Texas at Austin.

Schumacher, K.L. (1994). *Shifting patterns of self-care and caregiving during chemotherapy.* Unpublished doctoral dissertation, Rush University, College of Nursing.

Shaver, M.S. (1990). *The effects of motivation-based instruction on disabled persons' self-care behavior.* Unpublished doctoral dissertation, Fordham University.

Silko, B.J. (1993). *Midlife women's balanced health and ability to function through the process of self-care.* Unpublished doctoral dissertation, University of Washington.

Simmons. S.J. (1990). *Self-care agency and health-promoting behavior of a military population.* Unpublished doctoral dissertation, Medical College of Georgia.

Singleton, J.K. (1993). *Nursing interventions to encourage residents' self-care in long-term care: An ethnography.* Unpublished doctoral dissertation, Adelphi University.

Skelly, A.H. (1992). *Psychosocial determinants of self-care practices and glycemic control in black women with type II diabetes mellitus.* Unpublished doctoral dissertation, State University of New York at Buffalo.

Slusher, I.L. (1994). *Self-care agency and self-care practice of adolescent primiparas during the in-hospital postpartum period.* Unpublished doctoral dissertation, University of Alabama at Birmingham.

Spezia, M.A. (1991). *Family responses and self-care activities in school-age children with diabetes.* Unpublished doctoral dissertation, University of Alabama at Birmingham.

Stonebraker, D.H. (1991). *The relationship between self-care agency, self-care, and health in the pregnant adolescent.* Unpublished doctoral dissertation, Texas Women's University.

Thompson, K.O. (1992). *Perceived ability for self-care: A measurement study.* Unpublished doctoral dissertation, University of Maryland at Baltimore.

Urbancic, J.C. (1992). *The relationship between empowerment support, motivation, for self-care, mental health self-care, well-being, and incest trauma resolution in adult female survivors.* Unpublished doctoral dissertation, Wayne State University.

Villarruel, A.M. (1993). *Mexican-American cultural meanings, expressions, self-care and dependent-care actions associated with experiences of pain.* Unpublished doctoral dissertation, Wayne State University

West, P.P. (1993). *The relationship between depression and self-care agency in young adult women.* Unpublished doctoral dissertation, Wayne State University.

White, S.K. (1991). *Factors affecting adherence to self-care behaviors following myocardial infarction.* Unpublished doctoral dissertation, University of Alberta, Canada.

Widrow, L.A. (1995). *Self-care, compliance, and quality of life among patients receiving maintenance hemodialysis.* Unpublished doctoral dissertation, University of California, Los Angeles.

Wikblad, K.F. (1991). *Care and self-care in diabetes: A study in patients with onset of diabetes before 1975.* Unpublished doctoral dissertation, Uppsala University, Sweden.

Books

Chinn, P.L., & Jacobs, M.K. (1987). *Theory and nursing: A systematic approach.* St. Louis: Mosby.

Fitzpatrick, J., & Whall, A. (1983). *Conceptual models of nursing: Analysis and application.* Bowie, MD: Robert J. Brady.

Fitzpatrick, J.J., Whall, A.L., Johnston, R.L., & Floyd, J.A. (1982). *Nursing models and their psychiatric mental health applications.* Bowie, MD: Robert J. Brady

Hartweg, D.L. (1991). *Dorothea Orem: Self-care deficit theory.* Thousand Oaks, CA: Sage Publications.

Hill, L., & Smith, N. (1985). *Self-care nursing.* Englewood Cliffs, NJ: Prentice-Hall.

Horn, B.J., & Swain, M.A. (1977). *Development of criterion measures of nursing care* (Vols. 1 and 2). University of Michigan and National Center for Health Services Research. U.S. Department of Commerce (NTIS Publication No. 267-004 and 267-005).

Kin, H.S. (1983) *The nature of theoretical thinking in nursing.* Norwalk, CT.: Appleton-Century-Crofts.

Leddy, S., & Pepper, J.M. (1985). *Conceptual bases of professional nursing.* Philadelphia: J.B. Lippincott.

Meleis, A.J. (1985). *Theoretical nursing's development and progress.* Philadelphia: J.B. Lippincott.

National League for Nursing (1978). *Theory development: What, why, how?* (Publication 15-1708, pp. 73-74). New York: National League for Nursing.

Nursing Theories Conference Group, J.B. George, Chairperson, (1980). *Nursing theories: The base for professional practice.* Englewood Cliffs, NJ: Prentice Hall.

Parker, M.E. (1990). *Nursing theories in practice.* New York: National League for Nursing.

Parse, R.R. (1987). *Nursing science.* Philadelphia: W.B. Saunders.

Polit, D.F., & Hungler, B.P. (1987). *Nursing research principles and methods* (3rd ed.). Philadelphia: J.B. Lippincott.

Torres, G. (1986). *Theoretical foundations of nursing.* Norwalk, CT.: Appleton-Century-Crofts.

Winstead-Fry, P. (1986). *Case studies in nursing theory.* New York: National League for Nursing.

Book chapters

Berbiglia, V.A. (1997). Orem's self-care deficit theory in nursing practice. In M.R. Alligood & A. Marriner-Tomey (Eds.), *Nursing theory: utilization and application* (pp. 129-152). St. Louis: Mosby.

Calley, J.M., Dirksen, M., Engalla, M., & Hennrich, M.L. (1980). The Orem self-care nursing model. In J.P. Riehl & C. Roy (Eds.), *Conceptual models for nursing practice* (pp. 302-314). New York: Appleton-Century-Crofts.

Coleman, L.J. (1980). Orem's self-care nursing model. In J.P. Riehl & C. Roy (Eds.), *Conceptual models for nursing practice* (pp. 315-328). New York: Appleton-Century-Crofts.

Fawcett, J. (1984). Orem's self-care model. In J. Fawcett (Ed.), *Analysis and evaluation of conceptual models in nursing* (pp. 175-210). Philadelphia: F.A. Davis.

Foster, P.C., & Janssens, N.P. (1980). Dorothea E. Orem. In Nursing Theories Conference Group, J.B. George, Chairperson, *Nursing theories: The base for professional practice* (pp. 91-106). Englewood Cliffs, NJ: Prentice-Hall.

Goldstein, N., Zink, M., Stevenson, L., Anderson, M., Woolery, L., & DePompdo, T. (1983). Self-care: a framework for the future. In P.L. Chinn (Ed.), *Advances in nursing theory development* (pp. 107-121). Rockville, MD: Aspen Systems.

Horn, B.J. (1978). Development of criterion measures of nursing care (abstract). In *Communicating nursing research* (Vol. 11: New approaches to communicating nursing research). Boulder, CO: Western Interstate Commission for Higher Education.

Horn, B.J., & Swain, M.A. (1976). An approach to development of criterion measures for quality patient care. In *Issues in evaluation research.* Kansas City: American Nurses Association.

Johnston, R.L. (1982). Individual psychotherapy: Relationships of theoretical approaches to nursing conceptual models. In J. Fitzpatrick, A. Whall, R. Johnston, & J. Floyd, (Eds.), *Nursing models and their psychiatric mental health applications* (pp. 56-60). Bowie, MD: Robert J. Brady

Johnston, R.L. (1983). Orem self-care model of nursing. In J. Fitzpatrick & A. Whall (Eds.), *Conceptual models of nursing, analysis and application* (pp. 137-156). Bowie, MD: Robert J. Brady.

Kinlein, M.L. (1977). *Independent nursing practice with clients* (pp. 15-24). Philadelphia: J.B. Lippincott.

Meleis, A.I. (1985). Dorothea Orem. In A.I. Meleis (Ed.), *Dorothea Orem* (pp. 284-296). Philadelphia: J.B. Lippincott.

Roy, C. (1980). A case study viewed according to different models. In J.P. Riehl & C. Roy (Eds.), *Conceptual models for nursing practice* (pp. 385-386). New York: Appleton-Century-Crofts.

Spangler, Z.S., & Spangler, W.O. (1983). Self-care: A testable model. In P.L. Chinn (Ed.), *Advances in nursing theory development* (pp. 89-105). Rockville, MD: Aspen Systems.

Stanton, M. (1980). Nursing theories and the nursing process. In Nursing Theories Conference Group, J.B. George, Chairperson, *Nursing theories: The base for professional practice* (pp. 213-217). Englewood Cliffs, NJ: Prentice Hall.

Sullivan, T.J. (1980). Self-care model for nursing. In *Directions for nursing in the 80's*. Kansas City, MO: American Nurses Association.

Taylor, S.G. (1990). Nursing practice applications of self-care deficit nursing theory. In M. Parker (Ed.), *Nursing theories in practice* (pp. 61-70). Theory Conferences. New York: National League for Nursing.

Taylor, S.G., & Renpenning, K. (1995). Nursing in multiperson situations: family and community. In D.E. Orem, *Nursing: Concepts of practice* (pp. 348-380), 5th ed. St. Louis: Mosby.

Thibodeau, J.A. (1983). An eclectic model: The Orem model. In J.A. Thibodeau (Ed.), *Nursing models: Analysis and evaluation* (pp. 125-140). Monterey, CA: Wadsworth Health Sciences Division.

Underwood, P.R. (1980). Facilitating self-care. In P. Potheir (Ed.), *Psychiatric nursing: A basis text*. Boston: Little, Brown.

Other resources

Copies of papers presented at the Fifth, Sixth, and Seventh Annual Self-Care Deficit Nursing Theory Conferences and the First, Second, Third, and Fourth International Self-Care Deficit Nursing Theory Conferences are available. These include papers by Orem and others. Also available are introductory videotapes. Order from University of Missouri–Columbia, Sinclair School of Nursing, Continuing Nursing Education, S266 School of Nursing Building, Columbia, MO 65211; phone (573) 882-0216.

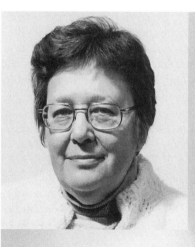

*M*yra Estrin Levine

The Conservation Model

Karen Moore Schaefer, Gloria S. Artigue, Karen J. Foli,
Tamara Johnson, Ann Marriner Tomey, Mary Carolyn Poat,
LaDema Poppa, Roberta Woeste, Susan T. Zoretich

CREDENTIALS AND BACKGROUND OF THE THEORIST

Myra Estrin Levine obtained a diploma from Cook County School of Nursing in 1944, an S.B. from the University of Chicago in 1949, and an M.S.N. from Wayne State University in 1962, and has taken postgraduate courses at the University of Chicago.[29] Hutchins's curriculum was being taught to undergraduate students at that time. All students took a year-long survey in the biological, physical, and social sciences and the humanities. The students read and analyzed primary work under the guidance of distinguished professors. Irene Beland became Levine's mentor while she was a graduate student at Wayne

The authors wish to express appreciation to Myra Levine for critiquing the original chapter.

State and directed her attention to many of the authors who greatly influenced her thinking.[31,33]

Levine has enjoyed a varied career. She has been a private duty nurse (1944), a civilian nurse in the U.S. Army (1945), a preclinical instructor in the physical sciences at Cook County (1947-1950), the director of nursing at Drexel Home in Chicago (1950-1951), and a surgical supervisor at the University of Chicago Clinics (1951-1952) and at Henry Ford Hospital in Detroit (1956-1962). She worked her way up the academic ranks at Bryan Memorial Hospital in Lincoln, Nebraska (1951), Cook County School of Nursing (1963-1967), Loyola University (1967-1973), Rush University (1974-1977), and the University of Illinois (1962-1963, 1977-1987). She chaired the Department of Clinical Nursing at Cook County School of Nursing (1963-1967) and coordinated the graduate nursing program in oncology at Rush University (1974-1977). Levine was the director of the Department of Continuing Education at Evanston Hospital (March-June 1974), and a consultant to the department (July 1974-1976). She was an adjunct associate professor of Humanistic Studies at the University of Illinois 1981-1987. In 1987 she became a Professor Emerita, Medical Surgical Nursing, University of Illinois at Chicago. In 1974 Levine went to Tel-Aviv University, Israel, as visiting associate professor and returned as a visiting professor in 1982. She was also a visiting professor at Recanati School of Nursing, Ben Gurion University of the Negev, Beer Sheva, Israel (March-April, 1982).

Levine has received numerous honors, including being a charter fellow of the American Academy of Nursing (1973), honorary member of the American Mental Health Aid to Israel (1976), and honorary recognition from the Illinois Nurses' Association (1977). She was the first recipient of the Elizabeth Russell Belford Award for excellence in teaching from Sigma Theta Tau (1977). Both the first and second editions of her book *Introduction to Clinical Nursing* received AJN Book of the Year awards, and her 1971 book, *Renewal for Nursing,* was translated into Hebrew.[29] Levine was listed in *Who's Who in American Women* (1977-1988) and in *Who's Who in American Nursing* (1987).[29,34] She was elected fellow of the Institute of Medicine of Chicago (1987-1991). Levine was recognized for her outstanding contributions to nursing by the Alpha Lambda Chapter of Sigma Theta Tau (1990). In January 1992, she was awarded an honorary doctorate of humane letters from Loyola University, Chicago.[40,43] Levine was an active leader in the American Nurses Association and the Illinois Nurses' Association. After her retirement in 1987, she remained active in theory development and encouraged questions and research about her theory.[47]

A dynamic speaker, she was a frequent presenter on programs, workshops, seminars, and panels and a prolific writer regarding nursing and education. Levine has also served as a consultant to hospitals and schools of nursing.[40,43] Although she never intended to develop theory, she provided an organizational structure for teaching medical-surgical nursing and a stimulus for theory development. "The

Four Conservation Principles of Nursing"[22] was the first statement of the conservation principles. Other preliminary work included "Adaptation and Assessment: A Rationale for Nursing Intervention,"[21] "For Lack of Love Alone,"[23] and "The Pursuit of Wholeness."[24] The first edition of her book using the conservation principles, *Introduction to Clinical Nursing,* was published in 1969. She addressed the consequences of the four conservation principles in "Holistic Nursing."[25] The second edition of the book was published[26] in 1973. Since then, Levine[27,28] has presented the conservation principles at nurse theory conferences, some of which have been audiotaped,[27] and at the Allentown College of St. Francis de Sales Conferences[28] in April 1984.

In 1989 substantial change and clarification about her theory were published in her chapter "Four Conservation Principles: Twenty Years Later" in Riehl's book *Conceptual Models for Nursing Practice.* Levine elaborates on how redundancy characterizes availability of adaptive responses when stability is threatened. Adaptation processes establish a body economy to safeguard the individual's stability. The outcome of adaptation is conservation.[37]

In 1991 she explicitly linked health to the process of conservation to clarify for her critics that the Conservation Model views health as one of its essential components.[39] Conservation, through treatment, focuses on integrity, the reclamation of oneness of the whole person.

Levine died on March 20, 1996, at the age of 75 years. She leaves a legacy as an educator, scholar, administrator, student, wife, mother, friend, and nurse.[48] Just before her untimely death she had the opportunity to assure her colleagues that spirituality was an implicit part of personhood, and essential to the maintenance of personal integrity.[45]

THEORETICAL SOURCES

Levine learned historical viewpoints of diseases and that the way people think about disease changes over time from Beland's presentation of the theory of specific causation and multiple factors.[2] Beland directed Levine's attention to numerous authors who became influential in her thinking, including Kurt Gold-

MAJOR CONCEPTS & DEFINITIONS

The three major concepts of the Conservation Model are wholeness, adaptation, and conservation. **Wholeness (Holism)** "Whole, health, hale are all derivations of the Anglo-Saxon word *hal*."[28] Levine based her use of wholeness on Erikson's description of wholeness as an open system. Levine[9:92;24:94;28] quotes Erikson, who says, "Wholeness emphasizes a sound, organic, progressive, mutuality between diversified functions and parts within an entirety, the boundaries of which are open and fluent." Levine believed that Erikson's definition set up the option of exploring the parts of the whole to understand the whole.[45] Integrity means the oneness of the individuals, emphasizing that they respond in an integrated yet singular fashion to environmental challenges.

Adaptation "Adaptation is a process of change whereby the individual retains his integrity within the realities of his internal and external environment."[26:11;33] Conservation is the outcome. Some adaptations are successful. Some are not. Adaptation is a matter of degree, not an all-or-nothing process.[26:11;33] There is no such thing as maladaptation.

Levine speaks of three characteristics of adaptation: historicity, specificity, and redundancy.[39] Levine[39:5] states: "... every species has fixed patterns of responses uniquely designed to ensure success in essential life activities, demonstrating that adaptation is both historical and specific." In addition, adaptive patterns may be hidden in the individual's genetic code. Redundancy represents the fail-safe options available to individuals to ensure adaptation. Loss of redundant choices either through trauma, age, disease, or environmental conditions makes it difficult for the individual to maintain life. Levine[39:6] suggests that "the possibility exists that aging itself is a consequence of failed redundancy of physiological and psychological processes."

Environment Environment is "where we are constantly and actively involved."[36] The person and his relationship to the environment is what counts.[29]

Levine also views each individual as having his own environment, both internally and externally. The internal environment can be related by nurses as the physiological and pathophysiological aspects of the patient. Levine uses a definition of the external environment from Bates[1] and suggests three levels: perceptual, operational, and conceptual. These levels give dimension to the interactions between individuals and their environments. The perceptual level includes the aspects of the world about us that we are able to intercept and interpret with our sense organs. The operational level contains things that affect us physically even though we cannot directly perceive them, such as microorganisms. At the conceptual level, the environment is constructed from cultural patterns, characterized by a spiritual existence, and mediated by the symbols of language, thought, and history.[26:12] There are four levels of integration that safeguard the end and help a person maintain his integrity or wholeness.[26:9]

Organismic response The capacity of the individual to adapt to his environmental condition has been called the organismic response. It can be divided into four levels of integration: fight or flight, inflammatory response, response to stress, and perceptual response. Treatment focuses on the management of these responses to illness and disease.

FIGHT OR FLIGHT The most primitive response is the fight or flight syndrome. The individual perceives that he is threatened, regardless of whether a threat actually exists. Hospitalization, illness, and new experiences elicit a response. The individual responds by being on the alert to find more information and to ensure his safety and well-being.

INFLAMMATORY RESPONSE This defense mechanism protects the self from insult in a hostile environment. It is a way of healing. The response uses available energy to remove or keep out unwanted irritants or pathogens. But it is limited in time because it drains the individual's energy reserves. Environmental control is important.

RESPONSE TO STRESS Selye[55] described the stress response syndrome to predictable, nonspecifically

Continued

MAJOR CONCEPTS & DEFINITIONS—cont'd

induced organismic changes. The wear and tear of life is recorded on the tissues and reflects long-term hormonal responses to life experiences that cause structural changes. It is characterized by irreversibility and influences the way patients respond to nursing care.

PERCEPTUAL RESPONSE This response is based on the individual's perceptual awareness. It occurs only as the individual experiences the world around him. This response is used by the individual to seek and maintain safety for himself. It is information seeking.[22:95-96; 23:33]

Trophicognosis Levine recommended trophicognosis as an alternative to nursing diagnosis. It is a scientific method to reach a nursing care judgment.[20]

Conservation
Conservation is from the Latin word *conservatio,* meaning to keep together.[17,26,27] "Conservation describes the way complex systems are able to continue to function even when severely challenged."[38:192] Through conservation, individuals are able to confront obstacles and adapt accordingly while maintaining their uniqueness. "The goal of conservation is health and the strength to confront disability" while ". . . the rules of conservation and integrity hold" in all situations where nursing is required.[38:193-195;21;45] The primary focus of conservation is on keeping together of the wholeness of the individual. Although nursing interventions may deal with one particular conservation principle, nurses must also recognize the influence of the other conservation principles.[38,39]

Levine's model[26,36] stresses nursing interactions and interventions that are intended "to keep together the unique and individual resources that each individual brings to his predicament." Those interactions are based on the scientific background of the conservation principles. Conservation focuses on achieving a balance of energy supply and demand within the biological realities unique to the individual. Nursing care is based on scientific knowledge and nursing skills. There are four conservation principles.

Conservation principles The goals of the Conservation Model are achieved through interventions that attend to the conservation principles.

CONSERVATION OF ENERGY The individual requires a balance of energy and a constant renewal of energy to maintain life activities. That energy is challenged by processes such as healing and aging. This second law of thermodynamics applies to everything in the universe, including people.

Conservation of energy has long been used in nursing practice even with the most basic procedures. Nursing interventions ". . . scaled to the individual's ability are dependent upon providing care that makes the least additional demand possible."[38:197,198]

CONSERVATION OF STRUCTURAL INTEGRITY Healing is a process of restoring structural and functional integrity[38] in defense of wholeness. The disabled are guided to a new level of adaptation.[45] Nurses should limit the amount of tissue involved in disease by early recognition of functional changes and by nursing interventions.

CONSERVATION OF PERSONAL INTEGRITY Self-worth and a sense of identity are important. The most vulnerable become patients. This begins with the erosion of privacy and the creation of anxiety. Nurses can show patients respect by calling them by name, respecting their wishes, valuing personal possessions, providing privacy during procedures, supporting their defenses, and teaching them. "The nurse's goal is always to impart knowledge and strength so that the individual can resume a private life—no longer a patient, no longer dependent."[38:199] The sanctity of life is manifested in all people. "The conservation of personal integrity includes recognition of the holiness of each person."[45:40]

CONSERVATION OF SOCIAL INTEGRITY Life gains meaning through social communities, and health is socially determined. Nurses fulfill professional roles, provide for family members, assist with religious needs, and use interpersonal relationships to conserve social integrity.[23;24:12-18;33] stein,[14] Edward T. Hall,[15] Sir Arthur Sherrington,[56] and Rene Dubos.[7,8] Levine uses James E. Gibson's definition[13] of perceptual systems, Erik Erikson's differentiation[9,10] between total and whole, Hans Selye's stress theory,[55] and M. Bates's models[1] of external environment. Levine is proud that Martha Rogers was her first editor.[31,33,52] Most recently she acknowledged Nightingale's contribution to her thinking about the "guardian activity" of observation used by nurses to "save lives and increase health and comfort."[41:42]

USE OF EMPIRICAL EVIDENCE

Levine believed that specific nursing activities could be deducted from scientific principles. The scientific theoretical sources have been well researched. She based much of her work on accepted science principles.[32,35]

MAJOR ASSUMPTIONS

Introduction to Clinical Nursing is a text for beginning nursing students that uses the conservation principles as an organizing framework. Therefore Levine does not specifically identify her assumptions.

Nursing

"Nursing is a human interaction."[26:1] "Professional nursing should be reserved for those few who can complete a graduate program as demanding as that expected of professionals in any other discipline.... There will be very few professional nurses."[19:214] "Nursing practice—and this includes the teaching of nurses—has always mirrored prevailing theories of health and disease."[18;22:240;40] "It is the nurse's task to bring a body of scientific principles on which decisions depend into the precise situation which she shares with the patient. Sensitive observation and the selection of relevant data form the basis for her assessment of his nursing requirements."[21:2452] "The nurse participates actively in every patient's environment, and much of what she does supports his adjustments as he struggles in the predicament of illness."[21:2452] The essence of Levine's theory is that "when nursing intervention influences adaptation

favorably, or toward renewed social well-being, then the nurse is acting in a therapeutic sense; when the response is unfavorable, the nurse provides supportive care."[26:13;21:2453;33] "The goal of nursing is to promote adaptation and maintain wholeness."[25:258]

Person

Person is who we know ourself to be or a sense of identity and self-worth.

Health

Health is socially determined by one's ability to function in a reasonably normal manner.[24] It is predetermined by social groups and is not just an absence of pathological conditions. Health is the return to selfhood where individuals are free and able to pursue their own interests within the context of their own resources. Levine stressed, "It is important to keep in mind that health is also culturally determined—it is not an entity on its own, but rather a definition imparted by the ethos and beliefs of the groups to which individuals belong."[44] Even for a single individual, the definition of health will change over time.

Environment

Environment is the "context in which we live our lives."[31] It is not a passive backdrop. "We are active participants in it."[31]

THEORETICAL ASSERTIONS

Because Levine's work was intended to provide an organizational structure for teaching medical-surgical nursing rather than to develop theory, she did not explicitly identify theoretical assertions. Although many theoretical assertions can be generated from her work, the four major ones follow:

1. "Nursing intervention is based on the conservation of the individual patient's energy."[26:13;22:47]
2. "Nursing intervention is based on the conservation of the individual patient's structural integrity."[26:13;22:53]

3. "Nursing intervention is based on the conservation of the individual patient's personal integrity."[26:13;22:53]
4. "Nursing intervention is based on the conservation of the individual patient's social integrity."[26:14;23:56]

LOGICAL FORM

Levine primarily uses deductive logic. In developing her model, Levine integrates theories and concepts from the humanities and the sciences of nursing, physiology, psychology, and sociology. She uses the information to analyze nursing practice situations and describe nursing skills and activities. With the assistance of many of her students and colleagues, as well as through her own personal health encounters, she has experienced the Conservation Model and its principles operating in practice.

ACCEPTANCE BY THE NURSING COMMUNITY

Practice

Levine helps define what nursing is by identifying the activities it encompasses while giving the scientific principles behind them. Conservation principles as a framework are not limited to nursing care in the hospital but can be generalized and used in every environment, hospital, or community.[38,39] Conservation principles, levels of integration, and other concepts can be used in numerous contexts.[38] Hirschfeld[17] has used the principles of conservation in the care of the older adult. Savage and Culbert used the Conservation Model to establish a plan of care for infants.[53] Dever based her care of children on the Conservation Model.[6] Roberts, Fleming, and Yeates/Giese designed interventions for women in labor on the basis of the Conservation Model.[51] Cooper developed a framework for wound care focusing on structural integrity while integrating all the integrities.[5] Webb used the Conservation Model to provide care for patients undergoing cancer treatment.[59] Roberts and coworkers[49,50] used the Conservation Model to study the boomerang pillow tech-

nique effect on respiratory capacity. Taylor[57,58] used them to measure outcomes of nursing care and then again in her textbook.

Conservation principles have been used as frameworks for numerous practice settings in cardiology, obstetrics, gerontology, acute care (neurology), pediatrics, long-term care, emergency care, primary care, neonatology, and critical care areas, as well as in the homeless community.[53,54]

Education

Levine wrote a textbook for beginning students that introduced new material into curricula. She presented an early discussion of death and dying and believed that women should be awakened after a breast biopsy and consulted about the next step.[26:356-359;31;33]

Introduction to Clinical Nursing provides an organizational structure for teaching medical-surgical nursing to beginning students. In both the 1969 and 1973 editions, Levine presents a model at the end of each of the first nine chapters. Each model contains objectives, essential science concepts, and nursing process to give nurses a foundation for nursing activities. These models are not part of the Conservation Model. The Conservation Model is addressed in the Introduction and in Chapter 10 of the introductory text. The teachers' manual written to accompany the text remains a timely source of educational principles that may be helpful to beginning teachers, as well as to seasoned teachers who may benefit from a review of our education roots.[31]

Critics argue that, although the text is labeled introductory, a beginning student would need a fairly extensive background in physical and social science to use it.[3] Another critic suggests a definite strength is the emphasis of scientific principles, but a weakness of the text is that it does not present adequate examples of pathological profiles when disturbances are discussed. For this reason, one reviewer recommends the text as supplementary or complementary, rather than as a primary text.[4]

Hall[16] indicates Levine's model is one used as a curriculum model. More recently the model has been successfully integrated into undergraduate and graduate curricula. Several graduate students are using Levine's model for theses and dissertations.[31,42,43,54]

Research

Fitzpatrick and Whall[12:115] state, "All in all, Levine's model served as an excellent beginning. Its contribution has added a great deal to the overall development of nursing knowledge." However, Fawcett[11:208] states that to establish credibility "more systematic evaluations of the use of the model in various clinical situations are needed, as are studies that test conceptual-theoretical-empirical structures directly derived from or linked with the conservation principles." Many research questions can be generated from Levine's model. Several graduate students are using the conservation principles as a framework for their research.[33,43]

FURTHER DEVELOPMENT

Levine and others have worked on using the conservation principles as the basis of a taxonomy of nursing diagnosis. However, further development of this concept has been deferred since the American Nurses Association took over nursing diagnosis.[42] Additional work is being done on its use in administration and with the frail elderly. It has great potential for work on sleep disorders and in the development of collaborative and primary care practices.

CRITIQUE
Clarity

Levine's model possesses clarity. Fitzpatrick and Whall[12] believe Levine's work to be both internally and externally consistent. Fawcett[11:208] states that "Levine's Conservation Model provides nursing with a logically congruent, holistic view of the person." The model has numerous terms; however, Levine adequately defines them for clarity.

Simplicity

Although the four conservation principles initially appear simple, they contain subconcepts and multi-

ple variables. Nevertheless, this model is still one of the simpler ones that has emerged.

Generality

The four conservation principles can be used in all nursing contexts.

Empirical Precision

Levine used deductive logic to develop her model, which can be used to generate research questions.

Derivable Consequences

Various authors disagree as to the level of contributions provided by Levine's model. The four conservation principles constituted one of the earliest models and seems to be receiving increasing recognition.

CRITICAL THINKING *Activities*

1 Keep a reflective journal about a health or illness experience of your own or of someone very close to you. Reflect on the experience and its consistence with the Conservation Model. Consider how you would modify, expand, or delimit the model to better provide a context within which the experience can be explained.

2 Levine said that "Every ethnic group defines health and illness in context of its cherished beliefs."[45:41] Visit a nearby museum and evaluate how artistic expression captures the beliefs of different ethnic groups. Explore how these beliefs may shape the definitions of health and compare it with Levine's approach to health and illness. On the basis of the ethnically derived definition of health, propose ethnically appropriate interventions using Levine's conservation principles.

3 Watch the movie *City of Joy*. Use examples from the movie to support or refute the propositional statements made by Levine about the environment and the relationships with person, nursing, and health/illness.

REFERENCES

1. Bates, M. (1967). A naturalist at large. *Natural History,* 76(6), 8-16.
2. Beland, I. (1971). *Clinical nursing: Pathophysiological and psychosocial implications* (2nd ed.). New York: Macmillan.
3. Book review. (1970, Jan.). *Canadian Nurse, 66,* 42.
4. Book review. (1974, May). *Canadian Nurse, 70,* 39.
5. Cooper, D.H. (1990). Optimizing wound healing: A practice within nursing domains. *Nursing Clinics of North America, 25*(1), 165-180.
6. Dever, M. (1991). Care of children. In K.M. Schaefer & J.B. Pond (Eds.), *The conservation model: A framework for nursing practice* (pp. 71-82). Philadelphia: F.A. Davis.
7. Dubos, R. (1961). *Mirage of health.* Garden City, NY: Doubleday.
8. Dubos, R. (1965). *Man adapting.* New Haven, CT: Yale University Press.
9. Erikson, E.H. (1964). *Insight and responsibility.* New York: W.W. Norton.
10. Erikson, E.H. (1968). *Identity: Youth and crisis.* New York: W.W. Norton.
11. Fawcett J. (1995). Levine's conservation model. In J. Fawcett, *Analysis and evaluation of conceptual models of nursing* (pp. 165-215). Philadelphia: F.A. Davis.
12. Fitzpatrick, J.J., & Whall, A.L. (1983). *Conceptual models of nursing: Analysis and application.* Bowie, MD: Robert J. Brady.
13. Gibson, J.E. (1966). *The senses considered as perceptual systems.* Boston: Houghton Mifflin.
14. Goldstein, K. (1963). *The organism.* Boston: Beacon Press.
15. Hall, E.T. (1966). *The hidden dimension.* Garden City, NY: Doubleday.
16. Hall, K.V. (1979). Current trends in the use of conceptual frameworks in nursing education. *Journal of Nursing Education, 18*(4), 26-29.
17. Hirschfeld, M.J. (1976). The cognitively impaired older adult. *American Journal of Nursing, 76,* 1981-1984.
18. Levine, M.E. (1963). Florence Nightingale: The legend that lives. *Nursing Forum, 2*(4), 24-35.
19. Levine, M.E. (1965, June). The professional nurse and graduate education. *Nursing Science, 3,* 206.
20. Levine, M.E. (1966). Trophicognosis: An alternative to nursing diagnosis. In *Exploring progress in medical-surgical nursing practice.* New York: American Nurses Association.
21. Levine, M.E. (1966, Nov.). Adaptation and assessment: A rationale for nursing intervention. *American Journal of Nursing, 66,* 2450.
22. Levine, M.E. (1967). The four conservation principles of nursing. *Nursing Forum, 6,* 45.
23. Levine, M.E. (1967, Dec.). For lack of love alone. *Minnesota Nursing Accent, 39,* 179.
24. Levine, M.E. (1969, Jan.). The pursuit of wholeness, *American Journal of Nursing, 69,* 93.
25. Levine, M.E. (1971, June). Holistic nursing. *Nursing Clinics of North America, 6,* 253.
26. Levine, M.E. (1973). *Introduction to clinical nursing* (2nd ed.). Philadelphia: F.A. Davis.
27. Levine, M.E. (1978). (Audiotape). Paper presented at the Second Annual Nurse Educators' Conference, New York.
28. Levine, M.E. (1984, April). *A conceptual model for nursing: The four conservation principles.* In the proceedings from Allentown College of St. Francis Conference.
29. Levine, M.E. (1984). Curriculum vitae.
30. Levine, M.E. (1984). Personal correspondence.
31. Levine, M.E. (1984). Telephone interviews.
32. Levine, M.E. (1985). Personal correspondence.
33. Levine, M.E. (1985). Telephone interviews.
34. Levine, M.E. (1988). Curriculum vitae.
35. Levine, M.E. (1988). Personal correspondence.
36. Levine, M.E. (1988). Telephone interviews.
37. Levine, M.E. (1989). The four conservation principles: Twenty years later. In J. Riehl (Ed.), *Conceptual models for nursing practice* (3rd ed.). New York: Appleton-Century-Crofts.
38. Levine, M.E. (1990). Conservation and integrity. In M. Parker (Ed.), *Nursing theories in practice* (pp. 189-201). New York: National League for Nursing.
39. Levine, M.E. (1991). The conservation principles: A model for health. In K. Schaefer & J. Pond (Eds.), *Levine's conservation model: A framework for nursing practice* (pp. 1-11). Philadelphia: F.A. Davis.
40. Levine, M.E. (1992). Curriculum vitae.
41. Levine, M.E. (1992). Nightingale redux. In B.S. Barnum (Ed.), *Nightingale's notes on nursing* (pp. 39-43). Philadelphia: J.B. Lippincott.
42. Levine, M.E. (1992). Personal correspondence.
43. Levine, M.E. (1992). Telephone interviews.
44. Levine, M.E. (1995). Personal correspondence.
45. Levine, M.E. (1996). The conservation principles: A retrospective. *Nursing Science Quarterly, 9*(1), 38-41.
46. Levine, M.E., & Levine, E.B. (1965, Dec.). Hippocrates: Father of nursing too. *American Journal of Nursing, 65,* 86.
47. *The nursing theorist: Portraits of excellence: Myra Levine* (1988). Oakland, CA: Studio III.
48. Pond, J.B. (1996). Myra Levine, nurse educator and scholar dies. *Nursing Spectrum, 5*(8), 8.
49. Roberts, K.L., Brittin, M., Cook, M., & deClifford, J. (1994). Boomerang pillows and respiratory capacity. *Clinical Nursing Research, 3*(2), 157-165.
50. Roberts, K.L., Britton, M., & deClifford, J. (1995). Boomerang pillows and respiratory capacity in frail elderly women. *Clinical Nursing Research,* 4(4):465-471.

51. Roberts, J.E., & Fleming, N., & Yeates-Giese, D. (1991). Perineal integrity. In K.M. Schaefer & J.B. Pond (Eds.), *The conservation model: A framework for nursing practice* (pp. 61-70). Philadelphia: F.A. Davis.

52. Rogers, M.E. (1970). *An introduction to the theoretical basis of nursing.* Philadelphia: F.A. Davis.

53. Savage, T.A., & Culbert C. (1989). Early intervention: The unique role of nursing. *Journal of Pediatric Nursing, 4*(5), 339-345.

54. Schaefer, K.M., & Pond, J.B. (Eds.) (1991). *Levine's conservation model: A framework for nursing practice.* Philadelphia: F.A. Davis.

55. Selye, H. (1956). *The stress of life.* New York: McGraw-Hill.

56. Sherrington, A. (1906). *Integrative function of the nervous system.* New York: Charles Scribner's Sons.

57. Taylor, J.W. (1974). Measuring the outcomes of nursing care. *Nursing Clinics of North America, 9,* 337-348.

58. Taylor, J., & Ballenger, S. (1980). *Neurological dysfunction and nursing interventions.* New York: McGraw-Hill.

59. Webb, H. (1993). Holistic care following a palliative Hartmann's procedure. *British Journal of Nursing, 2*(2), 128-132.

BIBLIOGRAPHY
Primary sources
Books

Levine, M.E. (1969). *Introduction to clinical nursing.* Philadelphia: F.A. Davis.

Levine, M.E. (1971). *Renewal for nursing.* Philadelphia: F.A. Davis.

Levine, M.E. (1973). *Introduction to clinical nursing* (2nd ed.). Philadelphia: F.A. Davis.

Book chapters

Levine, M.E. (1964). Nursing service. In M. Leeds & H. Shore, *Geriatric institutional management.* New York: G.J.P. Putnam & Sons.

Levine, M.E. (1966). Trophicognosis: An alternative to nursing diagnosis. In *ANA regional conference papers* (Vol. 2: Medical-Surgical Nursing).

Levine, M.E. (1972). Benoni. In *Comprehensive clinical papers* (Vol. 6: The nurse and the dying patient). American Journal of Nursing Company.

Levine, M.E. (1973). Adaptation and assessment: A rationale for nursing intervention. In M.E. Hardy (Ed.), *Theoretical foundations for nursing.* New York: Irvington.

Levine, M.E. (1988). Myra Levine. In T.M. Schorr & A. Zimmerman (Eds.), *Making choices, taking chances: Nursing leaders tell their stories.* St. Louis: Mosby.

Levine, M.E. (1989). The four conservation principles: Twenty years later. In J. Riehl (Ed.), *Conceptual models for nursing practice* (3rd ed.). New York: Appleton-Century-Crofts.

Levine, M.E. (1990). Conservation and integrity. In M. Parker (Ed.), *Nursing theories in practice* (pp. 189-201). New York: National League for Nursing.

Levine, M.E. (1991). The conservation principles: A model for health. In K. Schaefer & J. Pond (Eds.), *Levine's conservation model: A framework for nursing practice* (pp. 1-11). Philadelphia: F.A. Davis.

Levine, M.E. (1992). Nightingale redux. In B.S. Barnum (Ed.), *Nightingale's notes on nursing,* Commemorative edition with commentaries by nursing theorists. Philadelphia: J.B. Lippincott.

Levine, M.E. (1994). Some further thoughts on nursing rhetoric. In J.F. Kikuchi & H. Simmons (Eds.), *Developing a philosophy of nursing* (pp. 104-109). Thousand Oaks, CA: Sage.

Journal articles

Levine, M.E. (1963). Florence Nightingale: The legend that lives. *Nursing Forum, 2*(4), 24-35.

Levine, M.E. (1964, Feb.). Not to startle, though the way were steep. *Nursing Science, 2,* 58-67.

Levine, M.E. (1964, Dec.). There need be no anonymity. *First, 18*(9), 4.

Levine, M.E. (1965). Trophicognosis: An alternative to nursing diagnosis. *ANA Regional Clinical Conferences, 2,* 55-70.

Levine, M.E. (1965, June). The professional nurse and graduate education. *Nursing Science, 3,* 206-214.

Levine, M.E. (1966, Nov.). Adaptation and assessment: A rationale for nursing intervention. *American Journal of Nursing, 66*(11), 2450-2453.

Levine, M.E. (1967). The four conservation principles of nursing. *Nursing Forum, 6,* 45-59.

Levine, M.E. (1967, May). Medicine-nursing dialogue belongs at patient's bedside. *Chart, 64*(5), 136-137.

Levine, M.E. (1967, July). This I believe: About patient-centered care. *Nursing Outlook, 15,* 53-55.

Levine, M.E. (1967, Dec.). For lack of love alone. *Accent, 39*(7), 179-202.

Levine, M.E. (1968, Feb.). Knock before entering personal space bubbles (Part 1). *Chart, 65*(2), 58-62.

Levine, M.E. (1968, March). Knock before entering personal space bubbles (Part 2). *Chart, 65*(3), 82-84.

Levine, M.E. (1968, April). The pharmacist in the clinical setting: A nurse's viewpoint. *American Journal of Hospital Pharmacy, 25*(4), 168-171. (Also translated into Japanese and published in *Kyushu National Hospital Magazine for Western Japan.*)

Levine, M.E. (1969). Nursing for the 21st century. *National Student Association.*

Levine, M.E. (1969, Jan.). The pursuit of wholeness. *American Journal of Nursing, 69,* 93-98.

Levine, M.E. (1969, Feb.). Constructive student power. *Chart, 66*(2), 42FF.

Levine, M.E. (1969, Oct.). Small hospital—Big nursing. *Chart, 66,* 265-269.

Levine, M.E. (1969, Nov.). Small hospital—Big nursing. *Chart, 66,* 310-315.

Levine, M.E. (1970). Dilemma. *ANA Clinical Conferences,* pp. 338-342.

Levine, M.E. (1970, April). Breaking through the medications mystique. Published simultaneously in *American Journal of Nursing, 70*(4), 799-803, and *American Journal of Hospital Pharmacy, 27*(4), 294-299.

Levine, M.E. (1970, Oct.). The intransigent patient. *American Journal of Nursing, 70,* 2106-2111.

Levine, M.E. (1971, May). Consider implications for nursing in the use of physician's assistant. *Hospital Topics, 49,* 60-63.

Levine, M.E. (1971, June). Holistic nursing. *Nursing Clinics of North America, 6,* 253-264.

Levine, M.E. (1970, July-Dec.). Symposium on a drug compendium: View of a nursing educator. *Drug Information Bulletin,* pp. 133-135.

Levine, M.E. (1971, June). The time has come to speak of health care. *AORN Journal, 13,* 37-43.

Levine, M.E. (1972, Feb.). Nursing educators—An alienating elite? *Chart, 69*(2), 56-61.

Levine, M.E. (1972, March). Benoni. *American Journal of Nursing, 72*(3), 466-468.

Levine, M.E. (1972, March). Nursing grand rounds: Complicated case of CVA. *Nursing '72, 2*(3), 3-34 (with P. Moschel, J. Taylor, & G. Ferguson).

Levine, M.E. (1972, May). Nursing grand rounds: Insulin reactions in a brittle diabetic, *Nursing '72, 2*(5), 6-11 (with L. Line, A. Boyle, & E. Kopacewski).

Levine, M.E. (1972, June). Issues in rehabilitation: The quadriplegic adolescent. *Nursing '72, 2,* 6 (with M. Scanlon, P. Gregor, R. King, & N. Martin).

Levine, M.E. (1972, Sept.). Nursing grand rounds: Severe trauma, *Nursing '72, 2,* 9:33-38 (with J. Zoellner, B. Ozmon, & E. Simunek).

Levine, M.E. (1972, Oct.). Nursing grand rounds: Congestive failure. *Nursing '72, 2,* 10:18-23 (with C. Hallberg, M. Kathrein, & R. Cox).

Levine, M.E. (1973). On creativity in nursing. *Image, 3*(3), 15-19.

Levine, M.E. (1973, Nov.). A letter from Myra, *Chart, 70*(9) (also in *Israel Nurses' Journal,* December 1973, in English and Hebrew).

Levine, M.E. (1974, Oct.). The pharmacist's clinical role in interdisciplinary care: A nurse's viewpoint. *Hospital Formulary Management, 9,* 47.

Levine, M.E. (1975, Jan.-Feb.) On creativity in nursing. *Nursing Digest, 3,* 38-40.

Levine, M.E. (1977, May). Nursing ethics and the ethical nurse. *American Journal of Nursing, 77,* 845-849.

Levine, M.E. (1978, June). Cancer chemotherapy: A nursing model. *Nursing Clinics of North America, 13*(2), 271-280.

Levine, M.E. (1978, July). Kapklvoo and nursing, too (editorial). *Research in Nursing and Health, 1*(2), 51.

Levine, M.E. (1978, Nov.). Does continuing education improve nursing practice? *Hospitals, 52*(21), 138-140.

Levine, M.E. (1979). Knowledge base required by generalized and specialized nursing practice. *ANA Publications* (G-127), 57-69.

Levine, M.E. (1980). The ethics of computer technology in health care. *Nursing Forum, 19*(2), 193-198.

Levine, M.E. (1982, March-April). Bioethics of cancer nursing. *Rehabilitation Nursing, 7,* 27-31, 41.

Levine, M.E. (1982, March-April). The bioethics of cancer nursing. *Journal of Enterostomal Therapy, 9,* 11-13.

Levine, M.E. (1984, April). A conceptual model for nursing: The four conservation principles. In the proceedings from Allentown College of St. Francis Conference.

Levine, M.E. (1988, Feb.). Antecedents from adjunctive disciplines: Creation of nursing theory. *Nursing Science Quarterly,* Inaugural Issue.

Levine, M.E. (1988, June). What does the future hold for nursing? 25th Anniversary Address, 18th District, *Illinois Nurses Association Newsletter, XXIV*(6), 1-4.

Levine, M.E. (1989). Beyond dilemma. *Seminars in Oncology Nursing, 5,* 124-128.

Levine, M.E. (1989). The ethics of nursing rhetoric. *Image: The Journal of Nursing Scholarship, 21*(1), 4-5.

Levine, M.E. (1989). Ration or rescue: The elderly in critical care. *Critical Care Nursing, 12*(1), 82-89.

Levine, M.E. (1995). The rhetoric of nursing theory. *Image: The Journal of Nursing Scholarship, 27*(1), 11-14.

Levine, M.E. (1996). The conservation principles: A retrospective. *Nursing Science Quarterly, 9*(1), 38-41.

Audiotapes

Levine, M.E. (1978, Dec.). Paper presented at the Second Annual Nurse Educator Conference, New York: Audiotape available from Teach 'em Inc., 160 E. Illinois Street, Chicago, IL 60611.

Levine, M.E. (1979). Paper presented at nursing theory conference. Audiotapes (2 reels) available from Teach 'em Inc., 160 E. Illinois Street, Chicago, IL 60611.

Levine, M.E. (1984, May). Paper presented at Nursing Theory Conference, Boyle, Letoueneau Conference, Edmonton, Canada. Audiotapes available from Ed. Kennedy, Kennedy Recording, R.R.5, Edmonton, Alberta, Canada T5P4B7 (403-470-0013).

Videotape

The nursing theorist: Portraits of excellence: Myra Levine. (1988). Oakland: Studio III. Videotape available from Fuld Video Project, 370 Hawthorne Avenue, Oakland, CA 94609.

Proceedings

Levine, M.E. (1976, Jan.). On the nursing ethnic and the negative command. *Proceedings of the Intensive Conference* (Faculty of the University of Illinois Medical Center.) Philadelphia: Society for Health and Human Values.

Levine, M.E. (1977). History of nursing in Illinois. *Proceedings of the Bicentennial Workshop of the University of Illinois College of Nursing.* University of Illinois Press.

Levine, M.E. (1977). Primary nursing: Generalist and specialist education. *Proceedings of the American Academy of Nursing,* Kansas City, MO.

Levine, M.E. (1985). What's wrong about rights? In A. Carmi & S. Schneider (Eds.), *Proceedings of the 1st International Congress of Nursing Law and Ethics.* Berlin: Springer-Verlag.

Interviews

Levine, M. (1984). Telephone interviews.
Levine, M. (1985). Telephone interviews.
Levine, M. (1988). Telephone interviews.
Levine, M. (1992). Telephone interviews.

Correspondence

Levine, M. (1984). Curriculum vitae.
Levine, M. (1984). Personal correspondence.
Levine, M. (1985). Personal correspondence.
Levine, M. (1988). Personal correspondence.
Levine, M. (1992). Personal correspondence.

Secondary sources

Book reviews

Levine, M.E. (1969). *Introduction to clinical nursing.*
Bedside Nurse, 2, 4, Sept. - Oct. 1969.
Canadian Nurse, 66, 42, Jan. 1970.
American Journal of Nursing, 70, 99, Jan. 1970.
Nursing Outlook, 18, 20, Feb. 1970.
American Journal of Nursing, 70, 2220, Oct. 1970.
Nursing Mirror, 132, 43, April 2, 1971.
Bedside Nurse, 4, 2, Nov. 1971.
Canadian Nurse, 76, 47, Dec. 1971.
Nursing Mirror, 133, 16, Dec. 17, 1971.
American Journal of Nursing, 74, 347, Feb. 1974.
Canadian Nurse, 70, 39, May 1974.
Nursing Outlook, 22, 301, May 1974.
Levine, M.E. (1971). *Renewal for nursing.*
Supervisor Nurse, 2, 68, Aug. 1971.
Bedside Nurse, 4, 2, Nov. 1971.
AANA Journal, 49, 495, Dec. 1971.
Canadian Nurse, 67, 47, Dec. 1971.
Nursing Mirror, 133, 16, Dec. 1971.

Book chapters

Fawcett J. (1995). Levine's conservation model. In J. Fawcett, *Analysis and evaluating of conceptual models of nursing* (pp. 165-215). Philadelphia: F.A. Davis.

Griffith-Kenney, J.W., & Christensen, P. (1986). *Nursing process: Application of theories, frameworks, and models* (pp. 6, 24-25), St. Louis: Mosby.

Leonard, M.K. (1990). Myra Estrin Levine. In J.B. George (Ed.), *Nursing theories: The base for professional nursing practice* (pp. 181-192). Englewood Cliffs, NJ: Prentice Hall.

MacLean, S.L. (1989). Activity intolerance: Cues for diagnosis. In R.M. Carroll-Johnson (Ed.), *Classification proceedings of the eighth annual conference of North American Nursing Diagnosis Association* (pp. 320-327). Philadelphia: J.B. Lippincott.

McLane, A. (1987). Taxonomy and nursing diagnosis, a critical view. In A. McLane (Ed.). *Classification proceedings of the seventh annual conference of Nursing of North America.* St. Louis: Mosby.

Meleis, A.I. (1985). Myra Levine. In A.I. Meleis, *Theoretical nursing: Development and progress* (pp. 275-283). Philadelphia: J.B. Lippincott.

Peiper, B.A. (1983). Levine's nursing model. In J.J. Fitzpatrick & A.L. Whall, *Conceptual models of nursing: Analysis and application* (pp. 101-115). Bowie, MD: Robert J. Brady.

Pond, J.B. (1990). Application of Levine's conservation model to nursing the homeless community. In M.E. Parker (Ed.), *Nursing theories in practice* (pp. 203-215). New York: National League for Nursing.

Schaefer, K.M. (1990). A description of fatigue associated with congestive heart failure: Use of Levine's conservation model. In M.E. Parker (Ed.), *Nursing theories in practice* (pp. 217-237). New York: National League for Nursing.

Schaefer, K.M. (1996). Levine's conservation model: Caring for women with chronic illness. In P.H. Walker & B. Neuman (Eds.), *Blueprint for use of nursing models: Education, research, practice and administration* (pp. 187-228). New York: NLN Press.

Books

Barnum, B.J.S. (1994). *Nursing theory: Analysis application evaluation* (4th ed.). Philadelphia: J.B. Lippincott.

Chinn, P.L., & Kramer, M.K. (1995). *Theory and nursing: A systematic approach* (4th ed.). St. Louis: Mosby.

Dubos, R. (1961). *Miracle of health.* Garden City, NY: Doubleday.

Dubos, R. (1965). *Man adapting.* New Haven, CT: Yale University Press.

Erikson, E.H. (1964). *Insight and responsibility.* New York: W.W. Norton.

Erikson, E.H. (1968). *Identity: Youth and crisis.* New York: W.W. Norton.

Gibson, J.E. (1966). *The senses considered as perceptual systems.* Boston: Houghton Mifflin.

Goldstein, K. (1963). *The organism.* Boston: Beacon Press.

Hall, E. (1966). *The hidden dimension.* Garden City, NY: Doubleday.

Rogers, M.E. (1970). *An introduction to the theoretical basis of nursing.* Philadelphia: F.A. Davis.

Selye, H. (1956). *The stress of life.* New York: McGraw-Hill.

Sherrington, A. (1906). *Integrative function of the nervous system.* New York: Charles Scribner & Sons.

Taylor, J., & Ballenger, S. (1980). *Neurological dysfunction and nursing interventions.* New York: McGraw-Hill.

Journal articles

Bates, M. (1967). A naturalist at large. *Natural History, 76*(6), 8-16.

Brunner, M. (1985). A conceptual approach to critical care nursing using Levine's model. *Focus on Critical Care, 12*(2), 39-40.

Bunting, S.M. (1988, Nov.). The concept of perception in selected nursing theories. *Nursing Science Quarterly, 1*(4), 168-174.

Cooper, D.M. (1990, Mar.). Optimizing wound healing: A practice within nursing's domain. *Nursing Clinics of North America, 25*(1), 165-180.

Crawford-Gamble, P.E. (1986). An application of Levine's conceptual model. *Perioperative Nursing Quarterly, 2*(1), 64-70.

Foreman, M.D. (1989, Feb.). Confusion in the hospitalized elderly: Incidence, onset, and associated factors. *Research in Nursing & Health, 12*(1), 21-29.

Hall, K.V. (1979). Current trends in the use of conceptual frameworks in nursing education. *Journal of Nursing Education, 18*(4), 26-29.

Flaskerud, J.H., & Halloran, E.J. (1980). Areas of agreement in nursing theory development. *Advances in Nursing Science, 3*(1), 1-7.

Hirschfeld, M.J. (1976). The cognitively impaired older adult. *American Journal of Nursing, 76,* 1981-1984.

Langer, V.S. (1990, Oct.). Minimal handling protocol for the intensive care nursery. *Neonatal Network-Journal of Neonatal Nursing, 9*(3), 23-27.

Lynn-McHale, D.J., & Smith, A. (1991, May). Comprehensive assessment of families of the critically ill. *AACN Clinical Issues in Critical Care Nursing, 2*(2), 195-209.

Molchany, C.B. (1992). Ventricular septal and free wall rupture complicating acute MI. *Journal of Cardiovascular Nursing, 6*(4), 38-45.

Newport, M.A. (1984). Conserving thermal energy and social integrity in the newborn. *Western Journal of Nursing Reseach, 6*(2), 175-197.

O'Laughlin, K.M. (1986). Change in bladder function in the woman undergoing radical hysterectomy for cervical cancer. *Journal of Obstetrical, Gynecological and Neonatal Nursing, 15*(5), 380-385.

Roberts, K.L., Britton, M., Cook, M., & deClifford, J. (1994). Boomerang pillows and respiratory capacity. *Clinical Nursing Research, 3*(2), 157-165.

Roberts, K.L., Britton, M., & deClifford, J. (1995). Boomerang pillows and respiratory capacity in frail elderly women. *Clinical Nursing Research, 4*(4), 465-471.

Savage, T.V., & Culbert, C. (1989). Early intervention: The unique role of nursing. *Journal of Pediatric Nursing, 4*(5), 339-345.

Schaefer, K.M. (1997). Levine's conservation model in nursing practice. In M.R. Alligood and A. Marriner-Tomey (Eds.), *Nursing theory: Utilization and application* (pp. 89-107). St. Louis: Mosby.

Schaefer, K.M., & Shober-Potylycki, M.J. (1993). Fatigue in congestive heart failure: Use of Levine's conservation model. *Journal of Advanced Nursing, 18,* 260-268.

Schaefer, K.M., & Pond, J. (1994). Levine's conservation model as a guide to nursing practice. *Nursing Science Quarterly, 7*(2), 53-54.

Schaefer, K.M., Swavely, D., Rothenberger, C., Hess, S., & Willistin, D. (1996). Sleep disturbances post coronary artery bypass surgery. *Progress in Cardiovascular Nursing, 11*(1), 5-14.

Taylor, J.W. (1989). Levine's conservation principles: Using the model for nursing diagnosis in a neurological setting. In J.P. Riehl-Sisca (Ed.), *Conceptual models for nursing practice* (3rd ed.) (pp. 349-358). Norwalk, CT: Appleton & Lange.

Tillich, P. (1961). The meaning of health. *Perspectives in Biology and Medicine, 5,* 92-100.

Tompkins, E.S. (1980). Effect of restricted mobility and dominance on perceived duration. *Nursing Reseach, 29*(6), 333-338.

Tribotti, S. (1990). Admission to the neonatal intensive care unit: Reducing the risks. *Neonatal Network, 8*(4), 17-22.

Webb, H. (1993). Holistic care following a palliative Hartmann's procedure. *British Journal of Nursing, 2*(2), 128-132.

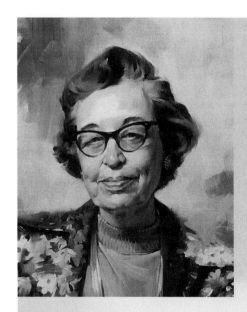

*M*artha E. Rogers

Unitary Human Beings

Kaye Bultemeier, Mary Gunther, Joann Sebastian Daily,
Judy Sporleder Maupin, Cathy A. Murray, Martha Carole Satterly,
Denise L. Schnell, Therese L. Wallace

CREDENTIALS AND BACKGROUND OF THE THEORIST

Martha Elizabeth Rogers, eldest of four children of Bruce Taylor Rogers and Lucy Mulholland Keener Rogers, was born May 12, 1914, in Dallas, Texas. Soon after her birth, her family returned to Knoxville, Tennessee, where she began her college education at the University of Tennessee, studying science from 1931 to 1933. She received her nursing diploma from Knoxville General Hospital School of Nursing in 1936. In 1937 she received a B.S. from

The authors wish to express appreciation to Dr. Lois Meier for her assistance and to Dr. Martha Rogers for critiquing the chapter.

George Peabody College in Nashville, Tennessee. Her other degrees include an M.A. in public health nursing supervision from Teachers College, Columbia University, New York, in 1945 and an M.P.H. in 1952 and a Sc.D. in 1954, both from Johns Hopkins University in Baltimore.

For 21 years, from 1954 to 1975, she was professor and head of the Division of Nursing at New York University. After 1975, she was professor, and in 1979 she became professor emerita, a title she held until her death, on March 13, 1994, at the age of 79.

Rogers's early nursing practice was in rural public health nursing in Michigan and in visiting nurse supervision, education, and practice in Connecticut.

Rogers subsequently established the Visiting Nurse Service of Phoenix, Arizona. Her publications include three books and more than 200 articles. She lectured in 46 states, the District of Columbia, Puerto Rico, Mexico, the Netherlands, China, Newfoundland, Columbia, Brazil, and other countries.[37]

Rogers received honorary doctorates from such renowned institutions as Duquesne University, University of San Diego, Iona College, Fairfield University, Emory University, Adelphi University, Mercy College, and Washburn University of Topeka. In addition, she received numerous awards and citations for her contributions and leadership in nursing, including citations for "Inspiring Leadership in the Field of Intergroup Relations" by Chi Eta Phi Sorority, "In Recognition of Your Outstanding Contribution to Nursing" by New York University, "For Distinguished Service to Nursing" by Teachers College, and many others. In 1996, Rogers was posthumously inducted into the American Nurses Association Hall of Fame. Many awards, funds, and scholarships have been established in her name.[37]

A verbal portrait of Rogers includes such descriptive terms as stimulating, challenging, controversial, idealistic, visionary, prophetic, philosophic, academic, outspoken, humorous, blunt, and ethical. Rogers was a widely recognized scholar honored for her contributions and leadership in nursing. Colleagues consider her one of the most original thinkers in nursing.[18]

THEORETICAL SOURCES

The origins of Rogerian science can be traced within nursing history to the writings of Florence Nightingale. During the midnineteenth century, Nightingale's proposals and statistical data placed the human being within the framework of the natural world, and "the foundation for the scope of modern nursing was laid."[32:30] This is the beginning of nursing's investigation of the relationship between human beings and the environment. Rogers was aware of the interrelatedness of knowledge and cites scientists from many fields as influencing the development of the Science of Unitary Human Beings.

Rogers's grounding in the liberal arts and sciences is apparent in both the origin and development of

her conceptual model published in 1970 as *An Introduction to the Theoretical Basis of Nursing*. In this book, she spoke to the Kuhnian revolution, the paradigm shift affecting all branches of science. Rogers believed that knowledge development within her model was a "never-ending process" using "a multiplicity of knowledge from many sources ... to create a kaleidoscope of possibilities."[35:4] Thus, Rogerian science emerged from a knowledge base gained from anthropology, psychology, sociology, astronomy, religion, philosophy, history, biology, physics, mathematics, and literature to create a model of unitary human beings and the environment as energy fields integral to the life process.[14:166] From this diverse knowledge, Rogers evolved philosophically to view the human being as a unified whole whose manifested characteristics are more than and different from the sum of the parts.

USE OF EMPIRICAL EVIDENCE

Being an abstract conceptual system, the Science of Unitary Human Beings does not directly identify testable empirical indicators. Rather it specifies a world view and philosophy used to identify the phenomena of concern to the discipline of nursing. As mentioned previously, Rogers's model emerged from multiple knowledge sources; the most readily apparent of these are the nonlinear dynamics of quantum physics and von Bertalanffy's general system theory.

Evident in her model is the influence of Einstein's theory of relativity in relation to space-time and Burr and Northrop's electrodynamic theory relating to electrical fields. By the time von Bertalanffy introduced general system theory in the 1950s, theories regarding a universe of open systems were beginning to affect the development of knowledge within all disciplines. With general system theory, the term *negentrophy* was brought into use to signify increasing order, complexity, and heterogeneity in direct contrast to the previously held belief that the universe was winding down. Rogers, however, refined and purified general system theory by denying hierarchal subsystems, the concept of single causation, and predictability of a system's behavior through investigations of its parts.

MAJOR CONCEPTS & DEFINITIONS

In 1970 Rogers's conceptual model of nursing rested on a set of basic assumptions that described the life process in human beings. The life process was characterized by wholeness, openness, unidirectionality, pattern and organization, sentience, and thought.[32]

Rogers postulates that human beings are dynamic energy fields integral with environmental fields. Both human and environmental fields are identified by pattern and characterized by a universe of open systems. From these concepts, in her 1983 paradigm, she postulated four building blocks for her model: energy field, a universe of open systems, pattern, and four dimensionality.[34]

Rogers consistently updated the conceptual model through revision of the homeodynamic principles. Such changes corresponded with scientific and technological advances. In 1983 Rogers changed her wording from that of *unitary man* to *unitary human being* to remove the concept of gender.[34] Additional clarification of *unitary human beings* as separate and different from the term *holistic* stressed the unique contribution of nursing to health care. In 1992, *four dimensionality* evolved into *pandimensionality*. Rogers's fundamental postulates have remained consistent since their introduction; her subsequent writings served to clarify the articulation of her original ideas.

Energy Field An energy field constitutes the fundamental unit of both the living and the nonliving. Field is a unifying concept, and energy signifies the dynamic nature of the field. Energy fields are infinite and pandimensional. Two fields are identified: the human field and the environmental field.[34] "Specifically human beings and environment are energy fields."[35:2] The *unitary human being* (human field) is defined as an irreducible, indivisible, pandimensional energy field identified by pattern and manifesting characteristics that are specific to the whole and that cannot be predicted from knowledge of the parts. The *environmental field* is defined as an irreducible, pandimensional energy field identified by pattern and integral with the human field. Each environmental field is specific to its given human field. Both change continuously, creatively, and integrally.[39]

Universe of Open Systems The concept of the universe of open systems holds that energy fields are infinite, open, and integral with one another.[34] The human and the environmental field are in continuous process and are open systems.

Pattern Pattern identifies energy fields. It is the distinguishing characteristic of an energy field and is perceived as a single wave. The nature of the pattern changes continuously, innovatively, and these changes give identity to the energy field. Each human field pattern is unique and is integral with the environmental field.[34] Manifestations emerge as a human-environmental mutual process. Pattern is an abstraction; it reveals itself through manifestation. "Manifestations of pattern have been described as unique and refer to behaviors, qualities, and characteristics of the field"; a sense of self is a field manifestation, the nature of which is unique to each individual.[11:30] Some variations in pattern manifestations have been described in phrases such as longer versus shorter rhythms, pragmatic versus imaginative, and time experienced as fast or slow. Pattern is continually changing and may manifest disease, illness, feelings, or pain.[43] Pattern change is continuous, innovative, and relative.

Pandimensionality Rogers defines *pandimensionality* as a nonlinear domain without spatial or temporal attributes. The term *pandimensional* provides for an infinite domain without limit. It best expresses the idea of a unitary whole.[39:31]

The introduction of the theory of relativity, of quantum theory, and of probability fundamentally challenged the prevailing absolutism. As new knowledge escalated, the traditional meanings of homeostasis, steady state, adaptation, and equilibrium were seriously questioned. The closed-system, entropic model of the universe was no longer adequate to explain phenomena, and evidence continued to accumulate in support of a universe of open systems.[40] Today, Rogers's model is validated by the continuing development within other disciplines of the acausal, nonlinear dynamics of life. Most notable of this development is that of chaos theory, quantum physics' contribution to the science of complexity (or wholeness) that is blurring the boundaries between the disciplines, allowing an exploration and deepening of the understanding of the totality of human experience.

MAJOR ASSUMPTIONS

Nursing

Nursing is a learned profession, both a science and an art. It is an empirical science and, like that of other sciences, lies in the phenomenon central to its focus. Rogerian nursing focuses on concern with people and the world in which they live. This area of concern is the natural fit for nursing care, encompassing people and their environments. The integrality of people and their environments, operating from a pandimensional universe of open systems, points to a new paradigm and initiates the identity of nursing as a science. The purpose of nursing is to promote health and well-being for all persons. The art of nursing, then, is the creative use of the science of nursing for human betterment.[40] "Professional practice in nursing seeks to promote symphonic interaction between human and environmental fields, to strengthen the integrity of the human field, and to direct and redirect patterning of the human and environmental fields for realization of maximum health potential."[32:122] Nursing exists for the care of people and the life process of humans.

Person

Rogers defines *person* as an open system in continuous process with the open system that is the envi-

ronment (integrality). She defines *unitary human being* as an "irreducible, indivisible, pandimensional energy field identified by pattern and manifesting characteristics that are specific to the whole."[39:29] Human beings "are not disembodied entities, nor are they mechanical aggregates. . . . Man is a unified whole possessing his own integrity and manifesting characteristics that are more than and different from the sum of his parts."[32:46-47] Within a conceptual model specific to nursing's concern, people and their environment are perceived as irreducible energy fields integral with one another and continuously creative in their evolution.

Health

Rogers uses *health* in many of her earlier writings without clearly defining the term. She uses the term *passive health* to symbolize wellness and the absence of disease and major illness.[32] Her promotion of positive health connotes direction in helping people with opportunities for rhythmic consistency.[32]

Health is used by Rogers as a value term defined by the culture or individual. Health and illness are manifestations of pattern and are considered "to denote behaviors that are of high value and low value."[18:248] Events manifested in the life process indicate the extent to which man achieves maximum health according to some value systems. In Rogerian science, the phenomena central to nursing's conceptual system is the human life process. The life process has its own dynamic and creative unity, inseparable from the environment, and is characterized by the whole.[32:85]

In *Dimensions of Health: A View from Space*, Rogers reaffirms the original theoretical assertions, adding philosophical challenges to the prevailing perception of health. Stressing a new world view that focuses on people and their environment, she lists iatrogenesis, nosocomial conditions, and hypochrondriasis as the major health problems in the United States. Rogers writes, "A new world view compatible with the most progressive knowledge available is a necessary prelude to studying human health and to determining modalities for its promotion whether on this planet or in the outer reaches of space."[36:2]

Environment

Rogers defines *environment* as "an irreducible, pandimensional energy field identified by pattern and manifesting characteristics different from those of the parts. Each environmental field is specific to its given human field. Both change continuously and creatively."[39:29]

Environmental fields are infinite, and change is continuously innovative, unpredictable, and characterized by increasing diversity. Environmental and human fields are identified by wave patterns manifesting continuous change. Environmental and human fields are in continuous and mutual process.[4:29]

THEORETICAL ASSERTIONS

The principles of homeodynamics postulate a way of perceiving unitary human beings. The evolution of these principles from 1970 to 1994 is depicted in Table 16-1. Rogers writes, "The life process is homeodynamic. . . . These principles postulate the way the life process is and predict the nature of its evolving."[32:96] Rogers identified the principles of helicy, resonancy, and integrality. The helicy principle describes *spiral development* in continuous, nonrepeating, and always innovative patterning. Rogers's articulation of the principle of helicy describing the nature of change evolved from *probabilistic* to *unpredictable* while remaining continuous and innovative. According to the principle of resonancy, patterning changes with development from lower to higher frequency. Resonancy embodies wave frequency and energy field pattern evolution. The third principle of homeodynamics, integrality, stresses the continuous mutual process of person and environment. The principles of homeodynamics evolved into a concise and clear description of the nature of change within human and environmental energy fields.

In 1970 Rogers identified five assumptions that are also theoretical assertions supporting her model derived from literature on human beings, physics, mathematics, and behavioral science:

1. Man is a unified whole possessing his own integrity and manifesting characteristics more than and different from the sum of his parts (energy field).[32:47]
2. Man and environment are continuously ex-

changing matter and energy with one another (openness).[32:54]
3. The life process evolves irreversibly and unidirectionally along the space-time continuum (helicy).[32:59]
4. Pattern and organization identify man and reflect his innovative wholeness (pattern and organization).[32:65]
5. Man is characterized by the capacity for abstraction and imagery, language and thought, sensation, and emotion (sentient, thinking being).[32:73]

LOGICAL FORM

Rogers uses a dialectic method as opposed to a logistic, problematic, or operational method; that is, Rogers explains nursing by referring to broader principles that explain human beings. She then explains human beings through principles that characterize the universe. The method is based on the perspective of a whole that organizes the parts.[28:21-22]

Rogers's model of unitary human beings is deductive and logical. The theory of relativity, general system theory, electrodynamic theory of life, and many other theories contributed ideas for Rogers's model. The central components of the model, unitary human beings and environment, are integral with one another. The basic building blocks of her model are energy field, openness, pattern, and pandimensionality providing a new world view. These concepts form the basis of an abstract conceptual system defining nursing and health. From the abstract conceptual system, Rogers derives the principles of homeodynamics, which postulate the nature and direction of human beings' evolution. While Rogers invents the words *homeodynamics* (similar state of change and growth), *helicy* (evolution), *resonancy* (intensity of change), and *integrality* (wholeness), all definitions are etymologically consistent and logical.

ACCEPTANCE BY THE NURSING COMMUNITY
Practice

The Rogerian model is an abstract system of ideas from which to approach the practice of nursing. Rogers's model, stressing the totality of experience

Table 16-1

Evolution of principles of homeodynamics: 1970, 1980, 1983, 1986, 1992

AN INTRODUCTION TO THE THEORETICAL BASIS OF NURSING 1970	NURSING: A SCIENCE OF UNITARY MAN 1980	SCIENCE OF UNITARY HUMAN BEINGS: A PARADIGM FOR NURSING 1983	DIMENSIONS OF HEALTH: A VIEW FROM SPACE 1986	NURSING SCIENCE AND THE SPACE AGE 1992
Resonancy—continuously propagating series of waves between man and environment	*Resonancy*—the continuous change from lower to higher frequency wave patterns in the human and environmental fields	*Resonancy*—the continuous change from lower to higher frequency wave patterns in human and environmental fields	*Resonancy*—the continuous change from lower to higher frequency wave patterns in human and environmental fields	*Resonancy*—the continuous change from lower to higher frequency wave patterns in human and environmental fields
Helicy—continuous, innovative change growing out of mutual interaction of man and environment along a spiralling longitudinal axis bound in space-time	*Helicy*—nature of change between human and environmental fields is continuously innovative, probabilistic, and increasingly diverse, manifesting nonrepeating rhythmicities	*Helicy*—the continuous, innovative, probabilistic, increasing diversity of human and environmental field patterns, characterized by nonrepeating rhythmicities	*Helicy*—the continuous innovative probabilistic, increasing diversity of human and environmental field patterns, characterized by nonrepeating rhythmicities	*Helicy*—the continuous innovative, unpredictable, increasing diversity of human and environmental field patterns
Reciprocy—continuous mutual interaction between the human field and environmental field				
Synchrony—change in the human field and simultaneous state of environmental field at any given point in space-time	*Complementarity*—the continuous, mutual, simultaneous interaction between human and environmental fields	*Integrality*—the continuous mutual human field and environmental field process	*Integrality*—the continuous mutual human field and environmental field process	*Integrality*—the continuous mutual human field and environmental field process

Conceptualized by Joann Daily from the following sources: Rogers, M.E. (1970). *An introduction to the theoretical basis of nursing.* Philadelphia: F.A. Davis; Riehl, J.P., & Roy, C. (Eds.). (1980). *Conceptual models for nursing practice* (2nd ed.). New York: Appleton-Century-Crofts; Rogers, M.E. (1983). Science of unitary human beings; A paradigm for nursing. In I.W. Clements & F.B. Roberts, *Family health: A theoretical approach to nursing care.* New York: John Wiley & Sons. Revised by Denise Schnell and Therese Wallace in 1988 to include: Rogers, M.E. (1986). *Dimensions of health: A view from space,* obtained through correspondence with Martha Rogers, March 1988. Updated by Cathy Murray from the following source: Rogers, M.E. (1992). Nursing science and the space age. *Nursing Science Quarterly, 5*(1), 27-34.

and existence, is relevant in today's health care system where continuum of care is more important than episodic illness and hospitalization. The model provides the abstract philosophical framework from which to view the unitary human-environmental field phenomenon. Within the Rogerian framework, nursing is based on theoretical knowledge that guides nursing practice. The professional practice of nursing is creative and imaginative and exists to serve people. It is rooted in intellectual judgment, abstract knowledge, and human compassion.

Historically, nursing has equated practice with the practical and theory with the impractical. More appropriately, theory and practice are two related components in a unified nursing practice. Alligood articulates how theory and practice direct and guide each other as they expand and increase nursing knowledge.[2] Nursing knowledge provides the framework for the emergent artistic application of nursing care.[32]

Within Rogers, the critical thinking process directing practice can be divided into three components: pattern appraisal, mutual patterning, and evaluation. Cowling introduced a template for pattern-based nursing practice.[12] This template emerged from Rogerian science and is widely accepted by nurses functioning within the Rogerian model. Further clarification of practice from the unitary perspective is outlined by Bultemeier, who expanded on the ideas of Cowling and articulated Rogerian nursing from a theoretical and practice stance.[6]

Cowling states that pattern appraisal is meant to avoid if not transcend reductionistic categories of physical, mental, spiritual, emotional, cultural, and social assessment frameworks.[13] Through observation and participation, the nurse focuses on human expressions of reflection, experience, and perception to form a profile of the patient. Mutual exploration of emergent patterns allows identification of unitary themes predominant in pandimensional human-environmental field process.

Noninvasive patterning modalities used within Rogerian practice include but are not limited to therapeutic touch, guided imagery, meditation, self-reflection, guided reminiscence, journal keeping, humor, hypnosis, sleep hygiene, dietary manipulation, and physical exercise.[1,5,26,30,31] Nurses participate in the lived experience of health in a multitude of roles, including "facilitators and educators, advocates, assessors, planners, coordinators, and collaborators" by accepting diversity, recognizing patterns, viewing change as positive, and accepting the connectedness of life.[26]

Evaluation centers on the perceptions emerging during mutual patterning. The appraisal process is continuous with intuitive emphasis on emergent patterns. The practice of nursing remains an ongoing emergent process. The Rogerian model provides a challenging and innovative framework from which to plan and implement nursing practice.

Education

Barrett calls Rogers a "consistent voice crying out against antieducationalism and dependency."[4:306] Rogers's model clearly articulates values and beliefs about human beings, health, nursing, and the educational process. As such, it has been used to guide curriculum development in all levels of nursing education.[4,22,27] Rogers said, "The only people competent to teach nursing or to teach what nurses are supposed to do are qualified nurses."[33:65] Her advocacies are evident in nursing education today; more nurses have been prepared to teach nurses at all levels of education.

Rogers, however, did advocate separate licensure for nurses prepared with an associate degree and those with a baccalaureate degree, recognizing that there is a difference between the technically oriented and the professional nurse. In her view, the professional nurse needs to be well rounded and educated in humanities and sciences as well as nursing. Such a program would include a basic education in language, mathematics, logic, philosophy, psychology, sociology, music, art, biology, microbiology, physics, and chemistry; elective courses could include economics, ethics, political science, anthropology, and computer science.[4] In regard to the research component of the curriculum, Rogers stated:

> Undergraduate students need to be able to identify problems, to have tools of investigation and to do studies that will allow them to use knowledge for

the improvement of practice, and they should be able to read the literature intelligently. People with master's degrees ought to be able to do applied research. . . . The theoretical research, the fundamental basic research is going to come out of doctoral programs of stature that focus on nursing as a learned field of endeavor.[40:34]

Barrett notes that with increasing use of technology and severity of illness of hospitalized patients, students may be limited to observational experiences in these institutions.[4] This will require that acquisition of manipulative technical skills be accomplished in practice laboratories and alternative sites, such as clinics and home health agencies. Other sites for education include health-promotion programs, managed-care programs, shelters for the homeless, and senior centers.[4:314]

Rogers clearly articulated guidelines for the education of nurses within the Science of Unitary Human Beings. Rogers discusses structuring the nursing education programs to teach nursing as a science and as a learned profession.

Research

Rogers's conceptual model provides a stimulus and direction for research and theory development in nursing science. The designation of the Science of Unitary Human Beings as a conceptual model rather than a grand theory is endorsed by Fawcett, who insists that the level of abstraction affects direct applicability.[15] She states clearly that it is the purpose of the work that determines its category. If, as in the case of the Science of Unitary Human Beings, the purpose of the work is to "articulate a body of distinctive knowledge," the work is a conceptual model.[15]

Emerging from Rogers's model are theories that explain human phenomena and direct nursing practice. The Rogerian model, with its implicit assumptions, provides broad principles that conceptually direct theory development. The conceptual model provides a stimulus and direction for scientific activity. Relationships among identified phenomena generate both grand (further development of one aspect of the model) and middle-range (description, explanation, or prediction of concrete aspects) theories.[15]

Two prominent grand nursing theories grounded in Rogers's model are Newman's Health as Expanding Consciousness and Parse's Human Becoming. Numerous middle-range theories have emerged out of Rogers's three homeodynamic principles: helicy, resonancy, and integrality. Exemplars of middle-range theories derived from the principles of Rogers's model include Power-as-Knowing-Participation-in-Change[3] (helicy), the Theory of Perceived Dissonance[5] (resonancy), and the Theory of Interactive Rhythms[19] (integrality) (Fig. 16-1).

New research methodologies arising out of a homeodynamic world view have become essential adjuncts to investigating unitary human beings and their experiences. Rogers maintains that research in nursing must examine unitary human beings as integral with their environment, and that new research tools are needed to accomplish this task.[35] The intent of nursing research, therefore, is to examine and understand a phenomenon and from this understanding design patterning activities that promote healing.

To obtain a clearer understanding of lived experiences, the person's perception and sentient awareness of what is occurring are imperative. The variety of events associated with human phenomena provide the experiential data for research, which is directed toward capturing the dynamic, ever-changing life experiences of human beings. Selecting the correct methodology for examining the person and the environment as health-related phenomena are experienced is the challenge of the Rogerian researcher. New research methodologies, arising out of a homeodynamic world view, have become essential adjuncts to investigating unitary human beings and their experiences. Methodologies based on description and explanation provide an avenue for exploration of human patterns and rhythms.[39]

Specific research methodologies emerging from midrange theories based on the Rogerian model capture the human-environment phenomena. Cowling describes the process of "pattern portrait" as a means of capturing the unitary human being.[13] Bultemeier introduced photodisclosure as a method of recording and entering the human-environmental field phenomenon.[7]

PRINCIPLES OF HOMEODYNAMICS

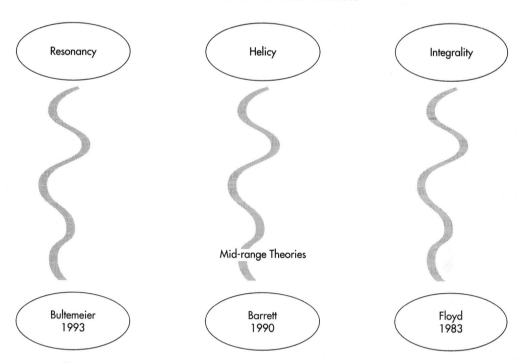

Fig. **16-1** Theory development within the Science of Unitary Human Beings.

Rogerian instrument development is extensive and ever evolving. A wide range of instruments for measuring human-environment field phenomena has emerged (Table 16-2). The continual emergence of midrange theories, methodologies, and instruments demonstrate recognition of the importance of Rogerian science to nursing.

CRITIQUE

Simplicity

Ongoing studies and work within the model have served to simplify and clarify some of the concepts and relationships, but when the model is examined in total perspective, some still classify it as complex. With its continued use in practice, research, and education, nurses will come to appreciate the model's elegant simplicity. As Whall notes, "With only three principles, a few major concepts, and five assump-

tions, Rogers has explained the nature of man and the life process."[42:154]

Generality

Rogers's conceptual model is abstract and therefore generalizable and powerful. It is broad in scope, providing a framework for the development of nursing knowledge.

Empirical Precision

Early criticisms of the model identified its major limitations as difficulty in understanding the principles, the lack of operational definitions, and inadequate tools for measurement.[9] Drawing on knowledge from a multitude of scientific fields, Rogers's conceptual model is deductive in logic with the inherent lack of immediate empirical support.[4] As Fawcett

Table 16-2

Instruments developed within Rogers's Science of Unitary Human Beings

INSTRUMENT	CONSTRUCT	AUTHOR
Power-as-Knowing-Participation-in-Change (PKPCT)	Power	E.A.M. Barrett (1990)[3]
Mutual Exploration of the Healing Human-Environment Field Relationship	Healing human-environmental mutual process	J.T. Carboni (1992)[10]
Human Field Motion Test (HFMT)	Human field motion	H.M. Ference (1986)[16,17]
Index of Field Energy (IFE)	Human field dynamics	S.H. Gueldner (1993)[20]
Diversity of Human Field Pattern Scale (DHFPS)	Human field pattern diversity	M. Hastings-Tolsma (1992)[21]
Human Field Image Metaphor Scale	Individual awareness of the infinite wholeness of the human field	L. Johnston (1994)[23]
Person-Environment Participation Scale (PEPS)	Experience of continuous human-environment mutual process	S. Leddy (1995)[24]
Leddy Healthiness Scale	Healthiness	S. Leddy (1996)[25]
Temporal Experience Scales (TES)	Subjective experience of temporal awareness	J. Paletta (1990)[29]
Assessment of Dream Experience	Dreaming as a beyond waking experience	J. Watson (1993)[41]
Perceived Field Motion Scale (PFM)	Human field motion	A. Yarcheski & N. Mahon (1991)[44]
Human Field Rhythms	Experience of rhythms in human-environmental field mutual process	A. Yarcheski & N. Mahon (1991)[44]

Modified from *Rogerian Nursing Science News, 8*(4), 9-12.

points out, failure to properly categorize the work as a conceptual model rather than a theory leads to "considerable misunderstandings and inappropriate expectations," which can result in the work being labeled inadequate.[15]

As was noted earlier, the development of the model by Rogerian scientists has resulted in the generation of testable theories accompanied by tools of measurement.

Derivable Consequences

Rogers's science has the fundamental intent of understanding human evolution and its potential. It "coordinates a universe of open systems to identify the focus of a new paradigm and initiate nursing's identity as a science."[38:182]

Although all the metaparadigm concepts are explored, the emphasis is on the integrality of human-environment field phenomena. Rogers suggested many ideas for future studies[17]; on the basis of this and the research of others, it can be said that the conceptual model is useful. Such utility has been proven in the arenas of practice, education, and research.

CONCLUSION

The Rogerian model emerged from a broad historical base and has moved to the forefront as scientific knowledge has evolved. Understanding the concepts and principles of the Science of Unitary Human Beings requires a foundation in general education, a willingness to let go of the traditional, and an ability to perceive the world in a new and creative way. Emerging from a strong educational base, the model provides a challenging framework from which to provide nursing care. The abstract ideas expounded in the Rogerian model and their congruence with modern scientific knowledge spur new and challenging theories that further the understanding of the unitary human being. Nursing scholars and practitioners are carrying Rogers's ideas into the next century.

CRITICAL THINKING *Activities*

1 Identify philosophical tenets from Nightingale that contributed to the basis for the development of the Rogerian model.

2 Discuss three main areas in which Rogerian science has had an impact on current nursing education.

3 Analyze your clinical practice and identify areas where practice based on Rogerian science would improve nursing care. Enumerate what the changes would be and identify anticipated positive outcomes.

4 Review two research articles grounded in Rogerian science. If possible, identify the midrange theory that guided the research process. What principle of homeodynamics was the midrange theory derived from?

REFERENCES

1. Alligood, M.R. (1991). Guided reminiscence: A Rogerian based intervention. *Rogerian Nursing Science News, 3*(3), 1-3.
2. Alligood, M.R. (1994). Toward a unitary view of nursing practice. In M. Madrid & E.A.M. Barrett (Eds.), *Rogers' scientific art of nursing practice* (pp. 223-240). New York: National League for Nursing.
3. Barrett, E.A.M. (1990). An instrument to measure power-as-knowing-participation-in-change. In O. Strickland & C. Waltz (Eds.), *The measurement of nursing outcomes: Measuring clients self-care and coping skills* (Vol 4) (pp. 159-180). New York: Springer.
4. Barrett, E.A.M. (1990). *Visions of Rogers' science-based nursing.* New York: National League for Nursing.
5. Bultemeier, K. (1993). *Photographic inquiry of the phenomenon premenstrual syndrome within the Rogerian derived theory of perceived dissonance.* Doctoral dissertation, University of Tennessee, Knoxville.
6. Bultemeier, K. (1996). Rogers' science of unitary human beings in nursing practice. In M.R. Alligood & A. Marriner-Tomey (Eds.), *Nursing theory: Utilization and application* (pp. 153-174). St. Louis: Mosby.
7. Bultemeier, K. (1997). Photo-disclosure: A research methodology for investigating the unitary human being. In M. Madrid (Ed.), *Patterns of Rogerian knowing.* New York: National League for Nursing Press. In press.
8. Butcher, H.K. (1993). Kaleidoscoping in life's turbulence: From Seurat's art of Rogers' nursing science. In M.E. Parker (Ed.), *Patterns of nursing theories in practice* (pp. 183-198). New York: National League for Nursing.
9. Butterfield, S.E. (1983). In search of commonalties: Analysis of two theoretical frameworks. *International Journal of Nursing Studies, 20*(1), 15-22.
10. Carboni, J.T. (1992). Instrument development and the measurement of unitary constructs. *Nursing Science Quarterly, 5,* 134-142.
11. Clarke, P.N. (1986). Theoretical and measurement issues in the study of field phenomena. *Advances in Nursing Science, 9*(1), 29-39.
12. Cowling, W.R. (1990). A template for nursing practice. In E.A.M. Barrett (Ed.), *Visions of Rogers' science-based nursing* (pp. 45-65). New York: National League for Nursing.
13. Cowling, W.R. (1993). Unitary knowing in nursing practice. *Nursing Science Quarterly, 6*(4), 201-207.
14. Falco, S.M., & Lobo, M.L. (1980). Martha E. Rogers. In Nursing Theories Conference Group, *Nursing theories: The base for professional practice* (pp. 164-183). Englewood Cliffs, NJ: Prentice Hall.
15. Fawcett, J. (1995). *Analysis and evaluation of conceptual models of nursing* (3rd ed.). Philadelphia: F.A. Davis.

16. Ference, H.M. (1986). Foundations of a nursing science and its evolution: A perspective. In V.M. Malinski (Ed.), *Explorations in Martha Rogers' science of unitary human beings* (pp. 35-44). Norwalk, CT: Appleton-Century-Crofts.

17. Ference, H.M. (1986). The relationship of time experience, creativity traits, differentiation, and human field motion. In V.M. Malinski (Ed.), *Explorations in Martha Rogers' science of unitary human beings* (pp. 95-106). Norwalk, CT: Appleton-Century-Crofts.

18. Fitzpatrick, J.J., & Whall, A.L. (1983). *Conceptual models of nursing: Analysis and application.* Bowie, MD: Robert J. Brady.

19. Floyd, J.A. (1983). Research using Rogers' conceptual system: Development of a testable theorem. *Advances in Nursing Science, 5*(2), 37-48.

20. Gueldner, S.H. (1993). *Index of field energy: A psychometric analysis.* Unpublished manuscript.

21. Hastings-Tolsma, M.T. (1992). The relationship of diversity of human field pattern to risk-taking and time experience: An investigation of Rogers' principles of homeodynamics. *Dissertation Abstracts International, 53,* 4029B.

22. Hellvig, S.D., & Ferrante, S. (1993). Martha Rogers' model in associate degree education. *Nurse Educator, 18*(5), 25-27.

23. Johnston, L.W. (1994). Psychometric analysis of Johnston's human field image metaphor scale. *Visions: The Journal of Rogerian Nursing Science, 2*(1), 7-11.

24. Leddy, S.K. (1995). Measuring mutual process: Development and psychometric testing of the person-environment participation scale. *Visions: The Journal of Rogerian Nursing Science, 3*(1), 20-31.

25. Leddy, S.K. (1996). Development and psychometric testing of the Leddy healthiness scale. *Research in Nursing and Health 19*(5), 431-440.

26. Malinksi, V.M. (1986). Explorations on Martha Rogers' science of unitary human beings. New York: Appleton-Century-Crofts.

27. Mathwig, G.M., Young, A.A., & Pepper, J.M. (1990). Using Rogerian science in undergraduate and graduate nursing education. In E.A.M. Barrett (Ed.), *Visions of Rogers' science-based nursing* (pp. 319-334). New York: National League for Nursing.

28. McHugh, M. (1986). Nursing process: Musings on the method. *Holistic Nursing Practice, 1*(1), 21-28.

29. Paletta, J.L. (1990). The relationship of temporal experience to human time. In E.A.M. Barrett (Ed.), *Visions of Rogers' science-based nursing* (pp. 239-254). New York: National League for Nursing.

30. Parker, K.P. (1989). The theory of sentience evolution: A practice-level theory of sleeping, waking, and beyond waking patterns based on the science of unitary human beings. *Rogerian Nursing Science News, 2*(1), 4-6.

31. Reed, P.G. (1991). Toward a nursing theory of self-transcendence: Deductive reformulation using developmental theories. *Advances in Nursing Science, 13*(4), 64-77.

32. Rogers, M.E. (1970). *An introduction to the theoretical basis of nursing.* Philadelphia: F.A. Davis.

33. Rogers, M.E. (1972). *Challenge to nursing . . . professional nursing practice . . . evaluation.* NLN Pub. No. 15-1456 (pp. 62-65). New York: National League for Nursing.

34. Rogers, M.E. (1983). Science of unitary human beings: A paradigm for nursing. In I.W. Clements & F.B. Roberts, *Family health: A theoretical approach to nursing care* (pp. 219-227). New York: John Wiley & Sons.

35. Rogers, M.E. (1986). Science of unitary human beings. In V.M. Malinski (Ed.), *Explorations in Martha Rogers' science of unitary human beings* (pp. 3-8). Norwalk, CT: Appleton-Century-Crofts.

36. Rogers, M.E. (1986, Sept.). Dimension of health: A view from space. Paper presented at the conference on "Law and Life in Space," September 12, 1986. Center for Aerospace Sciences, University of North Dakota.

37. Rogers, M.E. (1988, March). Personal correspondence.

38. Rogers, M.E. (1989). Nursing: A science of unitary human beings. In J.P. Riehl-Sisca (Ed.), *Conceptual models for nursing practice* (3rd ed., pp. 181-188). Norwalk, CT: Appleton-Century-Crofts.

39. Rogers, M.E. (1994). Nursing science evolves. In M. Madrid & E.A.M. Barrett (Eds.), *Rogers' scientific art of nursing practice* (pp. 3-9). New York: National League for Nursing.

40. Rogers, M.E. (1994). The science of unitary human beings: Current perspectives. *Nursing Science Quarterly, 7*(1), 33-35.

41. Watson, J. (1993). Relationship of sleep-wake rhythm, dream experience, human field motion, and time experience in older women. *Dissertation Abstracts International, 54*(12), 6137B.

42. Whall, A.L. (1987). A critique of Rogers' framework. In R.R. Parse (Ed.), *Nursing science: Major paradigms, theories, and critiques* (pp. 147-158). Philadelphia: W.B. Saunders.

43. Wright, S.M. (1987, Sept.). The use of therapeutic touch in the management of pain. *Nursing Clinics of North America, 22*(3), 705-713.

44. Yarcheski, A., & Mahon, N.E. (1991). An empirical test of Rogers' original and revised theory of correlates in adolescents. *Research in Nursing and Health, 14,* 447-455.

BIBLIOGRAPHY

Primary sources

Books

Rogers, M.E. (1961). *Educational revolution in nursing.* New York: Macmillan.

Rogers, M.E. (1964). *Reveille in nursing.* Philadelphia: F.A. Davis.

Rogers, M.E. (1970). *An introduction to the theoretical basis of nursing.* Philadelphia: F.A. Davis.

Book chapters

Rogers, M.E. (1980). Nursing: A science of unitary man. In J.P. Reihl & C. Roy, *Conceptual models for nursing practice.* New York: Appleton-Century-Crofts.

Rogers, M.E. (1981). Science of unitary man: A paradigm for nursing. In G.E. Laskar, *Applied systems and cybernetics* (Vol. IV). New York: Pergamon.

Rogers, M.E. (1983). Beyond the horizon. In N.L. Chaska, *The nursing profession: A time to speak.* New York: McGraw-Hill.

Rogers, M.E. (1983). The family coping with a surgical crisis: Analysis and application of Rogers' theory to nursing care. (Rogers's response). In I.W. Clements & F.B. Roberts, *Family health: A theoretical approach to nursing care.* New York: John Wiley & Sons.

Rogers, M.E. (1983). Science of unitary human beings: A paradigm for nursing. In I.W. Clements & F.B. Roberts, *Family health: A theoretical approach to nursing care.* New York: John Wiley & Sons.

Rogers, M.E. (1985). A paradigm for nursing. In R. Wood & J. Kekhababh, *Examining the cultural implications of Martha E. Rogers' science of unitary human beings.* Lecompton, KS: Wood-Kekhababh Associates.

Rogers, M.E. (1986). Science of unitary human beings. In V.M. Malinski, *Explorations on Martha Rogers: Science of unitary human beings.* Norwalk, CT: Appleton-Century-Crofts.

Rogers, M.E. (1987). Nursing research in the future. In J. Roode, *Changing patterns in nursing education.* New York: National League for Nursing.

Rogers, M.E. (1987). Rogers' science of unitary human beings. In R.R. Parse, *Nursing science: Major paradigms, theories, and critiques.* Philadelphia: W.B. Saunders.

Rogers, M.E. (1989). Nursing: A science of unitary human beings. In J.P. Riehl-Sisca (Ed.), *Conceptual models for nursing practice* (3rd ed., pp. 181-188). Norwalk, CT: Appleton & Lange.

Rogers, M.E. (1990). Nursing: Science of unitary, irreducible, human beings: Update 1990. In E.A.M. Barrett, *Visions of Rogers' science-based nursing.* New York: National League for Nursing.

Rogers, M.E. (1990). Space-age paradigm for new frontiers in nursing. In M.E. Parker (Ed.), *Nursing theories in practice.* New York: National League for Nursing.

Rogers, M.E. (1992). Nightingale's notes on nursing: Prelude to the 21st century. In F. Nightingale, *Notes on nursing: What it is and what it is not.* Philadelphia: J.B. Lippincott.

Rogers, M.E. (1994). Nursing science evolves. In M. Madrid & E.A.M. Barrett (Eds.), *Rogers' scientific art of nursing practice.* (pp. 3-9). New York: National League for Nursing.

Journal articles

Fulp, E.M., & Rogers, M.E. (1982, Nov.-Dec.). N.C. Nurses visit China health services for a billion people. *Tar Heel Nurse, 44*(6), 5, 8.

Keddy, B., Jones, G.M., Jacobs, P., Burton, H. & Rogers, M. (1986, Nov.). The doctor-nurse relationship: An historical perspective. Canada in the 1920s and/or 1930s. *Journal of Advanced Nursing, 11*(6), 745-753.

Lambertsen, E., et al. (1966, May). Action, reaction: Four New York State Nurses Association members react to the American Nurses Association position paper on education. *New York State Nurse, 38*(3), 6-8.

Rogers, M.E. (1953, May). Responses to talks on menstrual health. *Nursing Outlook, 1*(5), 272-274.

Rogers, M.E. (1959, Spring). Responses to talks on menstrual health [Abstract]. *Nursing Research, 8,* 114-115.

Rogers, M.E. (1963). Building a strong educational foundation. *American Journal of Nursing, 63,* 94-95.

Rogers, M.E. (1963). Some comments on the theoretical basis of nursing practice. *Nursing Science, 1,* 11-13, 60-61.

Rogers, M.E. (1963, June-July). The clarion call. *Nursing Science, 1,* 134-135.

Rogers, M.E. (1964, Feb.). Professional standards: Whose responsibility? *Nursing Science, 2,* 71-73.

Rogers, M.E. (1965). Legislative and licensing problems in health care. *Nursing Administration Quarterly, 2,* 71-78.

Rogers, M.E. (1965, Jan.). What the public demands of nursing today. *RN, 28,* 80.

Rogers, M.E. (1965, Oct.). Collegiate education in nursing [Editorial]. *Nursing Science, 3*(5), 362-365.

Rogers, M.E. (1965, Dec.). Higher education in nursing [Editorial]. *Nursing Science, 3*(6), 443-445.

Rogers, M.E. (1966). Doctoral education in nursing. *Nursing Forum, 5*(2), 75-82.

Rogers, M.E. (1966). New designs—Experiments in action. *National League for Nursing Conference Paper, 20,* 23-26.

Rogers, M.E. (1966, Winter). Quality nursing—Cliche or challenge? *Maine Nurse, 9*(1), 2-4.

Rogers, M.E. (1967, March). Teacher preparation. *NLN Department of Associate Degree Programs, 2,* 20-36.

Rogers, M.E. (1968, Feb.). Nursing science: Research and researchers, *Record, 69,* 469.

Rogers, M.E. (1969, March). Nursing research: Relevant to practice? *Nursing Research Conference, 5,* 352-359.

Rogers, M.E. (1969, Sept.). Nursing education for professional practice. *Catholic Nurse, 18*(1), 28-37, 63-64.

Rogers, M.E. (1969, Nov.-Dec.). Preparation of the baccalaureate degree graduate. *New Jersey State Nurses Association Newsletter, 25*(5), 32-37.

Rogers, M.E. (1970, Spring). Yesterday a nurse, tomorrow a manager: What now? *Journal of New York State Nurses Association, 1*(1), 15-21.

Rogers, M.E. (1972). *Challenge to nursing . . . professional nursing practice . . . evaluation.* NLN Pub. No. 15-1456. Dept. Baccalaureate Higher Education Degree Programs, pp. 62-65.

Rogers, M.E. (1972, Jan.). Nursing: To be or not to be? *Nursing Outlook, 20*(1), 42-46.

Rogers, M.E. (1972, Dec.). Nursing's expanded role . . . and other euphemisms. *Journal of New York State Nurses Association, 3*(4), 5-10.

Rogers, M.E. (1975). Euphemisms in nursing's future. *Image, 7,* 3-9.

Rogers, M.E. (1975). Forum: Professional commitment in nursing. *Image, 2,* 12-13.

Rogers, M.E. (1975). Yesterday a nurse, today a manager: What now? *Image, 2,* 12-13.

Rogers, M.E. (1975, Aug.). Reactions to the two foregoing presentations, in challenge to nursing . . . professional nursing practice . . . evaluation. NLN Pub. No. 15-1456. *Nursing Outlook, 20,* 436.

Rogers, M.E. (1975, Aug.). Research is a growing word. *Nursing Science, 31,* 283-294.

Rogers, M.E. (1975, Oct.). Nursing is coming of age . . . Through the practitioner movement. *American Journal of Nursing, 75*(10), 1834-1843, 1859.

Rogers, M.E. (1977). Legislative and licensing problems in health care. *Nursing Administration Quarterly, 2,* 71-78.

Rogers, M.E. (1978, Jan.-Feb.). A 1985 dissent [Peer review]. *Health PAC Bulletin, 80,* 32-35.

Rogers, M.E. (1979, Dec.). Contemporary American leaders in nursing: An oral history. An interview with Martha E. Rogers. *Kango Tenbo, 4*(12), 1126-1138.

Rogers, M.E. (1985, April). *Nursing education: Preparing for the future.* NLN Pub. No. 15-1974, pp. 11-14.

Rogers, M.E. (1985, Aug.). Euphemisms in nursing's future. *Kango, 37*(9), 101-113.

Rogers, M.E. (1985, Sept.). *High touch in a high-tech future.* Perspectives in nursing—1985-1987: Based on presentations at the seventeenth NLN biennial convention (pp. 25-31). NLN Pub. No. 41-1985.

Rogers, M.E. (1985, Nov.-Dec.). Classics from our heritage. The nature and characteristics of professional education for nursing. *Journal of Professional Nursing, 1*(6), 381-383.

Rogers, M.E. (1985, Nov.-Dec.). Classics from our heritage. The need for legislation for licensure to practice professional nursing. *Journal of Professional Nursing, 1*(6), 384.

Rogers, M.E. (1987, May). *Nursing research in the future* (pp. 121-123). NLN Pub. No. 14-2203.

Rogers, M.E. (1988). Nursing science and art: A prospective. *Nursing Science Quarterly, 1*(3), 99-102.

Rogers, M.E. (1989). Creating a climate for the implementation of a nursing conceptual framework. *Journal of Continuing Education in Nursing, 20*(3), 112-116.

Rogers, M.E. (1990). AIDS: Reason for optimism. *Philippine Journal of Nursing, 60*(2), 2-3.

Rogers, M.E. (1990). *Nurses in space* (pp. 213-220). NLN Pub. No. 41-2281.

Rogers, M.E. (1990). *A conversation with Martha Rogers on nursing in space* (pp. 375-386). NLN Pub. No. 15-2285.

Rogers, M.E. (1990). *Nursing: Science of unitary, irreducible, human beings: Update 1990* (pp. 5-11). NLN Pub. No. 15-2285.

Rogers, M.E. (1992). Nursing science and the space age. *Nursing Science Quarterly, 5*(1), 27-34.

Rogers, M.E. (1994). The science of unitary human beings: Current perspectives. *Nursing Science Quarterly, 7*(1), 33-35.

Rogers, M.E., & Malinski, V. (1989). Vital signs in the science of unitary human beings. *Rogerian Nursing Science News, 1*(3), 6.

Sanford, R., & Rogers, M. (1978, July). The SAIN alternative: An interview with Martha Rogers. *Journal of Nursing Care, 11*(7), 20-23.

Audiotapes

Rogers, M.E. (1978, Oct. 20). Nursing science: A science of unitary mass. Distinguished Lecture Series, Wright State University, Dayton, OH.

Rogers, M.E. (1978, Dec.). Paper presented at the Second Annual Nurse Educator Conference, New York. Audiotape available from Teach 'em Inc., 160 E. Illinois Street, Chicago, IL 60611.

Rogers, M.E. (1980). *The science of unitary man.* New York: Media for Nursing.

Rogers, M.E. (1984, May). Paper presented at Nurses Theorist Conference, Edmonton, Alberta, Canada. Audiotape available from Kennedy Recordings, R.R. 5, Edmonton, Alberta, Canada TSP 4B7 (403-470-0013).

Rogers, M.E. (1987, May). *Rogers' framework.* Nurse Theorist Conference held in Pittsburgh, PA. Audiotape available from Meetings International, 1200 Delor Avenue, Louisville, KY 40217.

Videotapes

Distinguished Leaders in Nursing—Martha Rogers (1982). Capitol Heights, Md. The National Audiovisual Center. Videotape available from National Institutes of Health, National Library of Medicine, Bethesda, MD 20894, and from Sigma Theta Tau International, 550 West North Street, Indianapolis, IN 46202.

The nurse theorist: Portraits of Excellence—Martha Rogers. (1988). Oakland, CA: Studio III. Videotape available from Fuld Video Project, Studio III, 370 Hawthorne Avenue, Oakland, CA 94609.

Nursing theory: A circle of knowledge. (1987). New York: National League for Nursing. Available from author, 10 Columbus Circle, New York, NY 10019.

Rogers, M.E. (1984, Oct.). *The science of unitary man.* An interview with Martha Rogers with E. Donnelly at Indiana University School of Nursing.

Rogers, M.E. (1987, May). *Rogers' framework.* Nurse Theorist Conference held in Pittsburgh, PA. Videotape available from Meetings International, 1200 Delor Avenue, Louisville, KY 40217.

Lectures

Rogers M.E. (1962, March). *Viewpoints—critical areas for nursing education in baccalaureate and higher degree programs.* An address given at the meeting of the Council of Member Agencies of the Department of Baccalaureate and Higher Degree Programs, Williamsburg, VA, March 26, 1962. New York: National League for Nursing, Department of Baccalaureate and Higher Degree Programs.

Rogers, M.E. (1984, Sept. 28.). *Current issues for nursing in the next decade.* Indiana Central University, Indianapolis.

Rogers, M.E. (1986, Sept.). *Dimensions of health: A view from space.* Paper presented at the Conference on Law and Life in Space, Sept. 12, 1986. Center for Aerospace Sciences, University of North Dakota.

Rogers, M.E. (1992, May). *Science and philosophy merge for a new reality.* Keynote speaker at the Fourth Annual Rosemary Ellis Scholars' Retreat, Case Western Reserve University, Cleveland, OH.

Rogers, M.E., et al. (1955). *Prenatal and paranatal factors in the development of behavior problems among the elementary school children.* Doctoral of Science dissertation. Baltimore: Johns Hopkins University.

Dissertation

Rogers, M.E. (1954). *The association of maternal and fetal factors with the development of behavior problems among elementary school children.* Doctor of Science dissertation. Baltimore: Johns Hopkins University.

Secondary sources

Books

Alligood, M.R., & Marriner-Tomey, A. (1996). *Nursing theory: Utilization and application.* St. Louis: Mosby.

Argyris, C., & Schon, D. (1974). *Theory in practice.* San Francisco: Jossey-Bass.

Barnum, B.J. (1994). *Nursing theory: Analysis, application, evaluation.* Philadelphia: J.B. Lippincott.

Barrett, E.A.M. (1990). *Visions of Rogers' science-based nursing.* New York: National League for Nursing.

de Chardin, T. (1961). *The phenomenon of man.* New York: Harper Torch.

Chaska, N.L. (1983). *The nursing profession: A time to speak.* New York: McGraw-Hill.

Chinn, P.L., & Kramer, M.K. (1991). *Theory and nursing: A systematic approach.* (3rd ed.). St. Louis: Mosby.

Directory of nurses with doctoral degrees. (1984). Kansas City, MO: American Nurses' Association.

Dossey, L. (1982). *Space, time, and medicine.* Boulder, CO: Shambhala Publications.

Einstein, A. (1961). *Relativity.* New York: Crown.

Fitzpatrick, J.J., & Whall, A.L. (1983). *Conceptual models of nursing: Analysis and application.* Bowie, MD: Robert J. Brady.

George, J.B. (1985). *Nursing theories: The base for professional nursing practice* (2nd ed.). Englewood Cliffs, NJ: Prentice-Hall.

Goldstein, K. (1939). *The organism.* New York: American Book.

Hanchett, E.S. (1979). *Community health assessment: A conceptual tool kit.* New York: John Wiley & Sons.

Herrick, C.J. (1956). *The evolution of human nature.* Austin: University of Texas Press.

Lewin, K. (1964). *Field theory in the social sciences.* New York: Harper Torch.

Lutjens, L.J.R. (1991). *Martha Rogers: The science of unitary human beings.* Sage Publications.

Madrid, M., & Barrett, E.A.M. (1994). *Rogers' scientific art of nursing practice.* New York: National League for Nursing.

Malinski, V.M. (Ed.). (1986). *Explorations on Martha Rogers' science of unitary human beings.* Norwalk, CT: Appleton-Century-Crofts.

Malinski, V.M., & Barrett, E.A.M. (1994). *Martha E. Rogers: Her life and her work.* Philadelphia: F.A. Davis.

Meleis, A.J. (1991). *Theoretical nursing: Development and progress* (2nd ed.). Philadelphia: J.B. Lippincott.

Newman, M.A. (1979). *Theory development in nursing.* Philadelphia: F.A. Davis.

Parse, R.R. (1981). *Man-living-health: A theory of nursing.* New York: John Wiley & Sons.

Polanyi, M. (1958). *Personal knowledge.* Chicago: University of Chicago Press.

Reynolds, P.D. (1971). *A primer in theory construction.* Indianapolis: Bobbs-Merrill.

Riehl-Sisca, J.P., & Roy, C. (Eds.). (1989). *Conceptual models for nursing practice* (3rd ed.). Norwalk, CT: Appleton & Lange.

Safier, G. (1977). *Contemporary American leaders: An oral history.* New York: McGraw-Hill.

Sarter, B. (1988). *The stream of becoming: A study of Martha Rogers' theory.* New York: National League for Nursing.

Sigma Theta Tau directory of nurse researchers. (1983). Indianapolis: Sigma Theta Tau.

Toffler, A. (1970). *Future shock.* New York: Random House.

Toffler, A. (1980). *The third wave.* New York: William Morrow.

von Bertalanffy, L. (1960). *General system theory: Foundations, developments, application.* New York: George Braziller.

Book chapters

Alligood, M.R. (1989). Rogers' theory and nursing administration: A perspective on health and environment. In B. Henry, C. Arndt, M. DeVincenti, & A. Marriner-Tomey (Eds.), *Dimensions of nursing administration: Theory, research, education, practice* (pp. 105-111). Boston: Blackwell Scientific.

Bultemeier, K. (1996). Rogers' science of unitary human beings in nursing practice. In M.R. Alligood & A. Marriner-Tomey (Eds.), *Nursing theory: Utilization and application* (pp. 153-174). St. Louis: Mosby.

Butcher, H.K. (1993). Kaleidoscoping in life's turbulence: From Seurat's art to Rogers' nursing science. In M.E. Parker (Ed.), *Patterns of nursing theories in practice* (pp. 183-198). New York: National League for Nursing.

Falco, S.M., & Lobo, M.L. (1980). Martha Rogers. In Nursing Theories Conference Group, J.B. George, Chairperson, *Nursing theories: The base for professional practice*. Englewood Cliffs, NJ: Prentice Hall.

Fawcett, J. (1995). Rogers' science of unitary human beings. In J. Fawcett (Ed.), *Analysis and evaluation of conceptual models of nursing* (3rd ed., pp. 375-436). Philadelphia: F.A. Davis.

Field, I., & Newman, M. (1982). Clinical application of the unitary man framework: Case study analysis (1980). In M.J. Kim & D.A. Moritz (Eds.), *Classification of nursing diagnosis: Proceedings of the third and fourth national conference*. New York: McGraw-Hill.

Madrid, M., & Winstead-Fry, P. (1986). Rogers' conceptual model. In P. Winstead-Fry (Ed.), *Case studies in nursing theory*. New York: National League for Nursing.

Meleis, A.I. (1985). Martha Rogers. In A.I. Meleis, *Theoretical nursing: Development and progress*. Philadelphia: J.B. Lippincott.

Whall, A.L. (1987). A critique of Rogers's framework. In R. R. Parse (Ed.), *Nursing science: Major paradigms, theories, and critiques* (pp. 147-158). Philadelphia: W.B. Saunders.

Journals

Nursing Science was published from 1961 to 1963 and edited by Martha Rogers. *Visions: The Journal of Rogerian Nursing Science* was first published in 1993.

Journal articles

Aggleton, P., & Chalmers, H. (1984, Dec.). Models and theories: Rogers' unitary field model. Within the bounds of the nursing process—part 4. *Nursing Times, 80*(50), 35-39.

Allanach, E.J. (1988). Perceived supportive behaviors and nursing occupational stress: An evolution of consciousness. *Advances in Nursing Science, 10*(2), 73-82.

Alligood, M.R. (1991). Guided reminiscence: A Rogers based intervention. *Rogerian Nursing Science News, 3*(3), 1-4.

Alligood, M.R. (1991). Testing Rogers' theory of accelerating change: The relationships among creativity, actualization, and empathy in persons 18 to 92 years of age. *Western Journal of Nursing Research, 13*(1), 84-96.

Anderson, M. (1980). A psychosocial screening tool for ambulatory health-care clients: A pilot study of validity. *Nursing Research, 29*(6), 347-351.

Anderson, M.D., & Smereck, G.A.D. (1992). The consciousness rainbow: An explication of Rogerian field pattern manifestations. *Nursing Science Quarterly, 5*(2), 72-79.

Anonymous. (1990). Mission statement of the Society of Rogerian Scholars. *Rogerian Nursing Science News, 3*(1), 6-7.

Armstrong, M.A., & Kelly, A.E. (1995). More than the sum of their parts: Martha Rogers and Hildegard Peplau. *Archives of Psychiatric Nursing, 9*(1), 40-44.

Atwood, J.R., & Gill-Rogers, B.P. (1984). Metatheory, methodology, and practicality: Issues in research uses of Rogers' science of unitary man. *Nursing Research, 33*(2), 88-91.

Barnard, K.E. (1977). Maternal-child nursing research: Review of past and strategies for future. *Nursing Research, 26*(3), 193-200.

Barnard, K.E. (1980). Knowledge for practice: Directions for the future. *Nursing Research, 29*(4), 208-212.

Barrett, E.A.M. (1988, May). Using Rogers' science of unitary human beings in nursing practice. *Nursing Science Quarterly, 1*(2), 50-51.

Bateau, J. (1985, May-June). Case study in family therapy: A Rogers/Minuchin reformation. *Michigan Nurse, 58*(3), 7-9.

Benedict, S.C., & Burge, J.M. (1990). The relationship between human field motion and preferred visible wavelengths. *Nursing Science Quarterly, 3*(2), 73-80.

Biley, F. (1990). Rogers' model: An analysis. *Nursing-Oxford, 4*(15), 31-33.

Biley, F.C. (1992). The perception of time as a factor in Rogers' science of unitary human beings: A literature review. *Journal of Advanced Nursing, 17*(9), 1141-1145.

Biley, F.C. (1993). Energy fields nursing: A brief encounter of a unitary kind. *International Journal of Nursing Studies, 30*(6), 519-525.

Blair, C. (1979). Hyperactivity in children: Viewed within the framework of synergistic man. *Nursing Forum, 18*, 293-303.

Boyd, C. (1985). Toward an understanding of mother-daughter identification using concept analysis. *Advances in Nursing Science, 7*(3), 78-86.

Bramlett, N.H., Gueldner, S.H. & Sowell, R.L. (1990). Consumer-centric advocacy: Its connection to nursing frameworks. *Nursing Science Quarterly, 3*(4), 156-61.

Brouse, S.H. (1985). Effect of gender role identity on patterns of feminine and self concept scores from late pregnancy to early postpartum. *Advances in Nursing Science, 7*(3), 32-48.

Buczny, B. (1990). Nursing care of the terminally ill client. Applying Martha Rogers' conceptual framework. *Home Health Nurse, 7*(4), 13-18.

Bullough, B. (1975). Barriers to nurse practitioner movement: Problems of women in a women's field. *International Journal of Health Services, 5*(2), 225-233.

Bullough, B. (1976). Influences on role expansion. *American Journal of Nursing, 76*(9), 1476-1481.

Burr, H.S., & Northrop, F.S.E. (1935). The electrodynamic theory of life. *Quarterly Review of Biology, 10*, 322-333.

Butcher, H.K., & Parker, N.I. (1988). Guided imagery within Rogers' science of unitary human beings: An experimental study. *Nursing Science Quarterly, 1*(3), 103-110.

Butterfield, S.E. (1983). In search of commonalities: Analysis of two theoretical frameworks. *International Journal of Nursing Studies, 20*(1), 15-22.

Carboni, J.T. (1991). A Rogerian theoretical tapestry. *Nursing Science Quarterly, 4*(3), 130-136.

Carboni, J.T. (1992). Instrument development and the measurement of unitary constructs. *Nursing Science Quarterly, 5*(3), 134-142.

Carboni, J.T. (1995). Enfolding health-as-wholeness-and-harmony: A theory of Rogerian nursing practice. *Nursing Science Quarterly, 8*(2), 71-78.

Carboni, J.T. (1995). A Rogerian process of inquiry. *Nursing Science Quarterly, 5*(1), 22-34.

Change through environmental interaction makes aging exciting: An interview with Martha Rogers (1985, Feb.). *Journal of Gerontological Nursing, 11*(2), 35-36.

Clarke, P.N. (1986). Theoretical and measurement issues in the study of field phenomena. *Advances in Nursing Science, 9*(1), 29-39.

Compton, M.A. (1989). A Rogerian view of drug abuse: Implications for nursing. *Nursing Science Quarterly, 2*(2), 98-105.

Conway, M.E. (1985). Toward greater specificity in defining nursing's metaparadigm. *Advances in Nursing Science, 7*(4), 73-81.

Cooperative nursing investigations: Role for everyone (1974). *Nursing Research, 23*(6), 452-456.

Cowling, W.R. (1993). Unitary knowing in nursing practice. *Nursing Science Quarterly, 6*(4), 201-207.

Craig, S.L. (1980). Theory development and its relevance for nursing. *Journal of Advanced Nursing, 5*(4), 349-355.

Crawford, G. (1985). A theoretical model of support network conflict experienced by new mothers. *Nursing Research, 34*(2), 100-102.

Cronenwett, L.R. (1983). Helping and nursing models. *Nursing Research, 32*(6), 342-346.

Davidson, A.W. (1992). Choice patterns: A theory of the human-environment relationship. *Rogerian Nursing Science News, 5*(1), 4-5.

DeFeo, D.J. (1990). Change: A central concern of nursing. *Nursing Science Quarterly, 3*(2), 88-94.

Denham, G. (1992). Toward the development of a theory of unitary perception. *Rogerian Nursing Science News, 5*(1), 7.

Donnelly, G.F. (1986). Nursing theory: Evolution of a sacred cow. *Holistic Nursing Practice, 1*(1), 1-7.

Duffey, M., & Muhlenkamp, A.F. (1974, Sept.). Framework for theory analysis. *Nursing Outlook, 22,* 570-574.

Dykeman, M.C., & Loukissa, D. (1993). The science of unitary human beings: An integrative review. *Nursing Science Quarterly, 6*(4), 179-188.

Ellis, R. (1968, May-June). Characteristics of significant theories. *Nursing Research, 17,* 217-222.

Fawcett, J. (1975). Family as a living open system: Emerging conceptual framework for nursing. *International Nursing Review, 22*(4), 113-116.

Fawcett, J. (1977). Relationship between identification and patterns of change in spouses' body images during and after pregnancy. *International Journal of Nursing Studies, 14*(4), 199-213.

Fawcett, J. (1984). The metaparadigm of nursing: Present status and future refinements. *Image, 16*(3), 84-87.

Flaskerud, J.H. (1986). On toward a theory of nursing action: Skills and competency in nurse-patient interaction. *Nursing Research, 35*(4), 250-252.

Floyd, J.A. (1983). Research using Rogers' conceptual system: Development of a testable theorem. *Advances in Nursing Science, 5*(2), 37-38.

Floyd, J.A. (1984). Interaction between personal sleep-wake rhythms and psychiatric hospital rest-activity schedule. *Nursing Research, 33*(5), 255-259.

Garon, M. (1991). Assessment and management of pain in the home care setting: Application of Rogers' science of unitary human beings. *Holistic Nursing Practice, 6*(1), 47-57.

Garon, M. (1992). Contributions of Martha Rogers to the development of nursing theory. *Nursing Outlook, 40*(2), 67-72.

Gill, B.P., & Atwood, J.R. (1981). Reciprocy and helicy used to relate MEGF and wound healing. *Nursing Research, 30*(2), 68-72.

Goldberg, W.G., & Fitzpatrick, J.J. (1980). Movement therapy with the aged. *Nursing Research, 29*(6), 339-346.

Greaves, F. (1980). Objectively toward curriculum improvement in nursing: Education in England and Wales. *Journal of Advanced Nursing, 5*(6), 591-599.

Greiner, D.S. (1991). Rhythmicities. *Nursing Science Quarterly, 4*(1), 21-23.

Gresham, F.M. (1981). Assessment of children's social skills. *Journal of School Psychology, 19*(2), 120-133.

Gunter, L.M., & Miller, J.C. (1977). Toward a nursing gerontology. *Nursing Research, 26*(3), 208-221.

Hanchett, E.S. (1990). Nursing models and community as client . . . public health/community health nursing. *Nursing Science Quarterly, 3*(2), 67-72.

Hanchett, E.S. (1992). Concepts from Eastern philosophy and Rogers' science of unitary human beings. *Nursing Science Quarterly, 5*(4), 164-170.

Hardin, S. (1990). *The caring imperative in education: A caring community.* NLN Pub. No. 15-2285, pp. 389-397.

Hardy, M.F. (1974, March-April). Theories: Components, development, evaluation. *Nursing Research, 23,* 100-107.

Hardy, M.F. (1978). Perspectives on nursing theory. *Advances in Nursing Science, 1,* 37-48.

Heggie, J.R., Schoenmehl, P.A., Chang, M.K., & Grieco, C. (1989). Selection and implementation of Dr. Martha Rogers' nursing conceptual model in an acute care setting. *Clinical Nurse Specialist, 3*(3), 143-147.

Heidt, P. (1981). Effect of therapeutic touch on anxiety level of hospitalized patients. *Nursing Research, 30*(1), 32-37.

Hellwig, S.D., & Ferrante, S. (1993). Martha Rogers' model in associate degree education. *Nurse Educator, 18*(5), 25-27.

Impact of physical-physiological activity on infants' growth and development. (1972). *Nursing Research, 21*(3), 210-219.

Interview with Dr. Rogers. (1984). *Kango, 36*(11), 48-51.

Iveson, J. (1982, Dec.). The four dimensional nurse. The Rogers' model of nursing. *Nursing Mirror, 155*(22), 52.

Johnson, D.E. (1974). Development of a theory: A requisite for nursing as a primary health profession. *Nursing Research, 23*(5), 372-377.

Johnston, L.W. (1994). Psychometric analysis of Johnston's human field image metaphor scale. *Visions: The Journal of Rogerian Nursing Science, 2*(1), 7-11.

Johnson, M. (1983). Some aspects of the relation between theory and research in nursing. *Journal of Advanced Nursing, 8*(1), 21-28.

Johnson, R.L., Fitzpatrick, J.J., & Donovan, M.D. (1982). Developmental stage: Relationship to temporal dimensions [abstract]. *Nursing Research, 31,* 120.

Jones, P.S. (1978). Adaptation model for nursing practice. *American Journal of Nursing, 78*(11), 1900-1906.

Joseph, L. (1990). *Nursing theories in practice. Practical application of Rogers' theoretical framework for nursing.* NLN Pub. No. 15-2350, pp. 115-125.

Joseph, L. (1991). *Caring: The compassionate healer: The energetics of conscious caring for the compassionate healer.* NLN Pub. No. 15-2401, pp. 51-60.

Katz, V. (1971). Auditory stimulation and developmental behavior of the premature infant. *Nursing Research, 20*(3), 196-201.

Keller, E., & Bzdek, V.M. (1986). Effects of therapeutic touch on tension headache pain. *Nursing Research, 35*(2), 101-106.

Ketefian, S. (1976). Curriculum change in nursing-education: Sources of knowledge utilized. *International Nursing Review, 23*(4), 107-115.

Ketefian, S. (1981). Critical thinking, educational preparation, and development of moral judgment among selected groups of practicing nurses. *Nursing Research, 30*(2), 98-103.

Ketefian, S. (1981). Moral reasoning and moral behavior among selected groups of practicing nurses. *Nursing Research, 30*(3), 171-176.

Kim, H.S. (1983). Use of Rogers' conceptual system in research: Comments. *Nursing Research, 32*(2), 89-91.

Kodiath, M.F. (1991). A new view of the chronic pain client. *Holistic Nursing Practice, 6*(1), 41-46.

Kontz, M. (1991). A proposed model for assessing compliance with the unitary man/human framework based on an analysis of the concept of compliance. *Classification of Nursing Diagnosis, Proceedings of the Conferences of the North American Nursing Diagnosis Association, Ninth Conference,* pp. 161-174.

Krieger, D. (1976). Healing by laying on of hands as a facilitator of bioenergetic change: The response of in vivo human hemoglobin. *International Journal of Psychoenergetic Systems, 1,* 121-129.

Kreiger, D. (1990). Compassion as power: Clinical implications of therapeutic touch. *Rogerian Nursing Science News, 3*(1), 1-5.

Lanara, V.A. (1976). Philosophy of nursing and current nursing problems. *International Nursing Review, 23*(2), 48-54.

Levine, N.H. (1976). A conceptual model for obstetric nursing. *Journal of Obstetric, Gynecologic, and Neonatal Nursing, 5*(2), 9-15.

Majesky, S.J., Brester, M.H., & Nishio, K.T. (1978). Development of a research tool: Patient indicators of nursing care. *Nursing Research, 27*(6), 365-371.

Malinski, V.M. (1991). The experience of laughing at oneself in older couples. *Nursing Science Quarterly, 4*(2), 69-75.

Malinski, V.M. (1994). Spirituality: A pattern manifestation of the human/environment mutual process. *Visions: The Journal of Rogerian Nursing Science, 2*(1), 12-18.

Mason, T., & Patterson, R. (1990). A critical review of the use of Rogers' model within a special hospital: A single case study. *Journal of Advanced Nursing, 15*(2), 130-141.

McCrae, J. (1979). Therapeutic touch in practice. *American Journal of Nursing, 79,* 664-665.

McFarlane, E.A. (1980). Nursing theory: Compassion of four theoretical proposals. *Journal of Advanced Nursing, 5*(1), 3-19.

McHugh, M. (1986). Nursing process: Musings on the method. *Holistic Nursing Practice, 1*(1), 21-28.

Miller, L.A. (1979). An explanation of therapeutic touch using the science of unitary man. *Nursing Forum, 18,* 278-287.

Moccia, P. (1985). A further investigation of "dialectical thinking as a means to understanding systems-in-development: Relevance to Rogers's principles." *Advances in Nursing Science, 7*(4), 33-38.

Moore, G. (1982). Perceptual complexity, memory and human duration experience [abstract]. *Nursing Research, 31*(3), 189.

Newman, M.A. (1994). Theory for nursing practice. *Nursing Science Quarterly, 7*(4), 153-157.

Nicoll, L.H., Meyer, P.A., & Abraham, I.L. (1985). Critique: External comparison of conceptual nursing models. *Advances in Nursing Science, 7*(4), 1-9.

Papowitz, L. (1986, April). During resuscitation, some patients face a life-or-death choice that no one else will know about—Unless they ask. *American Journal of Nursing, 86,* 416-418.

Parker, K.P. (1989). The theory of sentience evolution: A practice-level theory of sleeping, waking, and beyond waking patterns based on the science of unitary human beings. *Rogerian Nursing Science News, 2*(1), 4-6.

Parker, M.E. (1991). *Nursing theories in practice: South Florida Nursing Theorist conferences 1989.* NLN Pub. No. 15-2350, pp. v-305 overall.

Peterson, M. (1987). Time and nursing process. *Holistic Nursing Practice, 1*(3), 72-80.

Phillips, B.B., & Bramlett, M.H. (1994). Integrated awareness: A key to the pattern of mutual process. *Visions: The Journal of Rogerian Nursing Science, 2*(1), 19-34.

Phillips, J.R. (1989). Science of unitary human beings: Changing research perspectives. *Nursing Science Quarterly, 2*(2), 57-60.

Phillips, J.R. (1991). Human field research. *Nursing Science Quarterly, 4*(4), 142-143.

225
Martha E. Rogers

Porter, L.S. (1972). The impact of physical-physiological activity on infant growth and development. *Nursing Research, 21*(3), 210-219.

Porter, L.S. (1985). Is nursing ready for the year 2000? *Nursing Forum, 22*(2), 53-57.

Reed, P.G. (1986). Developmental resources and depression in the elderly. *Nursing Research, 35*(6), 368-374.

Reed, P.G. (1987, Feb.). Constructing a conceptual framework for psychosocial nursing. *Journal of Psychosocial Nursing and Mental Health Services, 25*(2), 24-28.

Reed, P.G. (1991). Toward a nursing theory of self-transcendence: Deductive reformulation using developmental theories. *Advances in Nursing Science, 13*(4), 64-77.

Reed, P.G., Fitzpatrick, J.J., Donovan, M.J., & Johnston, R.L. (1982). Suicidal crises: Relationship to the experience of time [Abstract]. *Nursing Research, 31,* 122.

Reeder, F. (1993). The science of unitary human beings and interpretive human science. *Nursing Science Quarterly, 6*(1), 13-24.

Rehabilitation workshops: Change in attitudes of nurses. (1972). *Nursing Research, 21*(2), 132-137.

Reiner, D.K. (1977). Persons in process: Model for professional education. *Archives of the Foundation of Thanatology, 6*(3), 24.

Rejoinder to commentary: Toward a clearer understanding of concept of nursing theory. (1972). *Nursing Research, 21*(1), 59-62.

Roberts, K.L. (1985). Theory of nursing as curriculum content. *Journal of Advanced Nursing, 10,* 209-215.

Roy, C., & Obloy, M. (1978). Practitioner movement: Toward a science of nursing. *American Journal of Nursing, 78*(10), 1698-1702.

Samarel, N. (1992). The experience of receiving therapeutic touch. *Journal of Advanced Nursing, 17*(6), 651-657.

Sarter, B. (1987). Evolutionary idealism: A philosophical foundation for holistic nursing theory. *Advances in Nursing Science, 9*(2), 1-9.

Sarter, B. (1988). Philosophical sources of nursing theory. *Nursing Science Quarterly, 1*(2), 52-59.

Sarter, B. (1989). Some critical philosophical issues in the science of unitary human beings. *Nursing Science Quarterly, 2*(2), 74-78.

Schodt, C.M. (1989). Parental-fetal attachment and couvade: A study of patterns of human-environment integrality. *Nursing Science Quarterly, 2*(2), 88-97.

Schoen, D.C. (1975). Comparing body systems and conceptual approaches to nursing education. *Nursing Research, 24*(5), 383-387.

Schroeder, C. (1991). Disembodiment or "where's the body in field theory?" *Nursing Science Quarterly, 4*(4), 146-148.

Sheahan, J. (1980). Some aspects of the teaching and learning in nursing. *Journal of Advanced Nursing, 5*(5), 491-511.

A science of unitary human beings—Paradigm for nursing. (1984). *Kango, 36*(11), 18-47.

Silva, M.C. (1986). Research testing nursing theory: State of the art. *Advances in Nursing Science, 9*(1), 1-11.

Silva, M.C., & Rothbart, D. (1984). An analysis of changing trends in philosophies of science on nursing theory development and testing. *Advances in Nursing Science, 6*(2), 1-13.

Skillman, L. (1991). A challenge to our current methods for studying and understanding human mutual processing. *Rogerian Nursing Science News, 3*(3), 4-7.

Smith, C.S. (1988, May). Testing propositions derived from Rogers' conceptual system. *Nursing Science Quarterly, 1*(2), 60-67.

Smith, D.W. (1994). Toward developing a theory of spirituality. *Visions: The Journal of Rogerian Nursing Science, 2*(1), 35-43.

Smith, D.W. (1995). Power and spirituality in polio survivors: A study based on Rogers' science. *Nursing Science Quarterly, 8*(3), 133-139.

Smith, M.C. (1991). Affirming the unitary perspective. *Nursing Science Quarterly, 4*(4), 148-152.

Smith, M.J. (1986, Oct.). Human-environment process: A test of Rogers' principle of integrality. *Advances in Nursing Science, 9*(1), 21-28.

Smith, M.J. (1989). Four-dimensionality: Where to go with it. *Nursing Science Quarterly, 2*(2), 56.

Taylor, S.D. (1975). Bibliography on nursing research: 1950-1974. *Nursing Research, 24*(3), 207-255.

Theiss, B.E. (1976). Investigation on perceived role functions and attitudes of nurse practitioner role in a primary care clinic. *Military Medicine, 141*(2), 85-89.

Thompson, J.E. (1990). Finding the borderline's border: Can Martha Rogers help? *Perspectives in Psychiatric Care, 26*(4), 7-10.

Ulys, L.R. (1987, May). Foundational studies in nursing: Orem, King, and Rogers. *Journal of Advanced Nursing, 12*(3), 275-280.

Walker, L.O., & Nicholson, R. (1980). Criteria for evaluating nursing process models. *Nurse Educator, 5*(5), 8-9.

Whall, A.L. (1981). Nursing theory and the assessment of families. *Journal of Psychiatric Nursing and Mental Health Services, 19*(1), 30-36.

Whelton, B.J. (1979). An operationalization of Martha Rogers' theory throughout the nursing process. *International Journal of Nursing Studies, 16*(1), 7-20.

White, E.J. (1986, May-June). Appraising the need for altered sexuality information. *Rehabilitation Nurse, 11*(3), 6-9.

Wilson, L.M., & Fitzpatrick, J.J. (1984). Dialectic thinking as a means of understanding systems-in-development: Relevance to Rogers' principles. *Advances in Nursing Science, 6*(2), 24-41.

Wright, S.M. (1987, Sept.). The use of therapeutic touch in the management of pain. *Nursing Clinics of North America, 22*(3), 705-713.

Yano, M., Onodera, T., & Higuchi, Y. (1980, Summer). Discussion on "An Introduction to the Theoretical Basis of Nursing" by Martha E. Rogers. *Kango-Kenkyu, 13*(3), 228-239.

Yarcheski, A., & Mahon, N.E. (1991). An empirical test of Rogers' original and revised theory of correlates in adolescents. *Research in Nursing & Health, 14*(6), 447-455.

Yarcheski, A., & Mahon, N.E. (1995). Rogers's pattern manifestations and health in adolescents. *Western Journal of Nursing Research, 17*(4), 383-397.

Young, A.A., & Keil, C. (1981, April). The Washburn nursing curriculum: Interpreting Martha Rogers in the Land of Oz. *Kansas Nurse, 56*(4), 7-8.

Doctoral dissertations

Barrett, E.A. (1983). *An empirical investigation of Rogers' principle of helicy: The relationship of human field complexity, human field motion, and power.* New York University.

Bays, C. (1995). *Older adults descriptions of hope after a stroke.* University of Cincinnati.

Bray, J.D. (1989). *The relationships of creativity, time experience and mystical experience.* New York University.

Bultemeier, K. (1993). *Photographic inquiry of the phenomenon premenstrual syndrome within the Rogerian derived theory of perceived dissonance.* University of Tennessee, Knoxville.

Conner, G.K. (1986). *The manifestations of human field motion, creativity, and time experience patterns of female and male parents.* University of Alabama, Birmingham.

Cowling, W.R. (1982). *The relationship of mystical experience, differentiation, and creativity in college students: An empirical investigation of the principle of helicy in Rogers' science of unitary man.* New York University.

De Sevo, M. (1991). *Temporal experience and the preference for musical sequence complexity: A study based on Martha Rogers' conceptual system.* New York University.

Doyle, M.B. (1995). *Mental health nurses' imagination, power, and empathy: A descriptive study using Rogerian nursing science.* New York University.

Ference, H. (1979). *The relationship of time experience, creativity traits, differentiation, and human field motion.* New York University.

Gabor, L.M. (1994). *Understanding the impact of chronically ill and/or developmentally disabled children on low-income, single parent families.* University of Nevada.

Girardin, B.W. (1990). *The relationship of lightwave frequency to sleepwakefulness frequency in well, full-term, Hispanic neonates.* Wayne State University.

Gueldner, S.H. (1983). *A study of the relationship between imposed motion and human field motion in elderly individuals living in nursing homes.* University of Alabama, Birmingham.

Hindman, M.L. (1993). *Humor and field energy in older adults.* Medical College of Georgia.

Johnston, L.W. (1993). *The development of the human field image metaphor scale.* Medical College of Georgia.

Kilker, M.J. (1994). *Transformational and transactional leadership styles: An empirical investigation of Rogers' principle of integrality.* Columbia University.

Kim, H. (1990). *Patterning of parent-fetal attachment during the experience of guided imagery: An experimental investigation of Martha Rogers' human-environment integrality.* Columbia University.

Krause, D.A. (1991). *The impact of an individually tailored nursing intervention on human field patterning in clients who experience dyspnea.* University of Miami.

Malinski, V. (1980). *The relationship between hyperactivity in children and perception of short wave length light: An investigation into the conceptual system proposed by Martha E. Rogers.* New York University.

Mellow, J.I. *The relationship of back massage to a person's patterning, using Martha Rogers' nursing theory.* University of Nevada.

Mersmann, C.A. (1993). *Therapeutic touch and milk letdown in mothers of non-nursing preterm infants.* New York University.

Muscari, M.E. (1992). *Binge/purge behaviors and attitudes as manifestation of relational patternings in a woman with bulimia nervosa.* Adelphi University.

McNiff, M. (1995). *A study of the relationship of power, perceived health, and life satisfaction in adults with long-term care need based on Martha E. Rogers' science of unitary human beings.* New York University.

Quinn, A.A. (1989). *Integrating a changing me: A grounded theory of the process of menopause for perimenopausal women.* University of Colorado.

Raile, M.M. (1982). *The relationship of creativity, actualization, and empathy in unitary human development: A descriptive study of Rogers' principle of helicy.* New York University.

Rawnsley, M. (1977). *Relationships between the perception of the speed of time and the process of dying: An empirical investigation of the holistic theory of nursing proposed by Martha Rogers.* Boston University.

Reeder, F. (1984). *Nursing research, holism, and philosophies of science: Points of congruence between Edmund Husserl and Martha E. Rogers.* New York University.

Rizzo, J.A. (1990). *An investigation of the relationships of life satisfaction, purpose in life, and power in individuals sixty-five years and older.* New York University.

Sarter, B.V. (1984). *The stream of becoming: A metaphysical analysis of Rogers' model of unitary man.* New York University.

Schodt, C.M. (1989). *Patterns of parent-fetus attachment and the couvade syndrome: An application of human-environment integrality as postulated in the science of unitary human beings.* New York University.

Straneva, J.A. (1992). *Therapeutic touch and in vitro erythropoiesis.* Indiana University School of Nursing.

Watson, J. (1993). *The relationships of sleep-wake rhythm, dream experience, human field motion, and time experience in older women.* New York University.

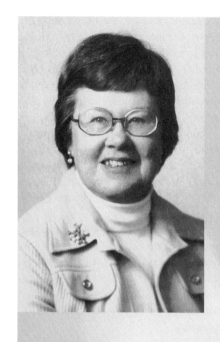

*D*orothy E. Johnson

Behavioral System Model

Victoria M. Brown, Sharon S. Conner, Linda S. Harbour,
Jude A. Magers, Judith K. Watt

CREDENTIALS AND BACKGROUND OF THE THEORIST

Dorothy E. Johnson was born Aug. 21, 1919, in Savannah, Georgia. She received her A.A. from Armstrong Junior College in Savannah, Georgia, in 1938; her B.S.N. from Vanderbilt University in Nashville, Tennessee, in 1942; and her M.P.H. from Harvard University in Boston in 1948.

Most of Johnson's professional experiences involved teaching, although she was a staff nurse at the

The authors wish to express appreciation to Dorothy E. Johnson for providing information through personal communication for this edition of the chapter.

Chatham-Savannah Health Council from 1943 to 1944. She had been an instructor and an assistant professor in pediatric nursing at Vanderbilt University School of Nursing. From 1949 until her retirement in 1978 and subsequent move to Florida, Johnson was an assistant professor of pediatric nursing, an associate professor of nursing, and a professor of nursing at the University of California in Los Angeles.

In 1955 and 1956 Johnson was a pediatric nursing advisor assigned to the Christian Medical College School of Nursing in Vellore, South India. In addition, from 1965 to 1967 she chaired the committee of the California Nurses' Association that developed a position statement on specifications for the clinical specialist. Johnson's publications[16] include four books, more than 30 articles in periodicals, and many report, proceedings, and monographs.

Of the many honors she has received, Johnson is proudest of the 1975 Faculty Award from graduate students, the 1977 Lulu Hassenplug Distinguished Achievement Award from the California Nurses' Association, and the 1981 Vanderbilt University School of Nursing Award for Excellence in Nursing.[18] She is pleased that her Behavioral System Model has been found useful in furthering the development of a theoretical basis for nursing and is being used as a model for nursing practice on an institution-wide basis, but she reports that her greatest source of satisfaction has come from following the productive careers of her students.[20]

THEORETICAL SOURCES

Johnson's Behavioral System Theory springs from Nightingale's belief that nursing's goal is to help individuals prevent or recover from disease or injury.[23:117] The science and art of nursing should focus on the patient as an individual and not on the specific disease entity.[19:25] Johnson reports that the Behavioral System Model is based on a preexistent body of knowledge developed over years by a number of different disciplines.

She used the work of behavioral scientists in psychology, sociology, and ethnology to develop her theory. Talcott Parsons is acknowledged specifically in early developmental writings presenting concepts of the behavioral system model.[9:3] She relies heavily on the systems theory and uses concepts and definitions from A. Rapoport, R. Chinn, and W. Buckley.[16:208] The structure of the Behavioral System Theory is patterned after a systems model; a system is defined as consisting of interrelated parts functioning together to form a whole. In her writings, Johnson conceptualizes man as a behavioral system in which the functioning outcome is observed behavior. An analogy to the Behavioral System Theory is the Biological System Theory, which states that man is a biological system consisting of biological parts and that disease is an outcome of biological system disorder.

Johnson notes that, although the literature indicates others support the idea that man is a behavioral system and that man's specific response patterns form an organized and integrated whole, as far as she knows, the idea is original with her. Just as the development of knowledge of the biological system as a whole was preceded by knowledge of the parts, the development of knowledge of behavioral systems has focused on specific behavioral responses. Empirical literature supporting the notion that the behavioral system is a whole has yet to be developed.[16:208]

Developing the Behavioral System Theory from a philosophical perspective, Johnson[16:207] writes that nursing contributes by facilitating effective behavioral functioning in the patient before, during, and after illness. She uses concepts from other disciplines, such as social learning, motivation, sensory stimulation, adaptation, behavioral modification, change process, tension, and stress to expand her theory for the practice of nursing.

USE OF EMPIRICAL EVIDENCE

Some of the concepts Johnson has identified and defined in her theory are supported in the literature. Leitch and Escolona point out that tension produces behavioral changes and that the manifestation of tension by an individual depends on both internal and external factors.[11:66] Johnson[8:292] uses the work of Selye, Grinker, Simmons, and Wolff to support the idea that specific patterns of behavior are reactions to stressors from biological, psychological, and sociological sources, respectively. Johnson[9:8] suggests a difference in her model from Selye's conception of stress. Johnson's concept of stress "follows rather closely Caudill's conceptualization; that is, that stress is a process in which there is interplay between various stimuli and the defenses erected against them. Stimuli may be positive in that they are present, or negative in that something desired or required is absent."[9:7-8] Selye "conceives stress as 'a state manifested by the specific syndrome which consists of all the nonspecifically induced changes within a biologic system.'"[9:8]

In *Conceptual Models for Nursing Practice*, Johnson describes seven subsystems that comprise her behavioral system. To support the attachment-affilia-tive subsystem, she uses the work of Ainsworth and Robson.[16:210] Heathers, Gerwitz, and Rosenthal have described and explained dependency behavior, an-other subsystem defined by Johnson.[16:212-213] The re-sponse systems of ingestion and elimination, as de-scribed by Walike, Mead, and Sears, are also parts of Johnson's behavior system.[16:213] The work of Kagan and Resnik is used to support the sexual subsys-tem.[16:213] The aggressive/protective subsystem, which functions to protect and preserve, is supported by Lorenz and Feshbach.[16:213] According to Atkinson, Feather, and Crandell, physical, creative, mechanical, and social skills are manifested by achievement be-havior, another subsystem identified by Johnson.[16:214]

Another subsystem, restorative, has been sug-gested by faculty and clinicians to include behaviors such as sleep, play, and relaxation.[5] Although John-son agrees that "there may be more or fewer subsys-tems" than originally identified, she does not accept restorative as a subsystem of the behavioral system model. She believes that sleep is primarily a biologi-cal force, not a motivational behavior. She suggests that many of the behaviors identified in infants dur-ing their first years of life, such as play, are actually achievement behaviors. Johnson states that there may be a need to examine the possibility of an eighth sub-system that addresses explorative behaviors: further investigation may delineate it as a subsystem separate from the achievement subsystem.[20]

MAJOR CONCEPTS & DEFINITIONS

Behavior Johnson accepts the definition of *be-havior* as expressed by the behavioral and biologi-cal scientists: the output of intraorganismic struc-tures and processes as they are coordinated and articulated by and responsive to changes in sensory stimulation. Johnson focuses on behavior affected by the actual or implied presence of other social beings that has been shown to have major adaptive significance.[16:207-208]

System Using Rapoport's 1968 definition of sys-tem, Johnson[16:208] states, "A system is a whole that functions as a whole by virtue of the interdepen-dence of its parts." She accepts Chinn's statement that there is "organization, interaction, interdepen-dency, and integration of the parts and ele-ments."[16:208] In addition, man strives to maintain a balance in these parts through adjustments and adaptations to the forces impinging on them.

Behavioral System A behavioral system encom-passes the patterned, repetitive, and purposeful ways of behaving. These ways of behaving form an organized and integrated functional unit that de-termines and limits the interaction between the person and his environment and establishes the re-lationship of the person to the objects, events, and situations within his environment. Usually the be-havior can be described and explained. Man as a behavioral system tries to achieve stability and bal-ance by adjustments and adaptations that are suc-cessful to some degree for efficient and effective functioning. The system is usually flexible enough to accommodate the influences affecting it.[16:208-209]

Subsystems Because the behavioral system has many tasks to perform, parts of the system evolve into subsystems with specialized tasks. A subsys-tem is "a minisystem with its own particular goal and function that can be maintained as long as its relationship to the other subsystems or the envi-ronment is not disturbed."[16:221] The seven subsys-tems identified by Johnson are open, linked, and interrelated. Input and output are components of all seven subsystems.[5]

Motivational drives direct the activities of these subsystems, which are continually changing be-cause of maturation, experience, and learning. The systems described appear to exist cross-culturally and are controlled by biological, psychological, and sociological factors. The seven identified subsys-

Continued

tems are attachment-affiliative, dependency, ingestive, eliminative, sexual, achievement, and aggressive/protective.[16:209-212]

Attachment-affiliative subsystem The attachment-affiliative subsystem is probably the most critical, because it forms the basis for all social organization. On a general level, it provides survival and security. Its consequences are social inclusion, intimacy, and formation and maintenance of a strong social bond.[16:212]

Dependency subsystem In the broadest sense, the dependency subsystem promotes helping behavior that calls for a nurturing response. Its consequences are approval, attention or recognition, and physical assistance. Developmentally, dependency behavior evolves from almost total dependence on others to a greater degree of dependence on self. A certain amount of interdependence is essential for survival of social groups.[16:213]

Ingestive subsystem The ingestive and eliminative subsystems should not be seen as the input and output mechanisms of the system. All subsystems are distinct subsystems with their own input and output mechanisms. The ingestive subsystem "has to do with when, how, what, how much, and under what conditions we eat."[16:213] "It serves the broad function of appetitive satisfaction."[16:213] This behavior is associated with social and psychological as well as biological considerations.[16:213]

Eliminative subsystem The eliminative subsystem addresses "when, how, and under what conditions we eliminate."[16:213] As with the ingestive subsystem, the social and psychological factors are seen as influencing the biological aspects of this subsystem and may be, at times, in conflict with it.[23:124]

Sexual subsystem The sexual subsystem has the dual functions of procreation and gratification. Including, but not limited to, courting and mating, this response system begins with the development of gender role identity and includes the broad range of sex role behaviors.[16:213]

Achievement subsystem The achievement subsystem attempts to manipulate the environment. Its function is control or mastery of an aspect of self or environment to some standard of excellence. Areas of achievement behavior include intellectual, physical, creative, mechanical, and social skills.[16:214]

Aggressive/protective subsystem The aggressive/protective subsystem's function is protection and preservation. This follows the line of thinking of ethologists such as Lorenz[22] and Feshbach[4] rather than the behavioral reinforcement school of thought, which contends that aggressive behavior is not only learned but has a primary intent to harm others. Society demands that limits be placed on modes of self-protection and that people and their property be respected and protected.[16:213]

Equilibrium Johnson states that equilibrium is a key concept in nursing's specific goal. It is defined "as a stabilized but more or less transitory, resting state in which the individual is in harmony with himself and with his environment."[11:65] "It implies that biological and psychological forces are in balance with each other and with impinging social forces."[10:11] It is "not synonymous with a state of health, since it may be found either in health or illness."[10:11]

Tension "The concept of tension is defined as a state of being stretched or strained and can be viewed as an end-product of a disturbance in equilibrium."[9:10] Tension can be constructive in adaptative change or destructive in inefficient use of energy, hindering adaptation and causing potential structural damage.[9:10] Tension is the cue to disturbance in equilibrium.[10:15]

Stressor Internal or external stimuli that produce tension and result in a degree of instability are called *stressors*. "Stimuli may be positive in that they are present; or negative in that something desired or required is absent. [Stimuli] . . . may be either endogenous or exogenous in origin [and] may play upon one or more of our linked open systems."[10:13] The open linked systems are in constant interchange. The open linked systems include the physiological, personality, and meaningful small group (e.g., the family) systems as well as the larger social system.[10:13]

MAJOR ASSUMPTIONS
Nursing

Nursing, as perceived by Johnson, is an external force acting to preserve the organization of the patient's behavior by means of imposing regulatory mechanisms or by providing resources while the patient is under stress.[23:118] An art and a science, it supplies external assistance both before and during system balance disturbance and therefore requires knowledge of order, disorder, and control.[16:209;13:207] Nursing activities do not depend on medical authority but are complementary to medicine.

Person

Johnson[16:209] views the person as a behavioral system with patterned, repetitive, and purposeful ways of behaving that link him to the environment. An individual's specific response patterns form an organized and integrated whole.[14:207] A person is a system of interdependent parts that requires some regularity and adjustment to maintain a balance.[16:208]

Johnson[16:208] further assumes that a behavioral system is essential to the individual, and when strong forces or lower resistance disturb behavioral system balance the individual's integrity is threatened.[23:126] A person's attempt to reestablish balance may require an extraordinary expenditure of energy, which leaves a shortage of energy to assist biological processes and recovery.[23:126]

Health

Johnson perceives health as an elusive, dynamic state influenced by biological, psychological, and social factors. Health is a desired value by health professionals and focuses on the person rather than the illness.[23:119]

Health is reflected by the organization, interaction, interdependence, and integration of the subsystems of the behavioral system.[16:208] An individual attempts to achieve a balance in this system, which will lead to functional behavior. A lack of balance in the structural or functional requirements of the subsystems leads to poor health. When the system requires a minimal amount of energy for maintenance, a larger supply of energy is available to affect biological processes and recovery.[23:126]

Environment

In Johnson's theory the environment consists of all the factors that are not part of the individual's behavioral system but influence the system, some of which can be manipulated by the nurse to achieve the health goal for the patient.[23:126] The individual links to and interacts with the environment.[7] The behavioral system attempts to maintain equilibrium in response to environmental factors by adjusting and adapting to the forces that impinge on it. Excessively strong environmental forces disturb the behavioral system balance and threaten the person's stability. An unusual amount of energy is required for the system to reestablish equilibrium in the face of continuing forces.[23:126] When the environment is stable, the individual is able to continue with successful behaviors.

THEORETICAL ASSERTIONS

Johnson's Behavioral System Theory addresses two major components: the patient and nursing. The patient is a behavioral system with seven interrelated subsystems (Fig. 17-1).

Each subsystem can be described and analyzed in terms of structure and functional requirements. The four structural elements that have been identified include (1) drive, or goal; (2) set, predisposition to act; (3) choice, alternatives for action: and (4) behavior.[16:210-211]

Each of the subsystems has the same functional requirements: protection, nurturance, and stimulation.[23:123] The system and subsystems tend to be self-maintaining and self-perpetuating as long as internal and external conditions remain orderly and predictable. If the conditions and resources necessary to their functional requirements are not met, or the interrelationships among the subsystems are not harmonious, dysfunctional behavior results.[16:212]

The responses by the subsystems are developed through motivation, experience, and learning and are influenced by biological, psychological, and social factors.[16:209] The behavioral system attempts to achieve

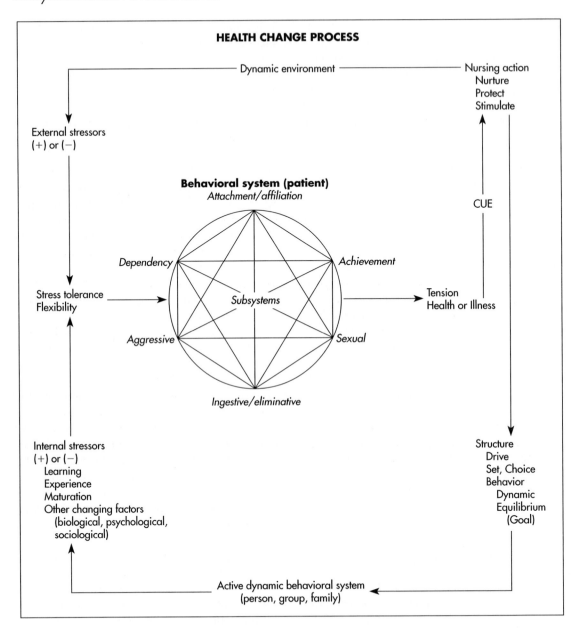

HEALTH CHANGE PROCESS

Dynamic environment

Nursing action
Nurture
Protect
Stimulate

External stressors
(+) or (−)

Behavioral system (patient)
Attachment/affiliation

Dependency

Achievement

Subsystems

CUE

Stress tolerance
Flexibility

Tension
Health or Illness

Aggressive

Sexual

Ingestive/eliminative

Internal stressors
(+) or (−)
Learning
Experience
Maturation
Other changing factors
(biological, psychological,
sociological)

Structure
Drive
Set, Choice
Behavior
Dynamic
Equilibrium
(Goal)

Active dynamic behavioral system
(person, group, family)

Fig. **17-1** Johnson's Behavioral System Model. *Conceptualized by Jude A. Magers.*

balance by adapting to internal and environmental stimuli. The behavioral system is made up of "all the patterned, repetitive, and purposeful ways of behaving that characterize each man's life."[16:209] This functional unit of behavior "determines and limits the interaction of the person and his environment and establishes the relationship of the person with the objects, events, and situations in his environment."[16:209] "The behavioral system manages its relationship with its environment."[16:209] The behavioral system appears to be active and not passive. The nurse is external to and interactive with the behavioral system.

A state of instability in the behavioral system results in a need for nursing intervention. Identification of the source of the problem in the system leads to appropriate nursing action that results in the maintenance or restoration of behavioral system balance.[23:129] Nursing is seen as an external regulatory force that acts to restore the balance in the behavioral system.[16:214]

LOGICAL FORM

By studying the literature of other disciplines and observing specifics in her practice, nursing literature, and research, Johnson used the logical forms of deductive and inductive reasoning to develop her theory. She states that a common core exists in nursing, a core that practitioners use in many settings and with varying populations.[7:200] Johnson used her observations of behavior over many years to formulate a general theory of man as a behavioral system.[15]

ACCEPTANCE BY THE NURSING COMMUNITY

Practice

According to Johnson,[16] the Behavioral System Theory provides direction for practice, education, and research. Because the goal of the theory is to maintain and restore balance in the patient by helping him achieve a more optimal level of functioning, a goal also valued by nursing, the theory is acceptable to nursing. Knowledge of the Behavioral System Theory allows the nurse to be aware of the importance of providing a constant supply of protection, nurturing, and stimulation.

In 1974 Grubbs[5:245,250] used the theory to develop an assessment tool and a nursing process sheet based on Johnson's seven subsystems. Questions and observations related to each subsystem provided powerful tools with which to collect important data. By using these tools, the nurse can discover other choices of behavior that will enable the patient to accomplish his goal of health.

That same year, Holaday[6:256] used the theory as a model to develop an assessment tool when caring for children. This tool allowed the nurse to objectively describe the child's behavior and to guide nursing action. Holaday concluded that the user of Johnson's theory was provided with a guide for planning and giving care based on scientific knowledge.

In 1980 Rawls[27:14-15] presented her attempt to use and evaluate the Johnson Behavioral System Theory in clinical practice. She used the theory to systematically assess a patient who was facing the loss of function in one arm and hand. Rawls concluded that Johnson's theory provided a theoretical base that predicted the results of nursing interventions, formulated standards for care, and administered holistic care.

Derdiarian investigated the effects of using two systematic assessment instruments on patient and nurse satisfaction. The Johnson Behavioral System Model was used to develop a self-report and observational instrument to be implemented with the nursing process. The results indicated that implementation of the instruments provided a more comprehensive and systematic approach to assessment and intervention, thereby increasing patient and nurse satisfaction with care.[2]

At the University of California, Los Angeles, Neuropsychiatric Hospital, the Johnson Behavioral System Model is being used by psychiatric nurses as the basis of practice. "Patients are assessed and behavioral data are classified by subsystem. Nursing diagnoses are formulated that reflect the nature of the ineffective behavior and its relationship to the regulators in the environment."[25:154] A study comparing the diagnostic labels generated from the Johnson Behavioral System Model to the North American Nursing Diagnosis Association list indicated that the Johnson Behavioral System Model was better at distinguishing the problems and the etiology.[25:159]

Johnson does not use the term *nursing process*. The concepts of assessment, disorders, treatment, and evaluation are referred to in a variety of works by Johnson. "For the practitioner, conceptual models provide a diagnostic and treatment orientation, and thus are of considerable practical import."[13:2]

The nursing process becomes applicable in the behavioral system model when behavioral malfunction occurs "that is in part disorganized, erratic, and dysfunctional. Illness or other sudden internal or external environmental change is most frequently responsible for such malfunctions."[16:212] "Assistance is appropriate at those times the individual is experiencing stress of a health-illness nature which disturbs equilibrium, producing tension."[9:6]

Johnson implies that the initial nursing assessment begins when the cue tension is observed and signals disequilibrium.[7:10] Sources for assessment data can be through history taking, testing, and structural observations.[16:211]

"The behavioral system is thought to determine and limit the interaction between the person and his environment."[13:3] This suggests that the accuracy and quantity of the data obtained during nursing assessment are not controlled by the nurse but by the patient (system). The only observed part of the subsystems structure is behavior. Six internal and external regulators have been identified that "simultaneously influence and are influenced by behavior" including biophysical, psychological, developmental, sociocultural, family, and physical environmental regulators.[25:157]

The nurse must be able to access information related to goals, sets, and choices that make up the structural subsystems. "One or more of [these] subsystems is likely to be involved in any episode of illness, whether in an antecedent or a consequential way or simply in association, directly or indirectly with the disorder or its treatment."[13:3] Accessing the data is critical to accurate statement of the disorder.

Johnson stated that nursing research would need to "identify and explain the behavioral system disorders which arise in connection with illness, and develop the rationale for the means of management."[13:7] Johnson does not define specific disorders but does state two general categories of disorders on the basis of the relationship to the biological system.[13:7]

Disorders are "those which are related tangentially or peripherally to disorder in the biological system; that is, they are precipitated simply by the fact of illness or the situational context of treatment; and . . . those [disorders] which are an integral part of a biological system disorder in that they are either directly associated with or a direct consequence of a particular kind of biological system disorder or its treatment."[13:7] Lachiocotte and Alexander[21] examined the use of Johnson's Behavioral System Model as a framework for nursing administrators to use when making decisions concerning the management of impaired nurses. They suggested that, by viewing all levels of the environment, the framework encouraged the nurse-administrators to assess the imbalance in the nursing system when nurse impairment exists and evaluate the "system's state of balance in relationship to the method chosen to deal with nurse impairment." The results of the study indicated that nurse-administrators preferred an assistive approach when dealing with nurse impairment. It was believed that "when the impaired nurse is confronted and assisted, equilibrium begins to be restored and balance brought back to the system" (p. 103).

The "means of management"[13:7] or interventions do consist in part of the provision of nurturance, protection, and stimulation.[16:212] The nurse may provide "temporary imposition of external regulatory and control mechanisms, such as inhibiting ineffective behavioral responses, and assisting the patient to acquire new responses."[13:6] Johnson suggests that techniques may include "teaching, role modeling, and counseling."[16:211] If a problem or disorder is anticipated, preventive nursing action is appropriate with adequate methodologies.[16:214] Nurturance, protection, and stimulation are as important for preventive nursing care or health promotion as they are for managing illness.

The outcome of nursing intervention is behavioral system equilibrium. "More specifically, equilibrium can be said to have been achieved at that point at which the individual demonstrates a degree of constancy in his pattern of functioning, both internally and interpersonally."[9:9] The evaluation of the nursing intervention is based on whether it made "a significant difference in the lives of the persons involved."[16:215] Johnson states that "the effective use of nurturance, protection, and stimulation during maternal contact at birth could significantly reduce the behavioral system problems we see today."[20]

Education

Loveland-Cherry and Wilkerson[23:133] analyzed Johnson's theory and concluded that it has utility in nursing education. A curriculum based on man as a behavioral system would have definite goals and straightforward course planning. Study would center on the patient as a behavioral system and its dysfunction, which would require use of the nursing process. In addition to an understanding of systems theory, the student would need knowledge from the social and behavioral disciplines and the physical and biological sciences.

Research

The Behavioral System Theory leads the researcher in one of two directions. One researcher might investigate the functioning of the system and subsystems by focusing on the basic sciences.[23:132] In addition to the growing body of knowledge concerning the patterning of behavior from infancy to adolescence and during aging, there is need for more knowledge about the response systems within the behavioral systems of individuals between adolescence and aging.[26:183] Another researcher might concentrate on investigating methods of gathering diagnostic data or problem-solving activities as they influence the behavioral system.[26:183]

Nurse researchers have demonstrated the usefulness of Johnson's theory in clinical practice. Small[29:264] used Johnson's theory as a conceptual framework to use when caring for visually impaired children. By evaluating and comparing the perceived body image and spacial awareness of normally sighted children with those of visually impaired children, Small found that the sensory deprivation of visual impairment affected the normal development of the child's body image and the awareness of his body in space. She concluded that when the human system is subjected to excessive stress, the goals of the system cannot be maintained.

Damus[1:276] tested the validity of Johnson's theory by comparing serum alanine aminotransferase (ALT) values in patients exposed to hepatitis B with the number of nursing diagnoses. Damus correlated the physiological disorder of elevated ALT values with behavioral disequilibrium and found that disorder in one area reflected disorder in another area.

Wilkie and coworkers examined cancer pain control behaviors with use of the Johnson Behavioral System Model. The results of the study demonstrated that with high pain intensity a person used known behaviors to protect himself or herself from the pain. This supported the assumption that "aggressive/protective subsystem behaviors are developed and modified over time to protect the individual from pain and these behaviors represent some of the patient's pain control choices."[32:729]

Believing the model to have potential in preventive care, Majesky, Brester, and Nishio[24] used it to construct a tool to measure patient indicators of nursing care. Holaday,[6] Rawls,[27] and Stamler[30] have conducted research using one subsystem.

Derdiarian examined the relationships between the aggressive/protective subsystem and the other subsystems. Findings supported the proposition that the subsystems are interactive, interdependent, and integrated; therefore, she supported Johnson's contention that "changes in a subsystem resulting from illness cannot be well understood without understanding their relationship to changes in the other subsystems."[3:219]

FURTHER DEVELOPMENT

Johnson believes people are active beings seeking constantly not only to adjust to their environments but also to adjust environments to the end of better functioning for themselves. She also views the behavioral system as active rather than merely reactive.[18] Because the model allows for this belief, it can be studied.

The theory has been associated primarily with individuals. Johnson believes groups of individuals can be considered as groups of interactive behavioral systems. Use of her theory with families and other groups needs more visibility.[12]

As a result of the current emphasis on health promotion and maintenance and on illness and injury prevention, the theory could be developed further by recognizing behavior disorders in these areas.

> It should be noted that preventive nursing, i.e., to prevent behavioral system disorder, is not the same as preventive medicine; i.e., to prevent biological system disorders; and that disorders in both cases must be identified and explicated before approaches to prevention can be developed. At this point not even medicine has developed very many specific preventive measures (immunizations for some infectious diseases, and protection against some vitamin deficiency diseases are notable exceptions). There are a number of general approaches to better health, of course—adequate nutrition, safe water, exercise, etc.—which are applicable contributing to prevention of some disorders. Small wonder then that preventive nursing remains to be developed, and this is true no matter what model or theory for nursing is used.[18]

Riegel reviewed the literature to identify major factors that predict "cardiac crippled behaviors or dependency following a myocardial infarction."[28:74] Social support, self-esteem, anxiety, depression, and perceptions of functional capacity were considered the primary factors affecting psychological adjustment to chronic coronary heart disease. This emphasized the effect of social support or nurturing on the structure and function of the dependency subsystem.[28]

Johnson states, "If care takers were aware of how their behaviors and family behaviors interact with patients to encourage dependency behaviors at the beginning of illness, they could easily prevent many dysfunctional problems."[20]

Further development could identify nursing actions that would facilitate appropriate functioning of the system toward disease prevention and health maintenance. Instead of expending energy developing nursing interventions in response to the consequences of disequilibrium, nurses need to learn how to identify precursors of disequilibrium and respond with preventive interventions.

Assuming that a community is a geographical area, a subpopulation, or any aggregate of people, and assuming that a community can benefit from

nursing interventions, the behavioral system framework can be applied to community health. A community can be described as a behavioral system with interacting subsystems that have structural elements and functional requirements. For example, mothers of chronically ill children have functional requirements needed to maintain stability within the achievement subsystem. The interaction of environmental factors such as "economic, educational, and employment influence mothers' caretaking skills."[31:97]

Communities have goals, norms, choices, and actions in addition to needing protection, nurturance, and stimulation. The community reacts to internal and external stimuli, which results in functional or dysfunctional behavior. An example of an external stimulus is health policy, and an example of dysfunctional behavior is a high infant mortality rate. The behavioral system consists of yet undefined subsystems that are organized, interacting, interdependent, and integrated. Physical, biological, and psychosocial factors also affect community behavior.

CRITIQUE

Simplicity

Johnson's theory is relatively simple in relation to the number of concepts. A person is described as a behavioral system composed of seven subsystems. Nursing is an external regulatory force. However, the theory is potentially complex because of the number of possible interrelationships between and among the behavioral system and its subsystems and the forces impinging on them. At this point, however, only a few of the potential relationships have been explored.

Generality

Johnson's theory is relatively unlimited when applied to sick individuals, but it has not been used as much with well individuals or groups. Johnson perceives man as a behavioral system comprised of seven subsystems, aggregates of interactive behavioral systems. Initially, Johnson did not clearly address nonillness situations or preventive nursing.[17:132] In later publications, Johnson emphasized the role of nurses in preventive health care of individuals and for society. She stated, "Nursing's special responsibility for health is derived from its unique social mission. Nursing needs to concentrate on developing preventive nursing to fulfill its social obligations."[19:26]

Empirical Precision

Empirical precision is difficult to achieve when a theory contains highly abstract concepts and has only potential generality. Empirical precision can improve when the subconcepts and the relationships between and among the subconcepts are well defined and reality indicators are introduced. The units and the relationships between the units in Johnson's theory are consistently defined and used. However, Johnson's theory has only a moderate degree of empirical precision because the highly abstract concepts need to be better defined. Throughout Johnson's writings terms such as *balance, stability and equilibrium, adjustments and adaptations, disturbances, disequilibrium, and behavioral disorders* are used interchangeably, which confounds their meanings. The introduction of subsystems improves the theory's empirical precision.

Derivable Consequences

Johnson's theory could guide nursing practice, education, and research; generate new ideas about nursing; and differentiate nursing from other health professions. By focusing on behavior rather than biology, the theory clearly differentiates nursing from medicine, although the concepts overlap with the psychosocial professions.

Johnson's Behavioral System Theory provides a conceptual framework for nursing education, practice, and research. The theory has directed questions for nursing research. It has been analyzed and judged to be appropriate as a basis for the development of a nursing curriculum. Practitioners and patients have judged the resulting nursing actions to be satisfactory.[16:215] The theory has potential for continued utility in nursing to achieve valued nursing goals.

CRITICAL THINKING *Activities*

1 In a practice setting, use Johnson's Behavioral System Model to guide your practice for 1 day. Describe how the use of this model affected your approach to assessing needs, making and prioritizing nursing decisions, and evaluating outcomes.

2 Identify the strengths and limitations of the model for preventive care.

3 With use of Johnson's Behavioral System Model, develop a teaching plan for a 45-year-old-black female diabetic client.

REFERENCES

1. Damus, K. (1980). An application of the Johnson behavioral system model for nursing practice. In J.P. Riehl & C. Roy (Eds.), *Conceptual models for nursing practice* (2nd ed.). New York: Appleton-Century-Crofts.
2. Derdiarian, A.K. (1990). Effects of using systematic assessment instruments on patient and nurse satisfaction with nursing care. *Oncology Nursing Forum, 17*(1), 95-100.
3. Derdiarian, A.K. (1991). Effects of using a nursing model–based assessment instrument on quality of nursing care. *Nursing Administration Quarterly, 15*(3), 1-16.
4. Feshbach, S. (1970). Aggression. In P. Mussen (Ed.), *Carmichael's manual of child psychology* (3rd ed.). New York: John Wiley & Sons.
5. Grubbs, J. (1980). *An interpretation of the Johnson behavioral system model for nursing practice* (2nd ed.). New York: Appleton-Century-Crofts.
6. Holaday, B. (1980). Implementing the Johnson model for nursing practice. In J.P. Riehl, & C. Roy (Eds.), *Conceptual models for nursing practice* (2nd ed.). New York: Appleton-Century-Crofts.
7. Johnson, D.E. (1959, April). A philosophy of nursing. *Nursing Outlook, 7,* 198-200.
8. Johnson, D.E. (1959, May). the nature of a science of nursing. *Nursing Outlook, 7,* 291-294.
9. Johnson, D.E. (1961, Jan.). Nursing's specific goal in patient care. Unpublished lecture. Faculty Colloquium, School of Nursing, University of California, Los Angeles.
10. Johnson, D.E. (1961, June). A conceptual basis for nursing care. Unpublished lecture. Third Conference, C.E. Program, University of California, Los Angeles.
11. Johnson, D.E. (1961, Nov.). The significance of nursing care. *American Journal of Nursing Studies, 61,* 63-66.
12. Johnson, D.E. (1965, April). Is nursing meeting the challenge of family needs? Unpublished lecture; Wisconsin League for Nursing. Madison, WI.

13. Johnson, D.E. (1968, April). One conceptual model of nursing. Unpublished lecture. Vanderbilt University, Nashville, Tennessee.

14. Johnson, D.E. (1968, May-June). Theory in nursing: Borrowed and unique. *Nursing Research, 17,* 206-209.

15. Johnson, D.E. (1974, Sept.-Oct.). Development of theory: A requisite for nursing as a primary health profession. *Nursing Research, 23,* 372-377.

16. Johnson, D.E. (1980). The behavioral system model for nursing. In J.P. Riehl & C. Roy (Eds.), *Conceptual models for nursing practice* (2nd ed.). New York: Appleton-Century-Crofts.

17. Johnson, D.E. (1984). Curriculum vitae.

18. Johnson, D.E. (1984). Personal correspondence.

19. Johnson, D.E. (1992). Origins of behavioral system model. In F. Nightingale (commemorative edition) (pp. 23-28). *Notes on nursing.* Philadelphia: J.B. Lippincott.

20. Johnson, D.E. (1996). Personal communication.

21. Lachicott, J.L., & Alexander, J.W. (1990). Management attitudes and nurse impairment. *Nursing Management, 21*(9), 102-110.

22. Lorenz, K. (1966). *On aggression.* New York: Harcourt.

23. Loveland-Cherry, C., & Wilkerson, S. (1983). Dorothy Johnson's behavioral systems model. In J. Fitzpatrick & A. Whall (Eds.), *Conceptual models of nursing: Analysis and application.* Bowie, MD: Robert J. Brady.

24. Majesky, S.J., Brester, M.H., & Nishio, K.T. (1978). Development of a research tool: Patient indicators of nursing care. *Nursing Research, 27*(6), 365-371.

25. Randell, B.P. (1991). NANDA versus the Johnson behavioral systems model: Is there a diagnostic difference? In R.M. Carroll-Johnson (Ed.), *Classification of nursing diagnosis: Proceedings of the ninth conference.* Philadelphia: J.P. Lippincott.

26. Randell, B.P. (1992). Nursing theory: The 21st century. *Nursing Science Quarterly, 5*(4), 176-184.

27. Rawls, A. (1980). Evaluation of the Johnson behavioral model in clinical practice: Report of a test and evaluation of the Johnson theory. *Image, 12,* 13-16.

28. Riegel, B. (1989). Social support and psychological adjustment to chronic coronary heart disease: Operalization of Johnson's behavioral system model. *Advances in Nursing Science, 11*(2), 74-84.

29. Small, B. (1980). Nursing visually impaired children with Johnson's model as a conceptual framework. In J.P. Riehl & C. Roy (Eds.), *Conceptual models for nursing practice* (2nd ed.). New York: Appleton-Century-Crofts.

30. Stamler, C. (1971). Dependency and repetitive visits to nurses' office in elementary school children. *Nursing Research, 20*(3), 254-255.

31. Turner-Henson, A. (1992). *Chronically ill children's mothers' perceptions of environmental variables.* Doctoral dissertation, University of Alabama at Birmingham.

32. Wilkie, D., Lovejoy, N., Dodd, M., & Tesler, M. (1988). Cancer pain control behaviors: Description and correlation with pain intensity. *Oncology Nursing Forum, 15*(6), 723-731.

BIBLIOGRAPHY

Primary sources

Book chapters

Johnson, D.E. (1964, June 19-26). Is there an identifiable body of knowledge essential to the development of a generic professional nursing program? In M. Maker (Ed.), *Proceedings of the first interuniversity faculty work conference.* Stowe, VT: New England Board of Higher Education.

Johnson, D.E. (1973). Medical-surgical nursing: Cardiovascular care in the first person. In *ANA Clinical Sessions* (pp. 127-134). New York: Appleton-Century-Crofts.

Johnson, D.E. (1976). Foreword. In J.R. Auger, *Behavioral systems and nursing.* Englewood Cliffs, NJ: Prentice-Hall.

Johnson, D.E. (1978). State of the art of theory development in nursing. In *Theory development: What, why, how?* New York, National League for Nursing. NLN Pub. No. 15-1708.

Johnson, D.E. (1980). The behavioral system model for nursing. In J.P. Riehl & C. Roy (Eds.), *Conceptual models for nursing practice* (2nd ed.). New York: Appleton-Century-Crofts.

Johnson, D.E. (1990). The Behavioral System Model for nursing. In M.E. Parker (Ed.), *Nursing theories in practice.* New York: National League for Nursing.

Johnson, D.E. (1992). Origins of behavioral system model. In F. Nightingale (commemorative edition). *Notes on nursing* (p. 23-28). Philadelphia: J.B. Lippincott.

Journal articles

Johnson, D.E. (1943, March). Learning to know people. *American Journal of Nursing, 43,* 248-252.

Johnson, D.E. (1954). Collegiate nursing education. *College Public Relations Quarterly, 5,* 32-35.

Johnson, D.E. (1959, April). A philosophy of nursing. *Nursing Outlook, 7,* 198-200.

Johnson, D.E. (1959, May). The nature of a science of nursing. *Nursing Outlook, 7,* 291-294.

Johnson, D.E. (1961, Oct.). Patterns in professional nursing education. *Nursing Outlook, 9,* 608-611.

Johnson, D.E. (1961, Nov.). The significance of nursing care. *American Journal of Nursing, 61,* 63-66.

Johnson, D.E. (1962, July-Aug.). Professional education for pediatric nursing. *Children, 9,* 153-156.

Johnson, D.E. (1964, Dec.). Nursing and higher education. *International Journal of Nursing Studies, 1,* 219-225.

Johnson, D.E. (1965, Sept.). Today's action will determine tomorrow's nursing. *Nursing Outlook, 13,* 38-41.

Johnson, D.E. (1965, Oct.). Crying in the newborn infant. *Nursing Science, 3,* 339-355.

Johnson, D.E. (1966, Jan. 16). Year round programs set the pace in health careers promotion. *Hospitals, 40,* 57-60.

Johnson, D.E. (1966, Oct.). Competence in practice: Technical and professional. *Nursing Outlook, 14,* 30-33

Johnson, D.E. (1967). Professional practice in nursing. *NLN Convention Papers, 23,* 26-33.

Johnson, D.E. (1967, April). Powerless: A significant determinant in patient behavior? *Journal of Nursing Educators, 6,* 39-44.

Johnson, D.E. (1968). Critique: Social influences on student nurses in their choice of ideal and practiced solutions to nursing problems. *Communicating Nursing Research, 1,* 150-155.

Johnson, D.E. (1968, April). Toward a science in nursing. *Southern Medical Bulletin, 56,* 13-23.

Johnson, D.E. (1968, May-June). Theory in nursing: Borrowed and unique. *Nursing Research, 17,* 206-209.

Johnson, D.E. (1974, Sept.-Oct.). Development of theory: A requisite for nursing as a primary health profession. *Nursing Research, 23,* 372-377.

Johnson, D.E. (1982, Spring). Some thoughts on nursing. *Clinical Nurse Specialist, 3,* 1-4.

Johnson, D.E. (1987, July-Aug.). Evaluating conceptual models for use in critical care nursing practice. *Dimensions of Critical Care Nursing, 6,* 195-197.

Johnson, D.E., Wilcox, J.A., & Moidel, H.C. (1967). The clinical specialist as a practitioner. *American Journal of Nursing, 67,* 2298-2303.

McCaffery, M., & Johnson, D.E. (1967). Effect of parent group discussion upon epistemic responses. *Nursing Research, 16,* 352-358.

Audiotape

Johnson, D.E. (1978, Dec.). Paper presented at the Second Annual Nurse Educator Conference, New York. Audiotape available from Teach 'em Inc., 160 E. Illinois Street, Chicago, IL 60611.

Videotape

The nurse theorists: Portraits of excellence: Dorothy Johnson. 1988, Oakland, CA: Studio III. Videotape available from Fuld Video Project, 370 Hawthorne Avenue, Oakland, CA 94609.

Unpublished lectures

Johnson, D.E. (1961). *A conceptual basis for nursing care.* Presentation given at the Third Conference, C.E. Program, at the University of California, Los Angeles.

Johnson, D.E. (1961). *Nursing's specific goal in patient care.* Presentation given at a Faculty Colloquium, University of California, Los Angeles.

Johnson, D.E. (1965). *Is nursing meeting the challenge of family needs?* Presentation given to the Wisconsin League for Nursing at Madison, WI.

Johnson, D.E. (1968). *One conceptual model of nursing.* Lecture given at Vanderbilt University.

Johnson, D.E. (1976). *The search for truth.* Presentation to Sigma Theta Tau, University of California, Los Angeles.

Johnson, D.E. (1977). *The behavioral system model for nursing.* Sigma Theta Tau conference. University of California, Los Angeles.

Johnson, D.E. (1978). *The behavioral system model: Then and now.* Presentation given to Vanderbilt University.

Johnson, D.E. (1982). *Conceptual frameworks or models.* Presentation at Wheeling College, West Virginia.

Johnson, D.E. (1986). *The search for truth.* Presentation to Sigma Theta Tau, University of Miami.

Correspondence

Johnson, D.E. (1984, Feb.). Curriculum vitae.

Johnson, D.E. (1984, Feb.). Personal correspondence.

Johnson, D.E. (1988, Mar.). Personal correspondence.

Johnson D.E. (1996, Aug.). Personal communication.

Secondary sources

Books

Auger, J.R. (1976). *Behavioral systems and nursing.* Englewood Cliffs, NJ: Prentice-Hall.

Chinn, P.L., & Kramer, M.K. (1995). *Theory and nursing: A systematic approach* (4th ed.). St. Louis: Mosby.

Fawcett, J. (1995). *Analysis and evaluation of conceptual models of nursing* (3rd ed.). Philadelphia: F.A. Davis.

Feshbach, S. (1970). Aggression. In P. Mussen (Ed.), *Carmichael's manual of child psychology* (3rd ed.). New York: John Wiley & Sons.

Fitzpatrick, J.J., & Whall, A.L. (1996). *Conceptual models of nursing: Analysis and application* (3rd ed.). Norwalk, CT: Appleton & Lange.

Fitzpatrick, J.J., Whall, A., Johnston, R., & Floyd, J. (1982). *Nursing models and their psychiatric mental health applications.* Bowie, MD: Robert J. Brady.

Hoeman, S.P. (1996). Conceptual bases for rehabilitation nursing. In S.P. Hoeman (Ed.), *Rehabilitation nursing: Process and application* (2nd ed., p.7). St. Louis: Mosby.

Infante, M.S. (1982). *Crisis theory: A framework for nursing practice.* Reston, VA: Reston Publishing.

Kim, H.S. (1983). *The nature of theoretical thinking in nursing.* Norwalk, CT: Appleton-Century-Crofts.

Parker, M.E. (1990). *Nursing theories in practice.* New York: National League for Nursing.

Riehl-Sisca, J.P. (1989). *Conceptual models for nursing practice.* New York: Appleton-Century-Crofts.

Dissertations

Dee, V. (1986). Validation of a patient classification instrument for psychiatric patients based on the Johnson model for nursing. *Dissertation Abstracts International, 47,* 4822B.

Lovejoy, N.C. (1981). *An empirical verification of the Johnson behavioral system model for nursing.* Doctoral dissertation, University of Alabama, Birmingham.

Riegal, B.J. (1991). *Social support and cardiac invalidism following myocardial infarction.* Doctoral dissertation, University of California, Los Angeles.

Turner-Henson, A. (1992). *Chronically ill children's mothers' perceptions of environmental variables.* Doctoral dissertation, University of Alabama at Birmingham.

Book chapters

Damus, K. (1974). An application of the Johnson behavioral system model for nursing practice. In J.P. Riehl & C. Roy (Eds.), *Conceptual models for nursing practice* (pp. 218-233). New York: Appleton-Century-Crofts.

Damus, K. (1980). An application of the Johnson behavioral system model for nursing practice. In J.P. Riehl & C. Roy (Eds.), *Conceptual models for nursing practice* (2nd ed.) (pp. 274-289). New York: Appleton-Century-Crofts.

Dee, B. (1990). Implementation of the Johnson model: One hospital's experience. In M.E. Parker (Ed.), *Nursing theories in practice.* New York: National League for Nursing.

Fawcett, J. (1995). Johnson's behavioral systems model. In J. Fawcett, *Analysis and evaluation of conceptual models of nursing* (3rd ed.) (pp. 67-107). Philadelphia: F.A. Davis.

Glennin, C.G. (1980). Formulation of standards of nursing practice using a nursing model. In J.P. Riehl & C. Roy (Eds.), *Conceptual models for nursing practice* (2nd ed.) (pp. 290-310). New York: Appleton-Century-Crofts.

Grubbs, J. (1974). An interpretation of the Johnson behavioral systems model for nursing practice. In J.P. Riehl & C. Roy (Eds.), *Conceptual models for nursing practice* (pp. 160-194). New York: Appleton-Century-Crofts.

Grubbs, J. (1980). An interpretation of the Johnson behavioral system model for nursing practice. In J.P. Riehl & C. Roy (Eds.), *Conceptual models for nursing practice* (2nd ed., pp. 217-249). New York: Appleton-Century-Crofts.

Holaday, B. (1974). Implementing the Johnson model for nursing practice. In J.P. Riehl & C. Roy (Eds.), *Conceptual models for nursing practice* (2nd ed., pp. 197-206). New York: Appleton-Century-Crofts.

Holaday, B. (1980). Implementing the Johnson model for nursing practice. In J.P. Riehl & C. Roy (Eds.), *Conceptual models for nursing practice* (2nd ed., pp. 255-263). New York: Appleton-Century-Crofts.

Holaday, B. (1997). Johnson's behavioral system model in nursing practice. In M.R. Alligood & A. Marriner-Tomey (Eds.), *Nursing theory: Utilization and application* (pp. 49-70). St. Louis: Mosby.

Lewis, C., & Randell, B.P. (1991). Alteration in self-care: An instance of ineffective coping in the geriatric patient. In R.M. Carroll-Johnson (Ed.), *Classification of nursing diagnoses: Proceedings of the ninth conference.* Philadelphia: J.B. Lippincott.

Loveland-Cherry, C., & Wilkerson, S.A. (1983). Dorothy Johnson's behavioral systems model. In J.P. Fitzpatrick & A.L. Whall (Eds.), *Conceptual models of nursing: Analysis and application* (pp. 117-135). Bowie, MD: Robert J. Brady.

Meleis, A.I. (1985). Dorothy Johnson. In A.I. Meleis, *Theoretical nursing: Development and progress* (pp. 195-205). Philadelphia: JB Lippincott.

Randell, B.P. (1991). NANDA versus the Johnson behavioral system model: Is there a diagnostic difference? In R.M. Carroll-Johnson (Ed.), *Classification of nursing diagnosis: Proceedings of the ninth conference.* Philadelphia: J.B. Lippincott.

Riehl, J.P., & Roy, C. (1980). Appendix: Nursing assessment tool using Johnson model. In J.P. Riehl & C. Roy (Eds.), *Conceptual models for nursing practice* (2nd ed., pp. 250-254). New York: Appleton-Century-Crofts.

Skolny, M.S., & Riehl, J.P. (1974). Hope: solving patient and family problems by using a theoretical framework. In J.P. Riehl & C. Roy (Eds.), *Conceptual models for nursing practice* (pp. 206-218). New York: Appleton-Century-Crofts.

Small, B. (1980). Nursing visually impaired children with Johnson's model as a conceptual framework. In J.P. Riehl & C. Roy (Eds.), *Conceptual models for nursing practice* (2nd ed., pp. 264-273). New York: Appleton-Century-Crofts.

Steven, B.J. (1979). Criteria for evaluating theories. In B.J. Stevens, *Nursing theory: Analysis, application, evaluation* (pp. 49-67). Boston: Little, Brown.

Wesley, R.L. (1991). Johnson's behavioral systems model. In D. Moreau & K. Zimmerman (Eds.), *Nursing theories and models* (pp. 60-63). Springhouse, PA: Springhouse.

Directional and biographical sources

Henderson, J. (1957-1959). *Nursing studies index* (vol. IV). Philadelphia: J.B. Lippincott.

Journal articles

Abdellah, F.G. (1969). Dept. HEW-Health administration center of health services research and development health services. *Nursing Research, 18*(5), 390-393.

Adam, E. (1983). Frontiers of nursing in the 21st century: Development of models and theories on the concept of nursing. *Journal of Advanced Nursing, 8*, 41-45.

Ainsworth, M. (1964). Patterns of attachment behavior shown by the infant in interaction with mother. *Merrill Palmer Quarterly, 10*(1), 51-58.

Arndt, C. (1970). Role sharing in diversified role set director of nursing service. *Nursing Research, 19*(3), 253-259.

Bates, B. (1970). Doctor and nurse, changing nurse, and relations. *New England Journal of Medicine, 283*, 129-130.

Botha, M.E. (1989). Theory development in perspective: The role of conceptual frameworks and models in theory development. *Journal of Advanced Nursing, 14*, 49-55.

Brandt, E.M. (1967). Comparison of on job performance of graduates with school of nursing objectives. *Nursing Research, 16*(1), 50-60.

Brester, M.H., Majesky, S.J., & Nishio, K.T. (1978, Nov.-Dec.). Development of a research tool: Patient indicators of nursing care. *Nursing Research, 27*, 365-371.

Broncatello, K.F. (1980). Anger in action: Application of the model. *Advances in Nursing Science, 2*(2), 13-24.

Bullough, B. (1976). Influences in role expansion. *American Journal of Nursing, 76*(9), 1476-1481.

Chance, K.S. (1982). Nursing models: A requisite for professional accountability. *Advances in Nursing Science, 4*(2), 57-65.

Conway, B. (1971). Effects of hospitalization on adolescence. *Adolescence, 6*(21), 77-92.

Crawford, G. (1982). The concept of pattern in nursing, conceptual development and measurement. *Advances in Nursing Science, 5*(1), 1-6.

Craig, S.L. (1980). Theory development and its relevance for nursing. *Journal of Advanced Nursing, 5*(4), 349-355.

Darnell, R.E. (1973). Promotion of interest in role of physician association as a potential career opportunity for nurses' alternative strategy. *Social Science and Medicine, 7*(7), 495.

Dee, U., & Auger, J.A. (1983, May). A patient classification system based on behavioral system model of nursing. Part II. *Journal of Nursing Administration, 13*, 18-23.

Derdiarian, A.K. (1983, July-Aug.). An instrument for theory and research development using the behavioral system model for nursing: The cancer patient. Part I. *Nursing Research, 32*, 196-201.

Derdiarian, A.K. (1990). Effects of using systematic assessment instruments on patient and nurse satisfaction with nursing care. *Oncology Nursing Forum, 17*(1), 95-100.

Derdiarian, A.K. (1991). Effects of using a nursing model–based assessment instrument on quality of nursing care. *Nursing Administration Quarterly, 15*(3), 1-16.

Derdiarian, A.K., & Forsythe, A.B. (1983, Sept.-Oct.). An instrument for theory and research development using the behavioral systems model for nursing: The cancer patient. Part II. *Nursing Research, 32*, 260-266.

Evans, R.T. (1969). Exploration of factors involved in maternal adaption to breastfeeding. *Nursing Research, 18*(1), 28-33.

Flint, R.T. (1969). Recent issues in nursing manpower review. *Nursing Research, 18*(3), 217-222.

Fritz, E. (1966). Baccalaureate nursing education: What is its job? *American Journal of Nursing, 66*(6), 1312-1316.

Georgopo, B.S. (1970). Nursing Kardex behavior in an experimental study of patient units with and without clinical nurse specialists. *Nursing Research, 19*(3), 196-218.

Godley, S.T. (1976). Community based orientation and mobility programs. *Nursing Outlook, 70*(10), 429-432.

Gortner, S.R. (1977). Overview of nursing research in United States. *Nursing Research, 26*(1), 16-23.

Gray, S.E. (1977). Do graduates of technical and professional nursing programs differ in practice? *Nursing Research, 26*(5), 368-373.

Greaves, F. (1980). Objectively toward curriculum improvement in nursing education in England and Wales. *Journal of Advanced Nursing, 5*, 591-599.

Hadley, B.J. (1969). Evolution of a conception of nursing. *Nursing Research, 18*(5), 400-405.

Hall, B.P. (1981). The change paradigm in nursing: Growth versus persistence. *Advances in Nursing Science, 3*(4), 1-6.

Hogstel, M.O. (1977). Associate degree and baccalaureate graduates: Do they function differently? *American Journal of Nursing, 77*(10), 1598-1600.

Holaday, B. (1974). Achievement behavior in chronically ill children. *Nursing Research, 23*, 25-30.

Holaday, B. (1981). Maternal response to their chronically ill infants' attachment behavior of crying. *Nursing Research, 30*, 343-348.

Holaday, B. (1982). Maternal conceptual set development: Identifying patterns of maternal response to chronically ill infant crying. *Maternal-Child Nursing Journal, 11*(1), 47-58.

Iveson-Iveson, J. (1982). Standards of behavior . . . theories of nursing practice . . . the Johnson model. *Nursing Mirror, 155*(20), 38.

Ketefian, S. (1981). Critical thinking: Educational preparation and development of moral judgment among selected groups of practicing nurses. *Nursing Research, 30*(2), 98-103.

Kohnk, M.F. (1973). Do nursing educators practice what is preached? *American Journal of Nursing, 73*(9), 1571.

Lovejoy, N. (1983). The leukemic child's perceptions of family behaviors. *Oncology Nursing Forum, 10*(4), 20-25.

Majesky, S.J. (1978). Development of a research tool: patient indicators of nursing care. *Nursing Research, 27*(6), 365-371.

Mauksch, I.G. (1972). Prescription for survival. *American Journal of Nursing, 72*(12), 2189-2193.

McCain, R.F. (1965, April). Systematic investigation of medical-surgical nursing content. *Journal of Nursing Education, 4*, 23-31.

McFarlane, E.A. (1980). Nursing theory: comparison of four theoretical proposals. *Journal of Advanced Nursing, 5*, 3-19.

McQuaid, E.A. (1979). How do graduates of different types of programs perform on state boards? *American Journal of Nursing, 79*(2), 305-308.

Newman, M.A. (1994). Theory for nursing practice. *Nursing Science Quarterly, 7*(4), 153-157.

Randell, B.P. (1992). Nursing theory: The 21st century. *Nursing Science Quarterly, 5*(4), 176-184.

Rawls, A.C. (1980, Feb.). Evaluation of the Johnson behavioral model in clinical practice. *Image, 12*, 13-16.

Reynolds, W., & Cormack, D. (1991). An evaluation of the Johnson behavioral system model of nursing. *Journal of Advanced Nursing, 16*(9), 1122-1130.

Rickelma, B.L. (1971). Bio-psycho-social linguistics conceptual approach to nurse-patient interaction. *Nursing Research, 20*(5), 398-403.

Riegel, B. (1989). Social support and psychological adjustment to chronic coronary heart disease: Operationalization of Johnson's behavioral system model. *Advances in Nursing Science, 11*(2), 74-84.

Rogers, C.G. (1973). Conceptual models as guides to clinical nursing specialization. *Journal of Nursing Education, 12*(4), 2-6.

Rogers, J.C. (1982, Jan.). Order and disorder in medicine and occupational Therapy. *American Journal of Occupational Therapy, 36,* 29-35.

Scher, M.E. (1975). Stereotyping and role conflicts between medical students and psychiatric nurses. *Hospital and Community Psychiatry, 26*(4), 219-221.

Secrest, H.P. (1968). Nurses and collaborative peritonatal research project. *Nursing Research, 17,* 292.

Smith, M.C. (1974). Perceptions of head nurses, clinical nurse specialists, nursing educators and nursing office personnel re: performance of selected nursing activities. *Nursing Research, 23*(6), 505-510.

Smith, M.C. (1976). Patient responses to being transferred during hospitalization. *Nursing Research, 25*(3), 192-196.

Smithern, C. (1969). Vocal behavior of infants as related to nursing procedures of rocking. *Nursing Research, 18*(3), 256-258.

Sorrentino, E.A. (1991). Making theories work for you. *Nursing Administration Quarterly, 15*(3), 54-59.

Stamler, C. (1971). Dependency and repetitive visits to nurses' offices in elementary school children. *Nursing Research, 20*(3), 254-255.

Stevens, B.J. (1971). Analysis of structural forms used in nursing curricula. *Nursing Research, 20*(5), 388-397.

Taylor, S.D. (1975). Bibliography on nursing research 1950-1975. *Nursing Research, 24*(3), 207-225.

Vaillot, M.C. (1970). Hope: restoration of being. *American Journal of Nursing, 10*(2), 268.

Waltz, C.F. (1978). Faculty influence on nursing students' preference in practice. *Nursing Research, 27*(2), 89-97.

Waters, V.H. (1972). Nursing practice: Implemental and supplemental. *Nursing Research, 21*(2), 124-131.

White, M.B. (1972). Importance of selected nursing activities. *Nursing Research, 21*(1), 4-14.

Wilkie, D., Lovejoy, N., Dodd, M., & Tesler, M. (1988). Cancer pain control behaviors: Description and correlation with pain intensity. *Oncology Nursing Forum, 15*(6), 723-731.

Zbilut, J.P. (1978). Epistemologic constraints to development of a theory of nursing. *Nursing Research, 27*(2), 128-129.

Other sources

Ainsworth, M. (1964). Patterns of attachment behavior shown by the infant in interaction with mother. *Merrill-Palmer Quarterly, 10*(1), 51-58.

Ainsworth, M. (1972). Attachment and dependency: A comparison. In J. Gewirtz (Ed.), *Attachment and dependency.* Englewood Cliffs, NJ: Prentice-Hall.

Atkinson, J.W. (1966). *Feather NT: A theory of achievement maturation.* New York: John Wiley & Sons.

Buckley, W. (Ed.). (1968). *Modern systems research for the behavioral scientist.* Chicago: Aldine.

Chin, R. (1961). The utility of system models and developmental models for practitioners. In K. Benne, W. Bennis, & R. Chin (Eds.), *The planning of change.* New York: Holt, Rinehart, & Winston.

Crandal, V. (1963). Achievement. In H.W. Stevenson (Ed.), *Child psychology.* Chicago: University of Chicago Press.

Feshbach, S. (1970). Aggression. In P. Mussen (Ed.), *Carmichael's manual of child psychology* (3rd ed., vol. 2). New York: John Wiley & Sons.

Gerwitz, J. (Ed.). (1972). *Attachment and dependency.* Englewood Cliffs, NJ: Prentice-Hall.

Grinker, R.R. (Ed.). (1956). *Toward a unified theory of human behavior.* New York: Basic Books.

Heathers, G. (1955). Acquiring dependence and independence: A theoretical orientation. *Journal of General Psychology, 87,* 277-291.

Kagan, J. (1964). Acquisition and significance of sex typing and sex role identity. In M.L. Hoffman & L.W. Hoffman, (Eds.), *Review of child development research.* New York: Russell Sage Foundation.

Leitch, M., & Escalona, E. (1949). The reaction of infants to stress. In *Psychoanalytic study of the child* (vols. 3-4). New York: International Universities Press.

Lorenz, K. (1966). *On aggression.* New York: Harcourt.

Mead, M. (1953). *Cultural patterns and technical change.* World Federation for Mental Health, UNESCO.

Rapoport, A. (1968). Foreword. In W. Buckley (Ed.), *Modern systems research for the behavioral scientist.* Chicago: Aldine.

Resnik, H.L.P. (1972). *Sexual behaviors.* Boston: Little, Brown.

Robson, K.S. (1967). Patterns and determinants of maternal attachment. *Journal of Pediatrics, 77,* 976-985.

Rosenthal, M. (1967). The generalization of dependency from mother to a stranger. *Journal of Child Psychology and Psychiatry, 8,* 177-183.

Sears, R., Macoby, E., & Levin, H. (1954). *Patterns of child rearing.* White Plains, NY: Row, Peterson.

Selye, H. (1956). *The stress of life.* New York: McGraw-Hill.

Simmons, L.W., & Wolff, H.G. (1954). *Social science in medicine.* New York: Russell Sage Foundation.

Walike, B., Jordan, H.A., & Stellar, E. (1969). Studies of eating behavior. *Nursing Research, 18,* 108-113.

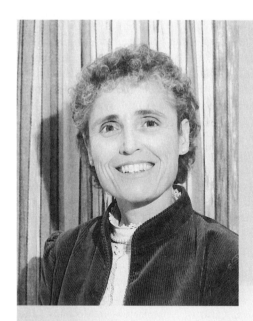

Sister Callista Roy

Adaptation Model

Kenneth D. Phillips, Carolyn L. Blue, Karen M. Brubaker, Julia M.B. Fine, Martha J. Kirsch, Katherine R. Papazian, Cynthia M. Riester, Mary Ann Sobiech

CREDENTIALS AND BACKGROUND OF THE THEORIST

Sister Callista Roy, a member of the Sisters of Saint Joseph of Carondelet, was born October 14, 1939, in Los Angeles, California. She received a Bachelor of Arts in Nursing in 1963 from Mount Saint Mary's College in Los Angeles and a Master of Science in nursing from the University of California, Los Angeles, in 1966. After earning her nursing degrees, Roy began her education in sociology, receiving both an

The authors wish to express their appreciation to Sister Callista Roy for critiquing the chapter.

M.A. in sociology in 1973 and a Ph.D. in sociology in 1977 from the University of California.

While working toward her master's degree, Roy was challenged in a seminar with Dorothy E. Johnson to develop a conceptual model for nursing. Roy had worked as a pediatric staff nurse and had noticed the great resiliency of children and their ability to adapt in response to major physical and psychological changes. Roy was impressed by adaptation as an appropriate conceptual framework for nursing. The basic concepts of the model were developed while Roy was a graduate student at the University of California, Los Angeles, from 1964 to 1966. Roy began operationalizing her model in 1968 when Mount Saint Mary's College adopted the adaptation framework as the philosophical foundation of the nursing curriculum. The Roy Adaptation Model was first presented in the literature in an article published in *Nursing Outlook* in 1970 entitled, "Adaptation: A Conceptual Framework for Nursing."

Roy was an associate professor and chairperson of the Department of Nursing at Mount Saint Mary's College until 1982. From 1983 to 1985, she was a Robert Wood Johnson Post Doctoral Fellow at the University of California, San Francisco, as a clinical nurse scholar in neuroscience. During this time she conducted research on nursing interventions for cognitive recovery in head injuries and on the influence of nursing models on clinical decision making. In 1988 Roy began the newly created position of graduate faculty nurse theorist at Boston College School of Nursing.[73]

Roy has published many books, chapters, and periodical articles and has presented numerous lectures and workshops focusing on her nursing adaptation theory. The most recent refinement and restatement of the Roy Adaptation Model (RAM) is published in her 1991 book, *The Roy Adaptation Model: The Definitive Statement.*[64]

Roy is a member of Sigma Theta Tau, and she received the National Founder's Award for Excellence in Fostering Professional Nursing Standards in 1981. Her achievements include a 1984 Honorary Doctorate of Humane Letters by Alverno College, a 1985 Honorary Doctorate from Eastern Michigan University, and a 1986 A.J.N. Book of the Year Award for *Essentials of the Roy Adaptation Model.* Roy has been recognized in the *World Who's Who of Women, Personalities of America,* and as a Fellow of the American Academy of Nursing.

Theoretical Sources

Roy's Adaptation Model for Nursing was derived in 1964 from Harry Helson's work in psychophysics. In Helson's Adaptation Theory, adaptive responses are a function of the incoming stimulus and the adaptive level. A stimulus is any factor that provokes a response. Stimuli may arise from either the inter-

nal or the external environment.[64] The adaptation level is made up of the pooled effect of three classes of stimuli: (1) focal stimuli, which immediately confront the individual; (2) contextual stimuli, which are all other stimuli present that contribute to the effect of the focal stimulus; and (3) residual stimuli, environmental factors whose effects are unclear in a given situation. Helson's work developed the concept of the adaptation level zone, which determines whether a stimulus will elicit a positive or negative response. According to Helson's theory, adaptation is a process of responding positively to environmental changes.[68]

Roy[68] combines Helson's work with Rapoport's definition of *system* and views the person as an adaptive system. With Helson's Adaptation Theory as a foundation, Roy[68] developed and further refined the model with concepts and theory from B.P. Dohrenwend, R.S. Lazarus, N. Malaznik, D. Mechanic, and H. Selye. Roy gave special credit to coauthors Driever, for outlining subdivisions of self-integrity, and Martinez and Sato, for identifying both common and primary stimuli affecting the modes. Other coworkers also elaborated the concepts: M. Pousch and J. Van Landingham for the interdependence mode and B. Randall for the role function mode.

After the development of her theory, Roy developed the model as a framework for nursing practice, research, and education.[86] According to Roy[52] more than 1500 faculty and students have contributed to the theoretical development of the adaptation model.

In *Introduction to Nursing: An Adaptation Model,* Roy discussed self-concept. She and her collaborators used the work of Coombs and Snygg regarding self-consistency and major influencing factors of self-concept. Social interaction theories provided a theoretical basis. Cooley indicates in Epstein's publication that self-perception is influenced by perceptions of other's responses. Mead expanded the idea by hypothesizing that self-appraisal uses the "generalized other." Sullivan suggests that self arises from social interaction. Gardner and Erickson provide developmental approaches.[61:263-265] The other modes—physiological, role functioning, and interdependence— were drawn similarly from biological and behavioral sciences for an understanding of the person.

Roy is developing the humanism value base of her model. The model uses concepts from A.H. Maslow to explore beliefs and values of persons. According to Roy, humanism in nursing is the belief in the person's own creative power or the belief that the person's own coping abilities will enhance wellness. Roy's holistic approach to nursing is grounded in humanism.[61]

USE OF EMPIRICAL EVIDENCE

The use of the Roy Adaptation Model (RAM) in nursing practice led to further clarification and refinement. A 1971 pilot research study and a survey research study from 1976 to 1977 led to some tentative confirmations of the model.[59]

From this beginning, the RAM has been supported through research in practice and in education.*

Rambo[47] and Randell, Tedrow, and Van Landingham[48] have expanded Roy's model for nursing implementation. According to Roy,[61] there is increasing testing through research related to the model.

*References 5, 14, 35, 36, 67, 85.

MAJOR CONCEPTS & DEFINITIONS

System A system "is a set of parts connected to function as a whole for some purpose, and it does so by the interdependence of its parts. In addition to having wholeness and related parts, systems also have *inputs, outputs,* and *control* and *feedback* processes."[3:7]

Adaptation Level A person's adaptation level is "a constantly changing point, made up of focal, contextual, and residual stimuli, which represent the person's own standard of the range of stimuli to which one can respond with ordinary adaptive responses."[61:27-28]

Adaptation Problems Adaptation problems are "the occurrences of situations of inadequate response to need deficits or excesses."[56:4] In the second edition of *Introduction to Nursing,* Roy states: "It can be noted at this point that the distinction being made between adaptation problems and nursing diagnosis is based on the developing work in both of these fields. At this point, adaptation problems are seen not as nursing diagnosis, but as areas of concern for the nurse related to adapting person or group (within each adaptive mode).[61:89-90]

Focal Stimulus "The focal stimulus is the internal or external stimulus most immediately confronting the person; the object or event that attracts one's attention."[3:8]

Contextual Stimuli Contextual stimuli "are all other stimuli present in the situation that contribute to the effect of the focal stimulus. That is, contextual stimuli are all the environmental factors that present to the person from within or without but which are not the center of the person's attention and/or energy."[3:9]

Residual Stimuli Residual stimuli "are environmental factors within or without the person whose effects in the current situation are unclear."[3:13]

Coping Mechanisms Coping mechanisms "are defined as innate or acquired ways of responding to the changing environment."[3:13]

Innate Coping Mechanisms Innate coping mechanisms "are genetically determined or common to the species and are generally viewed as automatic processes; the person does not have to think about them."[3:9]

Acquired Coping Mechanisms Acquired coping mechanisms "are developed through processes such as learning. The experiences throughout life contribute to customary responses to particular stimuli."[3:13-14]

Regulator Regulator is a coping subsystem that "responds automatically through neural, chemical, and endocrine processes."[3:14]

Continued

Major Concepts & Definitions—cont'd

Cognator Cognator is a coping subsystem that "responds through four cognitive-emotive channels: perceptual information processing, learning, judgment, and emotion."[3:14]

Adaptive Responses Adaptive responses "are those that promote the integrity of the person in terms of the goals of adaptation: survival, growth, reproduction, and mastery."[3:12]

Ineffective Responses Ineffective responses "are those that neither promote integrity nor contribute to the goals of adaptation."[3:12]

Physiological Adaptive Mode The physiological adaptive mode "is associated with the way the person responds as a physical being to stimuli from the environment. Behavior in this mode is the manifestation of the physiological activities of all the cells, tissues, organs, and systems comprising the human body.... Five needs are identified in the physiological mode relative to the basic need of physiologic integrity: oxygenation, nutrition, elimination, activity and rest, and protection."[3:16]

Self-Concept Adaptive Mode The self-concept adaptive mode "is one of the three psychosocial modes, and it focuses specifically on the psychological and spiritual aspects of the person. The basic need underlying the self-concept mode has been identified as psychic integrity—the need to know who one is so that one can be or exist with a sense of unity.... Self-concept is defined as the composite of beliefs and feelings that a person holds about him or herself at a given time. Formed from internal perceptions and perceptions of others, self-concept directs one's behavior."[3:16] Its components include (1) the physical self, which involves sensation and body-image and (2) the personal self, which is made up of self-consistency, self-ideal or expectancy, and the moral-ethical-spiritual self.[3]

Role Function Adaptive Mode The role function adaptive mode "is one of two social modes and focuses on the roles the person occupies in society. A role, as the functioning unit of society, is defined as a set of expectations about how a person occupying one position behaves toward a person occupying another position. The basic need underlying the role function mode has been identified as social integrity—the need to know who one is in relation to others so that one can act."[3:16] Persons perform primary, secondary, and tertiary roles. These roles are carried out with both instrumental and expressive behaviors. Instrumental behavior is "the actual physical performance of a behavior."[1:348] Expressive behaviors are "the feelings, attitudes, likes or dislikes that a person has about a role or about the performance of a role."[1:348] "The primary role determines the majority of behavior engaged in by the person during a particular period of life. It is determined by age, sex, and developmental stage."[1:349] "Secondary roles are those that a person assumes to complete the task associated with a developmental stage and primary role".[1:349] "Tertiary roles are related primarily to secondary roles and represent ways in which individuals meet their role associated obligations.... Tertiary roles are normally temporary in nature, freely chosen by the individual, and may include activities such as clubs or hobbies."[1:349] "The major roles that one plays can be analyzed by imagining a tree formation. The trunk of the tree is one's primary role, that is, one's developmental level—for example, generative adult female. Secondary roles branch off from this—for example, wife, mother, teacher. Finally, tertiary roles branch off from secondary roles—for example, the mother role might involve the role of PTA president for a given period of time (Malaznik, 1976). Each of these roles is seen as occurring in a dyadic relationship, that is with a reciprocal role."[68:44]

Interdependence Adaptive Mode The interdependence adaptive mode "focuses on interactions related to the giving and receiving of love, respect, and value. The basic need of this mode is termed affectional adequacy—the feeling of security in nurturing relationships. Two specific relationships are the focus of the interdependence mode: (1) significant others, persons who are the most important to the individual and (2) support systems, that is, others contributing to the meeting of interdependence needs."[1:17] Two types of behaviors characterize this mode: receptive behavior and contributive behavior. These behaviors refer to the "receiving and giving of love, respect and value in interdependent relationships."[1:17]

Perception "Perception is the interpretation of a stimulus and the conscious appreciation of it."[63:169] Perception links the regulator with the cognator and thus connects the adaptive modes.[64]

Tiedeman[75] assesses Roy's assumptions for soundness by classifying them into three levels according to their foundation in (1) previous research, (2) accepted theory, particularly theory with empirical substantiating data, or (3) personal experience. The first level is the strongest base, the third, the weakest. Roy's assumptions from systems theory and from stress-adaptation theories can be classified into the second level. However, Roy's assumption, which conceptualizes the person as having four modes of adaptation—physiological needs, self-concept, role function, and interdependence relations—is based on experience of Roy and others.[75] Roy[51,57,59] admits that the assumption needs empirical data for support. In a 1983 address, Roy noted that these categories have been refined and established as useful and valid for nursing assessment.

MAJOR ASSUMPTIONS

Roy discussed her scientific and philosophical assumptions at the International Nursing Theory Conference in Edmonton, Alberta, May 2-3, 1984, and at other conferences. Her assumptions, drawn from systems theory and Helson's adaptation level theory and philosophical assumptions from humanistic values, have been further refined in a recent National League for Nursing Press monograph.[65]

Assumptions From Systems Theory

1. Holism—A system is a set of units so related or connected as to form a unity or whole.

2. Interdependence—A system is a whole that functions as a whole by virtue of the interdependence of its parts.
3. Control processes—A system has inputs, outputs, and control and feedback processes.
4. Information feedback—Input, in the form of a standard or feedback, often is referred to as information.
5. Complexity of living systems—Living systems are almost infinitely more complex than mechanical systems and have standards and feedback to direct their function as a whole.[65:216-217]

Assumptions From Adaptation-Level Theory

1. Behavior as adaptive—Human behavior represents adaptation to environmental and organismic forces.
2. Adaptation as a function of stimuli and adaptation level—Adaptive behavior is a function of the stimulus and adaptation level, that is, the pooled effect of the focal, contextual, and residual stimuli.
3. Individual dynamic adaptation levels—Adaptation is a process of responding positively to environmental changes; this positive response decreases the responses necessary to cope with the stimuli and increases the sensitivity to respond to other stimuli.
4. Positive and active processes of responding—Responses reflect the state of the organism and the properties of stimuli and hence are regarded as active processes.[65:217]

Assumptions From Humanism

1. Creativity—Creativity is a person's own creative power.
2. Purposefulness—A person's behavior is purposeful and not merely a chain of cause and effect.
3. Holism—A person is holistic.
4. Interpersonal process—The interpersonal relationship is significant.[65:217-218]

Assumptions From Veritivity

Four assumptions may be made from veritivity:
1. The purposefulness of human existence
2. The unity of purpose
3. Activity and creativity
4. The value and meaning of life.[65:218]

Nursing

Nursing is defined broadly as a "theoretical system of knowledge which prescribes a process of analysis and action related to the care of the ill or potentially ill person."[56:4] "Nursing activities involve the assessment of behavior and the stimuli that influence adaptation. Nursing judgments are based on this assessment and interventions are planned to manage these stimuli. Roy[61:3-4] differentiates nursing as a science from nursing as a practice discipline. Nursing science is "a developing system of knowledge about persons that observes, classifies, and relates the processes by which persons positively affect their health status."[61:3-4] Nursing as a practice discipline is "nursing's scientific body of knowledge used for the purpose of providing an essential service to people, that is, promoting ability to affect health positively."[61:3-4] "Nursing acts to enhance the interaction of the person with the environment—to promote adaptation."[3:20]

Roy's goal[2,61] of nursing is to help the person adapt to changes in his physiological needs, his self-concept, his role function, and his interdependent relations during health and illness. Nursing fills a unique role as a facilitator of adaptation by assessing behavior in each of these four adaptive modes and intervening by managing the influencing stimuli.[2,61]

Person

According to Roy,[56] a person is a "biopsychosocial being in constant interaction with a changing environment." Roy[2,61,66] defined the person, the recipient of nursing care, as a living, complex, adaptive system with internal processes (the cognator and regulator) acting to maintain adaptation in the four adaptive modes (physiological needs, self-concept, role function, and interdependence).

The person's adaptive nature "means that the human system has the capacity to adjust effectively to changes in the environment and, in turn, affects the environment."[3:7] The person as a living system is "a whole made up of parts or subsystems that function as a unity for some purpose."[66:53]

Health

"Health is a state and a process of being and becoming an integrated and whole person. It is a reflection of adaptation, that is, the interaction of the person and the environment."[3:21] Roy[61:24] derived this definition from the thought that adaptation is a process of promoting physiological, psychological, and social integrity and that integrity implies an unimpaired condition leading to completeness or unity. In her earlier work, Roy viewed health along a continuum flowing from death and extreme poor health to high-level wellness and peak wellness. As a person moves along the health-illness continuum, the person encounters problems to which he or she must adapt.[5] However, Roy's recent writings have focused more on health as a process.

Health and illness are one inevitable dimension of the person's total life experience.[50] Nursing is concerned with this dimension. When mechanisms for coping are ineffective, illness results. Health ensues when man continually adapts. As people adapt to stimuli, they are free to respond to other stimuli. The freeing of energy from ineffective coping attempts can promote healing and enhance health.[61:26]

Environment

According to Roy,[61:22] environment is "all the conditions, circumstances, and influences surrounding and affecting the development and behavior of persons or groups." "It is the changing environment [that] stimulates the person to make adaptive responses."[3:18] Environment is the input into the person as an adaptive system involving both internal and external factors. These factors may be slight or large, negative or positive. However, any environmental change demands increasing energy to adapt to the situation. Factors in the environment that affect the person are categorized as focal, contextual, and residual stimuli.

THEORETICAL ASSERTIONS

Roy's model focuses on the concept of adaptation of the person. Her concepts of nursing, person, health, and environment are all interrelated to this central concept. The person continually scans the environment for stimuli. Ultimately, a response is made and adaptation occurs. That adaptive response may be either an effective or an ineffective response. Nursing has a unique goal to assist the person's adaptation effort by managing the environment. The result is attainment of an optimum level of wellness by the person.*

As an open, living system, the person receives inputs or stimuli from both the environment and the self. The adaptation level is determined by the combined effect of the focal, contextual, and residual stimuli. Adaptation occurs when the person responds positively to environmental changes. This adaptive response promotes the integrity of the person, which leads to health. Ineffective responses to stimuli leads to disruption of the integrity of the person.*

There are two interrelated subsystems in Roy's model (Fig. 18-1). The primary, functional, or control processes subsystem consists of the regulator and the cognator. The secondary, effector subsystem consists of four adaptive modes: physiological needs, self-concept, role-function, and interdependence.†

Roy views the regulator and cognator as methods of coping. The regulator coping subsystem, by way of the physiological adaptive mode, "responds automatically through neural, chemical, and endocrine coping processes."[3:14] The cognator coping subsystem, by way of the self-concept, interdependence, and role-function adaptive modes "responds through four cognitive-emotive channels: perceptual information processing, learning, judgment, and emotion."[3:14] Perception of the person links the regulator with the cognator in that "input into the regulator is transformed into perceptions. Perception is a process of the cognator. The responses following perception are feedback into both the cognator and the regulator."[23:67]

The four adaptive modes of the second subsystem in Roy's model provide form or manifestations of cognator and regulator activity. Responses to stimuli are carried out through these four modes. The mode's purpose is to achieve physiological, psychological, and social integrity. Interrelated propositions of the cognator and regulator subsystems link the systems of the adaptive modes.[14]

*References 2, 48, 51, 52, 59, 61, 66, 68.

*References 2, 48, 51, 52, 59, 61, 66.
†References 2, 32, 36, 37, 50, 52, 54.

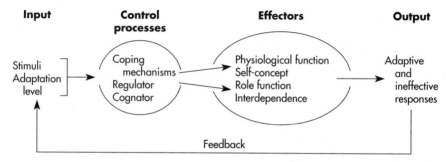

Fig. **18-1** Person as an adaptive system. *From Roy, C. (1984).* Introduction to nursing: An adaptation model *(2nd ed.). Englewood Cliffs, NJ: Prentice Hall, Inc., p. 30. Reprinted with permission.*

The person as a whole is made up of six subsystems. These subsystems—the regulator, cognator, and the four adaptive modes—are interrelated to form a complex system for the purpose of adaptation. Relationships among the four adaptive modes occur when internal and external stimuli affect more than one mode, when disruptive behavior occurs in more than one mode, or when one mode becomes the focal, contextual, or residual stimulus for another mode.[5,10,35]

LOGICAL FORM

Roy's Adaptation Model of nursing is both deductive and inductive. It is deductive in that much of Roy's theory is derived from Helson's psychophysics theory. Helson developed the concepts of focal, contextual, and residual stimuli, which Roy redefined within nursing to form a typology of factors related to adaptation levels of persons. Roy also uses other concepts and theory outside the discipline of nursing and relates these to her adaptation theory.

Roy's adaptation theory is inductive in that she developed the four adaptive modes from research and the practice experiences of herself, her colleagues, and her students. Roy[56,59,61] built on the conceptual framework of adaptation and as a result developed a step-by-step model by which nurses use the nursing process to administer nursing care to promote adaptation in situations of health and illness.

ACCEPTANCE BY THE NURSING COMMUNITY

Practice

With use of Roy's six-step nursing process, the nurse (1) assesses the behaviors manifested from the four adaptive modes; (2) assesses the stimuli for those behaviors and categorizes them as focal, contextual, or residual stimuli; (3) makes a statement or nursing diagnosis of the person's adaptive state; (4) sets goals to promote adaptation; (5) implements interventions aimed at managing the stimuli to promote adaptation; and (6) evaluates whether the adaptive goals have been met. By manipulating the stimuli and not

the patient, the nurse enhances "the interaction of the person with their environment, thereby promoting health."[2:51]

Brower and Baker[5] consider Roy's model useful for nursing practice because it outlines the features of the discipline and provides direction for practice as well as for education and research. The model considers goals, values, the client, and practitioner interventions. These authors view Roy's nursing process as well developed. The two-level assessment assisted in identification of nursing goals and diagnoses. They also note the need for continued work on a typology of nursing and on organizing categories of nursing interventions.

It is a valuable theory for nursing practice because it includes a goal that is specified as the aim for activity and prescription for activities to realize the goal.[11] The goal of the model is the person's adaptation in four adaptive modes in situations of health and illness. The prescriptions or interventions are the management of stimuli by removing, increasing, decreasing, or altering them. These prescriptions can be obtained by listing practice-related hypotheses generated by the model.[61]

The nursing process is well suited for use in a practice setting. The two-level assessment is unique to this model and leads to the identification of adaptation problems or nursing diagnosis. Beginning work is being done on a typology of nursing diagnoses.[61,68] Intervention is based specifically on the model, but there is a need to develop an organization of categories of nursing interventions.[68]

The model was used in practice by graduate nursing students as cited by Wagner[85] in 1976. They found some blurring in the categories of self-concept, role function, and interdependence when deciding where a given behavior belonged. They also found the nursing process lengthy and repetitive, taking much time to complete. The model was useful in inpatient settings, except in intensive care units where there were rapid changes in the patient's condition. The students also found it easier to use the model in outpatient settings such as clinics and physician's offices.[85] The model provided a system that accounted for physical needs as well as psychosocial needs. It was particularly useful in the pediatric setting, because it allowed for assessment of covert psychological needs of children.

Mitchell and Pilkington[38] are also of the notion that the complexity of the assessment process would not be useful in a rapidly changing environment such as labor and delivery or critical care. They have also discussed the linearity of the six-step nursing process in the model and that it is not realistic in practice settings. They do not believe that the model provides direction for priority setting for interventions.

Mitchell and Pilkington found Roy's model useful for patients receiving care because they could participate in care planning and problem solving. Patients learn about healthier behaviors and ineffective behaviors. The authors think that the patient is passive in the nursing process because the nurse is viewed as a change agent.

Hamner[26] in 1989 discussed the Roy model and how it could be applied to nursing care in a cardiac care unit (CCU). Hamner describes the model as enhancing care in the CCU and being consistent with the nursing process. Hamner found that the model assessed all patients' behavior, so that none were excluded. The author discovered that the Roy model provides a structure in which manipulation of stimuli are not overlooked. The model puts emphasis on identifying and reinforcing positive behavior, which speeds recovery.

Frank and Lang[22] used the RAM to analyze disturbances in the sexual role performance of alcoholics. In the physiological mode, alcohol use was shown to alter sex hormone function and depress sexual response. In the role performance mode, there was an inconsistency between alcoholic men and women about the effect of alcohol on sexual performance and the depressant effects alcohol has on sexual performance. For example, alcoholic men believe that their sexual pleasure increased with alcohol use even when their physiological response decreased (such as difficulty in maintaining an erection after increased alcohol consumption). In the self-concept role, alcoholics may use alcohol to increase their self-concept. In the interdependence mode, the decreased quality of a relationship as a result of alcohol use may prompt prolonged drinking bouts.

Giger, Davidhizar, and Miller[24] evaluated the RAM and the Nightingale theory as a means of providing care for patients in the operating room. They discovered many similarities between the models and some differences. Both described the metaparadigm of nursing in relation to the models and defined the interrelatedness among concepts. Both are deductive, both provide a systems model, and both provide an open systems model. However, while Roy's model is a practice theory and is testable, the Nightingale theory is a grand theory and is not testable. The main focus of Nightingale's theory is environment, whereas Roy's theory focuses on the person and the person's adaptation. Nightingale sees the person as having a passive role and the nurse an active role, whereas Roy sees the person as an active participant and the nurse more as a guide. The authors concluded that the operating room (OR) nurse should use various nursing theories and models to care for patients in the OR. Both the RAM and the Nightingale model can be applied easily.

Piazza and Foote[43] have found Roy's model useful for rehabilitation nursing practice. The rehabilitation patient frequently encounters changes in all adaptive modes. The model provides a holistic approach for the care of patients in all four modes.

Galligan[23] in 1979 reported that the model had been used by nurses who cared for young hospitalized children. Schmitz[69] in 1980 used the model in a community setting for patients receiving care in the home. The model enabled needs assessment, goal setting, and prioritization of goals. Interventions and evaluations were reported to be more efficient and effective.

In May 1979 three nursing administrators initiated a pilot study using the model in an 18-bed unit in Arlington, Virginia. Evaluation and revision of the nursing assessment tools were conducted. By April 1980, the model was in practice. Early research suggests that it enhanced patient satisfaction and improved health outcomes. Consistent with the model, the nurses began to enhance their professionalism by writing complete care plans and phrasing patient problems in terms of nursing diagnosis. A year after initiation, the model was still supported by the staff. The group directors admitted that the model's abstractness required diligence in applying it to practice. They also contended that further validation of the theory was needed.[36]

In September 1981, a research study was published that dealt with problems associated with nursing home applications for elderly persons. The research was performed within the framework of the adaptation model. The research design was used to identify adaptation problems, and hypotheses were formulated. The study concluded that, "As a broad conceptual framework, the Roy Adaptation Nursing Model served as a useful tool for systematically gathering responses regarding adaptation problems experienced by the elderly persons and their significant others."[14]

Fitzpatrick and others[21] also found Roy's model useful in the psychological assessment of the family. These authors used the model to analyze role function needs and interdependence needs, which may lead to maladaption in a troubled family system. The authors asserted that the nurse, as the environmental change agent, could thus improve a maladaptive family system.

Another research study, published in August 1983, used the model to analyze the content of 20 interviews of parents whose children had been recently diagnosed as having cancer. Although operational definitions of Roy's adaptation modes were used in the study, the origins of the definitions remain unclear. The authors of the study found the framework applicable as a result of its ability to treat multiple patient variables.[72]

In 1986 Logan[33] described the practical use of the model and explored its appropriateness for palliative care nursing and its applicability in improving care of the dying patient. Logan noted that basic assumptions to the Roy model seemed to correlate with the palliative care philosophy, except that terminology relating to goals differed. A utility index was used to assess the usefulness of the model on the basis of feasibility, practicality, compatibility, social benefit, and completeness. The Roy nursing process is well illustrated by Logan's application of the model with an oncology case study. The nursing care plan is described and includes analysis of diagnosis and behaviors. Logan suggests the need to perfect the model's language in the use of like words when describing like things.

In addition, the RAM has been evaluated for the care of clients with breast cancer,[39,44] cervical cancer,[42] ulcerative colitis,[7] colectomy,[6] depression,[8] quadriplegia,[25] dermatomyositis,[27] Alzheimer's disease,[73] leukemia,[87,88] and acquired immunodeficiency syndrome.[42] The RAM has been used as a theoretical basis and an organizing framework for group psychotherapy in a 15-bed acute inpatient psychiatric unit.[31] The RAM has been analyzed for use in accident and emergency nursing,[30] neonatal intensive care units,[28] rehabilitation nursing,[43] and a rehabilitation program for women with breast cancer.[39]

During the 1980s a number of health care agencies have begun implementing the RAM as a basis for nursing practice. Roy has compiled a list of experienced resource persons who can assist with this work in the United States and Canada.

Education

The adaptation model has also been useful in the educational setting and is currently in use at Mount Saint Mary's College Department of Nursing in Los Angeles.[61] Mount Saint Mary's program demonstrates the relationship of nursing theory to nursing education. Three vertical strands run throughout the curriculum: two theory strands (the adapting person and health-illness) and one practice strand (nursing management). There are two horizontal strands in the curriculum—nursing process and student adaptation/leadership. The horizontal strands enhance the theory and practice of the vertical strands. All strands within the curriculum build in complexity from one level to the next.[58] In addition, the model allows for increasing knowledge in the areas of both theory and practice.[53]

Roy[53,58] states that the model defines for students the distinct purpose of nursing, which is to promote man's adaptation in each of the adaptive modes in situations of health and illness. The model also distinguishes nursing science and medical science by having the content of these areas taught in separate courses. She stresses collaboration but delineates separate goals for nurses and physicians. The nurse's goal, according to Roy,[52] "is to help the patient put his energy into getting well," whereas the medical student focuses on "the patient's position on the health-illness continuum with the goal of causing movement along the continuum." She views the model as a valuable tool to analyze overlap and distinctions between the professions of nursing and medicine. Roy[58] believes that curriculum based on this model helps in theory development by the students, who also learn how to test theories and develop new theoretical insights. Roy[52] states that the model is advantageous for an integrated curriculum and that "it leads to objectives, points out content to be used and specifies patterns for learning and teaching."

In the early 1980s the School of Nursing at the University of Ottawa experienced a major curriculum change.[40] This change included incorporating a nursing model on which to base the new curriculum. The RAM was one of the models to be included in the first year of the baccalaureate program. The professors had to meet four challenges during this change: (1) adapting the course to be congruent with the Roy model, (2) developing teaching tools suitable for student learning, (3) sequencing of content for student learning, and (4) obtaining competent role models. These challenges were met, but the faculty continues to evaluate and modify the course.

In 1976 the model was used for curriculum development of a practitioner program at the University of Miami in Florida. Organization of curriculum content and selections of student learning experiences were derived from the model. Course objectives included identifying adaptive problems and distinguishing between effective and noneffective coping mechanisms. Application of the model resulted in decreased anxiety in the students and provided a framework to give direction to the education of practitioners.[5] Carveth[9] proposed the use of conceptual models as one means of improving the scientific knowledge base in nurse-midwifery. This author asserted that the use of Roy's model will assist nurse-midwives to systematically study, communicate, define, and describe their interdependent role.

Throughout the 1970s and 1980s, the Roy model was implemented as a basis for curriculum development in associate degree diploma, baccalaureate, and higher degree programs in many countries. Articles and books on Roy's model have been published in several languages, including Portuguese, Japanese, and French. Roy and her colleagues have provided consultation for this work in more than 30 schools in the United States, Canada, and abroad.

Research

Development and testing of theories. If research is to affect practitioners' behavior, it must be directed at testing and retesting conceptual models for nursing practice. Roy[61] has stated that theory development and the testing of developed theories are nursing's highest priorities. The model must be able to generate testable hypotheses for it to be researchable.

As previously stated, Roy's theory has generated a number of general propositions. From these general propositions, specific hypotheses can be developed and tested. B. J. Hill and C. S. Roberts[29] have demonstrated the development of testable hypotheses from the model, as had Roy. Data to validate or support the model would be created by the testing of such hypotheses, but to date there has been little research in this area.[75] Lutjens[34] derived a theory from the RAM and has applied this theory to social organizations.

Roy[51] has identified a set of concepts forming a model from which the process of observation and classification of facts would lead to postulates. The postulates concern the occurrence of adaptation problems, coping mechanisms, and interventions based on laws derived from factors making up the response potential of the focal, contextual, and residual stimuli. Roy[53-55] has outlined a typology of adaptation problems or nursing diagnoses. Research and testing are needed in the area of typology and categories of interventions that fit into the model. General propositions that need to be tested have been developed.[66]

Practice-based research. A group of graduate students at DePaul University tested the model in a number of practice situations. The students adapted an assessment tool and tested the model in episodic settings in a variety of units in different hospitals. They also used distributive settings in physicians' offices, industrial health settings, and outpatient clinics. The students concluded that the model provided a good framework for ordering a variety of observations and was flexible enough to be used in both episodic and distributive settings.[72] The study provided empirical support for the model only in the area of the process of assessment within the four adaptive modes.

Limadri[32] studied the model as a conceptual framework in her descriptive research study and in her practice with abused women in an outpatient setting. She identified patterns of help-seeking behaviors in a group of 40 abused women. From her experiences in practice, Limadri analyzed the model's construct interrelationships and expanded Roy's original model to illustrate a conceptualization of the abused women's adaptive response in help-seeking behaviors. Limadri did report difficulty with mode overlap but found that "the model proves a useful framework to identify the complex needs of the client."

In 1987, Silva[71] used the Roy model to structure the perceived needs of family members of patients undergoing surgery. The four modes were reflected in responses to a questionnaire, but the patterning of relationships was somewhat different from that suggested by the model. Some needs classified in the psychosocial modes were found to be interrelated, whereas other needs, theoretically related to these modes, appeared independent. Silva also found the physiological mode to be relatively independent of the psychosocial modes. She suggests further refinement of the modes to clarify the interdependent and interrelated areas of each. Roy,[62] in her response to this article, states that Silva's use of factor analysis in exploring and testing the model contributes to the basic science of adaptation nursing.

Brydolf and Segesten[6] used the RAM to assess long-term physiologic adaptation in 30 young persons with ulcerative colitis who had undergone a colectomy. Twenty-four of the young persons reported significant problems related to nutrition, elim-

ination, activity and rest, and protection, whereas six subjects reported no adaptation problems.

Pittman[45] studied wellness promotion behaviors among school-age children using a Q-sort methodology. Four factors related to wellness promotion behaviors represented the four adaptive modes. The self-concept adaptive mode was represented by the most enabling wellness promotion behaviors.

Development of programs of research. A program of research has been developed around various aspects of the childbirth experience.* Fawcett and Tulman[17,76] used the model for the design of studies measuring functional status after childbirth. They used the model for retrospective and longitudinal studies of variables associated with functional status during the postpartum period. The model was also used for ongoing studies of functional status during pregnancy and after the diagnosis of breast cancer. The model facilitated the selection of study variables and clarified thinking about the classification of study variables. The model was a useful guide for the design and conduct of studies of functional status.

Fawcett[15] used the RAM as a guide to design four studies. The first was a retrospective survey of cesarean birth parents, which revealed the need for detailed information about the events surrounding the cesarean birth. The second was a field test of a nursing intervention that consisted of a pamphlet with information about cesarean births with follow-up discussion of the pamphlet content. The third was a field test of a different version of the pamphlet intervention and focused discussion about cesarean birth. The fourth study is an ongoing experiment that tests the effects of nursing intervention on responses to unplanned cesarean birth. The purpose of all of the studies was to determine whether responses to unplanned cesarean birth are adaptive or ineffective. The survey and field tests provided support for the RAM "in as much as the modes of adaptation were sufficiently comprehensive to permit classification of all data."[15:1423]

Fawcett, Tulman, and Spedden[19] studied the perceptions of women who experienced a vaginal birth after cesarean birth (VBAC). The researchers compared the women's perceptions of the VBAC with

---

*References 12, 15, 16, 20, 77, 79-81.

their perception of the past cesarean by use of the Perception of the Birth Scale. While women reported positive perceptions of the VBAC, their perceptions were significantly less positive than for vaginally delivered women.

A program of research related to functional status in clients with cancer is being developed.[78] An instrument has been developed to measure functional status in this population of clients.[82]

Pollock[46] has developed a program of research around the concept of adaptation to chronic illness. Over a 7-year period, 597 adults with various chronic illnesses have participated. Significant differences related to physiological adaptation have been found; however, no differences in psychosocial adaptation have been identified.

Development of adaptation research instruments. The RAM has provided the theoretical basis for the development of a number of research instruments. An instrument has been developed to measure functional status during pregnancy[84] and childbirth[79] and after childbirth.[18] An instrument has been developed to measure role function changes exhibited by new fathers.[83] Tulman, Fawcett, and McEvoy[82] developed the Inventory of Functional Status–Cancer to measure functional status in women with cancer. Zhan and Shen[89] developed an instrument to measure self-consistency in elderly people with chronic conditions. By use of Roy's self-concept adaptive mode, Phillips[41] developed the Phillips Stigma Questionnaire–AIDS to measure internalized stigma in persons with human immunodeficiency virus infection. Research is underway to test the Phillips Stigma Questionnaire and to explore the nature of stigma in an obese population.

Need for further testing. Silva[70] points out that using the conceptual framework of a theory for a research study is not in itself a test of the theory. Most of the researchers who have used Roy's model have not actually tested the assumptions, propositions, or hypotheses of her model but have provided much face validity for its usefulness.

Some research has been conducted on the model, but more is needed for further validation. The model does generate many testable hypotheses related to practice and theory.

FURTHER DEVELOPMENT

The RAM is an approach to nursing that has made and can continue to make a significant contribution to nursing's body of knowledge, but a few needs remain in the development of the theory. Some assumptions about the model should be validated, such as the assumption that the person has four modes of adaptation. A more thoroughly defined typology of nursing diagnosis and an organization of categories of interventions are needed. There is some overlapping of the categories of self-concept, role function, and interdependence. Roy has sought to define health more clearly by deemphasizing the concept of a health-illness continuum and conceptualizing health as integration and wholeness of the person. This approach more clearly incorporates the adaptive mechanisms of the comatose patient in response to tactile and verbal stimuli.

There appear to be problems involved in using the model in an intensive care unit, where situations change rapidly. Roy notes that it is helpful to use a system for setting priorities with the model. When a priority-setting system is used in conjunction with the model, it might be better suited for use in a critical care setting.[57:690] For instance, the priority of nursing care for a patient having a cardiac arrest is the physiological adaptive mode. Whether the patient lives or dies, the other adaptive modes begin to emerge as a priority and nursing care begins to focus on the other modes. A chapter regarding life closure was added to the 1984 edition of *Introduction to Nursing: An Adaptation Model*. Support and encouragement of adaptation to the dying process is an integral component of nursing.

Of great significance is the use by Roy and Roberts[68] of elements of the model to construct for each subsystem and mode a series of propositions. They acknowledge that the propositions are too simplistic, implying linear bivariate relationships, and state that further work is necessary. This work gives starting points of theory-testing research to validate the subsystems of the model. Roy sees a possibility of combining these propositions into interrelated systems and thus building actual theory. Note that Roy classifies her model as a conceptualization of nursing, not as a theory, and calls for more middle-range theory development in nursing.[60]

Limadri[32] concluded that Roy and Roberts[68] obscured the regulator mechanism and the physiological mode by superimposing one on the other in forming propositions. She further suggested a rather sweeping modification: grouping the physiological mode into a category of the biological self and grouping the other three modes into the psychosocial self. Fitzpatrick and others[21] reformulated the model to include the alternative nursing intervention strategy of increasing the adaptation range as well as that of manipulating stimuli. Roy's model is useful and contributes to the science and practice of nursing.

Artinian[4] had attempted to strengthen the Roy model through conceptual problem solving. She believed that strengthening the model will aid in knowledge development. The author has identified four areas of conceptual problems in the model: health and adaptation, adaptation versus coping, the person as an adaptive system, and goals of adaptation. Artinian believed that the state of health is synonymous with the end state of adaptation and the process of health is synonymous with the process of adaptation. She thought that this overlap leads to confusion within the Roy framework. Artinian proposed that adaptation refers to the process by which health is obtained and health refers to a state of integration and wholeness.

In the Roy model, coping and adaptation are viewed as synonymous. Artinian believes this definition is a conceptual problem "because of its disparity with other traditional writings about coping and adaptation and because of its incongruity with the recent assumptions stated by Roy."[4] Artinian suggested the two terms be used synonymously and that the definition of adaptation include the meaning portrayed by Dubos. In this way the model is brought up to date and there is consistency between the definition of adaptation and the assumptions. Artinian believed that the positive feedback process is congruent with Roy's assumptions but that it has not been described in the adaptation mode. She suggested that positive as well as negative feedback processes should be incorporated into the model. Finally, Artinian thought that the goals of adaptation should be expanded to include self-actualization, carrying out role functions, and achieving affectional adequacy. These goals would incorporate Roy's holistic and humanistic view of the person.

CRITIQUE

Clarity

According to Chinn and Jacobs,[10:140] "clarity requires the semantic and structural organization of goals, assumptions, concepts, definitions, relationships, and structure into a logically coherent whole." Duldt and Giffin[13] state that Roy's arrangement of concepts is logical but that the development of definitions is inadequate related to her original format. Terms and concepts borrowed from other disciplines are not redefined for nursing. Roy's theory examples tend to use a biopsychosocial set as the principle for organizing, instead of the adaptive modes and the internal processors. One limitation these authors cite is that Roy claims to follow a holistic view but leaves out "spiritual, humanistic, and existential aspects of being a person." Instead, "man is defined as a survival-oriented, behaviorist (condition-response), amoral, living system."[13:246]

Mastal and Hammond[35:75] discussed difficulties with Roy's model in classifying certain behaviors because of overlapping of concept definitions. The problem identified dealt with theory conceptualization and the need for mutually exclusive categories to classify human behavior. Their problem with the person's position on the health-illness continuum has been clarified by Roy in the redefining of health as personal integration. However, other researchers[32:37] have also referred to difficulty in classifying behavior exclusively in one adaptive mode.

A part of the structural inconsistency of the model occurs because a series of assumptions borrowed from behavioristic thought and systems theory are difficult to reconcile with the assumptions of humanism. This combination of such divergent theoretical roots may be a basis for a part of the internal tension of the Roy model, but these assumptions of humanism are what makes the model applicable to nursing.

Simplicity

The Roy model includes the concepts of nursing, person, health-illness, environment, adaptation, and nursing activities. It also includes the subconcepts of regulator, cognator, and the four effector modes of physiological, self-concept, role function, and interdependence. Because this theory has several major concepts and subconcepts and numerous relational statements, it is complex.

Generality

Roy[61] defines her model as drawn from multiple middle-range theories and advocates multiple middle-range theories for use in nursing. Middle-range theories are testable but have sufficient generality to be scientifically interesting.[86] Roy's model has been classified as a grand theory. The broad scope is an advantage because the model may be used for other theory building and testing in studying smaller ranges of phenomena. Roy's model is generalizable to all settings in nursing practice but is limited in scope because it primarily addresses the concept of person-environment adaptation and focuses primarily on the client; information on the nurse is implied.

Empirical Precision

Increasing complexity within theories often helps increase empirical precision. When subcomponents are designated within the theory, the empirical precision increases, assuming the broad concepts are based in reality.[10]

Because Roy's broad concepts stem from theory in physiological psychology, psychology, sociology, and nursing, empirical data indicate that this general theory base has substance.

Roy[51,59] studied and analyzed 500 samples of patient behaviors collected by nursing students. From this analysis, Roy proposed her four adaptive models in man. This is the least supported of Roy's concepts.[75]

Roy's assumptions can also be analyzed to determine what type of statements they are. The eight

assumptions of the Adaptation Model of Nursing follow:

1. The person is a biopsychosocial being.
2. The person is in constant interaction with a changing environment.
3. To cope with a changing world, the person uses both innate and acquired mechanisms, which are biological, psychological, and sociological in origin.
4. Health and illness are one inevitable dimension of the person's life.
5. To respond positively to environmental changes, the person must adapt.
6. The person's adaptation is a function of the stimulus he is exposed to and of his adaptation level.
7. The person's adaptation level is such that it comprises a zone indicating the range of stimulation that will lead to a positive response.
8. The person is conceptualized as having four modes of adaptation: physiological needs, self-concept, role function, and interdependence relations.[59:180-182]

Of the eight basic assumptions presented in the model, assumptions 1 through 5 are existence statements. Assumptions 6 and 7 are associational statements. As defined by Reynolds,[49] relational statements can be either associational or causal. The relational statements are the relations that may be tested.

Roy[66,68] identifies many propositions in relation to the regulator and cognator mechanisms and the self-concept, role function, and interdependence modes. These propositions have varying degrees of support from general theory and empirical data. The majority of the propositions are relational statements and can also be tested.[75] Testable hypotheses have been derived from the model.[29]

Derivable Consequences

Derivable consequences refer to how practically useful, important, and generally sufficient the theory is in relation to achieving valued nursing outcomes. The theory needs to guide research and practice, generate ideas, and differentiate the focus of nursing from other service professions.[10]

The Roy adaptation model has a clearly defined nursing process and can be useful in guiding clinical practice. The model is also capable of generating new information through the testing of the hypotheses that have been derived from it.[72]

Conclusion

Meleis[37:180] asserts that there are three types of nursing theorists: those who focus on needs, those who focus on interaction, and those who focus on outcome. Roy's Adaptation Model is classified as an outcome theory, defined by this author as "a well-articulated conception of man as a nursing client and of nursing as an external regulatory mechanism." Roy, in applying the concepts of system and adaptation to man as a client of nursing, has presented her articulation of man for nurses to use as a tool in practice, education, and research. Her conceptions of person and of the nursing process contribute to the science and the art of nursing. The RAM deserves further study and development by nursing educators, researchers, and practitioners.

CRITICAL THINKING *Activities*

A 23-year-old male patient is admitted to your unit with a fracture of C6 and C7 that resulted in quadriplegia. He was injured during a football game at the university where he is currently a senior. His career as quarterback had been very promising. At the time of the injury, contract negotiations were in progress with a leading professional football team.

1 Use Roy's criteria to identify focal and contextual stimuli for each of the four adaptive modes.

2 Consider the adaptations that would be necessary in each of the four adaptive modes: physiological, self-concept, interdependence, and role function.

3 Create an intervention for each of the adaptive modes that will promote adaptation.

REFERENCES

1. Andrews, H. (1991). Overview of the role function mode. In C. Roy & H. Andrews (Eds.), *The Roy adaptation model: The definitive statement* (pp. 347-361). Norwalk, CT: Appleton & Lange.
2. Andrews, H., & Roy, C. (1986). *Essentials of the Roy adaptation model.* Norwalk, CT: Appleton-Century-Crofts.
3. Andrews, H., & Roy, C. (1991). Essentials of the Roy adaptation model. In C. Roy & H. Andrews (Eds.), *The Roy adaptation model: The definitive statement* (pp. 3-25). Norwalk, CT: Appleton & Lange.
4. Artinian, N. T. (1990). Strengthening the Roy adaptation model through conceptual clarification: Commentary and response. *Nursing Science Quarterly, 3*(2), 60-64.
5. Brower, H.T.F., & Baker, B.J. (1976, Nov.). The Roy adaptation model: Using the adaptation model in a practitioner curriculum. *Nursing Outlook, 24,* 686-689.
6. Brydolf, M., & Segesten, K. (1994). Physical health in young subjects after colectomy: An application of the Roy model. *Journal of Advanced Nursing, 20*(3), 500-508.
7. Brydolf, M., & Segesten, K. (1996). Living with ulcerative colitis: Experiences of adolescents and young adults. *Journal of Advanced Nursing, 23*(1), 39-47.
8. Campbell, J.M. (1992). Treating depression in well older adults: Use of diaries in cognitive therapy. *Issues in Mental Health Nursing, 13*(1), 19-27.
9. Carveth, J.A. (1987). Conceptual models in nurse-midwifery. *Journal of Nurse-Midwifery, 32*(1), 20-25.
10. Chinn, P., & Jacobs, M.K. (1987). *Theory and nursing: A systematic approach.* St. Louis: Mosby.
11. Dickoff, J., James, P., & Weidenbach, E. (1968, May). Theory in practice discipline. Part I, Practice oriented theory. *Nursing Research, 17,* 413-415.
12. Drake, M.L., Verhulst, D., & Fawcett, J. (1988). Physical and psychological symptoms experienced by Canadian women and their husbands during pregnancy and the postpartum. *Journal of Advanced Nursing, 13*(4), 436-440.
13. Duldt, B., & Giffin, K. (1985). *Theoretical perspectives for nursing,* pp. 242-247. Boston: Little, Brown.
14. Farkas, L. (1981, March). Adaptation problems with nursing home application for elderly persons: An application of the Roy adaptation nursing model. *Journal of Advanced Nursing, 6,* 363-368.
15. Fawcett, J. (1990). Preparation for caesarean childbirth: Derivation of a nursing intervention from the Roy adaptation model. *Journal of Advanced Nursing, 15*(2), 1418-1425.
16. Fawcett, J., Bliss-Holtz, V.J., Haas, M.B., Leventhal, M., & Rubin, M. (1986). Spouses' body image changes during and after pregnancy: A replication and extension. *Nursing Research, 35*(4), 220-223.

17. Fawcett, J., & Tulman, L. (1990). Building a program of research from the Roy adaptation model of nursing. *Journal of Advanced Nursing, 15*(6), 720-725.

18. Fawcett, J., Tulman, L., & Myers, S.T. (1988). Development of the Inventory of Functional Status after Childbirth. *Journal of Nurse Midwifery, 33*(6), 252-260.

19. Fawcett, J., Tulman, L., & Spedden, J.P. (1994). Responses to vaginal birth after cesarean section. *JOGNN: Journal of Obstetric, Gynecologic, and Neonatal Nursing, 23*(3), 253-259.

20. Fawcett, J., & York, R. (1986). Spouses' physical and psychological symptoms during pregnancy and the postpartum. *Nursing Research, 35*(3), 144-148.

21. Fitzpatrick, J., Whall, A., Johnston, R., & Floyd, J. (1982). *Nursing models and their psychiatric mental health application.* Bowie, MD: Brady.

22. Frank, D.I., & Lang, A.R. (1990). Disturbances in sexual role performance of chronic alcoholics: An analysis using Roy's adaptation model. *Issues in Mental Health Nursing, 11*(3), 243-254.

23. Galligan, A.C. (1979, Jan.). Using Roy's concept of adaptation to care for young children. *American Journal of Maternal Child Nursing, 4,* 24-28.

24. Giger, J.N., Davidhizar, R., & Miller, S.W. (1990). Nightingale & Roy: A comparison of nursing models. *Today's OR Nurse, 12*(4), 25-28.

25. Gless, P.A. (1995). Applying the Roy adaptation model to the care of clients with quadriplegia. *Rehabilitation Nursing, 20*(1), 11-16, 66.

26. Hamner, J.B. (1989). Applying the Roy adaptation model to the CCU. *Critical Care Nurse, 9*(3), 51-52.

27. Hartley, B., & Campion-Fuller, C. (1994). Juvenile dermatomyositis: A Roy nursing perspective. *Journal of Pediatric Nursing: Nursing Care of Children and Families, 9*(3), 175-182.

28. Haunt, C., Peddicord, K., & O'Brien, E. (1994). Supporting bonding in the NICU: A care plan for nurses. *Neonatal Network: Journal of Neonatal Nursing, 13*(8), 19-25.

29. Hill, B.J., & Roberts, C.S. (1981). Formal theory construction: An example of the process. In C. Roberts & S.L. Roberts (Eds.), *Theory construction in nursing: An adaptation model.* Englewood Cliffs, NJ: Prentice-Hall.

30. Ingram, L. (1995). Roy's adaptation model and accident and emergency nursing. *Accidental and Emergency Nursing, 3*(3), 150-153.

31. Kurek-Ovshinsky, C. (1991). Group psychotherapy in an acute inpatient setting: Techniques that nourish self-esteem. *Issues in Mental Health Nursing, 12*(1), 81-88.

32. Limadri, B.J. (1986). Research and practice with abused women, use of the Roy model as an explanatory framework. *Advances in Nursing Science, 8*(4), 52-61.

33. Logan, M. (1986). Palliative care nursing: Applicability of the Roy model. *Journal of Palliative Care, 1*(2), 18-24.

34. Lutjens, L.R.J. (1992). Derivation and testing of tenets of a theory of social organizations as adaptive systems. *Nursing Science Quarterly, 5*(2), 62-71.

35. Mastal, M., & Hammond, H. (1980, July). Analysis and expansion of the Roy model: A contribution to holistic nursing. *Advances in Nursing Science, 3,* 7-78.

36. Mastal, M., Hammond, H., & Roberts, M. (1982, June). Theory into hospital practice: A pilot implementation. *Journal of Nursing Administration, 12,* 9-15.

37. Meleis, A.I. (1986). *Theoretical nursing development and process* (pp. 206-218). Philadelphia: J.B. Lippincott.

38. Mitchell, G.J.., & Pilkington, B. (1990). Theoretical approaches in nursing practice: A comparison of Roy and Parse. *Nursing Science Quarterly, 3*(2), 81-87.

39. Mock, V., Burke, M.B., Sheehan, P., Creaton, E.M., Winningham, M.L., McKenney-Tedder, S., Schwager, L.P., & Liebman, M. (1994). A nursing rehabilitation program for women with breast cancer receiving adjuvant chemotherapy. *Oncology Nursing Forum, 21*(5), 899-908.

40. Morales-Mann, E.T., & Logan, M. (1990). Implementing the Roy model: Challenges for nurse educators. *Journal of Advanced Nursing, 15*(2), 142-147.

41. Phillips, K.D. (1994). *Biobehavioral adaptation in persons living with AIDS.* Unpublished doctoral dissertation, The University of Tennessee, Knoxville.

42. Phillips, K.D. (1997). Roy's adaptation model in nursing practice. In M. Alligood & A. Marriner-Tomey (Eds.), *Nursing theory utilization and application* (pp. 175-200). St. Louis: Mosby.

43. Piazza, D., & Foote, A. (1990). Roy's adaptation model: A guide for rehabilitation nursing practice. *Rehabilitation Nursing, 15*(5), 254-259.

44. Piazza, D., Foote, A., Holcombe, J., Harris, M.G., & Wright, P. (1992). The use of Roy's adaptation model applied to a patient with breast cancer. *European Journal of Cancer Care, 1*(4), 17-22.

45. Pittman, K.P. (1992). *A Q-analysis of the enabling characteristics of chronically ill school age children for the promotion of personal wellness.* Unpublished doctoral dissertation, University of Alabama, Birmingham.

46. Pollock, S.E. (1993). Adaptation to chronic illness: A program of research for testing nursing theory. *Nursing Science Quarterly, 6*(2), 86-92.

47. Rambo, B. (1983). *Adaptation nursing: Assessment and intervention.* Philadelphia: WB Saunders.

48. Randell, B., Tedrow, M.P., & Van Landingham, J. (1982). *Adaptation nursing: The Roy conceptual model applied.* St. Louis: Mosby.

49. Reynolds, P.D. (1971). *A primer in theory construction.* Indianapolis: Bobbs-Merrill.

50. Riehl, J.P., & Roy, C. (Eds.). (1980). *Conceptual models for nursing practice* (2nd ed.). New York: Appleton-Century-Crofts.

51. Roy, C. (1970, March). Adaptation: A conceptual framework in nursing. *Nursing Outlook, 18,* 42-45.

52. Roy, C. (1971, April). Adaptation: A basis for nursing practice. *Nursing Outlook, 19,* 254-257.

53. Roy, C. (1973, March). Adaptation: Implications for curriculum change. *Nursing Outlook, 21,* 163-168.

54. Roy, C. (1975, Feb.). A diagnostic classification system for nursing. *Nursing Outlook, 23,* 90-94.

55. Roy, C. (1976, Summer). The impact of nursing diagnosis. *Nursing Digest, 4,* 67-69.

56. Roy, C. (1976). *Introduction to nursing: An adaptation model.* Englewood Cliffs, NJ: Prentice-Hall.

57. Roy, C. (1976, Nov.). The Roy adaptation model: Comment. *Nursing Outlook, 24,* 690-691.

58. Roy, C. (1979, Feb.). Relating nursing theory to nursing education: A new era. *Nurse Educator, 4,* 16-21.

59. Roy, C. (1980). The Roy adaptation model. In J.P. Riehl & C. Roy (Eds.), *Conceptual models for nursing practice* (2nd ed.) (pp. 179-188). New York: Appleton-Century-Crofts.

60. Roy, C. (1983). Theory development in nursing: A proposal for direction. In N. Chaska (Ed.), *The nursing profession: A time to speak.* (pp. 453-467). New York: McGraw-Hill.

61. Roy, C. (1984). *Introduction to nursing: An adaptation model* (2nd ed.). Englewood Cliffs, NJ: Prentice-Hall.

62. Roy, C. (1987). Responses to "Needs of spouses of surgical patients, a conceptualization within the Roy adaptation model." *Scholarly Journal for Nursing Practice, 1*(1), 45-50.

63. Roy, C. (1991). Senses. In C. Roy & H. Andrews (Eds.), *The Roy adaptation model: The definitive statement* (pp. 165-189). Norwalk, CT: Appleton & Lange.

64. Roy, C., & Andrews, H. (1991). *The Roy adaptation model: The definitive statement.* Norwalk, CT: Appleton & Lange.

65. Roy, C., & Corliss, C.P. (1993). The Roy adaptation model: Theoretical update and knowledge for practice. In M.E. Parker (Ed.), *Patterns of nursing theories in practice* (pp. 215-229). New York: National League for Nursing.

66. Roy, C., & McLeod, D. (1981). Theory of the person as an adaptive system. In C. Roy & S.L. Roberts (Eds.), *Theory construction in nursing: An adaptation model.* Englewood Cliffs, NJ: Prentice-Hall.

67. Roy, C., & Obloy, M. (1978, Oct.). The practitioner movement. *American Journal of Nursing, 78,* 1698-1702.

68. Roy, C., & Roberts, S. (1981). *Theory construction in nursing: An adaptation model.* Englewood Cliffs, NJ: Prentice-Hall.

69. Schmitz, M. (1980). The Roy adaptation model: Application in a community setting. In J.P. Riehl & C. Roy (Eds.), *Conceptual models for nursing practice* (2nd ed.). New York: Appleton-Century-Crofts.

70. Silva, M.C. (1986). Research testing theory: State of the art. *Advanced Nursing Science, 9*(1), 1-11.

71. Silva, M.C. (1987). Needs of spouses of surgical patients, a conceptualization within the Roy adaptation model. *Scholarly Inquiry for Nursing Practice, 1*(1), 29-44.

72. Smith, C.E., Garvis, M.S., & Martinson, M.I. (1983, Aug.). Content analysis of interviews using a nursing model: A look at parents adapting to the impact of childhood cancer. *Cancer Nursing, 6,* 269-275.

73. Sr. Callista Roy to assume nurse theorist post at Boston College (1987). *Nursing and Health Care, 8*(9), 536.

74. Thornbury, J.M., & King, L.D. (1992). The Roy adaptation model and care of persons with Alzheimer's disease. *Nursing Science Quarterly, 5*(3), 129-133.

75. Tiedeman, M.E. (1983). The Roy adaptation model. In J. Fitzpatrick & A. Whall, *Conceptual models of nursing: Analysis and application* (pp. 157-180). Bowie, MD: Brady.

76. Tulman, L. (1990). Changes in functional status after childbirth. *Nursing Research, 39*(2), 70-75.

77. Tulman, L., & Fawcett, J. (1988). Return of functional ability after childbearing. *Nursing Research, 37*(2), 77-78.

78. Tulman, L., & Fawcett, J. (1990). A framework for studying functional status after diagnosis of breast cancer. *Cancer Nursing, 13*(2), 95-99.

79. Tulman, L., & Fawcett, J. (1990). Functional status during pregnancy and the postpartum: A framework for research. *Image: The Journal of Nursing Scholarship, 22*(3), 191-194.

80. Tulman, L., & Fawcett, J. (1990). Maternal employment following childbirth. *Research in Nursing and Health, 13*(3), 181-188.

81. Tulman, L., Fawcett, J., Groblewski, L., & Silverman, L. (1990). Changes in functional status after childbirth. *Nursing Research, 39*(2), 70-75.

82. Tulman, L., Fawcett, J., & McEvoy, M.D. (1991). Development of the Inventory of Functional Status–Cancer. *Cancer Nursing, 14*(5), 254-260.

83. Tulman, L., Fawcett, J., & Weiss, M. (1993). The Inventory of Functional Status–Fathers: Development and psychometric testing. *Journal of Nurse Midwifery, 38*(5), 276-282.

84. Tulman, L., Higgins, K., Fawcett, J., Nunno, C., Vansickel, C., Haas, M.B., & Speca, M.M. (1991). The Inventory of Functional Status–Antepartum Period: Development and testing. *Journal of Nurse Midwifery, 36*(2), 117-123.

85. Wagner, P. (1976, Nov.). The Roy adaptation model: Testing the adaptation model in practice. *Nursing Outlook, 24,* 682-685.

86. Walker, L.O., & Avant, K.C. (1983). *Strategies for theory construction in nursing.* Norwalk, CT: Appleton-Century-Crofts.

87. Wright, P.S., Holcombe, J., Foote, A., & Piazza, D. (1993). The Roy adaptation model used a guide for the nursing care of an 8-year-old child with leukemia. *Journal of Pediatric Oncology Nursing, 10*(2), 68-74.

88. Wright, P.S., Piazza, D., Holcombe, J., & Foote, A. (1994). A comparison of three theories of nursing used as a guide for the nursing care of an 8-year-old child with leukemia. *Journal of Pediatric Oncology Nursing, 11*(1), 14-19.

89. Zhan, L., & Shen, C. (1994). The development of an instrument to measure self-consistency. *Journal of Advanced Nursing, 20*(3), 509-516.

BIBLIOGRAPHY

Primary sources

Books

Andrews, H., & Roy, C. (1986). *Essentials of the Roy adaptation model.* Norwalk, CT: Appleton-Century-Crofts.

Riehl, J.P., & Roy, C. (Eds.). (1974). *Conceptual models for nursing practice.* Englewood Cliffs, NJ: Prentice-Hall.

Riehl, J.P., & Roy, C. (Eds.). (1980). *Conceptual models for nursing practice.* (2nd ed.). New York: Appleton-Century-Crofts.

Roy, C. (1976). *Introduction to nursing: An adaptation model.* Englewood Cliffs, NJ: Prentice-Hall.

Roy, C. (1982). *Introduction to nursing: An adaptation model.* Japanese translation by Yuriko Kanematsu. Japan: UNI Agency.

Roy, C. (1984). *Introduction to nursing: An adaptation model* (2nd ed.). Englewood Cliffs, NJ: Prentice-Hall.

Roy, C., & Andrews, H.A. (1991). *The Roy adaptation model: The definitive statement.* Norwalk, CT: Appleton & Lange.

Roy, C., & Roberts, S. (1981). *Theory construction in nursing: an adaptation model.* Englewood Cliffs, NJ: Prentice-Hall.

Book chapters

Roy, C. (1974). The Roy adaptation model. In J.P. Riehl & C. Roy (Eds.), *Conceptual models for nursing practice.* New York: Appleton-Century-Crofts.

Roy, C. (1975, June). Adaptation framework. In *Curriculum innovation through framework application.* Loma Linda, CA: Loma Linda University.

Roy, C. (1978, Jan. 12-13). Conceptual framework for primary care in baccalaureate programs. In *Primary care conference,* Denver, CO: U.S. Department of Health, Education, and Welfare.

Roy, C. (1978). The stress of hospital events: Measuring changes in level of stress. In M.V. Batey (Ed.), *Symposium on stress.* In Conference on Communicating Nursing Research. Boulder, CO: Western Interstate Commission on Higher Education (WICHE), Vol. 11.

Roy, C. (1979). Health-illness (powerlessness) questionnaire and hospitalized patient decision-making. In M.J. Ward & C.A. Linderman (Eds.), *Instruments for measuring practice and other health care variables* (Vol. 1). Hyattsville, MD: U.S. Department of Health, Education, and Welfare.

Roy, C. (1980). Exposé de Callista Roy sur theories. Exposé de Callista Roy sur l'utilisation de sa theories au nouveau de la recherche. In *Acta Nursological 3,* Ecole Genevoise D. Infirmieres Le Bon Secours, Geneva.

Roy, C. (1980). The Roy adaptation model. In J.P. Riehl & C. Roy (Eds.), *Conceptual models for nursing practice* (2nd ed.). New York: Appleton-Century-Crofts.

Roy, C. (1981). A systems model of nursing care and its effect on the quality of human life. *Proceedings of the International Congress on Applied Systems Research and Cybernetics.* London: Pergamon.

Roy, C. (1983). The expectant family: Analysis and application of the Roy adaptation model, and the family in primary care—Analysis and application of the Roy adaptation model. In I.W. Clements, & F. Roberts (Eds.), *Family health: A theoretical approach to nursing care.* New York: John Wiley & Sons.

Roy, C. (1983). The family in primary care: Analysis and application of the Roy adaptation model. In I.W. Clements & F.B.. Roberts (Eds.), *Family health: A theoretical approach to nursing care.* New York: John Wiley & Sons.

Roy, C. (1983). Foreword. In B.J. Rambo, *Adaptation nursing: Assessment and intervention.* Philadelphia: W.B. Saunders.

Roy, C. (1984). Framework for classification systems development: Progress and issues. *Proceedings of the fifth national conference on the classification of nursing diagnosis.* St. Louis: Mosby.

Roy, C. (1984). The Roy adaptation model: Applications in community health nursing. *Proceedings of the eighth annual community health nursing conference.* Chapel Hill, NC: University of North Carolina.

Roy, C. (1984, May 20-23). The Roy adaptation model: Applications in community health nursing. In *Proceedings of the annual community health nursing conference.* Chapel Hill, NC: University of North Carolina.

Roy, C. (1985). The future of the nursing science; Response of the Academy. *Scientific Session of the American Academy of Nursing.* Kansas City, MO: American Academy of Nursing.

Roy, C. (1988). Sister Callista Roy. In T.M. Schorr & A. Zimmerman (Eds.). *Making choices: Taking chances.* (pp. 291-298). St. Louis: Mosby.

Roy, C. (1987). The influence of nursing models on clinical decision making II. In K.J. Hannah, M. Reimer, W.C. Mills, & S. Letourneau (Eds.), *Clinical judgment and decision making: The future with nursing diagnosis* (pp. 42-47). New York: John Wiley & Sons.

Roy, C. (1987). Roy's adaptation model. In R.R. Parse, *Nursing science: Major paradigms, theories, and critiques.* Philadelphia: W.B. Saunders.

Roy, C. (1988). Human information processing and nursing research. In J. Fitzpatrick & R.L. Tauton (Eds.), *Annual Review of Nursing Research 6.* New York: Springer.

Roy, C. (1991). Altered cognition: An information processing approach. In P.H. Mitchell, L.C. Hodges, M. Muwaswes, & C.A. Walleck (Eds.), *AANN's neuroscience nursing: Phenomenon and practice—Human responses to neurological health problems* (pp. 185-211). Norwalk, CT: Appleton & Lange.

Roy, C. (1991). Structure of knowledge: Paradigm, model, and research specifications for differentiated practice. In I.E. Goertzen (Ed.), *Differentiating nursing practice: Into the twenty-first century.* Kansas City, MO: American Academy of Nursing, pp. 31-39.

Roy, C. (1992). Vigor, variables, and vision: Commentary of Florence Nightingale. In F. Nightingale, *Notes on nursing: What it is, and what it is not.* Philadelphia: J.B. Lippincott.

Roy, C., & Anway, J. (1988). Roy's adaptation model: Theories for nursing administration. In B. Henry, C. Arndt, M. DiVincenti, & A. Marriner-Tomey (Eds.), *Dimensions of nursing administration.* Boston: Blackwell Scientific.

Roy, C., & Corliss, C.P. (1993). The Roy adaptation model: Theoretical update and knowledge for practice. In M.E. Parker (Ed.), *Patterns of nursing theories in practice* (pp. 215-229). New York: National League for Nursing.

Roy, C., & McLeod, D. (1981). Theory of the person as an adaptive system. In C. Roy & S.L. Roberts (Eds.), *Theory construction in nursing: An adaptation model.* Englewood Cliffs, NJ: Prentice-Hall.

Roy, S.C. (1983). A conceptual framework for clinical specialist practice. In A. Harris & J. Spross (Eds.), *The clinical nurse specialist in theory and practice.* New York: Grune & Stratton.

Roy, S.C. (1983). Roy's adaptation model and application to family case studies. In I. Clements & F. Roberts (Eds.), *Theoretical approaches to family health.* New York: Wiley.

Roy, S.C. (1983). Theory development in nursing: a proposal for direction. In N. Chaska (Ed.), *The nursing profession: A time to speak.* New York: McGraw-Hill.

Roy, S.C. (1985). Practice in action: Clinical research. In K.E. Barnard & G.R. Smith (Eds.), *Faculty practice in action: Annual symposium on nursing faculty practice.* 2 (pp. 192-200). New York: American Academy of Nursing.

Journal articles

Roy, C. (1967, Feb.). Role cues and mothers of hospitalized children. *Nursing Research, 16,* 178-182.

Roy, C. (1970, March). Adaptation: A conceptual framework in nursing. *Nursing Outlook, 18,* 42-45.

Roy, C. (1971, April). Adaptation: A basis for nursing practice. *Nursing Outlook, 19,* 254-257.

Roy, C. (1973). Adaptation: Implications for curriculum change. *Nursing Outlook, 21,* 163-168.

Roy, C. (1975, Feb.). Adaptation: Implications for curriculum change. *Nursing Outlook, 23,* 90-94.

Roy, C. (1975, Feb.). A diagnostic classification system for nursing. *Nursing Outlook, 23,* 90-94.

Roy, C. (1976). Comment. *Nursing Outlook, 24,* 690-691.

Roy, C. (1976, Summer). The impact of nursing diagnosis. *Nursing Digest,* 467-469.

Roy, C. (1976, Nov.). The Roy adaptation model: Comment. *Nursing Outlook, 24,* 690-691.

Roy, C. (1979, Feb.). Relating nursing theory to nursing education: a new era. *Nurse Educator, 4,* 16-21.

Roy, C. (1979, Dec.). Nursing diagnosis from the perspective of a nursing model. *Nursing Diagnosis Newsletter, 6,* St. Louis School of Nursing.

Roy, C. (1983). To the editor. *Nursing Research, 23,* 320.

Roy, C. (1985). Acoustic neuroma: Notes. *Acoustic Neuroma Association, 13,* 8-9.

Roy, C. (1985). Nursing research makes a difference. *Newsletter of Nurses Educational Fund, Inc.* 4(1), 2-3.

Roy, C. (1987). Response to "Needs of spouses of surgical patients, a conceptualization within the Roy adaptation model." *Scholarly Journal for Nursing Practice, 1*(1), 45-50.

Roy, C. (1988). An explication of the philosophical assumptions of the Roy adaptation model. *Nursing Science Quarterly, 1*(1), 26-34.

Roy, C. (1990). Case reports can provide a standard for care in nursing practice. *Journal of Professional Nursing, 6*(3), 179-180.

Roy, C. (1990). Strengthening the Roy adaptation model through conceptual clarification. *Nursing Science Quarterly, 3*(2), 64-66.

Roy, C., & Obloy, M. (1978, Oct.). The practitioner movement. *American Journal of Nursing, 78,* 1698-1702.

Roy, S.C. (1975, May). The impact of nursing diagnosis. *AORN Journal, 21,* 1023-1030.

Gortner, S., Ellis, R., Roy, C., Williams, C., Benner, P., & Mercer, R. (1984). Explanation in nursing science. *Symposium abstract in Community Nursing Research, 17,* 101-103.

Dissertation

Roy, C. (1977). *Decision-making by the physically ill and adaptation during illness.* Unpublished doctoral dissertation, University of California, Los Angeles.

Booklet

Roy, S.C. (1978). *The future of nursing.* In Forum of Nursing Service, Administrators in the West. San Diego: National League for Nursing. Pub. No. 52-1805.

Audiotapes

Roy, C. (1978, Dec.). Paper presented at the second Annual Nurse Educator Conference. Audiotape available from Teach 'em Inc., 160 E. Illinois Street, Chicago, IL 60611.

Roy, C. (1984, May). Nurses' Theorist Conference at Edmonton, Alberta. Audiotape available from Kennedy Recordings, R.R. 5, Edmonton, Alberta, Canada TSP 4B7.

Correspondence

Roy, S.C. (1984, March 26), Curriculum vitae.

Roy, S.C. (1988, March 8). Curriculum vitae.

Interviews

Professional profile: "Sister Callista Roy: Influencing the direction of nursing" (1985). *Focus on Critical Care Nursing, 12*(3), 45-46.

Roy, S.C. (1984, March 25). Telephone interview.

Secondary sources

Book reviews

Riehl, J.P., & Roy, S.C. (1974). *Conceptual models for nursing practice.*
Nursing Outlook, 23, 457, July 1975.
Nursing Research, 24, 306-307, July-August 1975.

Roy, S.C. (1976). *Introduction to nursing: An adaptation model.* American Journal of Nursing, 77, 1359, August 1977. *Nursing Outlook, 25,* 658, October 1977.

Roy, S.C., & Roberts, S. (1981). *Theory construction in nursing. Nursing Outlook, 30,* 141, February 1982.

Books

Chinn, P.L., & Jacobs, M.K. (1987). *Theory and nursing; a systematic approach.* St. Louis: Mosby.

Fitzpatrick, J.J., & Whall, A.L. (1983). *Conceptual models of nursing: Analysis and application.* Bowie, MD: Robert J. Brady.

Fitzpatrick, J.J., Whall, A., Johnson, R., & Floyd, J. (1982). *Nursing models and their psychiatric mental health applications.* Bowie, MD: Robert J Brady.

Kim, H.S. (1983). *The nature of theoretical thinking in nursing.* Norwalk, CT: Appleton-Century-Crofts.

Lutjens, L.R.J. (1991). *Callista Roy: An adaptation model.* Newbury Park, CA: Sage.

Nicoll, L.H. (1986). *Perspectives on nursing theory.* Boston: Little, Brown.

Potter, D.O. (Ed.) (1984). *Practice nurses' reference library.* Springhouse, PA: Springhouse.

Rambo, B. (1983). *Adaptation nursing: Assessment and intervention.* Philadelphia: W.B. Saunders.

Randell, B., Tedrow, M.P., & Van Landingham, J. (1982). *Adaptation nursing: The Roy conceptual model applied.* St. Louis: Mosby.

Reynolds, P.D. (1971). *A primer in theory construction.* Indianapolis: Bobbs-Merrill.

Torres, G. (1986). *Theoretical foundations of nursing.* (pp. 151-165). Norwalk, CT: Appleton-Century-Crofts.

Walker, L.O., & Avant, K.C. (1983). *Strategies for theory construction in nursing.* Norwalk, CT: Appleton-Century-Crofts.

Book chapters

Blue, C.L., Brubaker, K.M., Fine, J.M., Kirsch, M.J., Papazian, K.R., Rieser, C.M., & Sobiech, M.A. (1989). Sister Callista Roy: Adaptation model. In A. Marriner-Tomey (Ed.), *Nursing theorists and their work* (2nd ed., pp. 325-344). St. Louis: Mosby.

Blue, C.L., Brubaker, K.M., Fine, J.M., Kirsch, M.J., Papazian, K.R., Rieser, C.M., Sobiech, M.A. (1994). Sister Callista Roy: Adaptation model. In A. Marriner-Tomey (Ed.), *Nursing theorists and their work* (3rd ed., pp. 246-268). St. Louis: Mosby.

Blue, C.L., Brubaker, K.M., Papazian, K.R., & Riester, C.M.. (1986). Sister Callista Roy: Adaptation model. In A. Marriner (Ed.), *Nursing theorists and their work* (pp. 297-312). St. Louis: Mosby.

Fawcett, J. (1981). Assessing and understanding the cesarean father. In C.F. Kehoe (Ed.), *The cesarean experience: Theoretical and clinical perspectives for nurses* (pp. 371-376). New York: Appleton-Century-Crofts.

Fawcett, J. (1984). Roy's adaptation model. In J. Fawcett, *Analysis and evaluation of conceptual models of nursing* (pp. 247-285). Philadelphia: F.A. Davis.

Fawcett, J. (1995). Roy's adaptation model. In J. Fawcett, *Analysis and evaluation of conceptual models of nursing* (pp. 437-515). Philadelphia: F.A. Davis.

Fitzpatrick, J.J., Whall, A., Johnson, R., & Floyd, J. (1982). *Nursing models: Applications to psychiatric mental health nursing.* Bowie, MD: Robert J. Brady.

Galbreath, J.G. (1980). Sister Callista Roy. In Nursing Theories Conference Group, J.B. George, Chairperson, *Nursing theories: The base for professional nursing practice* (pp. 199-212). Englewood Cliffs, NJ: Prentice-Hall.

Galbreath, J.G. (1985). Sister Callista Roy. In J.B. George (Ed.), *Nursing theories* (2nd ed., pp. 300-318). Englewood Cliffs, NJ: Prentice-Hall.

Germain, C.P. (1984). Power and powerlessness in the adult hospitalized cancer patient. In *Cancer Nursing in the 80's: Proceedings of the 3rd International Conference of Cancer Nursing* (pp. 158-162). Melbourne, Australia: The Cancer Institute/Peter MacCallum Hospital and the Royal Melbourne Hospital.

Gordon, J. (1974). Nursing assessment and care plan for a cardiac patient. In J.P. Riehl & C. Roy (Eds.), *Conceptual models for nursing practice.* New York: Appleton-Century-Crofts.

Hill, B.J., & Roberts, C.S. (1981). Formal theory construction: An example of the process. In C. Roy & S.L. Roberts (Eds.), *Theory construction in nursing: An adaptation model* (pp. 30-39). Englewood Cliffs, NJ: Prentice-Hall.

Idle, B.A. (1978). SPAL: A tool for measuring self-perceived adaptation level appropriate for an elderly population. In E.E. Bauwens (Ed.), *Clinical nursing research: Its strategies and findings.* Monograph series 1978: Two, pp. 56-63. Indianapolis: Sigma Theta Tau.

Kehoe, C.F. (1981). Identifying the nursing needs of the postpartum cesarean mother. In C.F. Kehoe (Ed.), *The cesarean experience: Theoretical and clinical perspectives for nurses* (pp. 85-141). New York: Appleton-Century-Crofts.

Kehoe, C.F., & Fawcett, J. (1981). An overview of the Roy adaptation model. In C.F. Kehoe (Ed.), *The cesarean experience: Theoretical and clinical perspectives for nurses* (pp. 79-84). New York: Appleton-Century-Crofts.

Leddy, S., & Pepper, J.M. (1985). Sister Callista Roy's adaptation model. In S. Leddy & J.M. Pepper, *Conceptual bases of professional nursing* (pp. 142-144). Philadelphia: J.B. Lippincott.

Levesque, L. (1980, Oct. 22-24). Rehabilitation of the chronically ill elderly: A method of operationalizing a conceptual model for nursing. In R.C. MacKay & E.G. Zilm (Eds.), *Research for practice: Proceedings of the National Nursing Research Conference,* Halifax, Nova Scotia, Canada.

Lewis, F., et al. (1978). Measuring adaptation of chemotherapy patients. In J.C. Krueger, A.H. Nelson, & M. Opal, *Nursing Research: Development, collaboration, utilization.* Rockville, MD: Aspen Systems.

Meleis, A.I. (1985). Sister Callista Roy. In A.I. Meleis, *Theoretical nursing: Development and progress* (pp. 206-218). Philadelphia: J.B. Lippincott.

Phillips. K.D. (1997). Roy's adaptation model in nursing practice. In M. Alligood & A. Marriner-Tomey (Eds.), *Nursing theory utilization and application* (pp. 175-200). St. Louis. Mosby.

Sato, M. (1986). The Roy adaptation model. In P. Winsted-Fry, (Ed.), *Case studies in nursing theory* (pp. 103-125). New York: National League for Nursing.

Schmitz, M. (1980. The Roy adaptation model: Application in a community setting. In J.P. Riehl & C. Roy (Eds.), *Conceptual models for nursing practice* (2nd ed., pp. 193-206). New York: Appleton-Century-Crofts.

Starr, S.L. (1980). Adaptation applied to the dying patient. In J.P. Riehl & C. Roy (Eds.), *Conceptual models for nursing practice* (2nd ed., pp. 189-192). New York: Appleton-Century-Crofts.

Tiedman, M.E. (1983). The Roy adaptation model. In J. Fitzpatrick & A. Whall (Eds.), *Conceptual models of nursing: Analysis and application* (pp. 157-180). Bowie, MD: Robert J. Brady.

Journal articles

Aggleton, P., & Chalmers, H. (1984, Oct.). The Roy Adaptation Model. *Nursing Times, 80,* 45-48.

Andreoli, K.G., & Thompson, C.E. (1977, June). The nature of science in nursing. *Image, 9*(2), 33-37.

Baker, A.C. (1993). The spouse's positive effect on the stroke patient's recovery. *Rehabilitation Nursing, 18*(1), 30-33, 67-68.

Barnfather, J.S., Swain, M.A.P., & Erickson, H.C. (1989). Evaluation of two assessment techniques for adaptation to stress. *Nursing Science Quarterly, 2*(4), 172-182.

Beckstrand, J. (1980). A critique of several conceptions of practice theory in nursing. *Research in Nursing and Health, 3,* 69-79.

Brower, H.T.F., & Baker, B.J. (1976, Nov.). The Roy adaptation model: Using the adaptation model in a practitioner curriculum. *Nursing Outlook, 24,* 686-689.

Calvillo, E.R., & Flaskerud, J.H. (1993). The adequacy of Roy's adaptation model to guide cross-cultural pain research. *Nursing Science Quarterly, 6*(3), 118-129.

Calvert, M.M. (1989). Human-pet interaction and loneliness: A test of concepts from Roy's adaptation model. *Nursing Science Quarterly, 2*(4), 194-202.

Camooso, C., Green, M., & Reilly, P. (1981). Students' adaptation according to Roy. *Nursing Outlook, 29,* 108-109.

Carveth, J.A. (1987). Conceptual models in nurse-midwifery. *Journal of Nurse-Midwifery, 32*(1), 20-25.

Chance, K.S. (1982). Nursing models: A requisite for professional accountability. *Advances in Nursing Science, 4*(2), 57-65.

Chen, H. (1994). Hearing in the elderly: Relation of hearing loss, loneliness, and self-esteem. *Journal of Gerontological Nursing, 20*(6), 22-28.

Coleman, P.M. (1993). Depression during the female climacteric period. *Journal of Advanced Nursing, 18*(10), 1540-1546.

Cottrel, B.H., & Shannaha, M.D. (1987). Effect of the birth chair in duration of second stage labor and maternal outcome. *Nursing Research, 35*(6), 364-367.

Dickoff, J., James, P., & Wiedenbach, E. (1968, May). Theory in a practice discipline. Part I. Practice oriented theory. *Nursing Research, 17,* 413-435.

Farkas, L. (1981, March). Adaptation problems with nursing home application for elderly persons: An application of the Roy adaptation nursing model. *Journal of Advanced Nursing, 6,* 363-368.

Fawcett, J. (1981). Needs of cesarean birth parents. *Journal of Obstetric, Gynecologic, and Neonatal Nursing, 10,* 371-376.

Fawcett, J. (1990). Preparation for caesarean childbirth: Derivation of a nursing intervention from the Roy adaptation model. *Journal of Advanced Nursing, 15*(12), 1418-1425.

Fawcett, J., & Buritt, J. (1985). An exploratory study of antenatal preparation for cesarean birth. *Journal of Obstetric, Gynecologic, and Neonatal Nursing, 14,* 224-230.

Friedmann, M., & Andrews, M. (1990). Family support and child adjustment in single-parent families . . . secondary analysis. *Issues in Comprehensive Pediatric Nursing, 13*(14), 289-301.

Frederickson, K., Jackson, B.S., Strauman, T., & Strauman, J. (1991). Testing hypotheses derived from the Roy adaptation model. *Nursing Science Quarterly, 4*(4), 168-174.

Florence, M.E., Lutzen, K., & Alexius, B. (1994). Adaptation of heterosexually infected HIV-positive women: A Swedish pilot study. *Health Care for Women International, 15*(4), 265-273.

Galligan, A.C. (1979, Jan.). Using Roy's concept of adaptation to care for young children. *American Journal of Maternal Child Nursing, 4,* 24-28.

Gamble, N., & Devanev, S. (1985). Application of the adaptation framework in an LPN program: A project. *Missouri Nurse, 54*(6), 10-13.

Gartner, S.R., & Nahm, H. (1977, Jan.-Feb.). An overview of nursing research in the United States. *Nursing Research, 26,* 10-29.

Germain, C.P. (1984). Sheltering abused women: A nursing perspective. *Journal of Psychological Nursing, 22*(9), 24-31.

Gerrish, C. (1989). From theory to practice: Applied Roy's model while caring for a woman with Hodgkin's disease. *Nursing Times, 85*(35), 42-45.

Glasper, A. (1986). Spotlight on children: Scaling down a model. *Nursing Times, 82*(43), 53-58.

Goodwin, J.O. (1980). A cross-cultural approach to integrating nursing theory and practice. *Nurse Educator, 5*(6), 15-20.

Gunderson, L.P. & Kenner, C. (1987, Aug.). Neonatal stress: Physiologic adaptation and nursing implications. *Neonatal Network,* 37-42.

Hammong, E., Roberts, M.P., & Silva, M.C. (1983, Spring). The effect of Roy's first level and second level assessment of nurses: Determination of accurate nursing diagnoses. *Virginia Nurse,* 14-17.

Harrison, L.L., Leeper, J.D., & Yoon, M. (1990). Effects of early parent touch on preterm infants' heart rates and arterial oxygen saturation levels. *Journal of Advanced Nursing, 15*(8), 877-885.

Heinrich, K. (1989). Growing pains: Faculty stages in adopting a nursing model. *Nurse Educator, 14*(1), 3-4.

Hoon, E. (1986). Game playing: A way to look at nursing models. *Journal of Advanced Nursing, 11*(4), 421-427.

Jackson, D.A. (1990). Roy in the postanesthesia care unit. *Journal of Post Anesthesia Nursing, 5*(3), 143-148.

Jackson, B.S., Strauman, J., Frederickson, K., & Strauman, T.J. (1991). Long-term biopsychosocial effects of interleukin-2 therapy. *Oncology Nursing Forum, 18*(4), 683-690.

Janelli, L.M. (1980). Utilizing Roy's adaptation model from a gerontological perspective. *Journal of Gerontological Nursing, 6*(3), 140-150.

Johnston, D.E. (1974, Sept.-Oct.). Development of theory: A requisite for nursing as a primary health profession. *Nursing Research, 23,* 372-377.

Kasemwatana, S. (1982). An application of Roy's adaptation model. *Thai Journal of Nursing, 31*(1), 25-46.

Kurek-Ovshinsky, C. (1991). Group psychotherapy in an acute inpatient setting: Techniques that nourish self-esteem. *Issues in Mental Health Nursing, 12*(1), 81-88.

LeMone, P. (1995). Assessing psychosexual concerns in adults with diabetes: Pilot project using Roy's modes of adaptation. *Issues in Mental Health Nursing, 16*(1), 67-78.

Limandri, B.J. (1986). Research and practice with abused women: Use of the Roy model as an explanatory framework. *Advanced Nursing Science, 8*(4), 52-61.

Laros, J. (1977). Deriving outcome criteria from a conceptual model. *Nursing Outlook, 25,* 333-336.

Lewis, F.M., Firsich, S.C., & Parsell, S. (1979). Clinical tool development for adult chemotherapy patients: Process and content. *Cancer Nursing, 2,* 99-108.

Logan, M. (1990). The Roy adaptation model: Are nursing diagnoses amendable to independent nurse functions? *Journal of Advanced Nursing, 15*(4), 468-470.

Mason, T. (1990). Nursing models in a special hospital: A critical analysis of efficacy. *Journal of Advanced Nursing, 15*(6), 667-673.

Mastal, M., & Hammond, H. (1980, July). Analysis and expansion of the Roy adaptation model: A contribution to holistic nursing. *Advances in Nursing Science, 2,* 71-81.

Mastal, M., Hammond, H., & Roberts, M. (1982, June). Theory into hospital practice: A pilot implementation. *Journal of Nursing Administration, 12,* 9-15.

McGill, J.S., & Paul, P.B. (1993). Functional status and hope in elderly people with and without cancer. *Oncology Nursing Forum, 20*(8), 1207-1213.

Meek, S.S. (1993). Effects of slow stroke back massage on relaxation in hospice clients. *Image: The Journal of Nursing Scholarship, 25*(1), 17-21.

Miller, F. (1991). Using Roy's model in a special hospital. *Nursing Standard, 5*(27), 29-32.

Newman, D.M.L., & Fawcett, J. (1995). Caring for a young child in a body cast: Impact on the care giver. *Orthopaedic Nursing, 14*(1), 41-46.

Norris, S., Campbell, L., & Brenkert, S. (1982). Nursing procedures and alterations in transcutaneous oxygen tension in premature infants. *Nursing Research, 31,* 330-336.

Park, K.O. (1982). Study of Roy's adaptation model. *Trehan Kanho, 21*(3), 49-58 (Japan).

Pepin, J., Ducharme, F., Kerouac, S., Levesque, L., Ricard, N., & Duquette, A. (1994). Development of a research program based on a conceptual model of the nursing discipline. *Canadian Journal of Nursing Research, 26*(1), 41-53.

Pollock, S.E., Frederickson, K., Carson, M.A., Massey, V.H., & Roy, C. (1994). Contributions to nursing science: Synthesis of findings from Adaptation Model research. *Scholarly Inquiry for Nursing Practice, 8*(4), 361-374.

Porth, C.M. (1977). Physiological coping: A model for teaching pathophysiology. *Nursing Outlook, 25,* 781-784.

Richard, L. (1982). Roy's adaptation model. *Infirmiere Canadienne (Montreal), 24*(9), 12-13.

Robinson, J.H. (1995). Grief responses, coping processes, and social support of widows: Research with Roy's model. *Nursing Science Quarterly, 8*(4), 158-164.

Robitaille-Tremblay, M. (1983). Les soins infirmiers en psychiatrie a l'ere d'un modele conceptuel. *L'infirmiere Canadienne, 6,* 37-40.

Robitaille-Tremblay, M. (1984, Aug.). A data collection tool for the psychiatric nurse. *Canadian Nurse, 31*(7), 26-31.

Rogers, M., Paul, L.J., Clarke, J., Mackay, C., Potter, M., & Ward, W. (1991). The use of the Roy adaptation model in nursing administration. *Canadian Journal of Nursing Administration, 4*(2), 21-26.

Samarel, N., & Fawcett, J. (1992). Enhancing adaptation to breast cancer: The addition of coaching to support groups. *Oncology Nursing Forum, 19*(4), 591-596.

Selman, S.W. (1989). Impact of total hip replacement on quality of life. *Orthopaedic Nursing, 8*(5), 43-49.

Sheppard, V.A., & Cunnie, K.L. (1996). Incidence of diuresis following hysterectomy. *Journal of Post Anesthesia Nursing, 11,* 20-28.

Short, J.D. (1994). Interdependence needs and nursing care of the new family. *Issues in Comprehensive Pediatric Nursing, 17*(1), 1-14.

Silva, M.C. (1977, Oct.). Philosophy science theory: Interrelationships and implications for nursing research. *Image, 9*(3), 59-63.

Silva, M.C. (1986). Research testing nursing theory, state of the art. [Published erratum appears in ANS1987, Jan. 9(2): ix.] *Advanced Nursing Science, 9*(1), 1-11.

Silva, M.C. (1987). Needs of spouses of surgical patients: A conceptualization within the Roy adaptation model. *Scholarly Inquiry for Nursing Practice, 1*(1), 29-44.

Smith, C.E., Garvis, M.S., & Martinson, I.M. (1983, Aug.). Content analysis of interviews using a nursing model: A look at parents adapting to the impact of childhood cancer. *Cancer Nursing, 6*, 269-275.

Strohmyer, L.L., Noroian, E.L., Patterson, L.M., & Carlin, B.P. (1993). Adaptation six months after multiple trauma: A pilot study. *Journal of Neuroscience Nursing, 25*(1), 270-276.

Torosian, L.C., DeStefano, M., & Deitrick-Gallagher, M. (1985). Day gynecologic chemotherapy unit: An innovative approach to changing health care systems. *Cancer Nursing, 8*, 221-227.

Tulman, L. (1990). Maternal employment after birth. *Research in Nursing and Health, 13*(3), 181-188.

Vicenzi, A.E., & Thiel, R. (1992). AIDS education on the college campus: Roy's adaptation model in practice: Nurses' perspectives. *Nursing Science Quarterly, 7*(2), 80-86.

Wagner, P. (1976, Nov.). The Roy adaptation model: Testing the adaptation model in practice. *Nursing Outlook, 24*(11), 682-685.

Weiss, M.E., Hastings, W.J., Holly, D.C., & Craig, D.I. (1994). Using Roy's adaptation model in practice: Nurses' perspectives. *Nursing Science Quarterly, 7*(2), 80-86.

Weiss, M.E., & Teplick, F. (1993). Linking perinatal standards, documentation, and quality monitoring. *Journal of Perinatal and Neonatal Nursing, 7*(2), 18-27.

Other sources

Coombs, A., & Snygg, D. (1959). *Individual behavior: A perceptual approach to behavior.* New York: Harper Brothers.

Dohrendwend, B.P. (1961). The social psychological nature of stress: A framework for causal inquiry. *Journal of Abnormal and Social Psychology, 62*(2), 294-302.

Driever, M.J. (1976). Theory of self-concept. In C. Roy (Ed.), *Introduction to nursing: An adaptation model.* Englewood Cliffs, NJ: Prentice-Hall.

Ellis, R. (1968, May-June). Characteristics of significant theories. *Nursing Research, 17*, 217-223.

Epstein, S. (1973, May). The self-concept revisited or a theory of a theory. *American Psychologist, 28*(5), 404-416.

Erikson, E.H. (1963). *Childhood and society* (2nd ed.). New York: W.W. Norton.

Gardner, B.D. (1964). *Development in early childhood.* New York: Harper & Row.

Helson, H. (19674). *Adaptational-level theory: An experimental and systematic approach to behavior.* New York: Harper & Row.

Lazarus, R.S. (1966). *Psychological stress and the coping process.* New York: McGraw-Hill.

Lazarus, R.S., Averill, J.R., & Opton, E.M., Jr. (1974). The psychology of coping: Issues of research and assessment. In G.V. Coelho, D.A. Hamburg, & J.E. Adams (Eds.), *Coping and adaptation.* New York: Basic Books.

Malaznik, N. (1976). Theory of role function. In C. Roy (Ed.), *Introduction to nursing: An adaptation model.* Englewood Cliffs, NJ: Prentice-Hall.

Maslow, A.H. (1968). *Toward a psychology of being* (2nd ed.). New York: Van Nostrand Reinhold.

Mead, G.H. (1934). *Mind, self, and society.* Chicago: University of Chicago.

Mechanic, D. (1974). Social structure and personal adaptation: Some neglected dimensions. In G.V. Coelho, D.A. Hamburg, & J.E. Adams (Eds.), *Coping and adaptation.* New York: Basic Books.

Mechanic, D. (1970). Some problems in developing a social psychology of adaptation to stress. In J. McGrath (Ed.), *Social and psychological factors in stress.* New York: Holt, Rinehart, & Winston.

Miller, J.G. (1965, July). Living systems: Basic concepts. *Behavioral Science, 10*, 193-237.

Pousch, M., & Van Landingham, J. (1977). *Interdependence mode module.* Class handout, Mount St. Mary's College, Los Angeles.

Randell, B. (1976). *Introduction to nursing: An adaptation model.* Englewood Cliffs, NJ: Prentice-Hall.

Reynolds, P.D. (1971). *A primer in theory construction.* Indianapolis: Bobbs-Merrill.

Selye, H. (1978). *The stress of life.* New York: McGraw-Hill.

Smith, B.J.A. (1989). *Caregiver burden and adaptation in middle-aged daughters of dependent elderly parents: A test of Roy's model,* (p. 177). Unpublished a doctoral dissertation, University of Pittsburgh.

Sullivan, H.S. (1953). *The interpersonal theory of psychiatry.* New York: W.W. Norton.

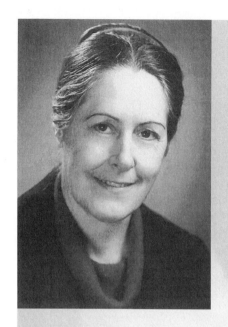

Betty Neuman

Systems Model

Barbara T. Freese, Sarah J. Beckman, Sanna Boxley-Harges,
Cheryl Bruick-Sorge, Susan Matthews Harris, Mary E. Hermiz,
Mary Meininger, Sandra E. Steinkeler

CREDENTIALS AND BACKGROUND OF THE THEORIST

Betty Neuman was born in 1924 on a farm near Low-ell, Ohio. Her father was a farmer and her mother a homemaker. She developed a love for the land while growing up in rural Ohio, and this rural background developed her compassion for people in need. Dr. Neuman's initial nursing education was completed

The authors wish to express appreciation to Dr. Betty Neuman, Rosalie Mirenda, and Dr. Lois Lowry for assistance with fourth edition revisions.

with double honors at Peoples Hospital School of Nursing (now General Hospital), Akron, Ohio, in 1947. She then moved to Los Angeles to live with relatives. In California she held various positions, including hospital staff and head nursing, school nursing, and industrial nursing. She was also involved in clinical teaching in what is now the USC Medical Center, Los Angeles, in the areas of medical-surgical, communicable disease, and critical care. Because she had always been interested in human behavior, she attended the University of California at Los Angeles with a double major in public health and psychology. She completed her baccalaureate degree with honors in nursing in 1957 and then helped establish and manage her husband's obstetrical and gynecological practice. In 1966 she received her master's degree in Mental Health, Public Health Consultation, from UCLA.[74,75] She received a doctoral degree in clinical psychology from Pacific Western University in 1985.[74]

Neuman was a pioneer of nursing involvement in mental health. She developed, taught, and refined a community mental health program for post–master level nurses at UCLA. Dr. Neuman and Donna Aquilina were the first two nurses to pioneer development of the nurse counselor role within Los Angeles–based community crisis centers.[81] She developed her first explicit teaching and practice model for mental health consultation in the late 1960s, before the creation of her systems model. This teaching and practice model is cited in her first book publication in 1971. Neuman then designed a conceptual model for nursing in 1970 in response to requests from UCLA graduate students who wanted a course emphasizing breadth rather than depth in understanding the variables in nursing. The model initially was developed to integrate student learning of client variables extending nursing beyond the medical model.[86:265] It included such behavioral science concepts as problem identification and prevention. Dr. Neuman first published her model in 1972.[79,81] She spent the following decade further defining and refining various aspects of the model in preparation for her book *The Neuman Systems Model: Application to Nursing Education and Practice.* Further development and revisions of the model are illustrated in the second (1989)[78] and third (1995)[83] editions.

Since developing the Neuman Systems Model, Neuman has been involved in a wide variety of professional international activities, including numerous publications, paper presentations, consultations, lectures, and conferences. Dr. Neuman has a wide range of teaching areas, having taught nurse continuing education at UCLA and community agencies for 14 years. She has remained an active private practice therapist as a licensed clinical member of the American Association of Marriage and Family Therapists since 1970. Dr. Neuman maintains her role as consultant internationally for nursing schools and practice agencies adopting the model.[78,80,81]

THEORETICAL SOURCES

The Neuman Systems Model has some similarity to Gestalt theory.[73:14] Gestalt theory maintains that the homeostatic process is the process by which an organism maintains its equilibrium, and consequently its health, under varying conditions. Neuman describes adjustment as the process by which the organism satisfies its needs. Because many needs exist and each may disturb client balance or stability, the adjustment process is dynamic and continuous. All life is characterized by this ongoing interplay of balance and imbalance within the organism. When the stabilizing process fails to some degree, or when the organism remains in a state of disharmony for too long and is consequently unable to satisfy its needs, illness may develop. When this compensatory process fails completely, the organism may die.[86:4] The Gestalt approach, then, considers the individual as a function of the organism-environmental field and views behavior as a reflection of relatedness within that field.[88:25]

The model is also derived from the philosophical views of Pierre Teihard deChardin and Bernard Marx.[73:14] Marxist philosophy suggests that the properties of parts are determined partly by the larger wholes within dynamically organized systems. Along with this view, Neuman[73:14] confirmed that the patterns of the whole influence awareness of the part, which is drawn from deChardin's philosophy of the wholeness of life. She used Hans Selye's definition of *Stress,* which is the nonspecific response of the body to any demand made on it.[102:14] Stress increases the demand for readjustment. This demand is nonspecific; it requires adaptation to a problem, irrespective of what the problem is. The essence of stress is therefore the nonspecific demand for activity.[102:15] Stressors are tension-producing stimuli with the potential for causing disequilibrium, such as situational or maturational crises.[72:14]

Neuman's model also reflects general systems theory, that is, the nature of living open systems.[7] This theory states that all the elements are in interaction in a complex organization.[73:3] From Caplan's conceptual model for levels of prevention, Neuman relates these prevention levels to nursing in the following manner: Primary prevention involves counteracting harmful environmental stressors before occurrence of illness.[17:26] Secondary prevention attempts to reduce the effect or possible effect of stressors through early diagnostic and effective treatment of illness symptoms. Tertiary prevention attempts to reduce the residual stressor effects after treatment.[17:113] The Neuman Systems Model is a synthesis of knowledge from several science disciplines and also incorporates Neuman's philosophic beliefs and earlier clinical nursing experience, particularly in mental health nursing.[26:36]

USE OF EMPIRICAL EVIDENCE

Neuman conceptualized the model from sound theories rather than from nursing research. She evaluated the utility of the model by submitting a tool to her nursing students who were beginning their master's program. The outcome data were published in the Spring 1972 issue of *Nursing Research.* Because the tool was for student evaluation rather than statistical evidence, the model originally lacked empirical support. Recent research, however, has produced considerable empirical evidence in support of the Neuman Systems Model. A research survey identified nearly 100 studies conducted between 1989 and 1993 for which the model provided the organizing framework.[57:475]

MAJOR CONCEPTS & DEFINITIONS

The major concepts identified in the model (Fig. 19-1) are wholistic client approach, open system, basic structure, environment, created environment, stressors, lines of defense and resistance, degree of reaction, prevention as intervention, and reconstitution.[73] Neuman's second edition included further development of the concepts of scholastic approach, content, process, input and output, feedback, negentropy, entropy, stability, wellness, and illness.[69,77,81]

Wholistic Client Approach The Neuman Systems Model is a dynamic, open, systems approach to client care originally developed to provide a unifying focus for nursing problem definition and for best understanding the client in interaction with the environment. The client as a system may be defined as a person, family, group, community, or issue.[77]

Wholistic Concept Clients are viewed as wholes whose parts are in dynamic interaction. The model considers all variables simultaneously affecting the client system: physiological, psychological, sociocultural, developmental, and spiritual. Neuman included the spiritual variable in the second book edition.[77] She changed the spelling of the term *holistic* to *wholisitc* in the second edition to enhance

understanding of the term as referring to the whole person.[77]

Open System A system is open when its elements are exchanging information energy within its complex organization. Stress and reaction to stress are basic components of an open system.[77]

Environment Internal and external forces affecting and being affected by the client at any time comprise the environment.[77]

Created Environment The created environment is the client's unconscious mobilization of all system variables toward system integration, stability, and integrity.[11:2;27:175]

Content The five variables (physiological, psychological, sociocultural, developmental, and spiritual) of man in interaction with the environment comprise the whole system of the client.[77]

Basic Structure "The basic structure consists of all variables as survival factors common to man, as well as unique individual characteristics."[77] The inner circle of the diagram (see Fig. 19-1) represents the basic survival factors or energy resources of the client.

Process or Function "The exchange of matter, energy, and information with the environment and the interaction of the parts and sub-parts of the

Continued

MAJOR CONCEPTS & DEFINITIONS—cont'd

system of man. A living system tends to move toward wholeness, stability, wellness, and negentropy."[77]

Input and Output "The matter, energy, and information exchanged between man and environment, which is entering or leaving the system at any point in time."[77]

Feedback "The process within which the matter, energy, and information, as system output, provides feedback for corrective action to change, enhance, or stabilize the system."[77]

Negentropy A process of energy utilization that assists system progression toward stability or wellness.[77]

Entropy A process of energy depletion and disorganization that moves the system toward illness or possible death.[77,88]

Stability The client or a system successfully copes with stressors; it is able to maintain an adequate level of health. Functional harmony or balance preserves the integrity of the system.[77]

Stressors Stressors are environmental forces that may alter system stability. Neuman[73:14] views stressors as:

1. Intrapersonal forces occurring within the individual (e.g., conditioned responses).
2. Interpersonal forces occurring between one or more individuals (e.g., role expectations).
3. Extrapersonal forces occurring outside the individual (e.g., financial circumstances).

Stressors are "stimuli which might penetrate both the client's flexible and normal lines of defense; the potential outcome of an interaction with a stressor may be beneficial (positive) or noxious (negative)."[27:176;77]

Wellness Wellness exists when the parts of the client system interact in harmony. System needs are met.[77,81]

Illness Disharmony among the parts of the system is considered illness in varying degrees reflecting unmet needs.[77,81]

Normal Line of Defense The normal line of defense is the model's outer solid circle. It represents a stability state for the individual, system, or the condition following adjustment made to stressors and maintained over time that is considered uniquely normal.[81]

"This is a result or composite of several variables and behaviors such as the individual's usual coping patterns, lifestyle, and developmental stage; it is basically the way in which an individual copes with stressors while functioning within the cultural pattern of birth and to which he attempts to conform."[73:15;81]

Flexible Lines of Defense The model's outer broken ring is called the flexible line of defense. It is dynamic and can be rapidly altered over a short time. It is perceived as a protective buffer for preventing stressors from breaking through the solid line of defense. The relationship of the variables (physiological, psychological, sociocultural, developmental, and spiritual)[77] can affect the degree to which individuals are able to use their flexible line of defense against possible reaction to a stressor or stressors, such as loss of sleep. It is important to strengthen this flexible line of defense to prevent a possible reaction.[73:15;81]

Lines of Resistance The series of broken rings surrounding the basic core structure are called the *lines of resistance*. These rings represent resource factors that help the client defend against a stressor. An example is the body's immune response system[73:15;81]

Degree of Reaction "The degree of reaction is the amount of system instability resulting from stressor invasion of the normal line of defense."[77]

Prevention as Intervention Interventions are purposeful actions to help the client retain, attain, and/or maintain system stability. They can occur before or after protective lines of defense and resistance are penetrated in both reaction and reconstitution phases. Neuman supports beginning inter-

MAJOR CONCEPTS & DEFINITIONS—cont'd

vention when a stressor is either suspected or identified.[73:15] Interventions are based on possible or actual degree of reaction, resources, goals, and the anticipated outcome. Neuman identifies three levels of intervention—primary, secondary, and tertiary.

Primary prevention Primary prevention is carried out when a stressor is suspected or identified. A reaction has not yet occurred, but the degree of risk is known. Neuman[73:15] states, "The actor or intervener would perhaps attempt to reduce the possibility of the individual's encounter with the stressor or in some way attempt to strengthen the individual's encounter with the stressor or attempt to strengthen the individual's flexible line of defense to decrease the possibility of a reaction."

Secondary prevention Secondary prevention involves interventions or treatment initiated after symptoms from stress have occurred. Both the client's internal and external resources would be used toward system stabilization to strengthen in-

ternal lines of resistance, reduce the reaction, and increase resistance factors.[73:15]

Tertiary prevention Tertiary prevention occurs after the active treatment or secondary prevention stage. It focuses on readjustment toward optimal client system stability. A primary goal is to strengthen resistance to stressors by reduction to help prevent recurrence of reaction or regression. This process leads back in a circular fashion toward primary prevention. An example would be avoidance of stressors known to be hazardous to the client.[73:16;81]

Reconstitution Reconstitution is the state of adaptation to stressors in the internal and external environment.[73:17] It can begin at any degree or level of reaction and may progress beyond or stabilize somewhat below the client's previous normal line of defense. Included in reconstitution are interpersonal, intrapersonal, extrapersonal, and environmental factors interrelated with client system physiological, psychological, sociocultural, developmental, and spiritual variables.[73:13;77]

MAJOR ASSUMPTIONS

Nursing

Neuman believes nursing is concerned with the whole person. She views nursing as a "unique profession in that it is concerned with all of the variables affecting an individual's response to stress."[73:14] Because the nurse's perception influences the care given, Neuman states that the caregiver's, as well as the client's, perceptual field must be assessed. She has developed an assessment and intervention tool to help with this task.

Person

The Neuman Systems Model presents the concept of person as a client/client system that may be an individual, family, group, community, or social issue. The client system is a dynamic composite of inter-

relationships among physiological, psychological, sociocultural, developmental, and spiritual factors. The client system is viewed as being in constant change or motion and is seen as an open system in reciprocal interaction with the environment.[27:172;30:225;73:9]

Health

Neuman considers her work as a wellness model. She views health as a continuum of wellness to illness that is dynamic in nature and constantly subject to change. "Optimal wellness or stability indicates that total system needs are being met. A reduced state of wellness is the result of unmet system needs. The client is in a dynamic state of either wellness or illness, in varying degrees, at any given point in time."[83:46]

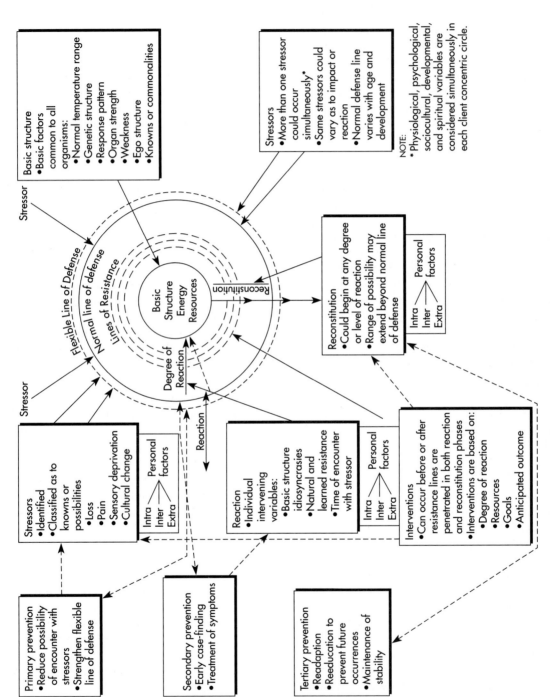

Fig. **19-1** The Neuman Systems Model. *Original copyright 1970, © by Betty Neuman. Used with permission.*

Environment

Environment and man are identified as the basic phenomena of the Neuman Systems Model, with the relationship between environment and man being reciprocal. Environment is defined as being all the internal and external factors that surround or interact with man/client. Significant to the concept of environment are stressors (intrapersonal, interpersonal, extrapersonal), which are identified as environmental forces that interact with and potentially alter system stability. Neuman has identified three relevant environments: internal, external, and created. Internal environment is intrapersonal with all interaction contained within the client. External environment is interpersonal or extrapersonal with all interactions occurring outside the client. Created environment is primarily intrapersonal but also encompasses the external environment and is subconsciously developed by the client as a "symbolic expression of system wholeness." Internal and external environments are both superseded by and contained within the created environment. The created environment mobilizes all system variables toward maintenance of client system integrity and stability. It is inherently purposeful as it acts to provide a protective, safe reservoir or arena for the client system. The created environment is in perpetual adjustment to an increase or decrease in the wellness state of the client.[12:2;27:175;83:31]

THEORETICAL ASSERTIONS

Theoretical assertions are the relationships among the essential concepts of a model.[89,109] The Neuman model depicts the nurse as an active participant with the client and as "concerned with all the variables affecting an individual's response to stressors."[73:14] The client is in a reciprocal relationship with the environment in that "he interacts with this environment by adjusting himself to it or adjusting it to himself."[73:14] Neuman links the four essential concepts of person, environment, health, and nursing in her statements regarding primary, secondary, and tertiary prevention. Earlier publications by Neuman stated basic assumptions that linked essential concepts of the model. These statements, listed in Box 19-1, have also been identified as propositions and

serve to define, describe, and link the concepts of the model.

LOGICAL FORM

Neuman used both deductive and inductive logic in developing her model. As previously discussed, Neuman derived her model from other theories and disciplines. The model is also a product of her philosophy and observations made in teaching mental health nursing and clinical counseling.[31:36]

ACCEPTANCE BY THE NURSING COMMUNITY

Neuman's model has been described by Walker and Avant as a grand nursing theory.[110:4] A grand theory consists of a global conceptual framework that defines broad perspectives for practice and includes diverse ways of viewing nursing phenomena based on these perspectives. As a grand theory, the Neuman Systems Model provides a comprehensive foundation for scientific nursing practice, education, and research.

The Neuman model has attained acceptance throughout the world and provides an ideal framework for health initiatives to address the World Health Organization goal of "Health for All by the Year 2000." The model is used throughout the United States and in Canada, Costa Rica, The Republic of China, Taiwan, Korea, Japan, Sweden, Finland, Wales, England, Denmark, Portugal, Spain, Ghana, Egypt, Australia, Puerto Rico, Iceland, Yugoslavia, New Zealand, and Brazil. As an example, the model has recently been used for structuring the World Health Organization Collaborative Center for Primary Health Care Nursing in Maribor, Yugoslavia (Slovenia).[82:688]

The model has been adapted equally well to all levels of nursing education and to a wide variety of practice areas. It adapts well transculturally and is used extensively for public health nursing in other countries. The model is the most widely accepted model for community health nursing in the United States and Canada.[60]

Ongoing development and universal appeal of the model are reflected in the biennial International Sym-

Box 19-1

Basic assumptions of the Neuman Systems Model

1. Although each individual client or group as a client system is unique, each system is a composite of common known factors or innate characteristics within a normal, given range of response contained within a basic structure.

2. Many known, unknown, and universal environmental stressors exist. Each differs in its potential for disturbing a client's usual stability level, or normal line of defense. The particular interrelationships of client variables—physiological, psychological, sociocultural, developmental, and spiritual—at any point in time can affect the degree to which a client is protected by the flexible line of defense against possible reaction to a single stressor or a combination of stressors.

3. Each individual client/client system has evolved a normal range of response to the environment that is referred to as a normal line of defense, or usual wellness/stability state. The normal line of defense can be used as a standard from which to measure health deviation.

4. When the cushioning, accordian-like effect of the flexible line of defense is no longer capable of protecting the client/client system against an environmental stressor, the stressor breaks through the normal line of defense. The interrelationships of variables—physiological, psychological, sociocultural, developmental, and spiritual—determine the nature and degree of system reaction or possible reaction to the stressor.

5. The client, whether in a state of wellness or illness, is a dynamic composite of the interrelationships of variables—physiological, psychological, sociocultural, developmental, and spiritual. Wellness is on a continuum of available energy to support the system in an optimal state of system stability.

6. Implicit within each client system are internal resistance factors known as lines of resistance, which function to stabilize and return the client to the usual wellness state (normal line of defense) or possibly to a higher level of stability following an environmental stressor reaction.

7. Primary prevention relates to general knowledge that is applied in client assessment and intervention in identification and reduction or mitigation of possible or actual risk factors associated with environmental stressors to prevent possible reaction. The goal of health promotion is included in primary prevention.

8. Secondary prevention relates to symptomatology following a reaction to stressors, appropriate ranking of intervention priorities, and treatment to reduce their noxious effects.

9. Tertiary prevention relates to the adjustive processes taking place as reconstitution begins and maintenance factors move the client back in a circular manner toward primary prevention.

10. The client as a system is in dynamic, constant energy exchange with the environment.

From Neuman, B. (1995). *The Neuman Systems Model* (3rd ed.). Norwalk, CT: Appleton & Lange, pp. 20-21. Copyright 1995 by Appleton & Lange; used with permission.

posia of the Neuman Systems Model. The first symposium was held at Neumann College in Aston, Pennsylvania (1986).[67,69,76] Subsequent symposia have been held in Kansas City (1988), Dayton, Ohio (1990), Rochester, New York (1993), Orlando, Florida (1995), and Boston (1997).* Each symposium shows increased participation from other countries.

Practice

The Neuman Systems Model has broad relevance for current and future nursing practice. Use of the model by nurses facilitates goal-directed, unified, wholistic approaches to client care. Yet it is also appropriate for interdisciplinary use to prevent fragmentation of client care. The model delineates a client system and classification of stressors that can be understood and used by all members of the health care team.[70:140] Other health disciplines are increasingly finding the work beneficial.

Neuman has developed several instruments to facilitate use of the model. These instruments include an assessment/intervention tool to assist nurses in collecting and synthesizing client data,[5:291-297] a format for prevention as intervention,[5:300] and a format for application of the nursing process within the framework of the Neuman Systems Model.[5:298-299] The Neuman Nursing Process Format comprises these three steps: nursing diagnosis, nursing goals, and nursing outcomes.[5:298-300] Nursing diagnosis consists of obtaining a broad, comprehensive database from which variances from wellness can be determined. Goals are then established by negotiation with the client for desired prescriptive changes to correct variances from wellness. Nursing outcomes are determined by nursing intervention through use of one or more of the three prevention-as-intervention modes. Evaluation then takes place either to confirm the desired outcome goals or to reformulate subsequent nursing goals.

Fawcett has incorporated Neuman's Nursing Process Format and Prevention as Intervention Format into an outline (Box 19-2) to illustrate steps of the nursing process based on the Neuman Systems Model.

The breadth of the Neuman model has resulted in its application and adaptation in a variety of nursing practice settings with individuals, families, groups, and communities. Numerous examples are cited in Neuman's books.[73,78,83] The model has been used successfully with clients in many settings, including hospitals, nursing homes, rehabilitation centers, hospices, and childbirth centers.* The model was selected for a comprehensive community nursing center[1] in Rochester, New York, because of the approach to client-centered care and also because of its proven strengths as a model for community practice.[16:1;60]

The model's systems perspective makes it particularly applicable for clients experiencing complex multidimensional stressors. Schlentz[100] applied the model as the organizing framework to plan care at primary, secondary, and tertiary levels for clients in a long-term care facility. Lile, Pase, Hoffman, and Mace[55] used the model as a wholistic approach to meet the needs of clients with multifaceted health problems including pressure ulcers. They described identification and management of stressors at the levels of primary (e.g., limited mobility), secondary (e.g., incontinence), and tertiary (e.g., reeducation of caregivers) prevention as intervention.

Neuman's model enables nurses to assess and care for the family unit as a client. Goldblum-Graff and Graff[41:217] adapted the model to family therapy. Issel[48] used it as the theoretical framework for a comprehensive case management program for obstetrical client families. Reed[92] used the model to describe the family as a client system based on clinical data and the experiences of practicing family nurses. Picton[90] used the model with emergency care clients to assist nurses to view clients wholistically as part of a family system. Bullock[13] used the model to enable obstetrical nurses to understand the effects of battering to improve the health of mothers and newborns.

The Neuman Systems Model is used in practice with groups and in public health nursing. Bowman[10:324] used it in the assessment of children's day

---

Box 19-2

The Neuman Systems Model: nursing process format

I. Nursing diagnosis
   A. Establish database that includes the simultaneous consideration of the dynamic interactions of physiological, psychological, sociocultural, developmental, and spiritual variables.
      1. Identify client/client system's perceptions
         a. Assess condition and strength of basic structure factors and energy resources
         b. Assess characteristics of the flexible and normal lines of defense, lines of resistance, degree of potential or actual reaction, and potential for reconstitution following a reaction
         c. Assess internal and external environments
            (1) Identify and evaluate potential or actual stressors that pose a threat to the stability of the client/client system
            (2) Classify stressors that threaten stability of client/client system
               (a) Deprivation
               (b) Excess
               (c) Change
               (d) Intolerance
         d. Identify, classify, and evaluate potential and/or actual intrapersonal, interpersonal, and extrapersonal interactions between the client/client system and the environment, considering all five variables
         e. Assess the created environment
            (1) Discover the nature of client/client system's created environment
               (a) Assess client/client system's perception of stressors
               (b) Identify client/client system's major problem, stress areas, or areas of concern
               (c) Identify client/client system's perception of how present circumstances differ from usual pattern of living
               (d) Identify ways in which client/client system handled similar problems in the past
               (e) Identify what client/client system anticipates for self in the future as a consequence of the present situation
               (f) Determine what client/client system is doing and what he or she can do to help himself or herself
               (g) Determine what client/client system expects caregivers, family, friends, or others to do for him or her
            (2) Determine degree of protection provided
            (3) Uncover cause of client/client system's created environment
         f. Evaluate influence of past, present, and possible future life process and coping patterns on client/client system stability
         g. Identify and evaluate actual and potential internal and external resources for optimal state of wellness
      2. Identify caregiver's perceptions (repeat 1 a, b, c, d, e, f, g from caregiver's perspective)
      3. Compare client/client system's and caregiver's perceptions
         a. Identify similarities and differences in perceptions

Box 19-2

The Neuman Systems Model: nursing process format—cont'd

      b. Facilitate client awareness of major perceptual distortions

      c. Resolve perceptual differences

  B. Variances from wellness

    1. Synthesize client database with relevant theories from nursing and adjunctive disciplines

    2. State a comprehensive nursing diagnosis

    3. Prioritize goals

      a. Consider client/client system wellness level

      b. Consider system stability needs

      c. Consider total available resources

    4. Postulate outcome goals and interventions that will facilitate the highest possible level of client/client system stability or wellness (i.e., maintain the normal line of defense and retain the flexible line of defense)

II. Nursing goals

  A. Negotiate desired prescriptive changes or outcome goals to correct variances from wellness with the client/client system

    1. Consider needs identified in I.B.3.b.

    2. Consider resources identified in I.B.3.c.

  B. Negotiate prevention as intervention modalities and actions with client/client system

III. Nursing outcomes

  A. Implement nursing interventions through use of one or more of three prevention modalities

    1. Primary prevention nursing action to retain system stability

      a. Prevent stressor invasion

      b. Provide information to retain or strengthen existing client/client system strengths

      c. Support positive coping and functioning

      d. Desensitize existing or possible noxious stressors

      e. Motivate toward wellness

      f. Coordinate and integrate interdisciplinary theories and epidemiological input

      g. Educate or reeducate

      h. Use stress as a positive intervention strategy

    2. Secondary prevention nursing actions to attain system stability

      a. Protect basic structure

      b. Mobilize and optimize internal/external resources to attain stability and energy conservation

      c. Facilitate purposeful manipulation of stressors and reactions to stressors

      d. Motivate, educate, and involve client/client system in health care goals

      e. Facilitate appropriate treatment and intervention measures

      f. Support positive factors toward wellness

      g. Promote advocacy by coordination and integration

      h. Provide primary prevention intervention as required

    3. Tertiary prevention nursing actions to maintain system stability

      a. Attain and maintain highest possible level of wellness and stability during reconstitution

Continued

Box 19-2

The Neuman Systems Model: nursing process format—cont'd

      b. Educate, reeducate, and/or reorient as needed

      c. Support client/client system toward appropriate goals

      d. Coordinate and integrate health service resources

      e. Provide primary and/or secondary preventive intervention as required

  B. Evaluate outcome goals

    1. Confirm attainment of outcome goals

    2. Reformulate goals

  C. Set intermediate and long-range goals for subsequent nursing action that are structured in relation to short-term goal outcomes

---

care centers. Anderson, McFarland, and Helton[1:220] adapted the model to develop a community health needs assessment in which the authors identified violence toward women as a major community health concern. Three Canadian provinces (Manitoba, Ontario, and Alberta) have accepted the model as the criteria on which to base their public health activities.

The Neuman Systems Model is used to promote advanced practice nursing. Russell and Hezel[98] applied it as the framework for role analysis of the clinical nurse specialist. Dwyer, Walker, Suchman, and Coggiola[24] used it as the basis for a collaborative practice by nurse practitioners and physicians at the University of Rochester community nursing center. Walker[112] described the quality and cost-effectiveness of care provided by advanced practice nurses using the model in a community nursing center.

The Neuman Systems Model is used equally well with clients as individuals, groups, or communities and the same principles apply for all. Its comprehensive systemic nature has allowed for a wide variety of clinical practice, research, and administrative applications worldwide.

Education

The model has also been well accepted in academic circles and is widely used as a curriculum guide oriented toward wellness. It is used at all levels of nursing education throughout the United States and in other countries, including Australia, Canada, Denmark, England, Korea, Kuwait, Portugal, and Taiwan.[5:301-302;47;54;71;84]

Its wholistic perspective provides an effective framework for education of generic nursing students from diploma, associate, and baccalaureate programs. Lowry and Newsome[64] reported on a study of 12 associate degree programs that use the model as a conceptual framework for curriculum development. Results indicated that graduates use the model most often in the roles of teacher and care provider and that they tend to continue practice from a Neuman Systems Model–based perspective following graduation.

Neuman's model has been selected for baccalaureate programs on the basis of its theoretical and comprehensive perspectives for a wholistic curriculum and its potential for use with the individual, family, small groups, and community. Neumann College Division of Nursing was the first school to select the Neuman Systems Model as its conceptual base for its curriculum and approach to client care in 1976. The faculty has developed an assessment/intervention tool based on Neuman's framework and clinical evaluation tools based on Neuman's model and Bondy's Evaluation Format. Mirenda[69] has formulated a set of questions related to graduates' perceptions and continued use of the model. The University of Pittsburgh in Pennsylvania had one of the first baccalaureate nursing programs to implement the model in an integrated curriculum.[52:117; 77] The model has been used at Lander University in Greenwood, South Carolina, as the framework for baccalaureate nursing education since 1987.[34] Its selection by the faculty was based on its wholistic perspective and its potential for use with community aggregate populations. The model is used as a comprehensive framework to organize data collected from maternity clients by undergraduate nursing students at the University of South Florida.[60] At the University of Texas–Tyler, the model is used as the unifying construct for the Bachelor of Science in Nursing program. Neuman's levels of prevention as intervention are used to level content throughout courses across the curriculum.[51] The Minnesota Intercollegiate Nursing Consortium (MINC), composed of three private church-related colleges, has developed a cooperative baccalaureate nursing program that used the Neuman Systems Model as its organizing curriculum framework. MINC faculty have engaged in evaluation over time of the utility of the model, affirming its value.[39]

The model has demonstrated its effectiveness in supporting the conceptual transition among levels of nursing education. Hilton and Grafton[44] discussed its application as the framework for the transition from diploma to associate degree education at the Los Angeles County Medical Center School of Nursing. Sipple and Freese[103] described the transition from associate degree to Neuman Systems Model–based baccalaureate education at Lander College in Greenwood, South Carolina. At the University of Tennessee at Martin, the model provided the curriculum framework for a Bachelor of Science in Nursing degree program initiated in 1988; Strickland-Seng[106] described its use as the basis for clinical evaluation of students in the new Bachelor of Science in Nursing degree program.

The Neuman Systems Model has been used effectively in post–basic nursing education and beyond. Bunn[14] described the development and implementation of a community mental health nursing course based on Canadian health care principles for registered nurses enrolled in a Bachelor of Science in Nursing program at the University of Ottawa. The model enabled students to study selected client populations (e.g., elderly Chinese) as a high-risk aggregate and to plan culturally relevant health prevention

activities at primary, secondary, and tertiary levels. At Northwestern State University in Shreveport, Louisiana, the faculty determined that a systems model approach was preferred for their master's program because of the universality of its application. They chose to adapt the Neuman model for their master's clinician program, with the clinician's major role being one of mediator between stressors and the various lines of defense and the resistance of the client as a system.[31:168-169]

Interdisciplinary use of the model continues to grow in health education; for example, it is currently being implemented beyond nursing in Kuwait and Jordan.[84] The model's emphasis on wholism, systems, prevention, and wellness prompted the Commission on Accreditation in Physical Therapy Education (CAPTE) to adapt it to conceptualize sections of the CAPTE evaluative criteria that address the organization and resources required for a physical therapy program.[108]

The model's inclusion of both client perception and nurse perception makes it particularly relevant for teaching culture concepts. The model is used at California State University, Fresno, to study the significance of culture and how culture influences each of the five client system variables.[105] Bloch and Bloch[9] described a format that uses the model to assist students to assess clients and provide culturally appropriate care across cultural barriers.

The Neuman Systems Model is used to provide the conceptual framework for multiple levels of nursing and health-related curricula around the world. Acceptance by the nursing community is clearly evident.

Research

For nursing to advance as a scientific discipline, testing of the efficacy and usefulness of nursing models through controlled research is imperative. Research on the components of the model for additional explication and generation of testable nursing theories through research are examples of the Neuman model's potential contribution to research activity and nursing knowledge.[28;29:461-470;70:139] Rules for Neuman Systems Model–based nursing research have been specified by Fawcett, a Neuman model trustee, based on the content of the model and related literature.[85:67]

Neuman reports that her model is one of the three most frequently used models for nursing research.[80,85] Increasing empirical use of the model is evident from research conducted in the nursing community. Louis and Koertvelyessy[59] conducted an international survey study in 1987 on the use of the Neuman model for nursing student research projects; they reported a total of 42 studies completed or in process. Abstracts of these studies are presented in the second edition of *The Neuman Systems Model*.[78]

Review of subsequently published research studies identified over 100 studies in which the Neuman Systems Model served as the organizing framework.[57,84] Studies conducted between 1989 and 1993 that used the model are listed in the third edition of *The Neuman Systems Model*.[57:490-495]

In research published since 1993 regarding the effects of using the Neuman model in practice, Beynon[8] reported that knowledge and experience by Canadian nurse managers in applying the model in practice had a positive impact on the nurse managers' attitudes. However, Mackenzie and Spence-Laschinger[65] examined the effect of experience with Neuman-based practice on the number and quality of nursing diagnoses generated by public health nurses and found that Neuman-based practice did not have a significant effect.

The model has been used extensively to guide research to enhance the nursing care of clients with specific physiological stressors. Flannery[33] reported a study using the model as a framework to adapt a cognitive functioning assessment tool for patients with traumatic brain injury; the purpose is to provide a tool for planning appropriate nursing care. Lowry and Anderson[62] conducted a pilot study in which mechanical ventilation was viewed as an extrapersonal stressor. The researchers studied how client variables were influenced by ventilation and the weaning process; they found that the ventilator itself was perceived as a stressor at the point of intubation but that over time it became part of the client's created environment as it relieved the work of breathing. Maligalig[66] studied the perceptions of stressors by parents whose children experience outpatient surgery and recommended nursing practice changes to help decrease stressors.

Rodrigues-Fisher, Bourguignon, and Good[93] used the model to study the effectiveness of dietary fiber in preventing constipation in older adults. Results identified nursing measures to strengthen the older adult client's normal line of defense to prevent constipation through the use of fiber and fluids. Waddell and Demi[110] used the model to study the effectiveness of a partial hospitalization program for clients with anxiety disorders; results indicated that the program was successful.

At the University of Portland, Oregon, international summer master's degree program, 75% of students used the Neuman Systems Model for their theses. Significant research is occurring on the model at the University of Alabama master's degree and doctoral level nursing programs.[81]

The biennial Neuman Systems Model Symposia provide a forum for presentation of research (completed and in progress) using the model. Extensive research projects were reported at the Fourth (1993) and Fifth (1995) Symposia. Nine studies were reported on health issues of the elderly.* Five studies were reported on perinatal nursing;[15,35,63,91,113] three, on women's health issues.[50,53,97] Two adult health studies,[18,32] two cardiac-related studies,[40,46] and one study of nurses' attitudes toward the terminally ill[42] were reported. Research was reported on the use of the model in nursing education[6,87] and in program evaluation.[20] Following identification of the spiritual variable as an area for further development,[5:279] two studies on this component of the model were reported.[36,38]

Most nursing models have not been researched adequately to establish their validity. Although the Neuman Systems Model has proved itself empirically, additional research is indicated to validate the lines of defense and of resistance.[84] Further research is also indicated regarding the spiritual variable, vulnerable aggregate client populations, using the model to provide culturally sensitive nursing care across cultural barriers,[84] and development and evaluation of primary prevention programs.[75-77]

*References 4, 19, 21, 43, 58, 61, 95, 100, and 101.

Fawcett[30] has set forth guidelines for research studies based on the Neuman Systems Model. Results of such studies will increase understanding of effectivenes of the model in enhancing client system stability.

FURTHER DEVELOPMENT

A conceptual model identifies relevant phenomena and describes the interrelationships in general and abstract terms, representing the initial step in the development of theoretical statements.[31:39] In 1983 the Neuman Systems Model was described as being at a very early stage of theory development.[111:142] However, findings from Louis and Koertvelyessy's 1987 study[59] and from subsequent research support increasing utility of the model for theory development in nursing.[12;29:242]

The model diagram has remained unchanged because of continuous positive feedback to Neuman on its completeness. The breadth of the model appeals to those in nursing because it allows for much creativity within its structure.[81]

Two areas identified for further development and clarification are Neuman's concept of health and her view of the relationship between client and environment.[30,77] Fawcett[30:238] suggests clarification of the concept of health by identification of wellness and illness as polar ends of a continuum rather than as dichotomous conditions. Further, Fawcett[30:238] states that viewing client-environment interactions as a dynamic equilibrium, as a steady state, and as homeostasis is logically incompatible and that Neuman should specify which view best represents her conceptualization of client-environment interaction.

Earlier evaluation of the model stated that two components needed further development—the spiritual variable and the created environment.[5:279] The spiritual variable is viewed by Neuman as an innate component of the basic structure; consideration of the spiritual variable is necessary for a wholistic perspective and caring concern for the client.[83:28-29] Description of the spiritual variable was expanded significantly in *The Neuman Systems Model,* third edition,[22,37] and is being researched.[36,38]

The created environment represents the client's unconsciously developed expression of system wholeness. It is dynamic in nature and pervades all client variables. The created environment provides an insulating effect to enable the client to cope with the threat of environmental stressors by changing the self and/or the situation. Examples are the use of denial (psychological variable) and life-cycle continuation of survival patterns (developmental variable).[83:30-31]

Future validity of the model depends on development and testing of middle-range theory from it. Neuman and Koertvelyessy[30:242] have identified two theories being generated from the model: the Theory of Optimal Client System Stability and the Theory of Prevention as Intervention. Breckenridge[12] has described use of the model to develop middle-range theory through research based on practice with nephrology clients.

The model is being used and studied in other disciplines, for example, physical therapy.[5:279;108] Further research is taking place to validate its applicability beyond nursing.

A Neuman Systems Model Trustee Group has been established to preserve, protect, and perpetuate the integrity of the model for the future of nursing. Its international members, personally selected by Neuman, are dedicated professionals.[77] The home of the Neuman Archives has been established at Neumann College Library at Aston, Pennsylvania.[68,69] Smith and Edgil[104] have proposed creation of an Institute for the Study of the Neuman Systems Model to formulate and test theories within the model. A web site has been placed on the Internet.

CRITIQUE

Neuman developed a comprehensive nursing conceptual model that operationalizes systems concepts for nursing relevant to the breadth of nursing phenomena. It should also remain relevant to future nursing needs as identified by the American Nurses Association and the World Health Organization. The model's wholistic perspective allows for a wide range of nurse creativity in its use. Neuman's own critique notes that prior criticisms, such as "its concepts are too broad," have been discounted. The model is congruent with the general trend toward wholistic systemic thinking in nursing. Its comprehensive and flexible nature will allow for future structuring of all nursing activities "as it has proven to do in the past."[81]

Clarity

Neuman presents abstract concepts that are familiar to nursing. The model's concepts of client, environment, health, and nursing are congruent with traditional values. Concepts defined by Neuman and those borrowed from other disciplines are used consistently throughout the model.

Simplicity

Multiple interactions and interrelationships comprise this broad systems-based model; they are organized in a complex yet logical manner, and variables tend to overlap to some degree. The concepts coalesce, but a loss of theoretical meaning would occur if they were completely separated. Neuman states that the concepts can be separated for analysis, specific goal setting, and interventions.[77] The model can be used to delineate further the systems concept for nursing and also to describe various other health care systems. It can be used to explain the client's dynamic state of equilibrium and the reaction or possible reaction to stressors. Using the prevention concept within the framework, one can predict the origin of stressors. The model can be used to describe, explain, or predict nursing phenomena. Because of the complex nature of the model, it cannot be described as a simple framework, yet nurses using the model describe it as easy to understand and to use across cultures and in a wide variety of settings.

Generality

The Neuman Systems Model has been used in a wide variety of nursing situations; it is readily adaptable and comprehensive enough to be useful in all health care settings, including administration and research. Other related health fields can use this framework because of its systemic nature and its emphasis on the client system as a whole. The social goals and utility of the model—for example, wholistic care, prevention, and systems concepts—are congruent with present social values.

Some concepts are broad and represent the phenomena of one person as client or a larger system, and others are more definitive and identify specific modes of action, such as primary prevention. The subgoals can be identified as broad nursing actions. Because of the broad scope of this model, it can be considered general enough to be useful to nurses and other health care professionals in working with individuals, families/groups, or communities in all health care settings.

Empirical Precision

Although the model has not been completely tested to date, nursing scientists are demonstrating major interest in and use of the model to guide nursing research. Early work by Hoffman[45:49-53] described a list of variables and selected operational definitions that were derived from the model. Louis and Koertvelyessy's 1987 survey on the use of the model in nursing research and subsequent research reports provide further documentation of increasing empiricism with the model. Continued testing and refinement will increase the model's empirical precision as the research process, analysis, and synthesis of findings from multiple studies are completed.[59]

Derivable Consequences

Neuman's conceptual model provides the professional nurse with important guidelines for assessment of the client system, utilization of the nursing process, and implementation of preventive intervention. The focus on primary prevention and interdisciplinary care facilities improved quality of care and is futuristic. Active client participation and negotiation of nursing goals illustrated in the Neuman nursing process fulfill current health mandates.[81]

Another derivable consequence of the model is its potential to generate nursing theory, for example, the theories of optimal client stability and prevention as intervention.[30:242] The model concepts are relevant to twenty-first-century health professional trends. With continued theory development through research with the model, nursing can expand its scientific knowledge. According to Fawcett,[27:187;30:243-245] the model meets social considerations of congruence, significance, and utility. The model is broad and systemically based. It lends itself well to a comprehensive view within which nursing can be responsive to the world's rapidly changing health care needs.

The Neuman Systems Model provides an appropriate nursing framework and a comprehensive approach to contemporary and future goal phenomena and concerns facing nursing and health care delivery in the twenty-first century.[70:155] A letter written to Dr. Neuman in 1991 by a recently deceased Manitoba Trustee member, Linda Drew, appropriately draws closure to this chapter and yet shares a flavor of the excitement felt as the discipline and science of nursing advances toward the next century:

> In my opinion, the Neuman model is not only alive and well, but will have a very long shelf life because it is so adaptable and continues to provide a very pragmatic framework for dealing with a whole host of issues in nursing practice, education, administration and research. This along with the commitment of nurses and other health care providers to continue using this framework will guarantee a very healthy, exciting future for the model.[16:4;81]

CRITICAL THINKING *Activities*

1 Identify a group of clients who share one or more characteristics—for example, the clients in your practice. Use the Neuman Systems Model to analyze this target group as an aggregate community client. What common stressors do they experience? How are their responses similar? How are they different? What is the nurse's role in health retention, attainment, and maintenance for these clients?

2 Identify a client care situation in your practice that has been particularly challenging or problematic. Analyze this situation from the per-

spective of the Neuman Systems Model. Who is the client? Describe the physiological, psychological, sociocultural, spiritual, and developmental variables. Describe the lines of resistance and the normal and flexible lines of defense. What is the specific problem or issue in this situation? Explain the points of view of all persons involved. What would be the *ideal* outcome to this situation? How can you intervene to support this outcome? What would happen if you took no action?

3 Use the Neuman Systems Model to analyze a specific client family from a culture different from your own, with emphasis on the sociocultural variable. Describe the family's central core, the lines of resistance, the normal line of defense, and the flexible lines of defense. Describe the client family as a system within the greater environment. Identify the stressors (actual and potential). How does culture impact on the family's perception of stressors and its responses to them? Identify culturally appropriate prevention as intervention strategies for this family at primary, secondary, and tertiary levels. Identify health care strategies that are appropriate in your culture but might not be appropriate for this family from another culture. Explain why they might not be appropriate.

REFERENCES

1. Anderson, E., McFarland, J., & Helton, A. (1986). Community-as-client: A model for practice. *Nursing Outlook, 34*(5), 220-224.
2. Babcock, P. (1984, June 10). Telephone interview.
3. Baker, N.A. (1982). Use of the Neuman model in planning for the psychological needs of the respiratory disease patient. In B. Neuman (Ed.), *The Neuman systems model: Application to nursing education and practice* (pp. 241-256). Norwalk, CT: Appleton-Century-Crofts.
4. Barnes, K.M. (1993, April 23). *The relationship between mistreatment of the elderly, quality of care, and demographic characteristics.* Paper presented at the Fourth International Neuman Systems Model Symposium, Rochester, NY.
5. Beckman, S.J., Boxley-Harges, S., Bruick-Sorge, C., Harris, S.M., Hermiz, M.E., Meininger, M., & Steinkeler, S.E. (1994). Betty Neuman Systems Model. In A. Marriner-

Tomey (Ed.), *Nursing theorists and their work* (3rd ed., pp. 269-304). St. Louis: Mosby.

6. Beckman, S.J., & Bruick-Sorge, C. (1995, Feb. 3). *Replication study: The efficacy of the Neuman systems model for associate degree nursing curriculum development.* Paper presented at the Fifth International Neuman Systems Model Symposium, Orlando, FL.

7. Bertalanffy, L. von. (1968). *General systems theory.* New York: George Braziller.

8. Beynon, C. (1993). Theory-based practice: Attitudes of nursing managers before and after educational sessions. *Public Health Nursing, 10*(3), 183-188.

9. Bloch, C., & Bloch, C. (1995). Teaching content and process of the Neuman systems model. In B. Neuman (Ed.), *The Neuman systems model* (3rd ed., pp. 175-182). Norwalk, CT: Appleton & Lange.

10. Bowman, G. (1982). The Neuman assessment tool adapted for child day-care centers. In B. Neuman (Ed.), *The Neuman systems model: Application to nursing education and practice* (pp. 324-334). Norwalk, CT: Appleton-Century-Crofts.

11. Breckenridge, D. (1992). A brief update on the Neuman systems model. *Neuman News, 3*(1), 2.

12. Breckenridge, D.M. (1995). Nephrology practice and directions for nursing research. In B. Neuman (Ed.), *The Neuman systems model* (3rd ed., pp. 499-507). Norwalk, CT: Appleton & Lange.

13. Bullock, L.F. (1993). Nursing interventions for abused women on obstetrical units. *AWHONN's Clinical Issues in Perinatal and Women's Health Nursing, 4*(3), 371-377.

14. Bunn, H. (1995). Preparing nurses for the challenge of the new focus on community mental health nursing. *The Journal of Continuing Education in Nursing, 26*(2), 55-59.

15. Cagle, R.H., & Reeb, R. (1993, April 24). *Perinatal management using the Neuman systems model.* Paper presented at the Fourth International Neuman Systems Model Symposium, Rochester, NY.

16. Capers, C. (Ed.) (1992). The Neuman Trustee Group, Inc. *Neuman News, 3*(1), 1-8.

17. Caplan, G. (1964). *Principles of preventive psychiatry.* New York: Basic Books.

18. Cotton, N.C. (1993, April 23). *An interdisciplinary high risk assessment tool for rehabilitation (in patient) falls.* Paper presented at the Fourth International Neuman Systems Model Symposium, Rochester, NY.

19. Craig, D. (1993, April 23). *An interdisciplinary high risk assessment tool for older adults' use of nursing services, life stress, ways of coping and health, mood and energy for living.* Paper presented at the Fourth International Neuman Systems Model Symposium, Rochester, NY.

20. Craig, D., & Morris-Coulter, C. (1995, Feb. 3). *Exploring partnerships in model implementation.* Paper presented at the Fifth International Neuman Systems Model Symposium, Orlando, FL.

21. Craig, D., & Timmings, C. (1995, Feb. 3). *Health promotion for older adults: Does it make a difference?* Paper presented at the Fifth International Neuman Systems Model Symposium, Orlando, FL.

22. Curran, G. (1995). The Neuman systems model revisited. In B. Neuman (Ed.), *The Neuman systems model* (3rd ed., pp. 93-99). Norwalk, CT: Appleton & Lange.

23. Darland, W. (1986). Congenital adrenocortical hyperplasia: Supportive nursing interventions. *Journal of Pediatric Nursing, 1*(2):117-123.

24. Dwyer, C.M., Walker, P.H., Suchman, A., & Coggiola, P. (1995). Opportunities and obstacles: Development of a true collaborative practice with physicians. In B. Murphy (Ed.), *Nursing centers: The time is now* (pp. 134-55). NLN Pub. No. 41-2629. New York: National League for Nursing.

25. Echlin, J.D. (1982). Palliative care and the Neuman model. In B. Neuman (Ed.), *The Neuman systems model: Application to nursing education and practice* (pp. 257-259). Norwalk, CT: Appleton-Century-Crofts.

26. Fawcett, J. (1989). *Analysis and evaluation of conceptual models of nursing.* Philadelphia: F.A. Davis.

27. Fawcett, J. (1989). *Analysis and evaluation of conceptual models of nursing* (2nd ed., pp. 172-177). Philadelphia: F.A. Davis.

28. Fawcett, J. (1990, Nov. 15). Keynote address presented at the Third International Neuman Systems Model Symposium, Dayton, OH.

29. Fawcett, J. (1995). Constructing conceptual-theoretical-empirical structures for research. In B. Neuman (Ed.), The *Neuman systems model* (3rd ed., pp. 459-471). Norwalk, CT: Appleton & Lange.

30. Fawcett, J. (1995). *Neuman's systems model: Analysis and evaluation of conceptual models of nursing* (3rd ed., pp. 217-275). Philadelphia: F.A. Davis.

31. Fawcett, J., Carpenito, L.J., Efinger, J., Goldblum-Graff, D., Groesbeck, M., Lowry, L.W., McCreary, C.S., & Wolf, Z.R. (1982). A framework for analysis and evaluation of conceptual models of nursing with an analysis of the Neuman systems model. In B. Neuman (Ed.), *The Neuman systems model: Application to nursing education and practice* (pp. 30-43). Norwalk, CT: Appleton-Century-Crofts.

32. Flannery, J. (1995, Feb. 3). *Application of the Neuman systems model in combination with cognitive recovery theory to assess TBI patients.* Paper presented at the Fifth International Neuman Systems Model Symposium, Orlando, FL.

33. Flannery, J. (1995). Cognitive assessment in the acute care setting: Reliability and validity of the levels of cognitive function assessment scale (LOCFAS). *Journal of Nursing Measurement, 3*(1), 43-58.

34. Freese, B.T., & Lander University Faculty (1995, Feb. 3). *Application of the Neuman systems model to education: Baccalaureate workshop.* Paper presented at the Fifth International Neuman Systems Model Symposium, Orlando, FL.

35. Freese, B.T., & Speer, I. (1995, Feb. 3). Nurse-managed childbearing in the U.K. and U.S.A.: A cross-cultural comparative study. Paper presented at the Fifth International Neuman Systems Model Symposium, Orlando, FL.

36. Fulton, R.A.B. (1993, April 23). *Spiritual well-being of baccalaureate nursing students and nursing faculty and their responses about spiritual well-being of persons.* Paper presented at the Fourth International Neuman Systems Model Symposium, Rochester, NY.

37. Fulton, R.A.B. (1995). The spiritual variable: Essential to the client system. In B. Neuman (Ed.), *The Neuman systems model* (3rd ed., pp. 77-92). Norwalk, CT: Appleton & Lange.

38. Fulton, R.A.B., & Moore, C.M. (1995, Feb. 3). *Spiritual well-being of parents of children with asthma.* Paper presented at the Fifth International Neuman Systems Model Symposium, Orlando, FL.

39. Glazebrook, D.S. (1995). The Neuman systems model in cooperative baccalaureate nursing education; The Minnesota Intercollegiate Nursing Consortium experience. In B. Neuman (Ed.), *The Neuman systems model* (3rd ed., pp. 227-230). Norwalk, CT: Appleton & Lange.

40. Gloss, E.F., & Crowe, R.L. (1993, April 24). *Coronary artery disease: Postmenopausal women, power, and anxiety.* Paper presented at the Fourth International Neuman Systems Model Symposium, Rochester, NY.

41. Goldblum-Graff, D., & Graff, H. (1982). The Neuman model adapted to family therapy. In B. Neuman (Ed.), *The Neuman systems model: Application to nursing education and practice* (pp. 217-222). Norwalk, CT: Appleton-Century-Crofts.

42. Hainsworth, D.S., & Grimes, J. (1993, April 23). *Use of the Neuman model as a framework for research and educational intervention for nurses who care for terminally ill patients and their families.* Paper presented at the Fourth International Neuman Systems Model Symposium, Rochester, NY.

43. Hamilton, E.M., & Schwieterman, I. (1995, Feb. 3). *The Neuman systems model in research data integration.* Paper presented at the Fifth International Neuman Systems Model Symposium, Orlando, FL.

44. Hilton, S.A., & Grafton, M.D. (1995). Curriculum transition based on the Neuman systems model: Los Angeles County Medical Center School of Nursing. In B. Neuman (Ed.), *The Neuman systems model* (3rd ed., pp. 163-174). Norwalk, CT: Appleton & Lange.

45. Hoffman, M.K. (1982). From model to theory construction: An analysis of the Neuman health-care system model. In B. Neuman (Ed.), *The Neuman Systems Model: Application to nursing education and practice* (pp. 44-54). Norwalk, CT: Appleton-Century-Crofts.

46. Hui-Tseng, Ting (1993, April 24). *Cognition and anxiety level of pre-cardiac catheterization patients before and after an education program.* Paper presented at the Fourth International Neuman Systems Model Symposium, Rochester, NY.

47. Indiana University–Purdue University at Fort Wayne, Ind. (1983). *Behavioral objectives for the associate degree program.*

48. Issel, L.M. (1995). Evaluating case management programs. *MCN, 29,* 67-74.

49. Kiernan, B.S., & Scoloveno, M.A. (1986). Assessment of the neonate. *Topics in Clinical Nursing, 8*(1):1-10.

50. Klinek, S.C. (1995, Feb. 4). *Effect of knowledge, attitudes, and beliefs on breast self care behavior.* Paper presented at the Fifth International Neuman Systems Model Symposium, Orlando, FL.

51. Klotz, L.D. (1995). Integration of the Neuman systems model into the BNS curriculum at the University of Texas at Tyler. In B. Neuman (Ed.), *The Neuman systems model* (3rd ed., pp. 183-190). Norwalk, CT: Appleton & Lange.

52. Knox, J.E., Kilchenstein, L., & Yakulis, I.M. (1982). Utilization of the Neuman model in an integrated baccalaureate program: University of Pittsburgh. In B. Neuman (Ed.), *The Neuman systems model: Application to nursing education and practice* (pp. 117-124). Norwalk, CT: Appleton-Century-Crofts.

53. Lancaster, D.R. (1995, Feb. 4). *Coping with appraised breast cancer threat among women at increased risk: A mid-range theory of primary prevention.* Paper presented at the Fifth International Neuman Systems Model Symposium, Orlando, FL.

54. Lebold, M.M., & Davis, L.H. (1982). A baccalaureate nursing curriculum based on the Neuman systems model: Saint Xavier College. In B. Neuman (Ed.), *The Neuman systems model: Application to nursing education and practice* (pp. 124-129). Norwalk, CT: Appleton-Century-Crofts.

55. Lile, J.L., Pase, N.M., Hoffman, R.G., & Mace, M.K. (1994). The Neuman systems model as applied to the terminally ill client with pressure ulcers. *Advances in Wound Care, 7*(4), 44-48.

56. Louis, M. (1988, Jan. 10). Personal communication.

57. Louis, M. (1995). The Neuman model in nursing research: An update. In B. Neuman (Ed.), *The Neuman systems model* (3rd ed., pp. 473-495). Norwalk, CT: Appleton-Lange.

58. Louis, M. (1995, Feb. 3). *Preferred other relationships, perceived health, and quality of life of elders.* Paper presented at the Fifth International Neuman Systems Model Symposium, Orlando, FL.

59. Louis, M., & Koertvelyessy, A. (1989). Neuman model: Use in research. In B. Neuman (Ed.), *The Neuman systems model* (2nd ed, pp. 93-114). Norwalk, CT: Appleton & Lange.

60. Lowry, L. (1992, June 4). Personal communication.

61. Lowry, L. (1993, April 23). *Using the Neuman systems model to guide research.* Paper presented at the Fourth International Neuman Systems Model Symposium, Rochester, NY.

62. Lowry, L., & Anderson, B. (1993). Neuman's framework and ventilator dependency: A pilot study. *Nursing Science Quarterly, 6*(4), 195-199.

63. Lowry, L.W. (1995, Feb. 3). *Client satisfaction with prenatal care and pregnancy outcomes.* Paper presented at the Fifth International Neuman Systems Model Symposium, Orlando, FL.

64. Lowry, L.W., & Newsome, G.G. (1995). Neuman-based associate degree programs: Past, present, and future. In B. Neuman (Ed.), *The Neuman systems model* (3rd ed., pp. 197-214). Norwalk, CT: Appleton & Lange.

65. Mackenzie, S., & Spence-Laschinger, H.K. (1995). Correlates of nursing diagnosis quality in public health nursing. *Journal of Advanced Nursing, 21,* 800-808.

66. Maligalig, R.M.L. (1994). Parents' perceptions of the stressors of pediatric ambulatory surgery. *Journal of Post Anesthesia Nursing, 9*(5), 278-282.

67. Mirenda, R. (1988, Jan. 10). Personal communication.

68. Mirenda, R. (1992, March 17). Personal communication.

69. Mirenda, R. (1992, June 16). Personal communication.

70. Mirenda, R.M. (1986). The Neuman systems model: Description and application. In P. Winstead-Fry (Ed.), *Case studies in nursing theory* (pp. 127-167). New York: National League for Nursing.

71. Moxley, P.A., & Allen, M.H. (1982). The Neuman systems model approach in a master's degree program: Northwestern State University. In B. Neuman (Ed.), *The Neuman systems model: Application to nursing education and practice* (pp. 168-175). Norwalk, CT: Appleton-Century-Crofts.

72. Neuman, B. (1977, Jan. 17). *An explanation of the Betty Neuman nursing model.* Paper presented at Indiana University-Purdue University at Fort Wayne, IN.

73. Neuman, B. (1982). *The Neuman systems model: Application to nursing education and practice.* Norwalk, CT: Appleton-Century-Crofts.

74. Neuman, B. (1983). Curriculum vitae.

75. Neuman, B. (1984, June 3). Personal communication.

76. Neuman, B. (1988, Jan. 10). Personal communication.

77. Neuman, B. (1988, Jan. 20). Personal communication.

78. Neuman, B. (1989). *The Neuman systems model* (2nd ed.). Norwalk, CT: Appleton & Lange.

79. Neuman, B. (1992, March 17). *Current status of the Neuman systems model.* Paper presented at Neuman Systems Model Theory Conference, Toledo, OH.

80. Neuman, B. (1992, June 17). Personal communication.

81. Neuman, B. (1992, June 21). Personal communication.

82. Neuman, B. (1995). In conclusion—Toward new beginnings. In B. Neuman (Ed.), *The Neuman systems model* (3rd ed., pp. 671-703). Norwalk, CT: Appleton & Lange.

83. Neuman, B. (1995). *The Neuman systems model* (3rd ed.). Norwalk, CT: Appleton & Lange.

84. Neuman, B. (1996, July 18). Personal communication.

85. Neuman, B. (1996). The Neuman systems model in research and practice. *Nursing Science Quarterly, 9*(2), 67-70.

86. Neuman, B., & Young, R.J. (1972, May-June). A model for teaching total person approach to patient problems. *Nursing Research, 21*:264-269.

87. Payne, P.L. (1995, Feb. 3). *A study of the teaching of primary prevention competencies as recommended by the report of the PEW Health Professions Commission in bachelor of science in nursing programs and associate in nursing programs.* Paper presented at the Fifth International Neuman Systems Model Symposium, Orlando, FL.

88. Perls, F. (1973). *The Gestalt approach: Eye witness to therapy.* Palo Alto, CA: Science and Behavior Books.

89. Reynolds, P.D. (1971). *A primer in theory construction.* Indianapolis: Bobbs-Merrill.

90. Picton, C.E. (1995). An explanation of family-centered care in Neuman's model with regard to the care of the critically ill adult in an accident and emergency setting. *Accident and Emergency Nursing, 3,* 33-37.

91. Poole, V.L. (1993, April 24). *Pregnancy wantedness, attitude toward pregnancy, and use of alcohol, tobacco, and street drugs during pregnancy.* Paper presented at the Fourth International Neuman Systems Model Symposium, Rochester, NY.

92. Reed, K.S. (1993). Adapting the Neuman systems model for family nursing. *Nursing Science Quarterly, 6*(2), 93-97.

93. Rodrigues-Fisher, L., Bourguignon, C., & Good, B.V. (1993). Dietary fiber nursing intervention: Prevention of constipation in older adults. *Clinical Nursing Research, 2*(4), 464-477.

94. Ross, M.M., & Bourbannais, F.F. (1985). The Neuman systems model in nursing practice; A case study approach. *Journal of Advanced Nursing, 10,* 199-207.

95. Rowles, C.J. (1993, April 23). *The relationship between selected personal and organizational variables and the tenure of directors in nursing homes.* Paper presented at the Fourth International Neuman Systems Model Symposium, Rochester, NY.

96. Russell, J. (1988, Jan. 10). Personal communication.

97. Russell, J. (1995, Feb. 4). *The lived experience of black women infected with HIV/AIDS.* Paper presented at the Fifth International Neuman Systems Model Symposium, Orlando, FL.

98. Russell, J., & Hezel, L. (1994). Role analysis of the advanced practice nurse using the Neuman health care systems model as a framework. *Clinical Nurse Specialist, 8*(4), 215-220.

99. Schlentz, M.D. (1993). The minimum data set and levels of prevention in the long term care facility. *Geriatric Nursing 14,* 79-83.

100. Schlentz, M.D. (1993, April 23). *The Neuman systems model in long term care.* Paper presented at the Fourth International Neuman Systems Model Symposium, Rochester, NY.

101. Schwieterman, I., Hamilton, E.M., & Braun, J.W. (1995, Feb. 3). *The Neuman systems model as a framework for describing physical mobility among the elderly.* Paper presented at the Fifth International Neuman Systems Model Symposium, Orlando, FL.

102. Selye, H. (1974). *Stress without distress.* Philadelphia: J.B. Lippincott.

103. Sipple, J.A., & Freese, B.T. (1989). Transition from technical to professional level education. In B. Neuman (Ed.), *The Neuman systems model* (2nd ed., pp. 193-200). Norwalk, CT: Appleton & Lange.

104. Smith, M.C., & Edgil, A.E. (1995). Future directions for research with the Neuman systems model. In B. Neuman (Ed.), *The Neuman systems model* (3rd ed., pp. 509-517). Norwalk, CT: Appleton & Lange.

105. Stittich, E.M., Flores, F.C., & Nuttall, P. (1995). Cultural considerations in a Neuman-based curriculum. In B. Neuman (Ed.), *The Neuman systems model* (3rd ed., pp. 147-162). Norwalk, CT: Appleton & Lange.

106. Strickland-Seng, V. (1995). The Neuman systems model in clinical evaluation of students. In B. Neuman (Ed.), *The Neuman systems model* (3rd ed., pp. 215-223). Norwalk, CT: Appleton & Lange.

107. Sullivan, J. (1986). Using Neuman's model in the acute phase of spinal cord injury. *Focus on Critical Care, 13*(5), 34-41.

108. Toot, J.L., & Schmull, B.J. (1995). The Neuman systems model and physical therapy educational curricula. In B. Neuman (Ed.), *The Neuman systems model* (3rd ed., pp. 231-246). Norwalk, CT: Appleton & Lange.

109. Torres, G. (1986). *Theoretical foundations of nursing.* Norwalk, CT: Appleton-Century-Crofts.

110. Waddell, K.L., & Demi, A.S. (1993). Effectiveness of an intensive partial hospitalization program for treatment of anxiety disorders. Archives of Psychiatric Nursing, 7(1), 2-10.

111. Walker, L.O., & Avant, K. (1983). *Strategies for theory construction in nursing.* Norwalk, CT: Appleton-Century-Crofts.

112. Walker, P.H. (1994). Dollars and sense in health reform: Interdisciplinary practice and community nursing centers. *Nursing Administration Quarterly, 19*(1), 1-11.

113. Walker, P.H., & Stone, P.L. (1995, Feb. 3). *Cost and quality outcomes of midwifery based on the Neuman systems model.* Paper presented at the Fifth International Neuman Systems Model Symposium, Orlando, FL.

BIBLIOGRAPHY

Primary sources

Books

Neuman, B. (1982). *The Neuman systems model: Application to nursing education and practice.* Norwalk, CT: Appleton-Century-Crofts.

Neuman B. (1989). *The Neuman systems model* (2nd ed.). Norwalk, CT: Appleton & Lange.

Neuman B. (1995). *The Neuman systems model* (3rd ed.). Norwalk, CT: Appleton & Lange.

Neuman, B., Deloughery, G.W., & Gebbie, M. (1971). *Consultation and community organization in community mental health nursing.* Baltimore: Williams & Wilkins.

Book chapters

Neuman, B. (1974). The Betty Neuman health care systems model: A total person approach to patient problems. In J.P. Riehl & C. Roy (Eds.), *Conceptual models for nursing practice* (pp. 94-104). New York: Appleton-Century-Crofts.

Neuman, B. (1980). The Betty Neuman health care systems model: A total person approach to patient problems. In J.P. Riehl & C. Roy (Eds.), *Conceptual models for nursing practice* (pp. 119-134). New York: Appleton-Century-Crofts.

Neuman, B. (1983). Analysis and application of Neuman's health care model. In I.W. Clements & F.B. Roberts, *Family health: A theoretical approach to nursing care* (pp. 239-254; 353-367). New York: John Wiley & Sons.

Neuman, B. (1986). The Neuman systems model explanation: Its relevance to emerging trends toward wholism in nursing. In I.B. Engberg (Ed.), *OMVARDNAD (Nursing Care Book).* Jonkoping, Sweden.

Neuman, B. (1989). The Neuman nursing process format: Adapted to a family case study. In J.P. Riehl & C. Roy (Eds.), *Conceptual models for nursing practice.* Norwalk, CT: Appleton & Lange.

Neuman, B. (1990). The Neuman systems model: A theory for practice. In M.E. Parker (Ed), *Nursing theories in practice.* New York: National League for Nursing.

Neuman, B. (1995). In conclusion—Toward new beginnings. In B. Neuman (Ed.), *The Neuman systems model* (3rd ed., pp. 671-703). Norwalk, CT: Appleton & Lange.

Neuman, B. (1995). The Neuman systems model. In B. Neuman (Ed.), *The Neuman systems model* (3rd ed., pp. 3-62). Norwalk, CT: Appleton & Lange.

Neuman, B., & Wyatt, M. (1980). The Neuman stress/adaptation systems approach to education for nurse administrators. In J.P. Riehl & C. Roy (Eds.), *Conceptual models for nursing practice* (2nd ed., pp. 142-150). New York: Appleton-Century-Crofts.

Journal articles

Neuman, B. (1985, Sept.). The Neuman Systems Model: its importance for nursing. *Senior Nurse, 3,* 3.

Neuman, B. (1990). Health: A continuum based on the Neuman Systems Model. *Nursing Science Quarterly, 3,* 129-135.

Neuman, B. (1996). The Neuman systems model in research and practice. *Nursing Science Quarterly, 9*(2), 67-70.

Neuman, B.M., Deloughery, G.W., & Gebbie, K.M. (1970, Jan.-Feb.). Levels of utilization: Nursing specialists in community mental health. *Journal of Psychiatric Nursing and Mental Health Services, 8*(1), 37-39.

Neuman, B.M., Deloughery, G.W., & Gebbie, K.M. (1970). Changes in problem solving ability among nurses receiving mental health consultation: A pilot study. *Communicating Nursing Research, 3,* 41-52.

Neuman, B.M., Deloughery, G.W., & Gebbie, K.M. (1971, Oct.). Nurses in community mental health: An informative interpretation for employees of professional nurses. *Public Personnel Review, 32*(4).

Neuman, B.M., Deloughery, G.W., & Gebbie, K.M. (1972, Feb.). Mental health consultation as a means of improving problem solving ability in work groups: A pilot study. *Comparative Group Studies, 3*(1), 81-97.

Neuman, B.M., & Young, R.J. (1972, May-June). A model for teaching total person approach to patient problems. *Nursing Research, 21,* 264-269.

Neuman, B., Deloughery, G.W., & Gebbie, K.M. (1974, Jan.). Teaching organizational concepts to nurses in community mental health. *Journal of Nursing Education, 13,* 1.

Neuman, B., & Wyatt, M.A. (1981, Jan.). Prospects for change: Some evaluative reflections by faculty members from one articulated baccalaureate program. *Journal of Nursing Education, 20,* 40-46.

Professional papers

Neuman, B. (1970, April-May). *A pilot study to measure change in problem solving ability among nurses receiving mental health consultation.* Paper presented at the Western Interstate Commission for Higher Education Conference on Communicating Research in Nursing, Salt Lake City, and at the State Department of Mental Health Center for Training in Community Psychiatry, Los Angeles, CA.

Neuman, B. (1970, Nov.). *Emerging leadership in mental health: Preparation of community mental health specialists.* Paper presented at the World Mental Health Assembly, Washington, DC.

Neuman, B. (1970, Nov.). *Improved utilization of nurses in community mental health.* Position paper presented to the Task Force for Development of the California State Plan for Health, Sacramento, CA.

Neuman, B. (1971, March). *Toward healthy, productive group interaction.* Paper presented to the Psychiatric Mental Health Conference Group, California Nurses' Association Convention, Anaheim, CA.

Neuman, B. (1977, Jan. 17). *An explanation of the Betty Neuman nursing model.* Paper presented at Indiana University–Purdue University at Fort Wayne, IN.

Neuman, B. (1980, Dec.). *A systems approach to the integrity of the client/client system based on the Neuman model.* Paper presented at the International Congress on Applied Systems Research and Cybernetics, Acapulco, Mexico.

Neuman, B. (1985, April). *The Neuman systems model for nursing.* Paper presented for the Royal College of Nursing and *Senior Nurse Magazine,* jointly sponsored, Models for Nursing Conference, University of Manchester, Manchester, England.

Neuman, B. (1985, April). *The Neuman systems model: Its relevance to nursing education, practice and research.* Paper presented to The Post Graduate School of Nursing, Aarhus and Copenhagen, Denmark, and to the Danish Institute for Health and Nursing Research, Copenhagen, Denmark.

Neuman, B. (1985, Aug.). *The Neuman systems model: Application to nursing education, practice and research.* Paper presented for the Nursing Theory in Action Conference, sponsored by Boyle, Letourneau & Associates, Inc., Edmonton, Alberta, Canada.

Neuman, B. (1986, Aug.). *The Neuman systems model: Usage in nursing education, practice and research.* Paper presented to the Nursing Theory Congress on Theoretical Pluralism: Direction for a Practice Discipline, sponsored by the Ryerson School of Nursing, Toronto, Ontario, Canada.

Neuman, B. (1986, Nov.). Keynote address for the First Biennial International Neuman Systems Model Symposium, sponsored by Neumann College, Division of Nursing, Aston, PA.

Neuman, B. (1988, Oct.). Keynote address for the Second Biennial International Neuman Systems Model Symposium, sponsored by the Neuman Trustee Group, Kansas City, MO.

Neuman, B. (1989, May). *Health on a continuum: The created environment and the Neuman Systems Model.* Paper presented at the Nurse Theorist Biennial Conference—The Meaning of Health in the Context of Nursing Science, sponsored by Discovery International, Inc.

Neuman, B. (1989, May). *The nursing model-research link.* Keynote address for the Eighth Annual Research Symposium, sponsored by the Edinburgh University School of Nursing and Honors Society, Edinburgh, Scotland.

Neuman, B. (1990, April). *The Neuman theoretical framework.* Paper presented at the Second South Florida Nursing Theorist Conference on Using Nursing Theory in Clinical Practice, sponsored by Cedars Medical Center, Miami, FL.

Neuman, B. (1990, May). *Bridging education and practice, simulated client interview and application of the Neuman model.* Paper presented at the 1990 Nursing Theory Conference, entitled Betty Neuman's Theory for Nursing: A System for practice, sponsored by Augsburg College, Minneapolis, MN.

Neuman, B. (1990, June). *Current status of the Neuman systems model.* Paper presented at the Neuman Systems Theory Conference: Understanding and Applying the Dr. Betty Neuman Systems Model, sponsored by Anna Maria College, Paxton, MA.

Neuman, B. (1990, Nov.). *Caring caregiving—An international model update, the Neuman Trustee Group, and future of the model.* Paper presented at the Third Biennial International Neuman Systems Model Symposium, sponsored by the Neuman Trustee Group, Wright State University, Miami Valley School of Nursing, and Dayton Area Nurse Educators, Dayton, OH.

Neuman, B. (1992, Feb.). *Understanding and applying the Neuman systems model.* Workshop presented at Center de Sorte, Elizabeth Bruyere Health Center, Ottawa, Ontario, Canada.

Neuman, B. (1992, March). *Current status of the Neuman systems model and future of the Neuman systems model.* Keynote presentations at the Neuman Systems Theory Conference, sponsored by the Toledo District Ohio Nursing Association, Medical College of Ohio Division of Continuing Education and School of Nursing, and Lourdes College, Toledo, OH.

Correspondence

Neuman, B. (1984, June 4). Personal correspondence.
Neuman, B. (1988, Jan. 20). Personal correspondence.
Neuman, B. (1988, Feb. 18). Personal correspondence.
Neuman, B. (1992, June 21). Personal correspondence and curriculum vitae.

Interviews

Neuman, B. (1984, June). Telephone interview.
Neuman, B. (1988, Jan.). Telephone interview.
Neuman, B. (1988, Feb.). Telephone interview
Neuman, B. (1988, May). Telephone interview.
Neuman, B.(1990, Nov.). Personal interview.
Neuman, B. (1992, Mar.). Personal interview.
Neuman, B. (1992, June). Telephone interview.
Neuman, B. (1995, Feb. 4). Personal communication.

Secondary sources

Books

Reed, K.S. (1993). *Betty Neuman: The Neuman systems model.* Newbury Park, CA: Sage.

Book reviews

Hawkins, J. (1983). [Review of *The Neuman systems model: Application to nursing education and practice.*] *Western Journal of Nursing Research, 5,* 182-183.
Varicchio, C.G. (1983). [Review of *The Neuman systems model: Application to nursing education and practice.*] *American Journal of Nursing, 83,* 963-964.

Book chapters

Arndt, C. (1982). Systems concepts for management of stress in complex health-care organizations. In B. Neuman, *The Neuman systems model: Application to nursing education and practice* (pp. 107-116). Norwalk, CT: Appleton-Century-Crofts.
Arndt, C. (1982). Systems theory and educational programs for nursing service administration. In B. Neuman, *The Neuman systems model: Application to nursing education and practice* (pp. 182-187). Norwalk, CT: Appleton-Century-Crofts.
Baker, N.A. (1982). The Neuman systems model as a conceptual framework for continuing education in the work place. In B. Neuman, *The Neuman systems model: Application to nursing education and practice* (pp. 260-266). Norwalk, CT: Appleton-Century-Crofts.
Baker, N.A. (1982). Use of the Neuman model in planning for the psychological needs of the respiratory disease patient. In B. Neuman, *The Neuman systems model: Application to nursing education and practice* (pp. 241-256). Norwalk, CT: Appleton-Century-Crofts.

Balch, C. (1974). Breaking the lines of resistance. In J.P. Riehl & C. Roy, *Conceptual models for nursing practice* (pp. 130-134). New York: Appleton-Century-Crofts.
Beckman, S.J., Boxley-Harges, S., Bruick-Sorge, C., Harris, S.M., Hermiz, M.E., Meininger, M., & Steinkeler, S.E. (1994). Betty Neuman systems model. In A. Marriner-Tomey (Ed.), *Nursing theorists and their work* (3rd ed., pp. 269-304). St. Louis: Mosby.
Beddome, G. (1995). Community-as-client assessment: A Neuman-based guide for education and practice. In B. Neuman (Ed.), *The Neuman systems model* (3rd ed., pp. 567-580). Norwalk, CT: Appleton & Lange.
Beitler, B., Tkachuck, B., & Aamodt, D. (1980). The Neuman model applied to mental health, community health, and medical-surgical nursing. In J.P. Riehl & C. Roy (Eds.), *Conceptual models for nursing practice* (2nd ed, pp. 170-178). New York: Appleton-Century-Crofts.
Benedict, M.B., & Sproles, J.B. (1982). Application of the Neuman model to public health nursing practice. In B. Neuman, *The Neuman systems model: Application to nursing education and practice* (pp. 223-240). Norwalk, CT: Appleton-Century-Crofts.
Beynon, C.E. (1995). Neuman-based experiences of the Middlesex-London health unit. In B. Neuman (Ed.), *The Neuman systems model* (3rd ed., pp. 537-549). Norwalk, CT: Appleton & Lange.
Bloch, C., & Bloch, C. (1995). Teaching content and process of the Neuman systems model. In B. Neuman (Ed.), *The Neuman systems model* (3rd ed., pp. 175-182). Norwalk, CT: Appleton & Lange.
Bonner, Sr. M. (1988). Proceedings. First Individual Nursing Symposium: Neuman Systems Model. Aston, PA: Neumann College Nursing Program.
Bower, F.L. (1982). Curriculum development and the Neuman model. In B. Neuman, *The Neuman systems model: Application to nursing education and practice* (pp. 223-240). Norwalk, CT: Appleton-Century-Crofts.
Bowman, G.E. (1982). The Neuman assessment tool adapted for child day-care centers. In B. Neuman, *The Neuman systems model: Application to nursing education and practice* (pp. 324-334). Norwalk, CT: Appleton-Century-Crofts.
Breckenridge, D.M. (1982). Adaptation of the Neuman systems model for the renal client. In B. Neuman, *The Neuman systems model: Application to nursing education and practice* (pp. 267-277). Norwalk, CT: Appleton-Century-Crofts.
Breckenridge, D.M. (1995). Nephrology practice and directions for nursing research. In B. Neuman (Ed.), *The Neuman systems model* (3rd ed., pp. 499-507). Norwalk, CT: Appleton & Lange.
Bueno, M.M., & Sengin, K.K. (1995). The Neuman systems model for critical care nursing: A framework for practice. In B. Neuman (Ed.), *The Neuman systems model* (3rd ed., pp. 275-292). Norwalk, CT: Appleton & Lange.

Campbell, V. The Betty Neuman health care systems model: An analysis. In J.P. Riehl-Sisca, *Conceptual models for nursing practice* (3rd ed., pp. 63-72). Norwalk, CT: Appleton & Lange.

Cardona, V.D. (1982). Client rehabilitation and the Neuman model. In B. Neuman, *The Neuman systems model: Application to nursing education and practice* (pp. 178-290). Norwalk, CT: Appleton-Century-Crofts.

Chiverton, P., & Flannery, J.C. (1995). Cognitive impairment: Use of the Neuman systems model. In B. Neuman (Ed.), *The Neuman systems model* (3rd ed., pp. 249-262). Norwalk, CT: Appleton & Lange.

Clark, F. (1982). The Neuman systems model: A clinical application for psychiatric nurse practitioners. In B. Neuman, *The Neuman systems model: Application to nursing education and practice* (pp. 335-354). Norwalk, CT: Appleton-Century-Crofts.

Clark, V.L. (1982). Teaching the Neuman systems model: An approach to student and faculty development. In B. Neuman, *The Neuman systems model: Application to nursing education and practice* (pp. 176-181). Norwalk, CT: Appleton-Century-Crofts.

Conners, V., Harmon, V.M., & Langford, R.W. (1982). Course development and implementation using the Neuman systems model as a framework: Texas Woman's University (Houston Campus). In B. Neuman, *The Neuman systems model: Application to nursing education and practice* (pp. 153-158). Norwalk, CT: Appleton-Century-Crofts.

Craddock, R.B., & Stanhope, M.K. (1980). The Neuman health care systems model: Recommended adaptation. In J.P. Riehl & C. Roy, (Eds.), *Conceptual models for nursing practice* (2nd ed.) (pp. 159-169). New York: Appleton-Century-Crofts.

Craig, D.M. (1995). Community/public health nursing in Canada: Use of the Neuman systems model in a new paradigm. In B. Neuman (Ed.), *The Neuman systems model* (3rd ed., pp. 521-528). Norwalk, CT: Appleton & Lange.

Craig, D.M., & Morris-Coulter, C. (1995). Neuman implementation in a Canadian psychiatric facility. In B. Neuman (Ed.), *The Neuman systems model* (3rd ed., pp. 397-406). Norwalk, CT: Appleton & Lange.

Cross, J. (1985). Betty Neuman. In J. George (Ed.), *Nursing theories: The base for professional nursing practice* (pp. 258-285). Englewood Cliffs, NJ: Prentice-Hall.

Cross, J. (1990). Betty Neuman. In J. George (Ed.), *Nursing theories: The base for professional nursing practice* (3rd ed.) (pp. 259-278). Norwalk, CT: Appleton & Lange.

Cunningham, S.G. (1982). The Neuman model applied to an acute care setting: Pain. In B. Neuman, *The Neuman systems model: Application to nursing education and practice* (pp. 291-296). Norwalk, CT: Appleton-Century-Crofts.

Curran, G. (1995). The Neuman systems model revisited. In B. Neuman (Ed.), *The Neuman systems model* (3rd ed., pp. 93-99). Norwalk, CT: Appleton & Lange.

Curran, G. (1995). The spiritual variable: A world view. In B. Neuman (Ed.), *The Neuman systems model* (3rd ed., pp. 581-590). Norwalk, CT: Appleton & Lange.

Damant, M. (1995). Community nursing in the United Kingdom: A case for reconciliation using the Neuman systems model. In B. Neuman (Ed.), *The Neuman systems model* (3rd ed., pp. 607-620). Norwalk, CT: Appleton & Lange.

Davies, P., & Proctor, H. (1995). In Wales: Using the model in community mental health nursing. In B. Neuman (Ed.), *The Neuman systems model* (3rd ed., pp. 621-628). Norwalk, CT: Appleton & Lange.

Davis, L.H. (1982). Aging: A social and preventive perspective. In B. Neuman, *The Neuman systems model: Application to nursing education and practice* (pp. 197-307). Norwalk, CT: Appleton-Century-Crofts.

Dunbar, S.B. (1982). Critical care and the Neuman model. In B. Neuman, *The Neuman systems model: Application to nursing education and practice* (pp. 297-307). Norwalk, CT: Appleton-Century-Crofts.

Dwyer, C.M., Walker, P.H., Suchman, A., & Coggiola, P. (1995). In *Nursing centers: The time is now* (pp. 135-155). NLN Pub. No. 41-2629. New York: National League for Nursing.

Echlin, D.J. (1982). Palliative care and the Neuman model. In B. Neuman, *The Neuman systems model: Application to nursing education and practice* (pp. 257-259). Norwalk, CT: Appleton-Century-Crofts.

Engberg, I.B. (1995). Brief abstracts: Use of the Neuman systems model in Sweden. In B. Neuman (Ed.), *The Neuman systems model* (3rd ed., pp. 653-656.) Norwalk, CT: Appleton & Lange.

Engberg, I.B., Bjalming, E., & Bertilson, B. (1995). A structure for documenting primary health care in Sweden using the Neuman systems model. In B. Neuman (Ed.), *The Neuman systems model* (3rd ed., pp. 637-654). Norwalk, CT: Appleton & Lange.

Fawcett, J. (1984). Neuman systems model. In J. Fawcett, *Analysis and evaluation of conceptual models of nursing* (pp. 154-174). Philadelphia: F.A. Davis.

Fawcett, J. (1989). Neuman systems model. In J. Fawcett, *Analysis and evaluation of conceptual models of nursing* (2nd ed., pp. 169-204). Philadelphia: F.A. Davis.

Fawcett, J. (1995). Constructing conceptual-theoretical-empirical structures for research: Future implications for use of the Neuman systems model. In B. Neuman (Ed.), *The Neuman systems model* (3rd ed., pp. 459-472). Norwalk, CT: Appleton & Lange.

Fawcett, J. (1995). Neuman's systems model. In J. Fawcett, *Analysis and evaluation of conceptual models of nursing* (3rd ed., pp. 217-275). Philadelphia: F.A. Davis.

Fawcett, J., Carpenito, L., Epinger, J., Goldblum-Graff, D., Groesbeck, M., Lowry, L., McCreary, C., & Wolf, Z. (1982). A framework for analysis and evaluation of conceptual models of nursing with an analysis and evaluation of the Neuman systems model. In B. Neuman, *The Neuman systems model: Application to nursing education and practice* (pp. 30-43). Norwalk, CT: Appleton-Century-Crofts.

Felix, M., Hinds, C., Wolfe, Sr. C., & Martin, A. (1995). The Neuman systems model in a chronic care facility: A Canadian experience. In B. Neuman (Ed.), *The Neuman systems model* (3rd ed., pp. 549-566). Norwalk, CT: Appleton & Lange.

Frioux, T.D., Roberts, A.G., & Butler, S.J. (1995). Oklahoma state public health nursing: Neuman-based. In B. Neuman (Ed.), *The Neuman systems model* (3rd ed., pp. 407-414). Norwalk, CT: Appleton & Lange.

Fulton, R.A.B. (1995). The spiritual variable: Essential to the client system. In B. Neuman (Ed.), *The Neuman systems model* (3rd ed., pp. 77-92). Norwalk, CT: Appleton & Lange.

Glazebrook, D.S. (1995). The Neuman systems model in cooperative baccalaureate nursing education: The Minnesota Intercollegiate Nursing Consortium experience. In B. Neuman (Ed.), *The Neuman systems model* (3rd ed., pp. 227-230). Norwalk, CT: Appleton & Lange.

Goldblum-Graff, D., & Graff, H. (1982). The Neuman model adapted to family therapy. In B. Neuman, *The Neuman systems model: Application to nursing education and practice* (pp. 217-222). Norwalk, CT: Appleton-Century-Crofts.

Gunter, L.M. (1982). Application of the Neuman systems model to gerontic nursing. In B. Neuman, *The Neuman systems model: Application to nursing education and practice* (pp. 196-210). Norwalk, CT: Appleton-Century-Crofts.

Harty, M.B. (1982). Continuing education in nursing and the Neuman model. In B. Neuman, *The Neuman systems model: Application to nursing education and practice* (pp. 100-106). Norwalk, CT: Appleton-Century-Crofts.

Hermiz, M.E., & Meininger, M. (1986). Betty Neuman: Systems model. In A. Marriner (Ed.), *Nursing theorists and their work* (pp. 313-331). St. Louis: Mosby.

Hilton, S.A., & Grafton, M.D. (1995). Curriculum transition based on the Neuman systems model: Los Angeles County Medical Center School of Nursing. In B. Neuman (Ed.), *The Neuman systems model* (3rd ed., pp. 163-174). Norwalk, CT: Appleton & Lange.

Hinton-Walker, P., & Raborn, M. (1989). Application of the Neuman model in nursing administration and practice. In B. Henry, C. Arndt, M. DiVencenti, & A. Marriner-Tomey (Eds.), *Dimensions of nursing administration* (pp. 711-723). Boston: Blackwell Scientific Publications.

Hoffman, M.K. (1982). From model to theory construction: An analysis of the Neuman health-care systems model. In B. Neuman, *The Neuman systems model: Application to nursing education and practice* (pp. 44-54). Norwalk, CT: Appleton-Century-Crofts.

Johnson, M., Vaughn-Wrobel, B., Ziegler, S.M., Hugh, L., Bush, H.A., & Kurtz, P. (1982). Use of the Neuman health-care systems model in the Master's curriculum: Texas Woman's University. In B. Neuman, *The Neuman systems model: Application to nursing education and practice* (pp. 130-152). Norwalk, CT: Appleton-Century-Crofts.

Kelley, J.A., & Sanders, N.F. (1995). A systems approach to the health of nursing and health care organizations. In B. Neuman (Ed.), *The Neuman systems model* (3rd ed., pp. 347-364). Norwalk, CT: Appleton & Lange.

Klotz, L.C. (1995). Integration of the Neuman systems model into the BSN curriculum at the University of Texas at Tyler. In B. Neuman (Ed.), *The Neuman systems model* (3rd ed., pp. 183-190). Norwalk, CT: Appleton & Lange.

Knox, J.E., Kilchenstein, L., & Yakulis, I.M. (1982). Utilization of the Neuman model in an integrated baccalaureate program: University of Pittsburgh. In B. Neuman, *The Neuman systems model: Application to nursing education and practice* (pp. 117-123). Norwalk, CT: Appleton-Century-Crofts.

Lebold, M., & Davis, L. (1980). A baccalaureate nursing curriculum based on the health systems model. In J.P. Riehl & C. Roy (Eds.), *Conceptual models for nursing practice* (2nd ed., pp. 151-158). New York: Appleton-Century-Crofts.

Leddy, S., & Pepper, J.M. (1985). Models of nursing. In S. Leddy & J.M. Pepper, *Conceptual bases of professional nursing* (pp. 135-149). Philadelphia: J.B. Lippincott.

Louis, M. (1989). An intervention to reduce anxiety levels for nurses working with long-term care clients using Neuman's model. In J.P. Riehl-Sisca, *Conceptual models for nursing practice* (3rd ed., pp. 95-103). Norwalk, CT: Appleton & Lange.

Louis, M. (1995). The Neuman model in nursing research: An update. In B. Neuman (Ed.), *The Neuman systems model* (3rd ed., pp. 473-495). Norwalk, CT: Appleton & Lange.

Louis, M., & Koertvelyessy, A. (1989). Neuman model: Use in research. In B. Neuman, *The Neuman systems model: Applications in nursing education and practice* (2nd ed.) Norwalk, CT: Appleton & Lange.

Lowry, L.W., & Jobb, M.C. An evaluation instrument for assessing an associate degree nursing curriculum based on the Neuman systems model, pp. 73-85.

Lowry, L.W., & Newsome, G.G. (1995). Neuman-based associate degree programs: Past, present, and future. In B. Neuman (Ed.), *The Neuman systems model* (3rd ed., pp. 197-214). Norwalk, CT: Appleton & Lange.

Lowry, L.W., Walker, P.H., & Mirenda, R. (1995). Through the looking glass back to the future. In B. Neuman (Ed.), *The Neuman systems model* (3rd ed., pp. 63-76). Norwalk, CT: Appleton & Lange.

Mayers, M.A., & Watson, A.B. (1982). Nursing care plans and the Neuman systems model. In B. Neuman, *The Neuman systems model: Application to nursing education and practice* (pp. 69-84). Norwalk, CT: Appleton-Century-Crofts.

McCulloch, S.J. (1995). Utilization of the Neuman systems model: University of South Australia. In B. Neuman (Ed.), *The Neuman systems model* (3rd ed., pp. 591-598). Norwalk, CT: Appleton & Lange.

McGee, M. (1995). Implications for use of the Neuman systems model in occupational health nursing. In B. Neuman (Ed.), *The Neuman systems model* (3rd ed., pp. 657-668). Norwalk, CT: Appleton & Lange.

McInerey, K.A. (1982). The Neuman systems model applied to critical care nursing of cardiac surgery clients. In B. Neuman, *The Neuman systems model: Application to nursing education and practice* (pp. 308-315). Norwalk, CT: Appleton-Century-Crofts.

Meleis, A.I. (1995). Theory testing and theory support: Principles, challenges, and a sojourn into the future. In B. Neuman (Ed.), *The Neuman systems model* (3rd ed., pp. 447-458). Norwalk, CT: Appleton & Lange.

Mirenda, R.M. (1986). The Neuman systems model: Description and application. In P. Winstead-Fry (Ed.), *Case studies in nursing theory* (pp. 127-167). New York: National League for Nursing.

Mischke-Berkey, K., Warner, P., & Hanson, S. (1989). Family health assessment and intervention. In P. Bomar (Ed.), *Nurses and family health promotion: Concepts, assessment, and interventions* (pp. 115-154). Baltimore: Williams & Wilkins.

Moxley, P.A., & Allen, L.M.H. (1982). The Neuman systems model approach in a master's degree program: Northwestern State University. In B. Neuman, *The Neuman systems model: Application to nursing education and practice* (pp. 168-175). Norwalk, CT: Appleton-Century-Crofts.

Moynihan, M.M. Implementation of the Neuman Systems Model in an acute care nursing department. In M.E. Parker (Ed.), *Nursing theories in practice* (pp. 263-273). New York: National League for Nursing.

Mrkonich, D.E., Hessian, M., & Miller, M.W. A cooperative process in curriculum development using the Neuman health-care systems model. In J.P. Riehl-Sisca, *Conceptual models for nursing practice* (3rd ed., pp. 87-94). Norwalk, CT: Appleton & Lange.

Neal, M.C. (1982). Nursing care plans and the Neuman systems model: II. In B. Neuman, *The Neuman systems model: Application to nursing education and practice* (pp. 85-93). Norwalk, CT: Appleton-Century-Crofts.

Neuman B. The Neuman nursing process format: Family. In J.P. Riehl-Sisca, *Conceptual models for nursing practice* (3rd ed., pp. 49-62). Norwalk, CT: Appleton & Lange.

Neuman, B. (1990). The Neuman Systems Model: A theory for practice. In M.E. Parker, *Nursing theories in practice* (pp 24-26). New York: National League for Nursing.

Pierce, A.G., & Fulmer, T.T. (1995). Application of the Neuman systems model to gerontological nursing. In B. Neuman (Ed.), *The Neuman systems model* (3rd ed., pp. 293-308). Norwalk, CT: Appleton & Lange.

Pinkerton, A. (1974). Use of the Neuman model in a home health-care agency. In J.P. Riehl & C. Roy (Eds.), *Conceptual models for nursing practice* (pp. 122-129). New York: Appleton-Century-Crofts.

Poole, V.L., & Flowers, J.S. (1995). Care management of pregnant substance abusers using the Neuman systems model. In B. Neuman (Ed.), *The Neuman systems model* (3rd ed., pp. 377-386). Norwalk, CT: Appleton & Lange.

Proctor, N.G. (1995). Nurses' role in world catastrophic events: War dislocation effects on Serbian Australians. In B. Neuman (Ed.), *The Neuman systems model* (3rd ed., pp. 119-132). Norwalk, CT: Appleton & Lange.

Purushotham, D., & Walker, G. (1994). The Neuman systems model: A conceptual framework for clinical teaching/learning process. In R.M. Carroll-Johnson & M. Paquette (Eds.), *Classification of nursing diagnosis: Proceedings of the tenth conference* (pp. 271-273). Philadelphia: J.B. Lippincott.

Reed, K. (1982). The Neuman systems model: A basis for family psychosocial assessment and intervention. In B. Neuman, *The Neuman systems model: Application to nursing education and practice* (pp. 188-195). Norwalk, CT: Appleton-Century-Crofts.

Rice, M.J. (1982). The Neuman systems model applied in a hospital medical unit. In B. Neuman, *The Neuman systems model: Application to nursing education and practice* (pp. 310-323). Norwalk, CT: Appleton-Century-Crofts.

Riehl-Sisca, J.P. (1989). *Conceptual models for nursing practice* (3rd ed.). Norwalk, CT: Appleton & Lange.

Rodriguez, M.L. (1995). The Neuman systems model adapted to a continuing care retirement community. In B. Neuman (Ed.), *The Neuman systems model* (3rd ed., pp. 431-442). Norwalk, CT: Appleton & Lange.

Russell, J., Hileman, J.W., & Grant, J.S. (1995). Assessing and meeting the needs of home caregivers using the Neuman systems model. In B. Neuman (Ed.), *The Neuman systems model* (3rd ed., pp. 331-342). Norwalk, CT: Appleton & Lange.

Scicchitani, B., Cox, J., Heyduk, L.J., Maglicco, P.A., & Sargent, N.A. (1995). Implementing the Neuman model in a psychiatric hospital. In B. Neuman (Ed.), *The Neuman systems model* (3rd ed., pp. 387-396). Norwalk, CT: Appleton & Lange.

Sipple, J.A., & Freese, B.T. (1989). Transition from technical to professional level education. In B. Neuman (Ed.), *The Neuman systems model* (2nd ed., pp. 193-200). Norwalk, CT: Appleton & Lange.

Smith, M.C., & Edgil, A.E. (1995). Future directions for research with the Neuman systems model. In B. Neuman (Ed.), *The Neuman systems model* (3rd ed., pp. 509-517). Norwalk, CT: Appleton & Lange.

Sohier, R. (1995). Nursing care for the people of a small planet: Culture and the Neuman systems model. In B. Neuman (Ed.), *The Neuman systems model* (3rd ed., pp. 101-118). Norwalk, CT: Appleton & Lange.

Sohier, R. (1997). Neuman's systems model in nursing practice. In M.R. Alligood & A. Marriner-Tomey (Eds.). *Nursing theory: Utilization and application* (pp. 109-127). St. Louis: Mosby.

Stittich, E.M., Flores, F.C., & Nuttall, P. (1995). Cultural considerations in a Neuman-based curriculum. In B. Neuman (Ed.), *The Neuman systems model* (3rd ed., pp. 147-162). Norwalk, CT: Appleton & Lange.

Strickland-Seng, V. (1995). The Neuman systems model in clinical evaluation of students. In B. Neuman (Ed.), *The Neuman systems model* (3rd ed., pp. 215-223). Norwalk, CT: Appleton & Lange.

Stuart, G.W., & Wright, L.K. (1995). Applying the Neuman systems model to psychiatric nursing practice. In B. Neuman (Ed.), *The Neuman systems model* (3rd ed., pp. 263-274). Norwalk, CT: Appleton & Lange.

Thibodeau, J.A. (1983). A systems model: the Neuman model. In J.A. Thibodeau, *Nursing models: Analysis and evaluation* (pp. 105-123). Monterey, CA: Wadsworth.

Tollett, S.M. (1982). Teaching geriatrics and gerontology: Use of the Neuman systems model. In B. Neuman, *The Neuman systems model: Application to nursing education and practice* (pp. 157-164). Norwalk, CT: Appleton-Century-Crofts.

Tomlinson, P.S., & Anderson, K.S. (1995). Family health and the Neuman systems model. In B. Neuman (Ed.), *The Neuman systems model* (3rd ed., pp. 133-144). Norwalk, CT: Appleton & Lange.

Toot, J.L., & Schmull, B.J. (1995). The Neuman systems model and physical therapy educational curricula. In B. Neuman (Ed.), *The Neuman systems model* (3rd ed., pp. 231-246). Norwalk, CT: Appleton & Lange.

Torres, G.(1986). Systems-oriented theories. In G. Torres, *Theoretical foundations of nursing* (pp. 112-165). Norwalk, CT: Appleton-Century-Crofts.

Trepanier, M.J., Dunn, S.J., & Sprague, A.E. (1995). Application of the Neuman systems model to perinatal nursing. In B. Neuman (Ed.), *The Neuman systems model* (3rd ed., pp. 309-329). Norwalk, CT: Appleton & Lange.

Vaughn, B., & Gough, P. (1995). Use of the Neuman systems model in England: Abstracts. In B. Neuman (Ed.), *The Neuman systems model* (3rd ed., pp. 599-606). Norwalk, CT: Appleton & Lange.

Venable J. (1974). The Neuman health-care systems model: An analysis. In J.P. Riehl & C. Roy (Eds.), *Conceptual models for nursing practice* (pp. 115-121). New York: Appleton-Century-Crofts.

Venable, J.F. (1980). The Neuman health-care systems model: An analysis. In J.P. Riehl & C. Roy (Eds.), *Conceptual models for nursing practice* (2nd ed.) (pp. 135-141). New York: Appleton-Century-Crofts.

Verbeck, F. (1995). In Holland: Application of the Neuman model in psychiatric nursing. In B. Neuman (Ed.), *The Neuman systems model* (3rd ed., pp. 629-636). Norwalk, CT: Appleton & Lange.

Vokaty, D.A. (1982). The Neuman systems model applied to the clinical nurse specialist role. In B. Neuman, *The Neuman systems model: Application to nursing education and practice* (pp. 165-167). Norwalk, CT: Appleton-Century-Crofts.

Walker, P.H. (1995). Neuman-based education, practice, and research in a community nursing center. In B. Neuman (Ed.), *The Neuman systems model* (3rd ed., pp. 415-430). Norwalk, CT: Appleton & Lange.

Walker, P.H. (1995). TQM and the Neuman systems model: Education for health care administration. In B. Neuman (Ed.), *The Neuman systems model* (3rd ed., pp. 365-376). Norwalk, CT: Appleton & Lange.

Walker, L.O., & Avant, K.C. (1983). Theory analysis: The Betty Neuman health care systems model: A total person approach to patient problems. In L.A. Walker & K.C. Avant, *Strategies for theory construction in nursing* (pp. 133-143). Norwalk, CT: Appleton-Century-Crofts.

Ware, L.A., & Shannahan, M.K. (1995). Using Neuman for a stable support group in neonatal intensive care. In B. Neuman (Ed.), *The Neuman systems model* (3rd ed., pp. 321-330). Norwalk, CT: Appleton & Lange.

Wesley, R.L. (1992). Neuman Systems Model. In *Springhouse notes: Nursing theories and models—a study and learning tool* (pp. 84-93). Springhouse, PA: Springhouse Corp.

Whall, L.O., & Avant, K.C. (1983). The Betty Neuman health care systems model. In J. Fitzpatrick & A. L. Whall (Eds.), *Conceptual models of nursing analysis and application* (pp. 204-219). Bowie, MD: Robert J. Brady.

Ziegler, S.M. (1982). Taxonomy for nursing diagnosis derived from the Neuman systems model. In B. Neuman, *The Neuman systems model: Application to nursing education and practice* (pp. 55-68). Norwalk, CT: Appleton-Century-Crofts.

Journal articles

Aggleton, P., & Chalmers, H. (1989). Neuman's systems model. *Nursing Times, 85*(51), 27-29.

Ali, N.S., & Khalil, H.Z. (1989). Effect of psychoeducational intervention on anxiety among Egyptian bladder cancer patients. *Cancer Nursing, 12,* 236-242.

Anderson, E., McFarland, J., & Helton, A. (1986). Community-as-client: A model for practice. *Nursing Outlook, 34*(5), 220-224.

Baerg, K.L. (1991). Using Neuman's model to analyze a clinical situation. *Rehabilitation Nursing, 16,* 38-39.

Barrett, M. (1991). A thesis is born. *Image: Journal of Nursing Scholarship, 23,* 261-262.

Beckingham, A.C., & Baumann, A. (1990). The aging family in crisis: Assessment decision-making models. *Journal of Advanced Nursing, 15,* 782-787.

Berkey, K.M., & Hanson, S.M.H. (1991). *Pocket guide to family assessment and intervention.* St. Louis: Mosby.

Beyea, S., & Matzo, M. (1989). Assessing elders using the functional health pattern assessment model. *Nurse Educator, 14*(5), 32-37.

Beynon, C. (1993). Theory-based practice: Attitudes of nursing managers before and after educational sessions. *Public Health Nursing, 10*(3), 183-188.

Biley, F. (1990). The Neuman Model: An analysis. *Nursing (London), 4*(4), 25-28.

Biley, F.C. (1989). Stress in high dependency units. *Intensive Care Nursing, 5,* 134-141.

Blank, J.J., Clark, L., Longman, A.J., & Atwood, J.R. (1989). Perceived home care needs of cancer patients and their caregivers. *Cancer Nursing, 12*, 78-84.

Bowdler, J.E., & Barrell, L.M. (1987). Health needs of homeless persons. *Public Health Nursing, 4*, 135-140.

Bowles, L., Oliver, N., & Stanley, S. (1995/Jan. 4). A fresh approach. *Nursing Times, 91*(1), 40-41.

Breckenridge, D.M., Cupit, M.C., & Raimond, J.N. (1982, Jan.-Feb.). Systematic nursing assessment tool for the CAPD client. *Nephrology Nurse, 24*, 26-27, 30-31.

Brown, M.W. (1988). Neuman's systems model in risk factor reduction. *Cardiovascular Nursing, 24*(6), 43.

Buchanan, B.F. (1987). Human-environment interaction: A modification of the Neuman systems model for aggregates, families, and the community. *Public Health Nursing, 4*(1), 52-64.

Bullock, L.F. (1993). Nursing interventions for abused women on obstetrical units. *AWHONN'S Clinical Issues in Perinatal and Women's Health Nursing, 4*(3), 371-377.

Bunn, H. (1995). Preparing nurses for the challenge of the new focus on community mental health nursing. *The Journal of Continuing Education in Nursing, 26*(2), 55-59.

Burke, S.O., & Maloney, R. (1986). The Women's Value Orientation Questionnaire: An instrument revision study. *Nursing Papers, 18*(1), 32-44.

Cantin, B., & Mitchell, M. (1989). Nurses' smoking behavior. *The Canadian Nurse, 85*(1), 20-21

Capers, C.F. (1991). Nurses' and lay African Americans' views about behavior. *Western Journal of Nursing Research, 13*, 123-135.

Carroll, T.L. (1989). Role deprivation in baccalaureate nursing students pre and post curriculum revision. *Journal of Nursing Education, 28*, 134-139.

Clark, C.C., Cross, J.R., Deane, D.M., & Lowry, L.W. (1991). Spirituality: Integral to quality care. *Holistic Nursing Practice, 5*, 67-76.

Courchene, V.S., Patalski, E., & Martin, J. (1991). A study of the health of pediatric nurses administering cyclosporine A. *Pediatric Nursing, 17*, 497-500.

Dale, J.L., & Savala, S.M. (1990). A new approach to the senior practicum. *Nursing Connections, 3*(1), 45-51.

Darland, N.W. (1986). Congenital adrenocortical hyperplasia: Supportive nursing interventions. *Journal of Pediatric Nursing, 1*(2), 117-123.

Delunas, L.R. (1990). Prevention of elder abuse: Betty Neuman health care systems approach. *Clinical Nurse Specialists, 4*, 54-58.

Evely, L. A model for successful breastfeeding. *Modern Midwife, 4*(12), 25-27.

Flannery, J. (1991). FAMLI-RESCUE: A family assessment tool for use by neuroscience nursing in the acute care setting. *Journal of Neuroscience Nursing, 23*, 111-115.

Flannery, J. (1995). Cognitive assessment in the acute care setting: Reliability and validity of the levels of cognitive function assessment scale (LOCFAS). *Journal of Nursing Measurement, 3*(1), 43-58.

Foote, A.W., Piazza, D., & Schultz, M. (1990). The Neuman Systems Model: Application to a patient with a cervical spinal cord injury. *Journal of Neuroscience Nursing, 22*, 302-306.

Fowler, B.A., & Risner, P.B. (1994). A health promotion program evaluation in a minority industry. *ABNF Journal, 5*(3), 72-76.

Galloway, D.A. (1993). Coping with a mentally and physically impaired infant: A self-analysis. *Rehabilitation Nursing 18*(1), 34-36.

Gavin, C.A.S., Hastings-Tolsma, M.T., & Troyan, P.J. (1988). Explication of Neuman's model: A holistic systems approach to nutrition for health promotion in the life process. *Holistic Nursing Practice, 3*(1), 26-38.

Gellner, P., Landers, S., O'Rouke, D., & Schlegal, M. (1994). Community health nursing in the 1990's: Risky business? *Holistic Nursing Practice, 8*(2), 15-21.

Goodman, H. (1995, Jun. 28-July 4). Patients' views count as well. *Nursing Standard, 9*(40), 55.

Grant, J.S., Kinney, M.R., & Davis, L.D. (1993). Using conceptual frameworks or models to guide nursing research. *Journal of Neuroscience Nursing, 25*(1), 52-56.

Gries, M., & Fernsler, J. (1988). Patient perceptions of the mechanical ventilation experience. *Focus on Critical Care, 15*, 52-59.

Haggart, M. (1993). A critical analysis of Neuman's systems model in relation to public health nursing. *Journal of Advanced Nursing, 18*(2), 1917-1922.

Heffline, M.S. (1991). A comparative study of pharmacological versus nursing interventions in the treatment of postanesthesia shivering. *Journal of Post Anesthesia Nursing, 6*, 311-320.

Herrick, C.A., & Goodykoonts, L. (1989). Neuman's systems model for nursing practice as a conceptual framework for a family assessment. *Journal of Child and Adolescent Psychiatric and Mental Health Nursing, 2*, 61-67.

Herrick, C.A., Goodykoonts, L., Herrick, R.H., & Kracket, B. (1991). Planning a continuum of care in child psychiatric nursing: A collaborative effort. *Journal of Child and Adolescent Psychiatric and Mental Health Nursing, 4*, 41-48.

Hitz, D. (1900). The Neuman Systems Model: An analysis of clinical situation. *Rehabilitation Nursing, 15*, 330-332.

Hinds, C. (1990). Personal and contextual factors predicting patients' reported quality of life: Exploring congruency with Betty Neuman's assumptions. *Journal of Advanced Nursing, 15*, 456-462.

Hoch, C.C. (1987). Assessing delivery of nursing care. *Journal of Gerontological Nursing, 13*(1), 10-17.

Hoeman, S.P., & Winters, D.M. (1990). Theory-based case management: High cervical spinal cord injury. *Home Healthcare Nurse, 8*, 25-33.

Huch, M.H. (1991). Perspective of health. *Nursing Science Quarterly, 4*, 33-40.

Issel, L.M. (1995). Evaluating case management programs. *MCN, 29*, 67-74.

Johns, C. (1991). The Burford Nursing Development Unit holistic model of nursing practice. *Journal of Advanced Nursing, 16,* 1090-1098.

Johnson, P.T. (1983). Black hypertension: A transcultural case study using the Betty Neuman model of nursing care. *Issues in Health Care, 4,* 191-210.

Kiernan, B.S., & Scoloveno, M.A. (1986). Assessment of the neonate. *Topics in Clinical Nursing, 8*(1), 1-10.

Knight, J.B. (1990). The Betty Neuman Systems Model applied to practice: A client with multiple sclerosis. *Journal of Advanced Nursing, 15,* 447-455.

Leja, A.M. (1989). Using guided imagery to combat postsurgical depression. *Journal of Gerontological Nursing, 15*(4), 6-11.

Lile, J.L., Pace, N.M., Hoffman, R.G., & Mace, M.K. (1994). The Neuman systems model as applied to the terminally ill client with pressure ulcers. *Advances in Wound Care, 7*(4), 44-48.

Lindell, J., & Olsson, H. (1991). Can combined oral contraceptives be made more effective by means of a nursing care model? *Journal of Advanced Nursing, 16,* 475-479.

Loescher, L.J., Clark, L., Attwood, J.R., Leigh, S., & Lamb, G. (1990). The impact of the cancer experience on long-term survivors. *Oncology Nursing Forum, 17*(2), 223-229.

Lowry, L. (1986). Adapted by degrees. *Senior Nurse, 5*(3), 25-26.

Lowry, L.W. (1988). Operationalizing the Neuman systems model: A course in concepts and process. *Nursing Educator, 13*(3), 19-22.

Lowry, L., & Anderson, B. (1993). Neuman's framework and ventilator dependency: A pilot study. *Nursing Science Quarterly, 6*(4), 195-199.

Mackenzie, S., & Spence-Laschinger, H.K. (1995). Correlates of nursing diagnosis quality in public health nursing. *Journal of Advanced Nursing, 21,* 800-808.

Maligalig, R.M.L. (1994). Parents' perceptions of the stressors of pediatric ambulatory surgery. *Journal of Post Anesthesia Nursing, 9*(5), 278-282.

Mann, A.H., Hazel, C., Geer, C., Hurley, C.M., & Podrapovic, T. (1993). Development of an orthopaedic case manager role. *Orthopaedic Nursing, 12*(4), 23-27.

Miner, J. (1995). Incorporating the Betty Neuman systems model into HIV clinical practice. *AIDS Patient Care, 9*(1), 37-39.

Mirenda, R.M. (1986). The Neuman model in practice. *Senior Nurse, 5*(3), 26-27.

Mirenda, R.M. (1986). The Neuman systems model: Description and application. NLN Pub. No. 15-2152, 127-166.

Moore, S.L., & Munro, M.F. (1990). The Neuman Systems Model applied to mental health nursing of older adults. *Journal of Advanced Nursing, 15,* 293-299.

Mynatt, S.L., & O'Brien, J. (1993). A partnership to prevent chemical dependency in nursing using Neuman's systems model. *Journal of Psychosocial Nursing and Mental Health Services, 31*(4), 27-34.

Mytka, S., & Beynon, C. (1994). A model for public health nursing in the Middlesex-London, Ontario, schools. *Journal of School Health, 64*(2), 85-86.

Orr, J.P. (1993). An adaptation of the Neuman systems model to the care of the hospitalized preschool child. *Curationis: South African Journal of Nursing, 16*(3), 37-44.

Owens, M. (1995). Care of a woman with Down's syndrome using the Neuman systems model. *British Journal of Nursing, 4*(13), 752-758.

Parr, M.S. (1993). The Neuman health care systems model: An evaluation. *British Journal of Theatre Nursing, 3*(8), 20-27.

Picton, C.E. (1995). An explanation of family-centered care in Neuman's model with regard to the care of the critically ill adult in an accident and emergency setting. *Accident and Emergency Nursing, 3,* 33-37.

Reed, K.S. (1993). Adapting the Neuman systems model for family nursing. *Nursing Science Quarterly, 6*(2), 93-97.

Ridgell, N.H. (1993). Home apnea monitoring: A systems approach to the family's home care needs. *Caring, 12*(2), 34-37.

Roberts, A.G. (1994). Effective inservice education process. *Oklahoma Nurse, 39*(4), 11.

Rodrigues-Fisher, L., Bourguignon, C., & Good, B.V. (1993). Dietary fiber nursing intervention: Prevention of constipation in older adults. *Clinical Nursing Research, 2*(4), 464-477.

Roggensack, J. (1994, Jun.-Aug.). The influence of perioperative theory and clinical in a baccalaureate nursing program on the decision to practice perioperative nursing. *Prairie Rose, 63*(2), 6-7.

Ross, M., & Bourbannais, F. (1985). The Neuman systems model in nursing practice: A case study approach. *Journal of Advanced Nursing, 10,* 199-207.

Ross, M.M., Bourbonnais, F.F., & Carroll, G. (1987). Curriculum design and the Betty Neuman systems model: A new approach to learning. *International Nursing Review, 34*(3), 75-79.

Russell, J., & Hezel, L. (1994). Role analysis of the advanced practice nurse using the Neuman health care systems model as a framework. *Clinical Nurse Specialist, 8*(4), 215-220.

Schare, B.L. (1993). A comparison of family needs based on the presence or absence of DNR orders. *DCCN, 11*(5), 286-292.

Schlentz, M.D. (1993). The minimum data set and levels of prevention in the long term care facility. *Geriatric Nursing 14,* 79-83.

Schorr, J. (1993). Music and pattern change in chronic pain. *Advances in Nursing Science, 15*(4), 27-36.

Smith, M.C. (1989). Neuman's model in practice. *Nursing Science Quarterly, 2,* 116-117.

Speck, B.J. (1990). The effect of guided imagery upon first semester nursing students performing their first injections. *Journal of Nursing Education, 29,* 346-350.

Story, E.L., & DuGas, B.W. (1988). A teaching strategy to facilitate conceptual model implementation in practice. *Journal of Continuing Education in Nursing, 19,* 244-247.

Sullivan, J. (1986). Using Neuman's model in the acute phase of spinal cord injury. *Focus on Critical Care, 13*(5), 34-41.

Tlaskund, J.H. (1980). Areas in theory development. *Advances in Nursing Science, 3,* 1-7.

Torkington, S. (1988). Nourishing the infant. *Senior Nurse, 8*(2), 24-25.

Utz, S.W. (1980). Applying the Neuman model to nursing practice with hypertensive clients. *Cardiovascular Nursing, 16,* 29-34.

Vaughn, M., Cheatwood, S., Sirles, A.T., & Brown, K.C. (1989). The effect of progressive muscle relaxation on stress among clerical workers. *American Association of Occupational Health Nursing Journal, 37,* 302-306.

Waddell, K.L., & Demi, A.S. (1993). Effectiveness of an intensive partial hospitalization program for treatment of anxiety disorders. *Archives of Psychiatric Nursing, 7*(1), 2-10.

Walker, P.H. (1994). Dollars and sense in health reform: Interdisciplinary practice and community nursing centers. *Nursing Administration Quarterly, 19*(1), 1-11.

Wallingford, P. (1989). The neurologically impaired and dying child: Applying the Neuman Systems Model. *Issues in Comprehensive Pediatric Nursing, 12,* 139-157.

Waters, T. (1993). Self-efficacy, change, and optimal client stability. *Addictions Nursing Network, 6*(2), 48-51.

Weinberger, S.L. (1901). Analysis of a clinical situation using the Neuman Systems Model. *Rehabilitation Nursing, 16,* 278-281.

Wormald, L. (1995). Samuel—The boy with tonsillitis: A care study. *Intensive and Critical Care Nursing, 11*(3), 157-160.

Wright, P.S., Piazza, D., Holcombe, J., & Foote, A. (1994). A comparison of three theories of nursing used as a guide for the nursing care of an 8-year-old child with leukemia. *Journal of Pediatric Oncology Nursing, 11*(1), 14-19.

Professional papers

Barnes, K.M. (1993, April 23). *The relationship between mistreatment of the elderly, quality of care, and demographic characteristics.* Paper presented at the Fourth International Neuman Systems Model Symposium, Rochester, NY.

Beckman, S.J., & Bruick-Sorge, C. (1995, Feb. 3). *Replication study: The efficacy of the Neuman systems model for associate degree nursing curriculum development.* Paper presented at the Fifth International Neuman Systems Model Symposium, Orlando, FL.

Cagle, R.H., & Reeb, R. (1993, April 24). *Perinatal management using the Neuman systems model.* Paper presented at the Fourth International Neuman Systems Model Symposium, Rochester, NY.

Cotton, N.C. (1993, April 23). *An interdisciplinary high risk assessment tool for rehabilitation in patient falls.* Paper presented at the Fourth International Neuman Systems Model Symposium, Rochester, NY.

Craig, D. (1993, April 23). *An interdisciplinary high risk assessment tool for older adults' use of nursing services, life stress, ways of coping and health, mood and energy for living.* Paper presented at the Fourth International Neuman Systems Model Symposium, Rochester, NY.

Craig, D., & Morris-Coulter, C. (1995, Feb. 3). *Exploring partnerships in model implementation.* Paper presented at the Fifth International Neuman Systems Model Symposium, Orlando, FL.

Craig, D., & Timmings, C. (1995, Feb. 3). *Health promotion for older adults: Does it make a difference?* Paper presented at the Fifth International Neuman Systems Model Symposium, Orlando, FL.

Flannery, J. (1995, Feb. 3). *Application of the Neuman systems model in combination with cognitive recovery theory to assess TBI patients.* Paper presented at the Fifth International Neuman Systems Model Symposium, Orlando, FL.

Freese, B.T., & Lander University Faculty. (1995, Feb. 3). *Application of the Neuman systems model to education: Baccalaureate workshop.* Paper presented at the Fifth International Neuman Systems Model Symposium, Orlando, FL.

Freese, B.T., & Speer, I. (1995, Feb. 3). *Nurse-managed childbearing in the U.K. and U.S.A.: A cross-cultural comparative study.* Paper presented at the Fifth International Neuman Systems Model Symposium, Orlando, FL.

Fulton, R.A.B. (1993, April 23). *Spiritual well-being of baccalaureate nursing students and nursing faculty and their responses about spiritual well-being of persons.* Paper presented at the Fourth International Neuman Systems Model Symposium, Rochester, NY.

Fulton, R.A.B., & Moore, C.M. (1995, Feb. 3). *Spiritual well-being of parents of children with asthma.* Paper presented at the Fifth International Neuman Systems Model Symposium, Orlando, FL.

Gloss, E.F., & Crowe, R.L. (1993, April 24). *Coronary artery disease: Postmenopausal women, power, and anxiety.* Paper presented at the Fourth International Neuman Systems Model Symposium, Rochester, NY.

Hainsworth, D.S., & Grimes, J. (1993, April 23). *Use of the Neuman model as a framework for research and educational intervention for nurses who care for terminally ill patients and their families.* Paper presented at the Fourth International Neuman Systems Model Symposium, Rochester, NY.

Hamilton, E.M., & Schwieterman, I. (1995, Feb. 3). *The Neuman systems model in research data integration.* Paper presented at the Fifth International Neuman Systems Model Symposium, Orlando, FL.

Hui-Tseng, Ting. (1993, April 24). *Cognition and anxiety level of pre-cardiac catheterization patients before and after an education program.* Paper presented at the Fourth International Neuman Systems Model Symposium, Rochester, NY.

Klinek, S.C. (1995, Feb. 4). *Effect of knowledge, attitudes, and beliefs on breast self care behavior.* Paper presented at the Fifth International Neuman Systems Model Symposium, Orlando, FL.

Lancaster, D.R. (1995, Feb. 4). *Coping with appraised breast cancer threat among women at increased risk: A mid-range theory of primary prevention.* Paper presented at the Fifth International Neuman Systems Model Symposium, Orlando, FL.

Louis, M. (1995, Feb. 3). *Preferred other relationships, perceived health, and quality of life of elders.* Paper presented at the Fifth International Neuman Systems Model Symposium, Orlando, FL.

Lowry, L. (1993, April 23). *Using the Neuman systems model to guide research.* Paper presented at the Fourth International Neuman Systems Model Symposium, Rochester, NY.

Lowry, L.W. (1995, Feb. 3). *Client satisfaction with prenatal care and pregnancy outcomes.* Paper presented at the Fifth International Neuman Systems Model Symposium, Orlando, FL.

Payne, P.L. (1995, Feb. 3). *A study of the teaching of primary prevention competencies as recommended by the report of the PEW Health Professions Commission in bachelor of science in nursing programs and associate in nursing programs.* Paper presented at the Fifth International Neuman Systems Model Symposium, Orlando, FL.

Poole, V.L. (1993, April 24). *Pregnancy wantedness, attitude toward pregnancy, and use of alcohol, tobacco, and street drugs during pregnancy.* Paper presented at the Fourth International Neuman Systems Model Symposium, Rochester, NY.

Rowles, C.J. (1993, April 23). *The relationship between selected personal and organizational variables and the tenure of directors in nursing homes.* Paper presented at the Fourth International Neuman Systems Model Symposium, Rochester, NY.

Russell, J. (1995, Feb. 4). *The lived experience of black women infected with HIV/AIDS.* Paper presented at the Fifth International Neuman Systems Model Symposium, Orlando, FL.

Schlentz, M.D. (1993, April 23). *The Neuman systems model in long term care.* Paper presented at the Fourth International Neuman Systems Model Symposium, Rochester, NY.

Schwieterman, I., Hamilton, E.M., & Braun, J.W. (1995, Feb. 3). *The Neuman systems model as a framework for describing physical mobility among the elderly.* Paper presented at the Fifth International Neuman Systems Model Symposium, Orlando, FL.

Walker, P.H., & Stone, P.L. (1995, Feb. 3). *Cost and quality outcomes of midwifery based on the Neuman systems model.* Paper presented at the Fifth International Neuman Systems Model Symposium, Orlando, FL.

Newsletters

Capers, C. (Ed.). (1992). *Neuman News.* The Neuman Trustee Group, Inc., 3, 1.

Capers, C. (Ed.). (1994, Spring/Summer). *Neuman News.* 1 (3).

Dissertations and theses

Al-Nagshabandi, E.A.H. (1993). An exploration of the physical and psychological responses of surgically-induced menopausal Saudi women using the Neuman systems model. *Dissertations Abstracts International,* 55-04B, 1374.

Averill, J.B. (1988). The impact of primary prevention as an interventions strategy. *Masters Abstracts International,* 27-01, 89.

Barnes, M.E. (1993). Knowledge, experiences, attitudes, and assessment practices of nurse practitioners with regard to stressors related to childhood sexual abuse. *Masters Abstracts International,* 32-01, 0223.

Baskin-Nedzelski, J. (1991). Job stressors among visiting nurses. *Masters Abstracts International,* 30-01, 0079.

Bittinger, J.P. (1995). Case management and satisfaction with nursing care of patients hospitalized with congestive heart failure. *Dissertations Abstracts International,* 56-07B, 3688.

Blount, K.R. (1988). The relationship between the parent's and five- to six-year-old child's perception of life events as stressors within the Neuman health care systems framework. *Masters Abstracts International,* 27-04, 0487.

Brown, F.A. (1994). The effects of an eight-hour affective education program on fear of AIDS and homophobia in student nurses. *Masters Abstracts International,* 33-05, 1487.

Burritt, J.E. (1988). The effects of perceived social support on the relationship between job stress and job satisfaction and job performance among registered nurses employed in acute care facilities. *Dissertations Abstracts International,* 49, 2123B.

Capers, C.F. (1986). Perceptions of problematic behavior as held by lay black adults and registered nurses. *Dissertations Abstracts International,* 47-11B, 4467.

Collins, A.S. (1991). *Effects of positional changes on selected physiological and psychological measurements in clients with atrial fibrillation.* Doctoral dissertation, University of Alabama at Birmingham.

Cullen, L.M. (1993). Nurses' perceptions of humor as a preventive intervention to promote the health of clients in a health care setting. *Masters Abstracts International,* 32-02, 0592.

Fields, W.L. (1987). The effects of the 12-hour shift on fatigue and critical thinking performance in critical care nurses. *Masters Abstracts International,* 26-02, 0237.

Flannery, J.C. (1988). Validity and reliability of levels of Cognitive Functioning Assessment Scale for adults with closed head injuries. *Dissertations Abstracts International,* 48, 3248B.

Fulton, B.J. (1992). *Evaluation of the effectiveness of the Neuman systems model as a theoretical framework for baccalaureate nursing programs.* Doctoral dissertation, University of Massachusetts.

Goble, D.S. (1991). A curriculum framework for the prevention of child sexual abuse. *Dissertations Abstracts International,* 52-06A, 2004.

Hanson, M.J.S. (1995). Beliefs, attitudes, subjective norms, perceived behavioral control, and cigarette smoking in white, African-American, and Puerto Rican–American teenage women. *Dissertations Abstracts International,* 56-08B, 4240.

Harbin, P.D.O. (1990). A Q-analysis of the stressors of adult female nursing students enrolled in baccalaureate schools of nursing. *Dissertations Abstracts International,* 50, 3919B.

Harper, B. (1992). Nurses' beliefs about social support and the effect of nursing care on cardiac clients' attitudes in reducing cardiac risk factors. *Masters Abstracts International,* 31-01, 0273.

Hayes, K.V.D. (1994). Diagnostic content validation and operational definitions of risk factors for the nursing diagnosis high risk for disuse syndrome. *Dissertations Abstracts International,* 55-12B, 5284.

Heaman, D.J. (1991). *Perceived stressors and coping strategies of parents with developmentally disabled children.* Doctoral dissertation, University of Alabama at Birmingham.

Henze, R.L. (1993). The relationship among selected stress variables and white blood count in severely head injured patients. *Dissertations Abstracts International,* 55-02B, 03365.

Herald, P.A. (1993). Relationship between hydration status and renal function in patients receiving aminoglycoside antibiotics. *Dissertations Abstracts International,* 55-02B, 0365.

Higgs, K.T. (1994). Preterm labor risk factors identified an an ambulatory perinatal setting with home uterine activity monitoring support. *Masters Abstracts International,* 33-05, 1490.

Holloway, C. (1995). Stress perceived among nurse managers in community health settings. *Masters Abstracts International,* 33-05, 1490.

Kazakoff, K.J. (1990). The evaluation of return to work and retention of employment of cardiac patients following cardiac rehabilitation programs. *Masters Abstracts International,* 29-03, 0450.

Lancaster, D.R.N. (1991). *Coping with appraised threat of breast cancer: Primary prevention coping behaviors utilized by women at increased risk.* Doctoral dissertation, Wayne State University.

Landry, K.A. (1994). *Relationship of serum levels of total cholesterol and selected risk factors in clients diagnosed with a cerebrovascular accident.* Master's thesis, Northwestern State University of Louisiana.

Lee, P.L. (1995). Caregiver stress as experienced by wives of institutionalized and in-home dementia husbands. *Dissertations Abstracts International,* 56-08B, 4241.

McDaniel, G.M.S. (1990). The effects of two methods of dangling on heart rate and blood pressure in postoperative abdominal hysterectomy patients. *Dissertations Abstracts International,* 50, 3923B.

Mirenda, R.M. (1995). A conceptual-theoretical strategy for curriculum development in baccalaureate nursing programs. *Dissertations Abstracts International,* 56-10B, 5421.

Moody, N.B. (1991). *Selected demographic variables, organizational characteristics, role orientation, and job satisfaction among nurse faculty.* Doctoral dissertation, University of Alabama at Birmingham.

Morris, D.C. (1991). Occupational stress among home care first line managers. *Masters Abstracts International,* 29-03, 0443.

Murphy, N.G. (1989). Factors associated with breastfeeding success and failure: A systematic integrative review. *Masters Abstracts International,* 28-02, 0275.

Nicholson, C.H. (1995). Clients' perceptions of preparedness for discharge home following total hip or knee replacement surgery. *Masters Abstracts International,* 33-03, 0873.

Norman, S.E. (1991). The relationship between hardiness and sleep disturbances in HIV-infected men. *Dissertations Abstracts International,* 51, 4780B.

Norris, E.W. (1990). Physiologic response to exercise in clients with mitral valve prolapse syndrome. *Dissertations Abstracts International,* 50, 5549B.

O'Neal, C.A.S. (1993). Effects of BSE on depression/anxiety in women diagnosed with breast cancer. *Masters Abstracts International,* 31-04, 1747.

Peoples, L.T. (1990). *The relationship between selected client, provider, and agency variables and the utilization of home care services.* Doctoral dissertation, University of Alabama at Birmingham.

Petock, A.M. (1990). Decubitus ulcers and physiological stressors. *Masters Abstracts International,* 29-02, 0267.

Pothiban, L. (1993). *Risk factor prevalence, risk status, and perceived risk for coronary heart disease among Thai elderly.* Doctoral dissertation, University of Alabama at Birmingham.

Rowe, M.L. (1989). *The relationship of commitment and social support to the life satisfaction of caregivers to patients with Alzheimer's disease.* Doctoral dissertation, The University of Texas at Austin.

Rowles, C.J. (1992). *The relationship of selected personal and organizational variables and the tenure of directors of nursing in nursing homes.* Doctoral dissertation, University of Alabama at Birmingham.

Scalzo Tarrant, T. (1992). Improving the frequency and proficiency of breast self examination. *Masters Abstracts International,* 31-03, 1211.

Schlosser, S.P. (1985). The effect of anticipatory guidance on mood state in primiparas experiencing unplanned cesarean delivery. *Dissertations Abstracts International,* 46-08B, 2627.

Sipple, J.E.A. (1990). A model for curriculum change based on retrospective analysis. *Dissertations Abstracts International,* 50, 1927A.

Tarmina, M.S. (1992). *Self-selected diet of adult women with families.* Doctoral dissertation, University of Utah.

Terhaar, M.F. (1989). The influence of physiologic stability, behavior stability, and family stability on the preterm infant's length of stay in the neonatal intensive care unit. *Dissertations Abstracts International,* 50, 1328B.

Vincent, J.L.M. (1988). A Q analysis of the stressors of fathers with an infant in an intensive care unit. *Dissertations Abstracts International,* 49, 3111B.

Watson, L.A. (1991). Comparison of the effects of usual, support, and informational nursing interventions on the extent to which families of critically ill patients perceive their needs were met. *Dissertations Abstracts International,* 52-06B, 2999.

Webb, C.A. (1989). A cross-sectional study of hope, physical status, cognitions and meaning and purpose of pre- and post-retirement adults. *Dissertations Abstracts International,* 50, 1922A.

Whatley, J.H. (1988). Effects of health locus of control and social network on risk-taking in adolescents. *Dissertations Abstracts International,* 50-01B, 0129.

Williamson, J.W. (1989). *The influence of self-selected monotonous sounds on the night sleep pattern of postoperative open heart surgery patients.* Doctoral dissertation, University of Alabama at Birmingham.

Wilkey, S.F. (1990). The effects of an eight-hour continuing education course on the death anxiety levels of registered nurses. *Masters Abstracts International,* 28-04, 0480.

Correspondence

Lowry, L. (1992, June 4). Personal correspondence.
Mirenda, R. (1992, June 16). Personal correspondence.

Interviews

Babcock, P. (1984, June 10). Telephone interview.
Louis, M. (1988, Jan. 10). Telephone interview.
Lowry, L. (1990, Nov. 15). Personal interview.
Mirenda, R. (1988, Jan. 10). Telephone interview.
Mirenda R. (1990, Nov. 15). Personal interview.
Mirenda, R. (1992, Mar. 17). Personal interview.
Mirenda, R. (1992, June 3). Telephone interview.
Russell, J. (1988, Jan. 10). Telephone interview.

Imogene King

Systems Framework and Theory of Goal Attainment

Christina L. Sieloff, Mary Lee Ackermann, Sallie Anne Brink,
Jo Anne Clanton, Cathy Greenwell Jones, Ann Marriner Tomey,
Sandra L. Moody, Gwynn Lee Perlich, Debra L. Price,
Beth Bruns Prusinski

CREDENTIALS AND BACKGROUND OF THE THEORIST

Imogene King earned a diploma in nursing from St. John's Hospital of Nursing in St. Louis in 1945. While working in a variety of staff nurse roles, she began course work toward a Bachelor of Science in Nursing Education, which she received from St. Louis University in 1948. From 1947 to 1958 King worked as an instructor in medical-surgical nursing and as an assistant director at St. John's Hospital School of

Nursing. She earned an M.S.N. (1957) from St. Louis University and a Doctor of Education (1961) from Teachers College, Columbia University, New York. King was awarded an honorary Ph.D. from Southern Illinois University in 1980.

From 1961 to 1966, King was an associate professor of nursing at Loyola University in Chicago, where she developed a master's degree program in nursing based on a nurse's conceptual framework. Her first theory article[28] appeared in 1964 in a journal edited by Dr. Martha Rogers titled *Nursing Science*. Between 1966 and 1968, King served as Assistant Chief of Research Grants Branch, Division of Nursing, in the United States Department of Health, Education, and Welfare. While she was in Washington, D.C., her ar-

The authors wish to thank Dr. Imogene King for her review of this chapter.
The authors and Dr. King strongly encourage all readers to read Dr. King's original materials in conjunction with this chapter.

ticle "A Conceptual Frame of Reference for Nursing" was published in *Nursing Research*.[29]

From 1968 to 1972, King was the director of the School of Nursing at The Ohio State University in Columbus. While at Ohio State, her book *Toward a Theory for Nursing*[30] was published. In this early work, King concluded "a systematic representation of nursing is required ultimately for developing a science to accompany a century or more of art in the everyday world of nursing."[30:129] This book subsequently was awarded the AJN Book of the year Award in 1973.[39]

King returned to Chicago in 1972 as a professor in the Loyola University graduate program. She also served as the Coordinator of Research in Clinical Nursing at the Loyola Medical Center, Department of Nursing (1978 to 1980).

From 1972 to 1975, she was a member of the Defense Advisory Committee on Women in the Services for the United States Department of Defense. She was elected "Alderman" in Ward 2, Wood Dale, Illinois, in 1975 and served until 1979.

In 1980, King moved to Tampa, Florida, where she was appointed professor at the University of South Florida College of Nursing. The manuscript for her second book, *A Theory for Nursing: Systems, Concepts, Process,*[34] was published in 1981. In addition to her first two books, she has authored multiple book chapters and articles in professional journals and a third book, *Curriculum and Instruction in Nursing,*[38] which was published in 1986.

King retired in 1990, is currently professor emeritus at the University of South Florida, and lectures at the University. She continues to provide community service and to help plan care through her framework and theory at a variety of health care organizations. She keynoted two Sigma Theta Tau theory conferences in 1992 and continues to present at local, national, and international nursing education conferences. She also consults with doctoral and master's students who are developing theories within the systems framework. She has contributed to the development of instruments to measure the power of a nursing group within an organization,[56] and patient satisfaction with professional nursing care.[27]

King has been an active member of the American Nurses Association, the Florida Nurses' Association, and Sigma Theta Tau International. She has held offices in a variety of organizations and has frequently served as a delegate from the Florida Nurses' Association to the American Nurses Association House of Delegates. In 1994, she was inducted into the American Academy of Nursing. Currently, she is one of the founding members of a nursing organization (King International Nursing Group) established to facilitate the dissemination and utilization of her systems framework and Theory of Goal Attainment. In 1996, she received the Jessie M. Scott Award at the American Nurses Association convention.

THEORETICAL SOURCES

King stated that the purpose of her first book was

> to propose a conceptual frame of reference for nursing. It is intended to be utilized specifically by students and teachers, and also by researchers and practitioners to identify and analyze events in specific nursing situations. The framework suggests that the essential characteristics of nursing are those properties that have persisted in spite of environmental changes.[30:ix]

King also stated that the framework served

> several purposes.... It is a way of thinking about the real world of nursing; ... an approach for selecting concepts perceived to be fundamental for the practice of professional nursing; [and] shows a process for developing concepts that symbolize experiences within the physical, psychological, and social environment in nursing.[30:125]

Theoretical sources are clearly identified and referenced throughout her 1981 book.[34]

USE OF EMPIRICAL EVIDENCE

King spoke of concepts as "abstract ideas that give meaning to our sense perceptions, permit generalizations, and tend to be stored in our memory for recall and use at a later time in new and different situations."[30:11-12] King defined theory as "a set of concepts, which, when defined, are interrelated and observable in the world of nursing practice,"[35:11] which serves to "build scientific knowledge for nursing."[33]

King identified at least two methods for developing theory. First, a theory can be developed and then tested in research. Second, research can provide data from which a theory may be developed. King stated, "It is my opinion that, in today's world of building knowledge for a complex profession such as nursing, one must consider these two strategies."[33]

Many research studies were cited in King's 1981 book,[34] especially with regard to the development of her concepts. Within the personal system, King examined studies related to "perception" by Allport,[3] Kelley and Hammond,[25] Ittleson and Cantril,[21] and others. In developing her definition of "space," she used Sommer's[57] and Ardrey's[4] studies, and noted Minckley's research.[46] For the concept of "time," Orme's work[48] was acknowledged.

Within the interpersonal system, King presented communication theories and models, and the studies of Watzlawick, Beavin, and Jackson[58] and Krieger[42] were noted. Studies by Whiting,[59] Orlando,[47] and Diers and Schmidt[11] were examined for information on "interaction." Dewey and Bentley's Theory of Knowledge, which deals with self-action, interaction, and transaction in *Knowing and the Known*,[10] and Kuhn's work[43] on transactions were also noted.

Commenting on research existing at that time, particularly operations research regarding patient care, King noted, "Most studies have centered on technical aspects of patient care and of the health care systems rather than on patient aspects directly. . . . Few problems have been stated that begin with what the patient's condition demands or what the patient wants."[32:9] In 1981 King further stated, "Several theoretical formulations about interpersonal relations and nursing process have been described in nursing situations,"[34:151-152] citing studies by Peplau,[50] Orlando,[47] Paterson and Zderad,[49] Yura and Walsh,[62] and herself.

Development of the Systems Framework

In preparation of her 1971 book,[30] King posed several questions:
1. What is the goal of nursing?

2. What are the functions of nurses?
3. How can nurses continue to expand their knowledge to provide quality care?[39:17]

As a result of a review of 20 years of nursing literature (prior to 1971), King identified multiple concepts used by nurses to describe nursing.

Fig. 20-1 demonstrates the systems framework, which provides "one approach to studying systems as a whole rather than as isolated parts of a system,"[39:18] and "was designed to explain (the) organized wholes within which nurses are expected to function."[40:23]

A systems approach was used in the development of her systems framework and the subsequent Theory of Goal Attainment. King stated that systems have been used in the past to comprehend and respond to "changes and complexity in health care organizations."[34:10] She added, "Some scientists who have been studying systems have noted that the only way to study human beings interacting with the en-

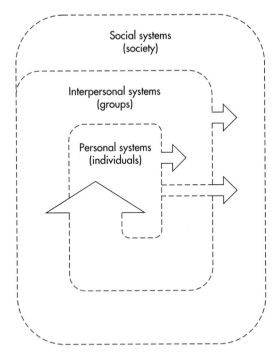

Fig. **20-1** Dynamic interacting systems. *From King, I. (1981). A theory for nursing: Systems, concepts, process (p. 11). New York: Delmar. Used with permission from I. King.*

vironment is to design a conceptual framework of interdependent variables and interrelated concepts."[34:10] King believes that her "framework differs from other conceptual schema in that it is concerned not with fragmenting human beings and the environment but with human transactions in different kinds of environments."[39:21]

"An awareness of the complex dynamics of human behavior in nursing situations prompted [King's] formulation of a conceptual framework that represents personal, interpersonal and social systems as the domain of nursing."[34:130] Each of the three systems identifies human beings as the basic element in the system. In addition, "the unit of analysis in [the] framework is human behavior in a variety of social environments."[39:18]

Individuals exist within personal systems, and King provided an example of a "total system" as being a patient or a nurse. King believes that it is necessary to understand the concepts of body image, growth and development, perception, self, space, and time to comprehend human beings as persons.

Interpersonal systems, or groups, are formed when two or more individuals interact, forming dyads (two people) or triads (three people). The dyad, nurse and client, is one type of interpersonal system. Families, when acting as small groups, would also be considered as interpersonal systems. Comprehension of the interpersonal system requires an understanding of the concepts of communication, interaction, role, stress, and transaction.

A comprehensive interacting system consists of groups that make up society and is referred to as a social system. Religious, educational, and health care systems are examples of social systems. The influential behavior of an extended family on an individual's growth and development in society is another example of the influence of a social system. Within a social system, the concepts of authority, decision making, organization, power, and status are essential for understanding this system.

"The concepts in the framework are the organizing dimensions and represent knowledge essential for understanding the interactions between the three systems."[39:18] Concepts were placed in the personal system because they primarily related to individuals, whereas concepts were placed in the interpersonal system because they "emphasized interactions between two or more persons."[39:18] Finally, concepts were placed in the social system because they "provided knowledge for nurses to function in larger systems."[39:18] However, King clearly stated that "the concepts in the framework are not limited to only one of the dynamic interacting systems but cut across all three systems."[39:19]

Development of the Theory of Goal Attainment

In 1981, King derived the Theory of Goal Attainment from her systems framework.[34] The question that "motivated [King] to develop a theory was, what is the nature of nursing?"[40:25] The answer, "It is the way in which nurses, in their role, do with and for individuals that differentiates nursing from other health professionals,"[40:26] guided the development of the Theory of Goal Attainment.

King used the following criteria to develop the theory:

1. What are the philosophical assumptions?
2. Are the concepts clearly identified and defined?
3. Are the concepts related in propositional statements or models?
4. Does the theory generate questions to be answered or hypotheses to be tested in research to generate knowledge and to affirm the theory?[40:26]

"The human process of interactions formed the basis for designing a model of transactions [Fig. 20-2] that depicts theoretical knowledge used by nurses to help individuals and groups attain goals."[39:27]

> Mutual goal setting [between a nurse and a client] is based on (a) nurses' assessment of a client's concerns, problems, and disturbances in health; (b) nurses' and client's perceptions of the interference; [and] (c) their sharing information whereby each functions to help the client attain the goals identified. In addition, nurses interact with family members when clients cannot verbally participate in the goal setting.[40:28]

To test her theory, King conducted research, identifying that her study varied from previous studies in

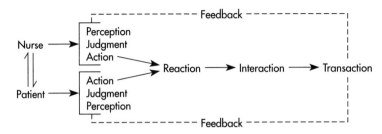

Fig. **20-2** A process of human interactions that lead to transactions: A model of transaction. *From King, I. (1981). A theory for nursing: Systems, concepts, process (p. 61). New York: Delmar. Used with permission from I. King.*

MAJOR CONCEPTS & DEFINITIONS

"Concepts give meaning to our sense perceptions and permit generalizations about persons, objects, and things."[39:16] A limited number of definitions based on the systems framework are listed below. The remainder of King's definitions can be found in her 1981 book.[34] To assist the reader, those concepts and the pages on which the definitions can be found from the systems framework and the theory are listed alphabetically in Table 20-1.

Health "Health is defined as dynamic life experiences of a human being, which implies continuous adjustment to stressors in the internal and external environment through optimum use of one's resources to achieve maximum potential for daily living."[34:5]

Nursing "Nursing is defined as a process of action, reaction, and interaction whereby nurse and client share information about their perceptions in the nursing situation."[34:2]

Self "The self is a composite of thoughts and feelings which constitute a person's awareness of his [/her] individual existence, his [/her] conception of who and what he [/she] is. A person's self is the sum total of all he [/she] can call his [/hers]. The self includes, among other things, a system of ideas, attitudes, values, and commitments. The self is a person's total subjective environment. It is a distinctive center of experience and significance. The self constitutes a person's inner world as distinguished from the outer world consisting of all other people and things. The self is the individual as known to the individual. It is that to which we refer when we say 'I.'"[22:9-10]

that it "described the nurse-patient interaction process that leads to goal attainment."[34:153] King's research described a process that leads to goal attainment and studied nurse-patient interactions to determine if nurses made transactions. A method of nonparticipant observation was used to collect information of nurse-patient interactions in a patient care unit in a hospital setting. Patients and nurses

volunteered to participate in the study. Graduate students were trained in the nonparticipant observation technique prior to collecting data. Multiple interactions were examined. Both verbal and nonverbal behaviors were recorded as raw data. A classification system was developed that can be used by nurses to determine if they make transactions that lead to goal attainment.[41]

Table 20-1

Location of concept definitions in I.M. King's A Theory for Nursing: Systems, Concepts, Process*

CONCEPTS	FROM SYSTEMS FRAMEWORK	FROM THEORY
Authority	p. 124	
Body image	p. 33	
Communication		p. 146
Decision making	p. 132	
Growth and development		p. 148
Interaction	p. 32	p. 145
Nursing situation	p. 2	
Organization (operational)	p. 119	
Perception	p. 24	p. 146
Power	p. 127	
Role	p. 93	
Space	pp. 37-38	
Status	p. 129	
Stress	p. 32	
Time	p. 44	
Transaction	p. 82	p. 147

*New York: John Wiley & Sons, 1981.

MAJOR ASSUMPTIONS

King's personal philosophy about human beings and life influenced her assumptions. Her assumptions include those related to the environment, health, nursing, individuals, and nurse-client interactions. Her systems framework and Theory of Goal Attainment were "based on an overall assumption that the focus of nursing is human beings interacting with their environment leading to a state of health for individuals, which is an ability to function in social roles."[34:143]

Nursing

"Nursing is an observable behavior found in the health care systems in society."[30:125] The goal of nursing "is to help individuals maintain their health so they can function in their roles."[34:3-4] Nursing is viewed as an interpersonal process of action, reaction, interaction, and transaction. Perceptions of a nurse and a client also influence the interpersonal process.

Person

Specific assumptions relating to persons or individuals are detailed in *A Theory for Nursing: Systems, Concepts, Process.*[34:143] In addition, the following assumptions have been detailed in King's subsequent works:

- Individuals are spiritual beings.[41]
- Individuals have the capacity to think, to know, to make choices, and to select alternative courses of action.
- Individuals have the ability through their language and other symbols to record their history and to preserve their culture.[38:56]
- Individuals are open systems in transaction with the environment. Transaction connotes

that there is no separateness between human beings and the environment.

- Individuals are unique (and) holistic (and are) of intrinsic worth who are capable of rational thinking and decision making in most situations.[40:26]
- Individuals differ in their needs, wants, and goals.[40:27]

Health

Health is viewed as a dynamic state in the life cycle; illness is an interference in the life cycle. Health "implies continuous adjustment to stress in the internal and external environment through optimum use of one's resources to achieve maximum potential for daily living."[34:5]

Environment

King stated that "an understanding of the ways that human beings interact with their environment to maintain health is essential for nurses."[34:2] Open systems imply interactions occur between the system and the system's environment, inferring that the environment is constantly changing. "Adjustments to life and health are influenced by [an] individual's interactions with environment . . . . Each human being perceives the world as a total person in making transactions with individuals and things in the environment."[34:141]

THEORETICAL ASSERTIONS

King's Theory of Goal Attainment[34] focuses on the interpersonal system and the interactions that take place between individuals, specifically in the nurse-client relationship. In the nursing process, each member of the dyad perceives the other, makes judgments, and takes actions. Together, these activities culminate in reaction. Interaction results and, if perceptual congruence exists and disturbances are conquered, transactions occur. The system is open to permit feedback because perception is potentially influenced by each phase of the activity.

Within King's Theory of Goal Attainment,[34] eight propositions were developed. These propositions are detailed in Box 20-1 and describe the relationships

---

Box **20-1**

Propositions Within King's Theory of Goal Attainment

1. If perceptual accuracy (PA) is present in nurse-client interactions (I), transactions (T) will occur.

$$\text{PA (I)} \xrightarrow{+} T$$

2. If nurse and client make transactions (T), goals will be attained (GA).

$$T \xrightarrow{+} GA$$

3. If goals are attained (GA), satisfactions (S) will occur.

$$GA \xrightarrow{+} S$$

4. If goals are attained (GA), effective nursing care (NC_e) will occur.

$$GA \xrightarrow{+} NC_e$$

5. If transactions (T) are made in nurse-client interactions (I), growth and development (GD) will be enhanced.

$$(I)T \xrightarrow{+} GD$$

6. If role expectations and role performance as perceived by nurse and client are congruent (RCN), transactions (T) will occur.

$$RCN \xrightarrow{+} T$$

7. If role conflict (RC) is experienced by nurse and client or both, stress (ST) in nurse-client interactions (I) will occur.

$$RC(I) \xrightarrow{+} ST$$

8. If nurses with special knowledge and skills communicate (CM) appropriate information to clients, mutual goal setting (T) and goal attainment (GA) will occur. [Mutual goal setting is a step in transaction and thus has been diagrammed as transaction.]

$$CM \xrightarrow{+} T \xrightarrow{+} GA$$

Reprinted from J.K. Austin and V.L. Champion, King's theory of nursing: Explication and evaluation. In P.L. Chinn (Ed.), *Advances in nursing theory development* (p. 55), with permission of Aspen Publishers, Inc., © 1983.

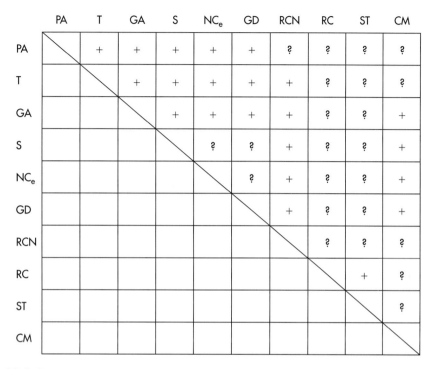

	PA	T	GA	S	NC$_e$	GD	RCN	RC	ST	CM
PA		+	+	+	+	+	?	?	?	?
T			+	+	+	+	+	?	?	?
GA				+	+	+	+	?	?	+
S					?	?	+	?	?	+
NC$_e$						?	+	?	?	+
GD							+	?	?	+
RCN								?	?	?
RC									+	?
ST										?
CM										

Fig. **20-3** Relationship table. *PA*, Perceptional accuracy; *T*, transactions; *GA*, goals attained; *S*, satisfactions; *NC*, effective nursing care; *GD*, growth and development; *RCN*, role congruency; *RC*, role conflict; *ST*, stress; *CM*, communicate. *From Austin, J.K., & Champion, V.L. (1983). King's theory for nursing: Explication and evaluation. In P.L. Chinn (Ed.),* Advances in theory development *(p. 58). Rockville, MD: Aspen. Used with permission of Aspen Publishers, copyright © 1983.*

between concepts. Diagrams follow each proposition. When the propositions were analyzed, 23 relationships were not specified; 22 relationships were positive, and no relationship was negative (Fig. 20-3). In addition, King derived seven hypotheses from the Theory of Goal Attainment, which are found in *A Theory for Nursing: Systems, Concepts, Process.*[34:156]

LOGICAL FORM

In the initial framework suggested in her 1968 article,[29] King identified four comprehensive concepts (health, interpersonal relationships, perceptions, and social systems) that centered around human beings. She stated that individuals are open systems and that energy exchange takes place within, and external to, human beings. Although King's original framework was abstract and dealt with "only a few elements of concrete situations,"[30:128] she believes her four "universal ideas, social systems, health, perception, and interpersonal relations, are relevant in every nursing situation."[30:128]

King then began further development of her systems framework and proposed the Theory of Goal Attainment to describe "the nature of nurse-client interactions that lead to achievement of goals."[34:142]

Nurses purposely interact with clients to mutually establish goals and to explore and agree on means to achieve goals. Mutual goal setting is based on nurses' assessment of clients' concerns, problems, and disturbances in health, their perceptions of problems, and their sharing information to move toward goal attainment.[34:142-143]

Later, in 1975, King identified that her "personal approach to synthesizing knowledge for nursing was to use data and information available from research in nursing and related fields and from 25 years in active practice, teaching, and research. From all the knowledge available, a theoretical framework relevant for nursing was formulated."[31:36] King, in 1978,[33] indicated that theory development is composed of inductive and deductive reasoning and that theory's primary purpose is to generate knowledge through research.

In her 1981 publication,[34] there was less dichotomy between health and illness, and illness was referred to as an interference in the life cycle. Through reformulation, King provided a more open system relationship between person and environment. King also revised her terminology, using *adjustment* instead of *adaptation,* and *person, human being,* and *individual* rather than *man.*

There was logical progression of development in the framework from 1971[30] to 1981[34] with King deriving her Theory of Goal Attainment from her systems framework. Her theory "organize[s] elements in the process of nurse-client interactions that result in outcomes, that is, goals attained."[34:143]

King initially stated:

> If nurses are to assume the roles and responsibilities expected of them, . . . the discovery of knowledge must be disseminated in such a way that they are able to use it in their practice . . . . Descriptive data collected systematically provide cues for generating hypotheses for research in human behavior in nursing situations.[30:128]

During a 1978 nursing theorist conference, King[33] indicated that if nurses were taught this process, they could begin to predict outcomes in nursing. Later, in 1981, she added, "This theory should serve as a standard of practice related to nurse-patient interactions, and is in this sense a normative theory."[34:145]

These ideas were expanded by Clements and Roberts[8] in 1983 to show the process of the theory in relation to a variety of nursing situations, including the health of families.

ACCEPTANCE BY THE NURSING COMMUNITY

Practice

King's early publication[30] led to nursing curriculum development and practice application at Ohio State and other universities. In her 1981 book King stated, "Theory, because it is abstract, cannot be immediately applied to nursing practice or to concrete nursing education programs. When empirical referents are identified, defined and described, . . . theory is useful and can be applied in concrete situations."[34:157] However, "knowledge of the concepts can be applied in concrete situations."[41]

Knowledge of the concepts of King's Theory of Goal Attainment[34] has been used in most specialty areas in nursing practice. Its relationship to practice is obvious because the profession of nursing functions primarily through interactions with individuals and groups within the environment.[17] Even before King's systems framework was published, Brown stated, "This proposed intrasystems model provides an approach for stimulating continued learning, for establishing innovative foundations for nursing practice, and for generating inquiry through research."[7:469] King stated, "Nurses who have knowledge of the concepts of this theory of goal attainment are able to accurately perceive what is happening to patients and family members and are able to suggest approaches for coping with the situations."[35:12]

King also developed a documentation system, a Goal Oriented Nursing Record (GONR), to accompany the Theory of Goal Attainment and record goals and outcomes. GONR is a method of collecting data, identifying problems, and implementing and evaluating care that has been used effectively in patient settings. The theory and the GONR are useful in practice, as nurses have the ability to provide individualized plans of care while encouraging active participation from clients in the decision-making phase.[35]

The GONR approach can be used to document the effectiveness of nursing care. "The major elements in this record system are: (a) data base, (b) nursing diagnosis, (c) goal list, (d) nursing orders, (e) flow sheets, (f) progress notes, and (g) discharge summary."[40:30-31]

King's systems framework and Theory of Goal Attainment[34] have been implemented in a variety of national and international practice settings. The following briefly identifies some of the settings. Jolly and Winker[23] described the application of the Theory of Goal Attainment within the context of nursing administration. Benedict and Frey[6] reported the implementation of theory-based practice in an emergency department. Alligood[1] applied the Theory of Goal Attainment to adult patients within orthopedic nursing settings. Laben, Sneed, and Seidel[44] used goal attainment in short-term group psychotherapy. Messmer[45] detailed the implementation of theory-based nursing practice in a large urban teaching hospital. Coker et al.[9] used the framework to implement nursing diagnoses in a Canadian community hospital, while Fawcett, Vaillancourt, and Watson[13] used the framework within a large Canadian tertiary care hospital.

Education

King's conceptual framework has been used at several universities (Ohio State, Loyola in Chicago, and University of Texas in Houston) for designing curriculum in nursing programs.[36] In 1980 Brown and Lee reported that King's concepts were useful in developing a framework for "use in nursing education, nursing practice, and for generating hypotheses for research . . . . [They] provide a systematic means of viewing the nursing profession, organizing a body of knowledge for nursing, and clarifying nursing as a discipline."[7:468] Rooke[51] described the use of King's system framework and the Theory of Goal Attainment in a Swedish educational setting.

Research

Many research projects have used King's work as a theoretical base. Several studies are mentioned here, and others are listed in the Bibliography.

Some research projects have used concepts from King's systems framework. Winker[61] developed a systems view of health. Rooke[52] identified the implications of space for nursing. Sieloff[54] defined the health of a social system.

Other research projects have used King's framework[34] as a theoretical base. This group of research includes the following studies:

1. Kemppainen[26] analyzed a case study of a patient who had HIV and was also experiencing psychotic symptoms.
2. Alligood, Evans, and Wilt[2] developed the concept of empathy within King's framework.
3. Hobdell[20] used King's framework[33] to work with parents of children with neural tube defects.
4. Sharts-Hopko[53] explored the perceived health status of women during the transition to menopause.
5. Doornbos[12] used King's framework to explore the health of families with young people who are chronically mentally ill.

Middle-range theories have also been developed using King's systems framework.[33] These include Frey's Theory of Families, Children, and Chronic Illness,[15] Killeen's Theory of Patient Satisfaction with Professional Nursing Care,[27] Sieloff's Theory of Departmental Power,[55] and Wicks's Theory of Family Health.[60]

Studies have also been done using the concepts of the Theory of Goal Attainment.[34] Hanucharurnkui and Vinya-nguag[19] used goal attainment to study the outcomes of self-care on postoperative patients' recovery and satisfaction. Froman[16] studied the perceptual congruency between nurses and clients experiencing medical-surgical conditions. Hanna's[18] use of the Theory of Goal Attainment promoted the health behavior of adolescents, and Kameoka[24] analyzed nurse-patient interactions.

FURTHER DEVELOPMENT

King has consistently demonstrated her belief in the need for further testing of the Theory of Goal Attainment. As early as 1971, she stated, "Any profession that has as its primary mission the delivery of social services requires continuous research to discover new knowledge that can be applied to improve practice. . . . The basis for the practice of nursing is knowledge; its activity is guided by the intellect, and applied in the practical realm."[30:112-113] "Because [the] systems framework has been synthesized from basic elements in nursing, it will persist into the 21st century despite professional and social changes."[39:15]

Fawcett and Whall[14] identified five major areas in which further development of King's work would be helpful. First, the concept of environment would benefit from additional definition and clarification. Second, King's views of illness, health, and wellness would also benefit from additional clarification and discussion. Third, middle-range theories that are currently implied, rather than explicit, such as those of Alligood, Evans, and Wilt[2] and Rooke,[51] would benefit from development into formal theories. Fourth, future linkages between King's systems framework[34] and other existing middle-range theories should continue to be done in a manner that assures congruency between the framework and the specific middle-range theory. And fifth, empirical testing should continue for both the Theory of Goal Attainment[34] and other middle-range theories developed within King's systems framework. Such testing would "add to the evidence regarding the empirical adequacy of the theories and their generalizability across various situations and client populations."[14:332]

CRITIQUE
Simplicity

King maintains that her definitions are clear and conceptually derived from research literature that existed at the time the definitions were published.

King's Theory of Goal Attainment[33] presented 10 major concepts, thus making the theory complex. However, these concepts are easily understood, and, with the exception of the concept of self, they have been derived from the research literature.

Generality

In the past, King's Theory of Goal Attainment[34] has been criticized for having limited application in areas of nursing where patients are unable to competently interact with the nurse.

King has responded that 70% of communication is nonverbal. She states the following:

> Try observing a good nurse interact with a baby or a child who has not yet learned the language. If you systematically recorded your observations, you would be able to analyze the behaviors and find many transactions at a nonverbal level. I have a beautiful example of that when I was working side by side with a graduate student in a neuro unit with a comatose patient. I was talking to the patient, explaining everything that was happening and showing the graduate student what I believe to be important in nursing care. When the patient regained consciousness a few days later, she asked the nurse in the unit to find that wonderful nurse who was the only one who explained what was happening to her. She wanted to thank her. I made transactions. I could observe her muscle movement. She was trying to help us as a physician poked a tube down her throat.
>
> A nurse midwife reports observing transactions between mothers and newborns. Psychiatric nurses have reported to me the value of my theory in their practice. So the need in nursing is to broaden nurses' knowledge of communication and that is what my theory is all about.[37]

Additional examples of the application of the Theory of Goal Attainment have been documented with psychiatric patients,[26,44] patients with acute orthopedic problems,[1] and developmentally disabled clients.[45]

King believes critics are assuming that a theory will address every person, event, and situation, which is impossible. She reminded critics that even Einstein's Theory of Relativity could not be tested completely until space travel made testing possible.[37]

Empirical Precision

King gathered empirical data on the nurse-patient interaction process that leads to goal attainment. A descriptive study was conducted to identify the characteristics of transaction and whether nurses made transactions with patients. From a sample of 17 patients, goals were attained in 12 cases (70% of the sample). King believes that if nursing students are taught the Theory of Goal Attainment and it is used in nursing practice, goal attainment can be measured and the effectiveness of nursing care can be demonstrated.[34]

King continues to serve as a consultant to researchers testing hypotheses derived from her theory. Since publication of her theory in 1981,[34] multiple research studies provide additional, and ongoing, evidence of the empirical precision of the Theory of Goal Attainment.

Froman[16] tested perceptual congruency between nurses and clients who were experiencing medical-surgical problems. Hanna[18] tested the Theory of Goal Attainment in promoting health behaviors of adolescents. Kameoka[24] analyzed interactions between nurses and patients, utilizing the Theory of Goal Attainment. Additional research projects are currently ongoing, and others are listed in the Bibliography.

Derivable Consequences

King's Theory of Goal Attainment focuses on all aspects of the nursing process (assessing, planning, implementing, evaluating). King believes one must assess to set mutual goals, plan to provide alternative means to achieve goals, and evaluate to determine if the goal was attained. King stated she is "the only [nurse theorist] who has provided a theory that deals with choice, alternatives, participation of all individuals in decision making and specifically deals with outcomes of nursing care."[37]

King's systems framework and Theory of Goal Attainment have been and continue to be used to implement theory-based practice in a variety of nursing practice settings in Canada, Japan, Sweden, and the United States. In addition, King's work has been demonstrated over time to be a comprehensive frame for curriculum development at various education levels. Finally, the framework has led to theory development at the grand and middle-range levels by King herself and other nurse researchers who have used her work.

CRITICAL THINKING *Activities*

1 Think about and write your personal definitions of environment, health, nursing, and person. Compare your definitions with King's definitions. How are they similar? How are they different? Are they more alike than different? If they are more alike, develop a plan to use King's framework and theory more extensively in your practice.

2 Analyze an interaction you have had with a patient. Were you able to achieve a transaction as King describes it? If so, why? If not, why not?

3 Does the philosophy of the organization in which you work encourage the involvement of the patients/clients in their care? If so, does mutual goal setting occur? If not, what changes would you suggest to more actively involve patients/clients in their own care?

4 Analyze the goal-setting process that occurs between the direct care staff and nursing management and administration in your organization. Is there mutual goal setting? Discuss changes that could be made in the organizational culture to facilitate mutual goal setting and attainment between nurse managers and administrators and registered nurses.

5 Develop a quality improvement plan to review patient outcomes based on whether the following occurs: mutual goal setting and attainment of client goals. Keep a record on the patients you care for to see the outcomes of the implementation of King's framework and theory in your nursing practice.

REFERENCES

1. Alligood, M.R. (1995). Theory of goal attainment: Application to adult orthopedic nursing. In M.A. Frey & C.L. Sieloff (Eds.), *Advancing King's systems framework and theory of nursing* (pp. 209-222). Thousand Oaks, CA: Sage.

2. Alligood, M.R., Evans, G.W., & Wilt, D.L. (1995). King's interacting systems and empathy. In M.A. Frey & C.L. Sieloff (Eds.), *Advancing King's systems framework and theory of nursing* (pp. 66-78). Thousand Oaks, CA: Sage.

3. Allport, F.H. (1955). *Theories of perception and the concept of structure.* New York: John Wiley & Sons.

4. Ardrey, R. (1966). *The territorial imperative.* New York: Atheneium.

5. Austin, J.K., & Champion, V.L. (1983). King theory for nursing: Explication and evaluation. In P. Chinn, *Advances in nursing theory development* (pp. 49-61). Rockville, MD: Aspen.

6. Benedict, M., & Frey, M.A. (1995). Theory-based practice in the emergency department. In M.A. Frey & C.L. Sieloff (Eds.), *Advancing King's systems framework and theory of nursing* (pp. 317-324). Thousand Oaks, CA: Sage.

7. Brown, S.T., & Lee, B.T. (1980). Imogene King's conceptual framework: A proposed model for continuing nursing education. *Journal of Advanced Nursing,* 5(5):467-473.

8. Clements, I.W., & Roberts, F.B. (1983). *Family health: A theoretical approach to nursing care.* New York: John Wiley & Sons.

9. Coker, E., Fradley, T., Harris, J., Tomarchio, D., Chan, V., & Caron, C. (1995). Implementing nursing diagnoses within the context of King's conceptual framework. In M.A. Frey & C.L. Sieloff (Eds.), *Advancing King's systems framework and theory of nursing* (pp. 161-175). Thousand Oaks, CA: Sage.

10. Dewey, J., & Bentley, A. (1949). *Knowing and the known.* Boston: Beacon Press.

11. Diers, D., & Schmidt, R. (1977). Interaction analysis in nursing research. In P. Verhonick (Ed.), *Nursing research II* (pp. 77-132). Boston: Little, Brown.

12. Doornbos, M.M. (1995). Using King's systems framework to explore family health in the families of the young chronically mentally ill. In M.A. Frey & C.L. Sieloff (Eds.), *Advancing King's systems framework and theory of nursing* (pp. 192-205). Thousand Oaks, CA: Sage.

13. Fawcett, J.M., Vaillancourt, V.M., & Watson, C.A. (1995). Integration of King's framework into nursing practice. In M.A. Frey & C.L. Sieloff (Eds.), *Advancing King's systems framework and theory of nursing* (pp. 176-191). Thousand Oaks, CA: Sage.

14. Fawcett, J., & Whall, A.L. (1995). State of the science and future directions. In M.A. Frey & C.L. Sieloff (Eds.), *Advancing King's systems framework and theory of nursing* (pp. 327-334). Thousand Oaks, CA: Sage.

15. Frey, M.A. (1995). Toward a theory of families, children, and chronic illness. In M.A. Frey & C.L. Sieloff (Eds.), *Advancing King's systems framework and theory of nursing* (pp. 109-125). Thousand Oaks, CA: Sage.

16. Froman, D. (1995). Perceptual congruency between clients and nurses: Testing King's theory of goal attainment. In M.A. Frey & C.L. Sieloff (Eds.), *Advancing King's systems framework and theory of nursing* (pp. 223-238). Thousand Oaks, CA: Sage.

17. Gonot, P.J. (1989). Imogene M. King: A theory for nursing. In J. Fitzpatrick & A. Whall, *Conceptual model of nursing: Analysis and application.* Bowie, MD: Robert J. Brady.

18. Hanna, K.M. (1995). Use of King's theory of goal attainment to promote adolescents' health behavior. In M.A. Frey & C.L. Sieloff (Eds.), *Advancing King's systems framework and theory of nursing* (pp. 239-250). Thousand Oaks, CA: Sage.

19. Hanucharurnkui, S., & Vinya-nguag, P. (1991). Effects of promoting patients' participation in self-care on postoperative recovery and satisfaction with care. *Nursing Science Quarterly,* 4(1):14-20.

20. Hobdell, E.F. (1995). Using King's interacting systems framework for research on parents of children with neural tube defect. In M.A. Frey & C.L. Sieloff (Eds.), *Advancing King's systems framework and theory of nursing* (pp. 126-136). Thousand Oaks, CA: Sage.

21. Ittleson, W., & Cantril, H. (1954). *Perception: A transactional approach.* Garden City, NY: Doubleday.

22. Jersild, A.T. (1952). *In search of self.* New York: Teachers College Press.

23. Jolly, M.L., & Winker, C.K. (1995). Theory of goal attainment in the context of organizational structure. In M.A. Frey & C.L. Sieloff (Eds.), *Advancing King's systems framework and theory of nursing* (pp. 305-316). Thousand Oaks, CA: Sage.

24. Kameoka, T. (1995). Analyzing nurse-patient interactions in Japan. In M.A. Frey & C.L. Sieloff (Eds.), *Advancing King's systems framework and theory of nursing* (pp. 251-260). Thousand Oaks, CA: Sage.

25. Kelley, K.J., & Hammond, K.R. (1964). An approach to the study of clinical inference. *Nursing Research,* 13(4):314-322.

26. Kemppainen, J.K. (1990). Imogene King's theory: A nursing case study of a psychotic client with human immunodeficiency virus infection. *Archives of Psychiatric Nursing,* 4(6):384-388.

27. Killeen, M.B. (1996). *Patient-consumer perceptions and responses to professional nursing care: Instrument development.* Unpublished doctoral dissertation, Wayne State University, Detroit.

28. King, I.M. (1964). Nursing theory: Problems and prospects. *Nursing Science, 1*(3):394-403.

29. King, I.M. (1968). A conceptual frame of reference for nursing. *Nursing Research, 17*(1):27-31.

30. King, I.M. (1971). *Toward a theory for nursing: General concepts of human behavior.* New York: John Wiley & Sons.

31. King, I.M. (1975). A process for developing concepts for nursing through research. In P. Verhonick, *Nursing research.* Boston: Little, Brown.

32. King, I.M. (1975). Patient aspects. In L.J. Schumann, R.D. Spears, Jr., & J.P. Young (Eds.), *Operations research in health care: A critical analysis.* Baltimore: Johns Hopkins University Press.

33. King, I.M. (Speaker). (1978). *Speech presented at Second Annual Nurse Educators' Conference.* Chicago: Teach 'Em.

34. King, I.M. (1981). *A theory for nursing: Systems, concepts, process.* New York: John Wiley & Sons.

35. King, I.M. (1984). Effectiveness of nursing care: Use of a goal oriented nursing record in end stage renal disease. *American Association of Nephrology Nurses and Technicians Journal, 11*(2):11-17, 60.

36. King, I.M. (1984). Telephone interview.

37. King, I.M. (1985). Personal correspondence.

38. King, I.M. (1986). *Curriculum and instruction in nursing: Concepts and process.* Norwalk, CT: Appleton-Century-Crofts.

39. King, I.M. (1995). A systems framework for nursing. In M.A. Frey & C.L. Sieloff (Eds.), *Advancing King's systems framework and theory of nursing* (pp. 14-22). Thousand Oaks, CA: Sage.

40. King, I.M. (1995). The theory of goal attainment. In M.A. Frey & C.L. Sieloff (Eds.), *Advancing King's systems framework and theory of nursing* (pp. 23-32). Thousand Oaks, CA: Sage.

41. King, I.M. (1996, July 11). Personal communication.

42. Krieger, D. (1975). Therapeutic touch: The imprimatur of nursing. *American Journal of Nursing, 75*(5):784-787.

43. Kuhn, A. (1975). *Unified social science.* Homewood, IL: Dorsey.

44. Laben, J.K., Sneed, L.D., & Seidel, S.L. (1995). Goal attainment in short-term group psychotherapy settings: Clinical implications for practice. In M.A. Frey & C.L. Sieloff (Eds.), *Advancing King's systems framework and theory of nursing* (pp. 261-277). Thousand Oaks, CA: Sage.

45. Messmer, P.R. (1995). Implementation of theory-based nursing practice. In M.A. Frey & C.L. Sieloff (Eds.), *Advancing King's systems framework and theory of nursing* (pp. 294-304). Thousand Oaks, CA: Sage.

46. Minckley, B.B. (1968). Space and place in patient care, *American Journal of Nursing, 68*(3):510-516.

47. Orlando, I.J. (1961). *The dynamic nurse-patient relationship: Functions, process, principles.* New York: G.P. Putnam's Sons.

48. Orme, J.E. (1969). *Time, experience and behavior.* New York: American Elsevier.

49. Paterson, J., & Zderad, L. (1976). *Humanistic nursing.* New York: John Wiley & Sons.

50. Peplau, H.E. (1952). *Interpersonal relations in nursing.* New York: G.P. Putnam's Sons.

51. Rooke, L. (1995). Focusing on King's theory and systems framework in education by using an experiential learning model: A challenge to improve the quality of nursing care. In M.A. Frey & C.L. Sieloff (Eds.), *Advancing King's systems framework and theory of nursing* (pp. 278-293). Thousand Oaks, CA: Sage.

52. Rooke, L. (1995). The concept of space in King's systems framework: Its implications for nursing. In M.A. Frey & C.L. Sieloff (Eds.), *Advancing King's systems framework and theory of nursing* (pp. 79-96). Thousand Oaks, CA: Sage.

53. Sharts-Hopko, N.C. (1995). Using health, personal, and interpersonal system concepts within the King's systems framework to explore perceived health status during the menopause transition. In M.A. Frey & C.L. Sieloff (Eds.), *Advancing King's systems framework and theory of nursing* (pp. 147-160). Thousand Oaks, CA: Sage.

54. Sieloff, C.L. (1995). Defining the health of a social system within Imogene King's framework. In M.A. Frey & C.L. Sieloff (Eds.), *Advancing King's systems framework and theory of nursing* (pp. 137-146). Thousand Oaks, CA: Sage.

55. Sieloff, C.L. (1995). Development of a theory of departmental power. In M.A. Frey & C.L. Sieloff (Eds.), *Advancing King's systems framework and theory of nursing* (pp. 46-65). Thousand Oaks, CA: Sage.

56. Sieloff, C.L. (1996). *Development of an instrument to estimate the actualized power of a nursing department.* Unpublished doctoral dissertation, Wayne State University, Detroit.

57. Sommer, R. (1969). *Personal space.* Englewood Cliffs, NJ: Prentice-Hall.

58. Watzlawick, P., Beavin, J.W., & Jackson, D.D. (1967). *Pragmatics of human communication.* New York: Norton.

59. Whiting, J.F. (1955). Q-sort technique for evaluating perceptions of interpersonal relationship. *Nursing Research, 4*:71-73.

60. Wicks, M.N. (1995). Family health as derived from King's framework. In M.A. Frey & C.L. Sieloff (Eds.), *Advancing King's systems framework and theory of nursing* (pp. 97-108). Thousand Oaks, CA: Sage.

61. Winker, C.K. (1995). A systems view of health. In M.A. Frey & C.L. Sieloff (Eds.), *Advancing King's systems framework and theory of nursing* (pp. 35-45). Thousand Oaks, CA: Sage.

62. Yura, H., & Walsh, M. (1978). *The nursing process.* New York: Appleton-Century-Crofts.

BIBLIOGRAPHY

Primary sources

Books

King, I.M. (1971). *Toward a theory for nursing: General concepts of human behavior.* New York: John Wiley & Sons.

King, I.M. (1981). *A theory for nursing: Systems, concepts, process.* New York: John Wiley & Sons.

King, I.M. (1986). *Curriculum and instruction in nursing: Concepts and process.* Norwalk, CT: Appleton-Century-Crofts.

Book chapters

King. I.M. (1976). The health care systems: Nursing intervention subsystem. In H.H. Werley, A. Zuzick, M.N. Zaikowski, & A.D. Zagornik (Eds.), *Health research: The systems approach* (pp. 51-60). New York: Springer.

King, I.M. (1983). King's theory of nursing. In I.W. Clements & F. B. Roberts (Eds.), *Family health: A theoretical approach to nursing care* (pp. 177-188). New York: John Wiley & Sons.

King, I.M. (1984). A theory for nursing: King's conceptual model applied in community health nursing. In M.K. Asay & C.C. Ossler (Eds.), *Proceedings of the Eighth Annual Community Health Nursing Conference: Conceptual models of nursing applications in community health nursing.* Chapel Hill: University of North Carolina.

King, I.M. (1988). Imogene M. King. In T.A. Schorr & A. Zimmerman (Eds.), *Making choices, taking chances* (pp. 146-153). St. Louis: Mosby.

King, I.M. (1988). King's system framework for nursing administration. In B. Henry, C. Arndt, M. DiVincenti, A. Marriner-Tomey (Eds.), *Dimensions of nursing administration* (pp. 35-45). Boston: Blackwell Scientific.

King, I.M. (1988). Measuring health goal attainment in patients. In C.F. Waltz & O.L. Strickland (Eds.), *Measurement of nursing outcomes: Vol. 4. Measuring client outcomes* (pp. 108-127). New York: Springer.

King, I.M. (1989). King's general systems framework and theory. In J.P. Riehl-Sisca (Ed.), *Conceptual models for nursing practice* (3rd ed.) (pp. 149-166). Norwalk, CT: Appleton & Lange.

King, I.M. (1990). King's conceptual framework and theory of goal attainment. In M.E. Parker (Ed.), *Nursing theories in practice* (pp. 73-84). New York: National League for Nursing.

Journal articles

Daubenmire, M.J., & King, I.M. (1973). Nursing process models: A systems approach. *Nursing Outlook, 21*(8):512-517.

Gulitz, E.A., & King, I.M. (1988, Aug.). King's general systems model: Application to curriculum development. *Nursing Science Quarterly, 1*(3):128-132.

King, I.M. (1970). A conceptual frame of reference for nursing. *Japanese Journal of Nursing Research, 3*:199-204.

King, I.M. (1970). Planning for change. *Ohio Nurses Review, 45*:4-7.

King, I.M. (1978). U.S.A.: Loyola University of Chicago School of Nursing. *Journal of Advanced Nursing, 3*(4):390.

King, I.M., & Tarsitano, B. (1982). The effect of structured and unstructured preop teaching: A replication. *Nursing Research, 31*(6):324-329.

King, I.M. (1984). Effectiveness of nursing care: Use of a goal-oriented nursing record in end-stage renal disease. *American Association of Nephrology Nurses and Technicians Journal, 11*(2):11-17, 60.

King, I.M. (1984). Philosophy of nursing education: A national survey. *Western Journal of Nursing Research, 6*(4):387-406.

King, I.M. (1985). Collaborative relationship in nursing research. *Florida Nurse, 33*(2):3, 15.

King, I.M. (1985). Patient education: Barriers and gateways. *Florida Nurse, 33*(5):4, 15.

King, I.M. (1987). Concepts: Essential elements of theories. *Nursing Science Quarterly, 1*(1):22-25.

King, I.M. (1987). Translating nursing research into practice. *Journal of Neuroscience Nursing, 19*(1):44-48.

King, I.M. (1990, Fall). Health as the goal for nursing. *Nursing Science Quarterly, 3*(3):123-128.

King, I.M. (1994). Quality of life and goal attainment. *Nursing Science Quarterly, 7*(1):29-32.

King, I.M. (1996). The theory of goal attainment in research and practice. *Nursing Science Quarterly, 9*(2):61-66.

Samples, J., Vancott, M.L., Long, C., King, I.M., & Kersenbrock, A. (1985). Circadian rhythms: Basis for screening for fever. *Nursing Research, 34*(6):377-379.

NLN publications

King, I.M. (1978). *How does the conceptual framework provide structure for the curriculum? Curriculum process for developing or revising baccalaureate nursing programs.* NLN Pub. No. 15-1700, pp. 23-34. New York: National League for Nursing.

King, I.M. (1978). The "why" of theory development. In *Theory development: What, why, how?* (pp. 11-16). NLN Pub. No. 15-1708. New York: National League for Nursing.

King, I.M. (1986). *King's theory of goal attainment.* NLN Pub. No. 15-2152, pp. 197-213. New York: National League for Nursing.

Letter to the editor

King, I.M. (1975). Reaction to "The patient rights advocate," by G.J. Annas & J. Healey. *Journal of Nursing Administration, 5*(1):40-41.

Foreword

King, I.M. (1969). Symposium on neurologic and neurosurgical nursing. *Nursing Clinics of North America, 4*(2):199-200.

Audiotapes

King, I.M. (1978, Dec. 4-6). *Nursing theory.* Wakefield, MA: Nursing Resources, Inc.

King, I.M. (1978). *Second Annual Nurse Educators' Conference,* held in New York City. Audiotape available from Teach 'em, Inc., 160 E. Illinois Street, Chicago, IL 60611.

King, I.M. (1984, 1986). *Nurse Theorist Conference* held at Edmonton, Alberta. Audiotapes available from Kennedy Recording, R.R. 5, Edmonton, Alberta, T5P 487 Canada.

King, I.M. (1985, 1987). King's theory. *Nurse Theorist Conference* held in Pittsburgh, PA. Audiotape available from Meetings International, 1200 Delor Ave., Louisville, KY 40217.

Videotapes

King, I.M. (1987). King's theory. *Nurse Theorist Conference* held in Pittsburgh, PA. Videotape available from Meetings International, 1200 Delor Ave., Louisville, KY 40217.

The Nurse Theorist: Portraits of Excellence: Imogene King. (1989). Oakland: Studio III from Fuld Video Project, 370 Hawthorne Ave., Oakland, CA 94609.

Presented paper

King, I.M. (1980, April 21). *Theory development in nursing.* Paper presented at Georgia State University, Atlanta.

Secondary sources

Book reviews

King, I.M. (1971). *Toward a theory for nursing: General concepts of human behavior.*
*Association of Operating Room Nurses' Journal, 14:*126, 1971.
*Canadian Nurse, 67:*40, 1971.
*Nursing Outlook, 19:*513, 1971.
*Nursing Research, 20:*462, 1971.
*American Journal of Nursing, 72:*1153, 1972.
*Journal of Nursing Administration, 2:*63, 1972.
*South African Nursing Journal, 40:*32, 1973.

King, I.M. (1981). *A theory for nursing: Systems, concepts, process.*
*American Association of Nurses and Nephrology Technicians Journal, 3:*39-40, 1981.

*Nursing Mirror, 154:*32, 1982.
*Nursing Outlook, 30:*414, 1982.
*Nursing Times, 78:*331, 1982.
*Research in Nursing and Health, 5:*166-167, 1982.
*Today's OR Nurse, 4:*62, 1982.
*Western Journal of Nursing Research, 4:*103-104, 1982.
Australian Nurses Journal, 12(7):33-34, 1983.

Books

Barnum, B.J. (1994). *Nursing theory: Analysis, application, evaluation* (4th ed.). Philadelphia: J.B. Lippincott.

Bevis, E.O. (1982). *Curriculum building in nursing: A process.* St. Louis: Mosby.

Chinn, P.L. (Ed.). (1983). *Advances in nursing theory development.* Rockville, MD: Aspen.

Chinn, P.L., & Jacobs, M.K. (1995). *Theory and nursing: A systematic approach.* St. Louis: Mosby.

Fitzpatrick, J.J., & Whall, A.L. (1995). *Conceptual models of nursing: Analysis and application.* Bowie, MD: Robert J. Brady.

Fitzpatrick, J.J., Whall, A., Johnston, R., & Floyd, J. (1982). *Nursing models and their psychiatric mental health applications.* Bowie, MD: Robert J. Brady.

George, J.B. (1995). *Nursing theories: The base for professional nursing practice.* Englewood Cliffs, NJ: Prentice-Hall.

Polit, D., & Hungler, B. (1995). *Nursing research: Principles and methods* (5th ed.). Philadelphia: J.B. Lippincott.

Steele, S. (1981). *Child health and the family: Nursing concepts and management.* New York: Masson.

Walker, L.O., & Avant, K.C. (1995). *Strategies for theory construction in nursing.* Norwalk, CT: Appleton-Century-Crofts.

Who's Who in America. (43rd ed.) (1984). Chicago: Marquis.

Who's Who in the Midwest. (1984). Chicago: Marquis.

Who's Who in American Women. (1986).

Who's Who in American Nursing. (1987, 1988).

Book chapters

Austin, J.K., & Champion, V.L. (1983). King theory for nursing: Explication and evaluation. In P. Chinn, *Advances in nursing theory development* (pp. 49-61). Rockville, MD: Aspen.

Chinn, P.L., & Jacobs, M.K. (1983). Theory in nursing: A current overview. In *Theory and nursing: A systematic approach* (pp. 190-191). St. Louis: Mosby.

Coker, E.B., & Schreiber, R. (1990). Implementing King's conceptual framework at the bedside. In M.E. Parker (Ed.), *Nursing theories in practice* (pp. 85-102). New York: National League for Nursing.

Secondary sources
Book chapters

Daubenmire, M.J. (1989). A baccalaureate nursing curriculum based on King's conceptual framework. In J.P. Riehl-Sisca (Ed.), *Conceptual models for nursing practice* (3rd ed.) (pp. 167-178). Norwalk, CT: Appleton & Lange.

DiNardo, P.B. (1989). Evaluation of the nursing theory of Imogene M. King. In J.P. Riehl-Sisca (Ed.), *Conceptual models for nursing practice* (3rd ed.) (pp. 159-166). Norwalk, CT: Appleton & Lange.

Elberson, E. (1989). Applying King's model to nursing administration. In B. Henry, C. Arndt, M. DiVincenti, & A. Marriner-Tomey (Eds.), *Dimensions of nursing administration* (pp. 47-53). Boston: Blackwell Scientific.

Fawcett, J. (1984). King's open systems model. In *Analysis and evaluation of conceptual models of nursing* (pp. 83-113). Philadelphia: F.A. Davis.

Fitzpatrick, J., Whall, A., Johnston, R., & Floyd, J. (1982). Nursing models. In *Nursing models and their psychiatric mental health application* (pp. 62-64). Bowie, MD: Robert J. Brady.

Frey, M.A., & Norris, D. (1997). King's systems framework and theory in nursing practice. In M.R. Alligood & A. Marriner-Tomey (Eds.), *Nursing theory: Utilization and application* (pp. 71-88). St. Louis: Mosby.

George, J.B. (1980). Imogene M. King. In Nursing Theories Conference Group, J.B. George, Chairperson, *Nursing theories: The base for professional nursing practice* (pp. 184-198). Englewood Cliffs, NJ: Prentice-Hall.

Gonot, P.J. (1983). Imogene M. King: A theory for nursing. In J. Fitzpatrick & A. Whall, *Conceptual models of nursing: Analysis and application* (pp. 221-243). Bowie, MD: Robert J. Brady.

Hanchett, E.S. (1988). Community assessment: King's conceptual framework—dynamic interacting systems. In *Nursing frameworks and community as client: Bridging the gap* (pp. 89-107). Norwalk, CT: Appleton & Lange.

Hanchett, E.S. (1988). King's general system framework. In *Nursing frameworks and community as client: Bridging the gap* (pp. 83-87). Norwalk, CT: Appleton & Lange.

Meleis, A.I. (1985). Imogene King. In *Theoretical nursing: Development and progress* (pp. 230-237). Philadelphia: J.B. Lippincott.

Pearson, A., & Vaughan, B. (1986). An interaction model for nursing. In A. Pearson & B. Vaughan, *Nursing models for practice* (pp. 124-139).

Thibodeau, J.A. (1983). History of the development of nursing models. In *Nursing models: Analysis and evaluation* (pp. 37-38). Monterey, CA: Wadsworth.

Journal articles

Brown, S.T., & Lee, B.T. (1980). Imogene King's conceptual framework: A proposed model for continuing nursing education. *Journal of Advanced Nursing, 5*(5):467-473.

Bunting, S.M. (1988, Nov.). The concept of perception in selected nursing theories. *Nursing Science Quarterly, 1*(4):168-174.

Burney, M.A. (1992). King and Neuman: In search of the nursing paradigm. *Journal of Advanced Nursing, 17*:601-603.

Byrne, E., & Schreiber, R. (1989, Feb.). Concept of the month: Implementing King's conceptual framework at the bedside [tables/charts]. *Journal of Nursing Administration, 19*(2):28-32.

Byrne-Coker, E., Fradley, T., Harris, J., Tomarchio, D., Chan, V., & Caron, C. (1990, July-Sept.). Implementing nursing diagnoses within the context of King's conceptual framework. *Nursing Diagnosis, 1*(3):107-114.

Byrne-Coker, E., & Schreiber, R. (1990, Jan.). King at the bedside. *Canadian Nurse, 86*(1):24-26.

Carter, K.F., & Dufour, L.T. (1994). King's theory: A critique of the critiques. *Nursing Science Quarterly, 7*(3):128-133.

Chance K.S. (1982). Nursing models: A requisite for professional accountability. *Advances in Nursing Science, 4*(2):46-65.

Connelly, C.E. (1986). Replication research in nursing. *AORN, 23*(1):71-77.

Craig, S. (1980). Theory development and its relevance for nursing. *Journal of Advanced Nursing, 5*(4):349-355.

Daubenmier, M.J., & King, I.M. (1973). Nursing process models: A systems approach. *Nursing Outlook, 21*:512-517.

DeFeo, D.J. (1990, Summer). Change: A central concern of nursing. *Nursing Science Quarterly, 3*(2):88-94.

DeHowitt, M.C. (1992). King's conceptual model and individual psychotherapy. *Perspectives in Psychiatric Care, 28*(4):11-14.

Flaskerud, J.H. (1986). On "Toward a theory of nursing action: Skills and competency in nurse-patient interaction." *Nursing Research, 35*(7):250-252.

Frey, M.A. (1989, Fall). Social support and health: A theoretical formulation derived from King's conceptual framework [research, tables/charts]. *Nursing Science Quarterly, 2*(2):138-148.

Gortner, S.R., & Nahm, H. (1977). An overview of nursing research in the U.S. *Nursing Research, 26*(1):10-33.

Hampton, D.C. (1994). King's theory of goal attainment as a framework for managed care implementation in a hospital setting. *Nursing Science Quarterly, 7*(4):170-173.

Hanchett, E.S. (1990, Summer). Nursing models and community as client . . . public health/community health nursing. *Nursing Science Quarterly, 3*(2):67-72.

Hanna, K. (1993). Effect of nurse-client transaction on female adolescents' oral contraceptive use. *Image, 25*(4):285-290.

Hanucharurnkui, S., & Vinya-nguag, P. (1991, Spring). Effects of promoting patients' participation in self-care on postoperative recovery and satisfaction with care [research, tables/charts]. *Nursing Science Quarterly, 4*(1):14-20.

Hanucharurnkul, S. (1989, May). Comparative analysis of Orem's and King's theories. *Journal of Advanced Nursing, 14*(5):365-72.

Husband, A. (1988, July). Application of King's theory of nursing to the care of the adult with diabetes. *Journal of Advanced Nursing, 13*(4):484-488.

Jacono, J., Hicks, G., Antonioni, C., O'Brien, K., & Rasi, M. (1990). Comparison of perceived needs of family members between registered nurses and family members of critically ill patients in intensive care and neonatal intensive care units. *Heart & Lung: Journal of Critical Care, 19*(1):72-78.

Jonas, C.M. (1987). King's goal attainment theory: Use in gerontological nursing practice. *Perspectives, 11*(4):9-12.

Kasch, C.R. (1986). Toward a theory of nursing action: Skills and competency in nurse-patient interaction. *Nursing Research, 35*(4):226-230.

Kenny, T. (1990). Erosion of individuality in care of elderly people in hospital—an alternative approach. *Journal of Advanced Nursing, 15*(5):571-576.

Kneeshaw, M.F. (1990). Nurses' perception of co-worker responses to smoking cessation attempts. *Journal of the New York State Nurses Association, 21*(1):9-13.

Kohler, P. (1988). Model of shared control. *Journal of Gerontological Nursing, 14*(7):21-25, 37-38.

Laben, J.K., Dodd, D., & Sneed, L. (1991). King's theory of goal attainment applied in group therapy for inpatient juvenile sexual offenders, maximum security state offenders, and community parolees, using visual aids. *Issues in Mental Health Nursing, 12*(1):51-64.

Levine, C.D., Wilson, S.F., & Guido, G.W. (1988, July). Personality factors of critical care nurses. *Heart & Lung: Journal of Critical Care, 17*(4):392-398.

Martin, J.P. (1990). Male cancer awareness: Impact of an employee education program [research, tables/charts]. *Oncology Nursing Forum, 17*(1):59-64.

McGirr, M., Rukholm, E., Salmoni, A., O'Sullivan, P., & Koren, I. (1990). Perceived mood and exercise behaviors of cardiac rehabilitation program referrals. *Canadian Journal of Cardiovascular Nursing, 1*(4):14-19.

Messner, R., & Smith, M.N. (1986). Neurofibromatosis: Relinquishing the masks; a quest for quality of life. *Journal of Advanced Nursing, 11*:459-464.

Norris, D.M., & Hoyer, P.J. (1993). Dynamism in practice: Parenting within King's framework. *Nursing Science Quarterly, 6*(2):79-85.

Rawlins, P.S., Rawlins, T.D., & Horner, M. (1990). Development of the family needs assessment tool. *Western Journal of Nursing Research, 12*(2):201-214.

Reed, P.G. (1986). A model for constructing a conceptual framework for education in clinical speciality. *Journal of Nursing Education, 25*(7):295-329.

Rooke, L., & Norberg, A. (1988). Problematic and meaningful situations in nursing interpreted by concepts from King's nursing theory and four additional concepts. *Scandinavian Journal of Caring Sciences, 2*(2):80-87.

Rossi, K., & Heikkinen, M. (1990). A view of occupational health nursing practice: Current trends and future prospects. *Recent Advances in Nursing, 26*:1-34.

Schreiber, R. (1991). Psychiatric assessment—"A la King." *Nursing Management, 22*(5):90.

Sirles, A.T., & Selleck, C.S. (1989). Cardiac disease and the family: Impact, assessment, and implications. *Journal of Cardiovascular Nursing, 3*(2):23-32.

Smith, M.C. (1988). King's theory in practice. *Nursing Science Quarterly, 1*(4):145-146.

Smith, M.J. (1988). Perspectives on nursing science. *Nursing Science Quarterly, 1*(2):80-85.

Strauss, S.S. (1981). Abuse and neglect of parents by professionals. *MCN, 6*:157-160.

Swindale, J.E. (1989). The nurse's role in giving preoperative information to reduce anxiety in patients admitted to hospital for elective minor surgery. *Journal of Advanced Nursing, 14*(11):899-905.

Symanski, M.E. (1991, March). Use of nursing theories in the care of families with high-risk infants: Challenges for the future. *Journal of Perinatal & Neonatal Nursing, 4*(4):71-77.

Takahashi, T. (1992). Perspectives on nursing knowledge. *Nursing Science Quarterly, 5*(2):86-91.

Temple, A., & Fawdry, K. (1992). King's theory of goal attainment: Resolving filial caregiver role strain. *Journal of Gerontological Nursing, 18*(3):11-15.

Villeneuve, M.J., & Ozolins, P.H. (1991, March). Sexual counselling in the neuroscience setting: Theory and practical tips for nurses. *AXON, 12*(3):63-67.

Weikel, C. (1987). Informed consent: An ethical dilemma . . . the nurse's role. *Today's OR Nurse, 9*(1):10-15.

Wheeler, K. (1989). Self-psychology's contributions to understanding stress and implications for nursing. *Journal of Advanced Medical-Surgical Nursing, 1*(4):1-10.

Woods, E.C. (1994). King's theory in practice with elders. *Nursing Science Quarterly, 7*(2):65-69.

Master's theses

Allan, N.J. (1995). Goal attainment and life satisfaction among frail elderly. *Master's Abstracts International, 35-05*, 1486.

Batchelor, S.G. (1994). Relationship of budgetary knowledge and staff nurses' attitudes towards cost-effectiveness. *Master's Abstracts International, 32-05,* 1365.

Davis, S.M. (1992). Patient outcome documentation: Development and implementation. *Master's Abstracts International, 30-04,* 1288.

Dawson, B.W. (1996). The relationship between functional social support, social network and the adequacy of prenatal care. *Master's Abstracts International, 35-01,* 0361.

Dispenza, J.M. (1990). Relationship of husband and wife perceptions of the coping responses of the female spouse of males in high level stress. *Master's Abstracts International, 28-03,* 407.

Monti, A. (1992). Members' perceptions of the transactions within their psychosocial club. *Master's Abstracts International, 30-04,* 1296.

O'Shall, M.L. (1989). The relationship congruency of role conception between head nurse and staff nurse and staff nurse job satisfaction. *Master's Abstracts International, 27-03,* 379.

Phillips, E.L. (1995). Diploma nursing students' attitudes toward poverty. *Master's Abstracts International, 33-06,* 1846.

Tawil, T.M.P. (1993). Gender differences in frequency of assistance and perceived elderly patients' level of need by spouse primary caregivers with the activities of daily living: Dressing and bathing. *Master's Abstracts International, 32-04,* 1172.

White-Linn, V.M. (1994). Perceived quality of life of adults aged 30-50 years with type I and type II diabetes. *Master's Abstracts International, 33-05,* 1496.

Doctoral dissertations

Brooks, E. (1995). *Exploring the perception and judgment of senior baccalaureate student nurses in clinical decision-making from a nursing theoretical perspective.* Unpublished doctoral dissertation, AAI9609336, The University of Tennessee–Knoxville.

Giovinco, G. (1985). Using patient care situations to apply Kohlberg's moral development theory to nursing. *Dissertation Abstracts International, 46-08A,* 2333.

Hanna, K.M. (1991). Effect of nurse-client transaction on female adolescents' contraceptive perceptions and adherence. *Dissertation Abstracts International, 51-07B,* 3323.

Killeen, M. (1996). Patient-consumer perceptions and responses to professional nursing care: Instrument development. *Dissertation Abstracts International, 57-04B,* 2479.

Krassa, T.J. (1994). A study of political participation by registered nurses in Illinois. *Dissertation Abstracts International, 56-02B,* 0743.

O'Connor, P. (1990). Service in nursing: Correlates of patient satisfaction. *Dissertation Abstracts International, 50-11B,* 4985.

Omar, M.A. (1990). Relationship of family processes to family life satisfaction in stepfamilies and biological families during pregnancy. *Dissertation Abstracts International, 51-03B,* 1196.

Rooke, L. (1990). Nursing and theoretical structures of nursing: A didactic attempt to develop the practice of nursing. *Dissertation Abstracts International, 51-04C,* 579.

Sieloff, C.L. (1996). Development of an instrument to estimate the actualized power of a nursing department. *Dissertation Abstracts International, 57-04B,* 2484.

Whetlon, B.T.B. (1996). A philosophy of nursing practice: An application of the Thomistic-Aristotelian concept of nature to the science of nursing. *Dissertation Abstracts International, 57-03A,* 1176.

Winker, C. (1996). A descriptive study of the relationship of interaction disturbance to the organizational health of a metropolitan general hospital. *Dissertation Abstracts International 57-07B,* 4306.

Zurakowski, T.L. (1991). Interpersonal factors and nursing home resident health (anomia). *Dissertation Abstracts International, 51-07B,* 4281.

Other sources

Allport, F.H. (1955). *Theories of perception and the concept of structure.* New York: John Wiley & Sons.

Bruner, J., Goodnow, J., & Austin, G. (1956). *A study in thinking.* New York: John Wiley & Sons.

Bruner, J.S., & Krech, W. (Eds.). (1968). *Perception and personality.* New York: Greenwood Press.

Buber, M. (1970). *I and thou.* New York: Scribner.

Churchman, C.W. (1968). *The systems approach.* New York: Delacorte Press.

Churchman, C.W., Ackoff, R., & Arnoff, E.L. (1957). *Introduction to operations research.* New York: John Wiley & Sons.

Dewey, J., & Bentley, A. (1949). *Knowing and the known.* Boston: Beacon Press.

Dubin, R. (1978). *Theory building.* New York: Free Press.

Dubos, R. (1961). *Mirage of health: Utopias, progress and biological change.* Garden City, NY: Doubleday.

Dubos, R. (1965). *Man adapting.* New Haven: Yale University Press.

Erikson, E. (1950). *Childhood and society.* New York: Norton.

Fawcett, J. (1978). The "what" of theory development. In *Theory development: What, why, how?* (pp. 17-33). NLN Pub. No. 15-1708. New York: National League for Nursing.

Feigl, H., & Brodbeck, M. (Eds.). (1953). *Readings in the philosophy of science.* New York: Appleton-Century-Crofts.

Freud, S. (1965). *Introductory lectures on psychoanalysis.* New York: Norton.

Gesell, A.L. (1952). *Infant development: The embryology of early human behavior.* New York: Harper.

Hall, J.E., & Weaver, B.R. (1977). *Distributive nursing: A system approach to community health.* Philadelphia: J.B. Lippincott.

Ittleson, W.H., & Cantril, H. (1954). *Perception: A transactional approach.* Garden City, NY: Doubleday.

Kelley, K.J., & Hammond, K.R. (1964). An approach to the study of clinical inference. *Nursing Research, 13*(4):314-322.

Knutson, A. (1965). *The individual, society, and health behavior.* New York: Russell Sage Foundation.

Linton, R. (1936). *The study of man: An introduction.* New York: Appleton-Century-Crofts.

Orlando, I.J. (1972). *The discipline and teaching of nursing process.* New York: G.P. Putnam's Sons.

Parsons, T. (1964). *The social system.* New York: Free Press of Glencoe.

Seyle, H. (1974). *Stress without distress.* Philadelphia: J.B. Lippincott.

Spiegel, J.P. (1971). *Transactions: The interplay between individual, family, and society.* New York: Science House.

von Bertalanffy, L. (1968). *General system theory: Foundations, development, application* (rev. ed.). New York: Braziller.

Weed, L.L. (1969). *Medical records, medical education, and patient care.* Cleveland: Press of Case Western Reserve University.

Wiener, N. (1967). *The human use of human beings: Cybernetics and society.* New York: Avon Books.

Woods, E.C. (1994). King's theory in practice with elders. *Nursing Science Quarterly, 7*(2):65-69.

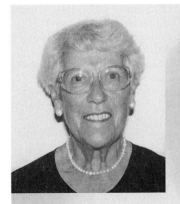

Nancy Roper

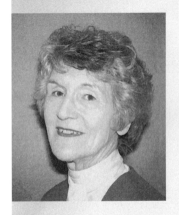

Winifred W. Logan

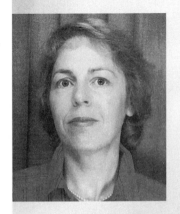

Alison J. Tierney

The Elements of Nursing: A Model for Nursing Based on a Model of Living

Ann Marriner Tomey

CREDENTIALS AND BACKGROUND OF THE THEORISTS

Nancy Roper

Nancy Roper was born in the United Kingdom on September 29, 1918. After completing a general education program, she left school in 1936 and became a student nurse for 3 years at a hospital for sick children, thereby gaining the qualification Registered Sick Children's Nurse (R.S.C.N.). During training she acknowledged her commitment to nursing by joining the Students' Association of the Royal College of Nursing.

World War II was declared as Roper moved into a 3-year program for general nursing, and she gained the qualification Registered General Nurse (R.G.N.). Career options were curtailed because conscription to the armed services was in force; but a teaching post was "reserved," and the principal invited Roper to accept the post as a staff nurse. After 2 years she was able to pursue the usual career of staff nurse posts in a variety of wards, followed by posts as a ward sister.

In 1950, Roper gained the London University's

The author wishes to express appreciation to Nancy Roper, Winifred W. Logan, and Alison J. Tierney for critiquing the chapter.

Teaching Diploma; thereafter, she taught for 15 years. During this period she acted as an examiner for the General Nursing Council and won a scholarship to investigate nurse education in the United States and Canada. Also during this time she edited *Churchill Livingstone Nurses' Dictionary*[7] and *Churchill Livingstone Pocket Medical Dictionary*.[5] Her writing during this period resulted in a book in which subjects were integrated; the book was called *Man's Anatomy, Physiology, Health and Environment*.[2] Toward the end of 1963, a choice had to be made between teaching and writing. In January 1964 Roper became self-employed as a writer, the first British nurse to do this.

For more than 30 years Roper has had the privilege of spending her time reading, writing, and thinking about nursing and observing the ever-changing scene related to practice, education, management, and research. The first edition of *Principles of Nursing*[3] was published in 1967, and the title of the fourth edition (1988) was *Principles of Nursing in Process Context*.[6]

In 1970, she was awarded a fellowship, which she used to pursue an M.Phil. at the University of Edinburgh. She investigated whether a core of nursing is required by patients wherever the patients are located. She defined this core of nursing and designed a Model of Living and a Model for Nursing. Her research monograph *Clinical Experience in Nurse Edu-*

cation was published in 1976.[4] Since it is now out of print, Roper has provided a synopsis of the recommendations, updating words where necessary:

> The model could be used for curriculum planning. Knowledge about each AL [activity of living] could be taught in the context of healthy people in a healthy environment. Knowledge about "the normal" would be assimilated before introduction to "the abnormal." The gap between theory and practice would be reduced if the model informed nursing education in such a way that it could guide nursing practice.
>
> The purpose of education programs is to help students to think in the way of the particular subject (discipline), for example, theologically. Our subject is nursing, and the suffix-*ology* means the study of, so logically the study of nursing is nursingology, and the objective of education programs should be to encourage nurses to think nursingologically.
>
> The literature refers to nursing as a practice discipline, and the two major components of practice disciplines are theory and practice. The practice of assessing, planning, implementing, and evaluating related to each patient needs to be supported by nursing's body of knowledge, a characteristic of a discipline, and this could be structured using the framework of the ALs.[4]

From 1974 to 1978, Roper was employed by the Scottish Home and Health Department in a newly created post of Nursing Research Officer. This enabled her to carry out several short-term assignments for the World Health Organization (WHO) European Office in Copenhagen and the Eastern Mediterranean Office in Alexandria, giving an international dimension to her nursing experience. She continues to collaborate with Logan and Tierney in refining the Roper/Logan/Tierney (R/L/T) Model for Nursing based on a Model of Living.[8]

Winifred W. Logan

Winifred Logan qualified as a nurse at the Royal Infirmary, Edinburgh. She had previously gained an M.A. degree at the University of Edinburgh and returned there in 1961 to take a teaching qualification. In 1966, on a WHO Fellowship, she completed an M.A. in Nursing and Allied Fields at Columbia University, New York. She was greatly influenced by her studies at Columbia; while there she was actively involved in discussions of concepts, models, definitions of nursing, and the nursing process, which she incorporated into her later work. She has an honorary degree from the University of Surrey.

Logan has enjoyed a varied career. Her nursing experience included periods in a diabetic unit and in thoracic and general surgery in the United Kingdom, Canada, and the United States.

While working in a thoracic surgery unit in Canada, the importance of considering the client's psychological and sociocultural circumstances made a profound impact when about 200 Eskimos (often whole families including grandparents) were airlifted from Baffinland to Hamilton to have treatment for tuberculosis. Inevitably there was considerable "culture shock" coming from igloos and skin tents to a modern hospital, and after a 2-year stay, of returning home to resume a nomadic existence in their arctic environment. Staff was almost forced to be aware of the psychological reactions of the Eskimos not only to illness but also to illness treated in an alien environment. Nurses also had to be responsive to the sociocultural differences between the Eskimos and most of the other patients and staff at the hospital. Shortly after, when Logan wrote the final year dissertation for a teaching qualification, this experience certainly contributed to her choice of the subject "Psychological and Sociocultural Aspects of Nursing." Later experiences reinforced these interests.

In 1956, a novel development in the United Kingdom was the creation of the Department of Nursing Studies at the University of Edinburgh. Logan was appointed to the staff in 1962 and became course coordinator for the first basic degree in Europe that included nursing as a graduating subject (almost 50 years after the first such course in the United States). She also taught in and at times was course organizer for the postbasic programs to prepare nurse educators and administrators, some of whom were recruited to the International School, located in the department, and sponsored by WHO. As a member of staff over a 12-year period, she was involved in promoting master's degrees and research degrees within the department.

During 1971 and 1972, Logan was granted a leave of absence from the University to take an appointment as the first Director of Nursing Services in the newly created Ministry of Health in Abu Dhabi, where she was responsible for setting up the Nursing Division.

In 1974, she moved to the Scottish Office to a newly created position as Nursing Officer for Education and Research. Later in the year the research commitment became a separate post, to which Roper was appointed. Then in 1978, Logan was appointed as Executive Director to the International Council of Nurses in Geneva, which permitted invaluable communication and cooperation with nurses on a worldwide scale. Her final post before retirement was as Head of Department of Health and Nursing at what is now Glasgow Caledonian University. At different points in her career, she was invited to act as a WHO Short-term Consultant in various countries (e.g., Malaysia, Iraq, Finland, Denmark, and Germany).

Logan has written a number of articles in a variety of journals and as co-author with Roper and Tierney has written several textbooks and articles. She has given lectures in various countries, participated in many nursing conferences nationally and internationally, and served on a number of nursing and academic committees.[1]

Alison J. Tierney

Alison Tierney decided at an early age that she wanted to become a nurse. Like many Scottish girls, she fancied the idea of going to London to train at one of the most famous schools of nursing. However, her parents persuaded her to go to a university because she had done well academically, and they thought she could do better than nursing. In the mid-1960s, nursing was still old-fashioned in outlook, and nurses were poorly paid. Her father learned that the University of Edinburgh combined university study with nurse training. So Tierney started as an undergraduate student in the Department of Nursing Studies at the University of Edinburgh in the autumn of 1966. Logan was one of the lecturers who taught Tierney.

The 4½-year integrated degree–nursing course contained enough clinical experience to satisfy Tierney's interest in "real" nursing. She found that the academic aspects opened up new and challenging

perspectives on nursing. Tierney found that, compared to other subjects that she studied as part of her integrated Social Sciences–Nursing degree such as psychology and social anthropology, nursing was very underdeveloped in terms of its own literature and research. After graduating in 1969 with a degree with distinction (B.Sc.:Soc.Sc.) and then registering as a general nurse (R.G.N.) early in 1971, Tierney worked as a Staff Nurse in London, where she quickly became frustrated by the highly routinized approach to patient care and the lack of opportunity to apply theoretical knowledge to practice.

Tierney returned home later that year to get married and to move to central Scotland, where her husband was pursuing his Ph.D. in the area of psychology at the University of Stirling. She had the opportunity to pursue a government-funded Nursing Research Training Fellowship. The Department of Nursing Studies at the University of Edinburgh was the only academic nursing center in Scotland. Consequently, Tierney registered there as a postgraduate research student to get supervision for her research. She commuted to Edinburgh for academic supervision and study while doing her research fieldwork near her home. She was exploring the application of behavioral therapy in nursing practice.

When her fellowship period expired in the autumn of 1973, Tierney was appointed to a junior lectureship in the department. She also continued working on her doctoral thesis and in 1976 was awarded her Ph.D., becoming one of the United Kingdom's first few graduate nurses to obtain this higher research degree. It was at this time that Tierney started working with Roper and Logan to further develop the Roper model. Tierney found this to be a valuable opportunity because at the time she was revising the first year undergraduate nursing curriculum and finding this difficult in the absence of a conceptual framework.

Tierney and her husband had moved back to Edinburgh. During the process of writing *The Elements of Nursing*,[9] she gave birth to their son. Soon after the publication of the book in 1980, she gave birth to their daughter. Tierney took a career break while both children were small and returned to work in 1984 as the Director of the Nursing Research Unit at the University of Edinburgh. That unit was the first government-funded center for nursing research in Europe when first established in 1971. After 10 years Tierney was tenured and then promoted in 1995 to Reader in Nursing Studies. Tierney was also honored that year with a Fellowship of the Royal College of Nursing (F.R.C.N.) and elected to this position in recognition of her "outstanding contribution to nursing research."

Tierney's extensive and varied involvement in nursing and health services research in the United Kingdom is evident in the many journal articles she has published and is reflected in the many invitations to present papers at international nursing research conferences. Because of her research background, her contribution to new editions of *The Elements of Nursing* are most concerned with the research content of the book. Tierney does not focus her own writing or conference presentations on the model. Roper is the group's ambassador. However, in 1997, Tierney presented a paper at a major International Conference on Nursing Theories in Germany, using that occasion for a critical appraisal of the relevance and role of the R/L/T model in Europe's fast-changing health care systems.[16]

THEORETICAL SOURCES

The original Roper models were based on research and an extensive review of the literature. They are now only of historical interest as they have been su-perseded by R/L/T models first published in 1980, followed by a second edition in 1985, a third in 1990, and a fourth in 1996.

USE OF EMPIRICAL EVIDENCE

When Roper was a principal of a teaching department preparing students for general registration, she arranged for various medical consultants to give lectures in their specialty. The nurse teachers then gave lectures about and practical demonstrations of the nursing procedures relevant to each consultant's lectures. Discussions with students who had practiced on each of the consultants' wards revealed there were more similarities than differences in the nursing activities on the various wards. Roper noticed that the similarities seemed to center around the patient's personal living, which was not medically prescribed. She began to see "nursing" and "doctoring" as complementary with distinct identities. She felt challenged to identify "nursing" and in 1964 became self-employed to pursue this "identification."

In 1970, she initiated a research project to investigate whether there was a "core of nursing." A literature review revealed a few projects about a core of nursing, but they had not collected data about actual patients; so a Patient Profile was used to collect data about patients in all the clinical areas to which one college of nursing allocated its students. Seven hundred seventy-four profiles were analyzed and re-

Text continued on p. 328.

MAJOR CONCEPTS & DEFINITIONS

A diagram of the Model of Living is presented in Fig. 21-1, and a diagram of the Model for Nursing is presented in Fig. 21-2. A comparison of the main concepts of the Model of Living and the Model for Nursing is presented in Table 21-1.

Four major concepts are common to both models and they are:
Activities of living (ALs)
Lifespan
Dependence/independence continuum

Five groups of factors influencing these:
Biological
Psychological
Sociocultural (including spiritual/religious/ ethical
Environmental
Politicoeconomic (including legal)
The interaction of these concepts produces the fifth main concept, which in the Model of Living is "individuality in living." To individualize nursing,

nurses need to know about the patient's individuality in living, which is accomplished by using the four phases of the nursing process dynamically and interactively. Furthermore, beginning students can imagine themselves at the center of the model and explore how the five concepts relate to their own lifestyle. Such knowledge about their own individuality in living can then influence their nursing practice.[14:51]

Activities of Living (ALs)
The person at the center of the models is characterized by 12 ALs, namely[14:20-23]:

Maintaining a safe environment
Communicating
Breathing
Eating and drinking
Eliminating
Personal cleansing and dressing
Controlling body temperature
Mobilizing
Working and playing
Expressing sexuality
Sleeping
Dying

Each AL has many dimensions, and it can be likened to a compound that comprises many elements.[14:20] The more one analyzes the ALs, the more one realizes just how complex each AL is. Compounding this complexity is the fact that the ALs are so closely related; we prioritize them in our daily living, and the concept of priority is of prime importance in nursing. The concept of relevance is also of importance, especially when people are being treated in day surgery units and short stay wards. Consequently, data about all 12 ALs may not need to be collected for every patient/client. Only relevant ALs need to be considered.[14:37] The experienced nurse can make decisions about "relatedness," "priorities," and "relevance" with speed and relative ease. The student, however, must learn to blend knowledge plus reflection on practice experience before being able to make such professional judgments.

Lifespan
The lifespan is defined as the temporal span of life on this earth from birth to death. Most countries have registry offices where births, deaths, and causes of death must be recorded, and from these data several predictions can be made about the population.[14:23] The relevance of the lifespan to nursing in general is discussed on p. 37 of the fourth edition of *The Elements of Nursing*,[14] and its relevance to each particular AL is discussed in the same book in the chapter about that AL.

Dependence/Independence Continuum
The dependence/independence continuum ranges from total dependence to total independence. Applying the continuum to the person as a whole is too broad, so it is directly applied to each AL. It acknowledges that there are stages when a person cannot yet (or can no longer) perform certain ALs independently.[14:23-24] The continuum is therefore bidirectional, an important concept in its application to nursing.[14:41-42] Its relevance to a particular AL is discussed in the appropriate chapter of *The Elements of Nursing*.

Factors Influencing ALs
There are many factors that have influenced or continue to influence the way in which an individual enacts the ALs. For the purpose of this model they are grouped under five headings[14:24-31, 42-51]:

Biological
Psychological
Sociocultural
Environmental
Politicoeconomic

In the Model of Living they are discussed on pp. 24 to 31 of *The Elements of Nursing*,[14] and in the Model for Nursing they are discussed on pp. 42 to 51 of the same book. They are applied to each particular AL in the appropriate chapter.

Individuality in Living
Individuality in living is manifested by the style in which individuals attend to each of their ALs according to the achieved stage on the lifespan and place on the dependence/independence continuum, which have all been, and still are being, influenced by the interacting five groups of factors. A schema of questions is proposed on p. 31 of *The Elements of Nursing*[14] to help the beginning student to conceptualize "individuality in living."

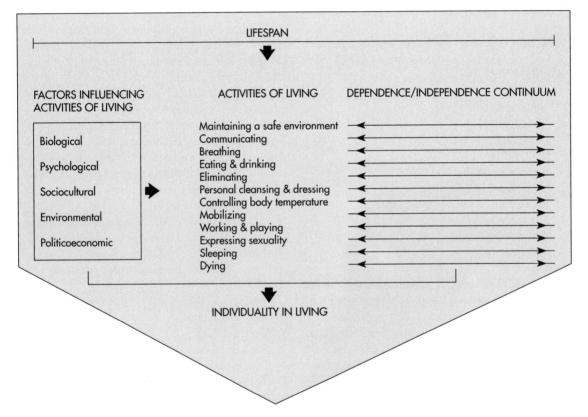

Fig. **21-1** Diagram of the Model of Living. *From Roper, N., Logan, W.W., & Tierney, A.J. (1996). The elements of nursing: A model for nursing based on a model of living (4th ed.) (p. 20). Edinburgh: Churchill Livingstone. Used with permission of Churchill Livingstone.*

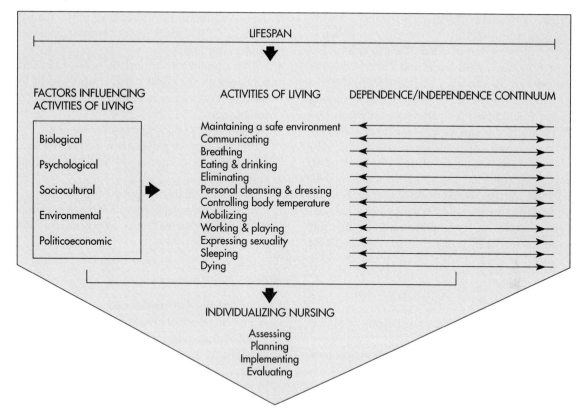

Fig. **21-2** **Diagram of the Model for Nursing.** *From Roper, N., Logan, W.W., & Tierney, A.J. (1996).* The elements of nursing: A model for nursing based on a model of living *(4th ed.) (p. 34). Edinburgh: Churchill Livingstone. Used with permission of Churchill Livingstone.*

Table **21-1**

Comparison of the main concepts in the Model of Living and the Model for Nursing

MODEL OF LIVING	MODEL FOR NURSING
12 Activities of living (ALs)	12 Activities of living (ALs)
Lifespan	Lifespan
Dependence/independence continuum	Dependence/independence continuum
Factors influencing the ALs	Factors influencing the ALs
Individuality in living	Individualizing nursing

From Roper, N., Logan, W.W., & Tierney, A. (1996). *The elements of nursing: A model for nursing based on a model of living* (4th ed.) (p. 33). Edinburgh: Churchill Livingstone. Used with permission of Churchill Livingstone.

vealed a core of everyday living activities. From the data and the literature review she developed a "Model of Living" and a "Model for Nursing."[4]

In 1976, she invited Logan and Tierney to refine and develop the models. Each member of the trio contributed her particular experiences of nursing practice, education, management, and research, and after frequent discussions and numerous drafts, the first combined R/L/T models were revised and published in 1980 in a book entitled *The Elements of Nursing.*[9] The title did not include the word "model," so library searches related to models for nursing did not retrieve this publication. For the second and subsequent editions of the book, however, the title was expanded to *The Elements of Nursing: A Model for Nursing Based on a Model of Living.*[12-14]

MAJOR ASSUMPTIONS[14:34-35]

- Living can be described as an amalgam of Activities of Living (ALs)
- The way ALs are carried out by each person contributes to individuality in living
- The individual is valued at all stages of the lifespan
- Throughout the lifespan until adulthood, the individual tends to become increasingly independent in the ALs
- While independence in the ALs is valued, dependence should not diminish the dignity of the individual
- An individual's knowledge, attitudes, and behavior related to the ALs are influenced by a variety of factors which can be categorized broadly as biological, psychological, sociocultural, environmental, and politicoeconomic factors
- The way in which an individual carries out the ALs can fluctuate within a range of normal for that person
- When the individual is "ill," there may be problems (actual or potential) with the ALs
- During the lifespan, most individuals experience significant life events which can affect the way they carry out ALs, and may lead to problems, actual or potential
- The concept of potential problems incorporates the promotion and maintenance of health, and

the prevention of disease, and identifies the role of the nurse as a health teacher, even in illness settings
- Within a health care context, nurses work in partnership with the client/patient, who, except for special circumstances, is an autonomous, decision-making person
- Nurses are part of a multiprofessional health care team who work in partnership for the benefit of the client/patient, and for the health of the community
- The specific function of nursing is to assist the individual to prevent, alleviate or solve, or cope positively with problems (actual or potential) related to the ALs

Nursing

Nursing is defined as helping people to:
- Prevent potential problems related to their ALs, becoming actual problems (This is particularly applicable to the work of midwives, health visitors, and school and occupational health nurses.)
- Alleviate or solve problems[14:35]
- Prevent recurrence of treated problems
- Cope in a positive way with any problems including death, dying, and bereavement[14:395]

Person

An individual person is central to both models and is conceptualized as attending to 12 ALs according to dependence/independence status for each of them and stage on the lifespan against the contextual background of biological, psychological, sociocultural, environmental, and politicoeconomic factors. The terms *person, patient,* and *client* are used interchangeably and sometimes include the family and significant others, who are also individuals.[14:31]

Health

The question "What is health?" is discussed by describing the WHO definition of health, health/illness continuum, lay perceptions of health, health as coping, personal responsibility for health, and current health targets.[14:5-6] Aided independence is also discussed; a person may feel healthy even when he or she has a significant disability, which may be mental or physical.[14:6]

Obviously the expected outcome when preventing potential problems from becoming actual ones is acquisition and maintenance of a positive health status. At appropriate places throughout the text, activities to prevent such conditions as dental caries, lung cancer, malnutrition, and sexually transmitted disease are discussed.

Environment

The environment is conceptualized in a broad dimension and includes all that is physically external to a person.[14:28-29, 47-49] This of course includes other people in the environment, highlighting the interaction of psychological and sociocultural factors with environmental factors. So important is the environment that "maintaining a safe environment" is featured as one of the 12 ALs[14:65-101] and is discussed in each of the other ALs in the appropriate chapter of *The Elements of Nursing*.[14]

THEORETICAL ASSERTIONS

"Individuality in living" is a product of the constant interaction of the model's other four main concepts, namely the 12 ALs, the lifespan, the dependence/independence continuum, and the five groups of factors influencing all of these.[14:31] People have to go on "living" while they require "nursing"; consequently, nurses need to know about a person's "individuality in living" before individualized nursing can be planned, implemented, and evaluated with the objectives of[14:33]:

  Preventing potential problems from becoming actual ones

  Alleviating or solving actual problems

  Coping in a positive way with problems that cannot be solved

  Preventing recurrence of treated problems

  Coping in a positive way with death, dying, and bereavement

LOGICAL FORM

Roper, Logan, and Tierney have used inductive logic by observing particular care situations and analyzing them to develop general theoretical statements.

ACCEPTANCE BY THE NURSING COMMUNITY

The Model for Nursing based on a Model of Living is used widely throughout Europe in a wide range of clinical areas. Nursing communities have asked for translation of *The Elements of Nursing* into Dutch, Estonian, Finnish, German, Italian, Lithuanian, Portuguese, and Spanish. Susan Whittam[17] has described use of the model, and Steve Smith[15] has received a grant to produce a booklet about providing nursing care based on the R/L/T model for people with Huntington's disease.

The model has provoked some negative criticism. When the first edition was published in 1980, "expressing sexuality" was still a taboo subject in the United Kingdom, whereas now it is discussed freely, even in lay magazines. The 1980 version was also criticized as still retaining the medical model flavor. In fact, psychological, sociocultural, environmental, and politicoeconomic factors were discussed in addition to the biological or physical factor, but their importance was underscored as long ago as the second edition (1985) when the five factors were presented as a separate concept in the diagram of the model and discussed as such within each AL chapter.

Practice

The Model for Nursing can be used by nurses in any specialty. The model is only a guideline, a reflection of reality. Nurses must make it real for each patient/client. There are numerous instances in the United Kingdom and in other countries where ward documentation has been based on the R/L/T model.

Education

The models are used widely in the United Kingdom in nursing education programs.

Research

Susan Whittam, of Bury Healthcare NHS Trust, Bury General Hospital, Walmersley Road, Bury, Lancashire, BL96PG, is doing current studies related to the models in nursing practice and education.

FURTHER DEVELOPMENT

The models can continue to be enlarged, changed, and refined. Concepts that are no longer useful in nursing practice can and should be deleted.

CRITIQUE

Simplicity

The model appears to be simple because of the use of everyday language, but the concepts are complex. John Ruskin indicated that it is more difficult to be simple than to be complex.[14:34]

Generality

The models can be adapted to any nursing situation,[14:33] including but not limited to:

Health promotion
Health maintenance
Prevention of disease
In relation to illness, acute or chronic
In relation to relationships
Helping to die with dignity
Any age group
Irrespective of dependence/independence status
Irrespective of culture, social class, environmental conditions, or politicoeconomic circumstances

Two of the authors' publications, *Learning to Use the Process of Nursing*[10] and *Using a Model for Nursing*,[11] illustrate the application of the first (1980) R/L/T models when providing nursing care for people of different age groups in different health settings (e.g., in the home, in medical, surgical, psychiatric and maternity units) who have a variety of health problems (actual and potential), such as postnatal management, diabetes mellitus, the aftermath of head injury, or coping with lung cancer. Articles by other nurse authors also demonstrate the use of the R/L/T models (in some instances, the more recent versions) in a range of settings.

Empirical Precision

The model initially looks simple, but the concepts are complex and may be difficult to measure. However, the concept of "activities of living" was selected in preference to "needs" because ALs are observable and can be explicitly described and, in some instances, objectively measured.[14:36]

Derivable Consequences

It is not necessary for a model to attempt to exhaust every aspect of a discipline. It is a guideline amenable to the creativity of the user. These models can be used in any nursing situation.

CRITICAL THINKING *Activities*

1 Identify the four major concepts common to both the Model of Living and the Model for Nursing.

2 List the 12 ALs down the side of a piece of paper and the five factors influencing ALs across the top of the page to form a grid. Create a case study addressing the items on the grid.

3 Plan care based on the case study you developed, one that your classmates developed, or a real situation using the Model for Nursing.

REFERENCES

1. Logan, W. (1996). Personal correspondence.
2. Roper, N. (1963). *Man's anatomy, physiology, health and environment.* Edinburgh: Churchill Livingstone.
3. Roper, N. (1967). *Principles of nursing.* Edinburgh: Churchill Livingstone.
4. Roper, N. (1976) *Clinical experience in nurse education* (research monograph). Edinburgh: Churchill Livingstone.
5. Roper, N. (1987). *Churchill Livingstone pocket medical dictionary* (14th ed.). Edinburgh: Churchill Livingstone.
6. Roper, N. (1988). *Principles of nursing in process context* (4th ed.). Edinburgh: Churchill Livingstone.

7. Roper, N. (1989). *Churchill Livingstone nurses' dictionary* (16th ed.). Edinburgh: Churchill Livingstone.
8. Roper, N. (1996). Personal correspondence.
9. Roper, N., Logan, W., & Tierney, A. (1980). *The elements of nursing.* Edinburgh: Churchill Livingstone.
10. Roper, N., Logan, W., & Tierney, A. (1981). *Learning to use the process of nursing.* Edinburgh: Churchill Livingstone.
11. Roper, N., Logan, W., & Tierney, A. (Eds.). (1983). *Using a model for nursing.* Edinburgh: Churchill Livingstone.
12. Roper, N., Logan, W., & Tierney, A. (1985). *The elements of nursing: A model for nursing based on a model of living* (2nd ed.). Edinburgh: Churchill Livingstone.
13. Roper, N., Logan, W., & Tierney, A. (1990). *The elements of nursing: A model for nursing based on a model of living* (3rd ed.). Edinburgh: Churchill Livingstone.
14. Roper, N. Logan, W., & Tierney, A. (1996). *The elements of nursing: A model for nursing based on a model of living* (4th ed.). Edinburgh: Churchill Livingstone.
15. Smith, S. (1983). Grant from National Board for Nursing Midwifery and Health Visiting Scotland, Education Fund to investigate Huntington's disease and (1994) grant from The Borders Health Board Research and Development to study Huntington's disease.
16. Tierney, A. (1996). Personal correspondence.
17. Whittam, S. (1993). *Introduction to Roper/Logan/Tierney model into practice* [unpublished paper].

BIBLIOGRAPHY
Primary sources
Books

Roper, N. (1976). *Clinical experience in nurse education* (research monograph). Edinburgh: Churchill Livingstone.
Roper, N. (1976). *Man's anatomy, physiology, health and environment* (5th ed.). Edinburgh: Churchill Livingstone.
Roper, N. (1987). *Churchill Livingstone pocket medical dictionary* (14th ed.). Edinburgh: Churchill Livingstone.
Roper, N. (1988). *New American pocket medical dictionary* (2nd ed.). Edinburgh: Churchill Livingstone.
Roper, N. (1988). *Principles of nursing in process context* (4th ed.). Edinburgh: Churchill Livingstone.
Roper, N. (1989). *Churchill Livingstone nurses' dictionary* (16th ed.). Edinburgh: Churchill Livingstone.
Roper, N., Logan, W., & Tierney, A. (1980). *The elements of nursing.* Edinburgh: Churchill Livingstone.
Roper, N., Logan, W., & Tierney, A. (1981). *Learning to use the process of nursing.* Edinburgh: Churchill Livingstone.
Roper, N., Logan, W., & Tierney, A. (Eds.). (1983). *Using a model for nursing.* Edinburgh: Churchill Livingstone.
Roper, N., Logan, W., & Tierney, A. (1985). *The elements of nursing: A model for nursing based on a model of living* (2nd ed.). Edinburgh: Churchill Livingstone.
Roper, N., Logan, W., & Tierney, A. (1990). *The elements of nursing: A model for nursing based on a model of living* (3rd ed.). Edinburgh: Churchill Livingstone.

Roper, N., Logan, W., & Tierney, A. (1996). *The elements of nursing: A model for nursing based on a model of living* (4th ed.). Edinburgh: Churchill Livingstone.

Book chapters

Roper, N. (1979). Nursing based on a model of living. In M. College & D. Jones (Eds.), *Readings in nursing.* Edinburgh: Churchill Livingstone.
Roper, N., Logan, W., & Tierney, A. (1986). Nursing models: A process of construction and refinement. In B. Kershaw & J. Salvage (Eds.), *Models for nursing.* Chichester: John Wiley.
Roper, N., Logan, W., & Tierney, A. (1996). The Roper-Logan-Tierney model: A model in nursing practice. In P. Hinton-Walker, B. Newman (Eds.), *Blueprint for use of nursing models.* New York: NLN Press.

Journal articles

Kilgour, D., & Logan, W. (1985). A model for health: Its use in an undergraduate nursing programme. *Nurse Education Today, 82*(35), 215-220.
Logan, W. (1981). A model for imitation [Janforum; The nursing process and standards of care]. *Journal of Advanced Nursing, 6,* 505-506.
Logan, W. (1987). Part of the plan: A degree programme in India (based on the R/L/T model). *Senior Nurse, 6*(6), 30-32.
Roper, N. (1976, April 29, May 6). An image of nursing for the 1970s. *Nursing Times* [Occasional papers], *72,* 17, 18.
Roper, N. (1976, May). A model for nursing and nursology. *Journal of Advanced Nursing, 1*(3), 219-227.
Roper, N. (1983, Nov. 30). A model for nursing. *Nursing Mirror, 157*(22), 21-23.
Roper, N. (1986). The Roper/Logan/Tierney model for nursing: Part II. *Irish Nursing Forum and Health Sciences, 3*(4), 32-34.
Roper, N. (1994, April 14). Definition of nursing . . . Part 1. *British Journal of Nursing, 3*(7), 355-357.
Roper, N. (1994, May 12). Definition of nursing . . . Part 2. *British Journal of Nursing, 3*(9), 460-462.
Roper, N., Logan, W., & Tierney, A. (1983, March 2). A model for nursing. *Nursing Times, 79*(9), 24-27.
Roper, N., Logan, W., & Tierney, A. (1983, May 25). A nursing model: Nursing process 1. *Nursing Mirror, 156*(21), 17-19.
Roper, N., Logan, W., & Tierney, A. (1983, June 1). Is there a danger of "processing" patients? Nursing process 2. *Nursing Mirror, 156*(22), 32-33.
Roper, N., Logan, W., & Tierney, A. (1983, June 8). Problems or needs? Nursing process 3. *Nursing Mirror, 156*(23), 43-44.
Roper, N., Logan, W., & Tierney, A. (1983, June 15). Identifying the goals: Nursing process 4. *Nursing Mirror, 156*(24), 22-23.
Roper, N., Logan, W., & Tierney, A. (1983, June 22). Endless paperwork: Nursing process 5. *Nursing Mirror, 156*(25), 34-35.
Roper, N., Logan, W., & Tierney, A. (1983, June 29). Unity—with diversity: Nursing process 6. *Nursing Mirror, 156*(26): 35.

Roper, N., Logan, W., & Tierney, A. (1985, July). The Roper-Logan-Tierney model. *Senior Nurse, 3*(2), 20-26.

Tierney, A. (1984). A response to Professor Mitchell's "Simple guide to the nursing process." *British Medical Journal, 288,* 835-838.

Tierney, A. (1984, May 16). Defending the process. *Nursing Times, 80*(20), 38-41.

Secondary sources

Books

Jamieson, E., McCall, J., Blythe, R., with Logan, W., as consultant. (1992). *Guidelines for clinical nursing practices: Related to a nursing model* (2nd ed.). Edinburgh: Churchill Livingstone.

Newton, C. (1991). The Roper-Logan-Tierney model in action. Basingstoke, Hampshire: Macmillan.

Book chapters

Chew, A., & Williams, A.P.M. (1988). Care plan for a woman with cardiac failure using Roper's activities of living mode. In H. Chalmers (Ed.), *Choosing a model: Caring for patients with cardiovascular and respiratory problems* (pp. 57-69). London: Edward Arnold.

Pearson, A., Vaughn, B., Fitzgerald, M. (1996). The activities of living model for nursing. In *Nursing models for practice* (2nd ed.) (pp. 72-89). Oxford: Butterworth-Heinemann.

Journal articles

Allan, D. (1986, Oct.). Nursing the unconscious patient. *The Professional Nurse,* pp. 15-17.

Allan, S. (1987). Arms extended (development of a tool to measure dependence/independence in people with multiple sclerosis). *Nursing Times, 83*(43), 44-45.

Bagnall, P., & Heslop, A. (1987, June). Chronic respiratory disease: Educating patients at home. *The Professional Nurse, 2*(9), 293-296.

Barr, A. (1992, Nov. 12). Care of a patient with breathing difficulties. *British Journal of Nursing, 1*(13), 660-665.

Bellman, L.M. (1996, July). Changing nursing practice through reflection on the Roper, Logan, and Tierney model. *Journal of Advanced Nursing, 24*(1), 129-138.

Davis, M. (1993, Jan. 27). Two contrasting nursing models. *Nursing Times, 89*(Suppl. 4), 1-8.

Dunn, C. (1986, Aug. 13). An holistic approach to intensive care. *Nursing Times, 82*(33), 36-38.

Ford, S. (1987). Into the outside. (Preparation of a mentally handicapped man to be discharged from hospital into the community.) *Nursing Times, 83*(20), 40-42.

Harrison, A. (1986, June 25). Compression fractures of the thoracic vertebrae. *Nursing Times, 82*(26), 40-42.

Heslop, A.P., & Bagnall, P. (1988). A study to evaluate the intervention of a nurse visiting patients with disabling chest disease in the community. *Journal of Advanced Nursing, 13,* 71-77.

James, G. (1986, April). Planning for terminal care. *Nursing Times, 23,* 24-27.

Jukes, M. (1987, March). Assessing the whole person (mental handicap). *Senior Nurse, 6*(3), 14-16.

Ledger, S.D. (1986). Management of a patient in respiratory failure due to chronic bronchitis. *Intensive Care Nursing, 2,* 30-43.

Mantle, F. (1996, Feb. 7). Safe practices. *Nursing Times, 92*(6), 36-38.

McCaugherty, D. (1992, Sept. 10). The Roper nursing model as an educational and research tool. *British Journal of Nursing, 1*(9), 455-459.

Mitchell, J.R.A. (1984). Is nursing any business of doctors? A simple guide to the nursing process. *British Medical Journal, 288,* 216-219.

Moir, S. (1986, May-June). Introducing a model for nursing to the community. *Irish Nursing Forum and Health Services,* pp. 26-28.

Page, M. (1995, Feb.). Tailoring nursing models to clients' needs. *Professional Nurse, 10*(5), 284-288.

Rhodes, K. (1990, May 23). Parkinson's disease using the Roper model. *Nursing Times, 86*(21), 36-39.

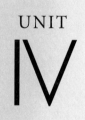

Middle-Range Nursing Theories

- *Nursing theories have been derived from works in other disciplines related to nursing, from earlier works in nursing such as philosophies and theories, and from nursing conceptual models and grand theories.*

- *Nursing theories propose outcomes that are less abstract than grand theories and more specific to practice.*

- *Middle-range theories are specific to nursing practice and specify the area of practice, age range of the client, the nursing action or intervention, and the proposed outcome.*

- *This section includes early nursing theories and current theoretical works.*

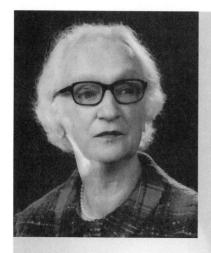

*H*ildegard E. Peplau

Psychodynamic Nursing

Chérie Howk, Gail H. Brophy, Elizabeth T. Carey, John Noll,
LyNette Rasmussen, Bryn Searcy, Nancy L. Stark

CREDENTIALS AND BACKGROUND OF THE THEORIST

Hildegard E. Peplau was born September 1, 1909, in Reading, Pennsylvania. She graduated from Pottstown, Pennsylvania, Hospital School of Nursing in 1931. Peplau received a B.A. in interpersonal psychology from Bennington College, Vermont, in 1943, an M.A. in psychiatric nursing from Teachers College, Columbia, New York, in 1947, and an Ed.D. in curriculum development from Columbia in 1953.[3]

Peplau's professional and teaching experiences have been broad and varied. She was operating room supervisor at Pottstown Hospital and later headed the staff of the Bennington infirmary while pursuing her undergraduate degree.

The authors wish to express appreciation to Hildegard E. Peplau for critiquing the original chapter.

Peplau did clinical work at Bellevue and White Institute psychiatric facilities, during which time she studied with renowned psychiatrists Eric Fromm, Freida Fromm-Riechman, and Harry Stack Sullivan. As a member of the Army Nurse Corps during World War II, Peplau worked in a neuropsychiatric hospital in England.

After obtaining her master's degree at Columbia, Peplau was invited to develop and teach in the graduate program in psychiatric nursing. She remained on the faculty 5 years. In 1954, Peplau went to Rutgers, where she developed and chaired the graduate psychiatric nursing program until her retirement in 1974.[14]

In 1969, Peplau became executive director of the American Nurses Association. She served as president of the ANA from 1970 to 1972, and as second vice-president from 1972 to 1974.[35] She has also served as director of the New Jersey State Nurses' Association; a member of the Expert Advisory Council of WHO; the National Nurse Consultant to the Surgeon General of the Air Force; and a nursing consultant to the United States Public Health Service, the National Institute of Mental Health, and various foreign countries.[3] She chaired the editorial board of *Perspectives in Psychiatric Care* when the journal was founded and served as chief advisor of *Nursing 74*. She is on the editorial board of the *Journal of Psychosocial Nursing* and the *Journal of Psychiatric and Mental Health Nursing*. In 1987, she was honored as the first psychosocial nurse of the year by the *Journal of Psychosocial Nursing*.

In 1994, Peplau's career was highlighted by her induction into the American Academy of Nursing Living Legends Hall of Fame. In 1995, Peplau was selected as one of the 50 Great Americans chosen to be included in the 50th Edition of *Who's Who in America*. At 87 years old, Peplau continues to occasionally lecture and present her work throughout the United States, Canada, Africa, and South America. Peplau's publications have continued consistently from 1952 to 1996, where enhancement and development of her work continues.[34]

Peplau has greatly contributed to the profession of nursing, in particular the specialty of psychiatric nursing, with the publishing of her book *Interpersonal Relations in Nursing*. Throughout the 1950s and 1960s, Peplau conducted workshops, "abundantly sharing her knowledge and clinical skills . . . [and] encouraged nurses to use their competence . . . in a continuous, experiential and educative process."[28;31:123] Peplau analyzed verbatim notes of sessions with medical and psychiatric patients to develop numerous lectures, articles, and workshops.

William E. Field, Jr., perpetuated Peplau's work by publishing *The Psychotherapy of Hildegard E. Peplau*.[7] In this book, Field compiled copious notes on the numerous lectures Peplau delivered to psychiatric nurses. Ultimately, Field's book presented Peplau's theory and method of investigative psychotherapy as it was developed from 1948 to 1974.

Peplau's archives are deposited in the Arthur and Elizabeth Schlesinger Library on the History of Women in America, Radcliffe College, Cambridge, Massachusetts.

THEORETICAL SOURCES

Peplau was committed to incorporating established knowledge into her conceptual framework, thus developing a theory-based nursing model. Peplau's theory of interpersonal relations integrated existing theories into her model at a time when nursing theory development was relatively new.

The nature of science in nursing refers to the "body of verified knowledge found within the discipline of nursing . . . [that is] mainly knowledge from the biological and behavioral sciences."[1:35] The "synthesis, reorganization, or extension of concepts drawn from the basic and applied sciences, which in their reformation tend to become new concepts," has led to the growth of nursing science[18:292]

Peplau used knowledge borrowed from behavioral science and what can be termed the *psychological model* to develop her theory of interpersonal relations. Borrowing from the psychological model "enabled the nurse to begin to move away from a disease orientation to one whereby the psychologic meaning of events, feelings, and behaviors could be explored and incorporated into nursing interventions. It gave nurses an opportunity to teach patients how to experience their feelings and to explore with clients how to bear their feelings."[35:6] The conceptual framework of interpersonal relations seeks to develop the nurse's skill in using these concepts. Harry Stack Sullivan,[42] Percival Symonds,[43] Abraham Maslow and Bela Mittleman,[21] and Neal Elgar Miller[23] are some of the major sources Peplau used in developing her conceptual framework. Some of the therapeutic conceptions devised by these theorists arose directly from the works of Freud[11] and Fromm.[12]

Peplau studied Freud extensively during her college days but rejected his theories as not very useful in her work with patients or clinical work in general.

USE OF EMPIRICAL EVIDENCE

Theories available when Peplau developed her theory described behavior within the prospectives of psychoanalytic theory, the principles of social learning, the concept of human motivation, and the concept of personality development. Peplau combined the various ideas of Maslow, Sullivan, Miller, and

Symonds. These theories were initiated by the genius of Freud, Fromm, and Pavlov.[26]

Although Peplau found Freud's theory by itself not very useful, particularly in clinical work with patients, Freud's hypotheses were a rich source of research study. Freud emphasized the importance of motivation, conflict, and the role of the family in early childhood and discovered the significance of the unconscious. Freudian principles have been tested extensively, and his influence on later theorists' hypotheses is obvious.

Maslow's theory of human motivation is well known, and a great deal of sound research has followed its publication. Maslow states, "The present theory must be considered to be a suggested program for future research and must stand or fall, not so much on facts available or evidence presented, as upon research yet to be done."[21:371]

Miller's work focused on personality theory, adjustment mechanisms, psychotherapy, and principles of social learning. Pavlov's stimulus-response model influenced Miller's principles of social learning. Most of Miller's work consisted of developing hypotheses, the basis for research, rather than proving principles. Miller based his hypotheses on experimental studies.

Sullivan was a pioneer in the field of modern psychiatry. A comprehensive evaluation of Sullivan's work regarding personality development and interpersonal relations was written by Patrick Mullahy in 1945. Sullivan's theoretical positions in *Conceptions of Modern Psychiatry* were tested by the Washington School of Psychiatry, and this work led to the further refinement of the theoretical positions of Sullivan.

MAJOR CONCEPTS & DEFINITIONS

Psychodynamic Nursing Peplau defines psychodynamic nursing because her model evolves through this type of nursing. "Psychodynamic nursing is being able to understand one's own behavior to help others identify felt difficulties, and to apply principles of human relations to the problems that arise at all levels of experience."[27:xiii]

Peplau develops the model by describing the structural concepts of the interpersonal process, which are the phases of the nurse-patient relationship. She holds this to be basic to psychodynamic nursing.

Nurse-Patient Relationship Peplau describes four phases of the nurse-patient relationship. Although separate, they overlap and occur over the time of the relationship.

Orientation During the orientation phase, the individual has a "felt need" and seeks professional assistance. The nurse helps the patient recognize and understand his problem and determine his need for help.[27:18-30]

Identification The patient identifies with those who can help him (relatedness). The nurse permits exploration of feelings to aid the patient in undergoing illness as an experience that reorients feelings and strengthens positive forces in the personality and provides needed satisfaction.[27:31-37]

Exploitation During the exploitation phase, the patient attempts to derive full value from what is offered him through the relationship. New goals to be achieved through personal effort can be projected, and power shifts from the nurse to the patient as the patient delays gratification to achieve the newly formed goals.[27:37-39]

Resolution Old goals are gradually put aside and new goals adopted. This is a process in which the patient frees himself from identification with the nurse.[27:39-41]

Nursing Roles Peplau[27] describes six different nursing roles that emerge in the various phases of the nurse-patient relationship (Fig. 22-1).

Continued

MAJOR CONCEPTS & DEFINITIONS—cont'd

Role of the stranger The first role is the role of the stranger. Peplau states that because the nurse and patient are strangers to each other, the patient should be treated with ordinary courtesy. In other words, the nurse should not prejudge the patient but accept him as he is. During this nonpersonal phase the nurse should treat the patient as emotionally able, unless evidence indicates otherwise. This coincides with the identification phase.[27:44-47]

Role of resource person In the role of the resource person, the nurse provides specific answers to questions, especially health information, and interprets to the patient the treatment or medical plan of care. These questions often arise within the context of a larger problem. The nurse determines what type of response is appropriate for constructive learning, either giving straightforward factual answers or providing counseling.[27:47-48]

Teaching role The teaching role is a combination of all roles and "always proceeds from what the patient knows and . . . develops around his interest in wanting and ability to use . . . information."[27:48]

Peplau[30] expands on the role of teacher in later writings. She separates teaching into two categories: *instructional*, which consists largely of giving information and is the form explained in educational literature, and *experiential*, which is "using the experience of the learner as a basis from which learning products are developed."[30:98] The products of learning are generalizations and appraisals the patient makes about his experiences. This concept of learning used in the teaching role overlaps with the nurse counselor role, because the concept of learning is carried out through psychotherapeutic techniques.[28]

Leadership role The leadership role involves the democratic process. The nurse helps the patient meet the tasks at hand through a relationship of cooperation and active participation.[27:49-51.]

Surrogate role The patient casts the nurse in the surrogate role. The nurse's attitudes and behaviors create *feeling tones* in the patient that reactivate feelings generated in a prior relationship. The nurse's function is to assist the patient in recognizing similarities between herself and the person recalled by the patient. She then helps the patient see the differences in her role and that of the recalled person. In this phase, both patient and nurse define areas of dependence, independence, and finally interdependence.[27:51-61]

Counseling role Peplau believes the counseling role has the greatest emphasis in psychiatric nursing.[29] Counseling functions in the nurse-patient relationship by the way nurses respond to patient demands. Peplau[27:64] says the purpose of interpersonal techniques is to help "the patient remember and understand fully what is happening to him in the present situation, so that the experience can be integrated rather than dissociated from other experiences in life" (Fig. 22-2).

Psychobiological Experiences Peplau describes four psychobiological experiences: needs, frustration, conflict, and anxiety. These experiences provide energy that is transformed into some form of action. Peplau uses nonnursing theoretical concepts to identify and explain these experiences that compel destructive or constructive responses from nurses and patients. This understanding provides a basis for goal formation and nursing interventions.[27]

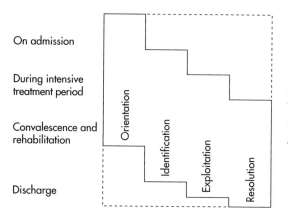

On admission

During intensive
treatment period

Convalescence and
rehabilitation

Discharge

Fig. **22-1** **Overlapping phases in nurse-patient rela-**
tionships. *From Peplau, H.E. (1952).* Interpersonal relations
in nursing *(p. 21). New York: G.P. Putnam & Sons. Used with
permission.*

Patient: personal goals ———————————————————————— Patient

| Entirely separate goals and interests. Both are strangers to each other. | Individual preconceptions on the meaning of the medical problem, the roles of each in the problematic situation. | Partially mutual and partially individual understanding of the nature of the medical problem. | Mutual understanding of the nature of the problem, roles of nurse and patient, and requirements of nurse and patient in the solution of the problem. Common, shared health goals. | Collaborative efforts directed toward solving the problem together, productively. |

Nurse

Nurse: professional goals

Fig. **22-2** **Continuum showing changing aspects of nurse-patient relationships.** *From Peplau, H.E. (1952).* Interpersonal relations in nursing *(p. 10). New York: G.P. Putnam & Sons. Used with
permission.*

Major Assumptions

Peplau[27:xii] identifies two explicit assumptions:

1. The kind of person the nurse becomes makes a substantial difference in what each patient will learn as he receives nursing care.
2. Fostering personality development toward maturity is a function of nursing and nursing education. Nursing uses principles and methods that guide the process toward resolution of interpersonal problems.

One implicit assumption was, "The nursing profession has legal responsibility for the effective use of nursing and for its consequences to patients."[27:6]

Nursing

Nursing is described as "a significant, therapeutic, interpersonal process. It functions cooperatively with other human processes that make health possible for individuals in communities." When professional health teams offer health services, nurses participate in the organization of conditions that facilitate natural ongoing tendencies in human organisms. "Nursing is an educative instrument, a maturing force that aims to promote forward movement of personality in the direction of creative, constructive, productive, personal, and community living."[27:16]

Person

Peplau defines person in terms of a man. Man is an organism that lives in an unstable equilibrium.[27:82]

Health

Peplau defines health as "a word symbol that implies forward movement of personality and other ongoing human processes in the direction of creative, constructive, productive, personal, and community living."[27:12]

Environment

Peplau[27:163] implicitly defines the environment in terms of "existing forces outside the organism and in the context of culture," from which mores, customs, and beliefs are acquired. "However, general conditions that are likely to lead to health always include the interpersonal process."[27:14]

THEORETICAL ASSERTIONS

Peplau makes theoretical relationships throughout her book. In summarizing these relationships, Peplau addresses the patient-nurse relationship, the patient and his awareness of feelings, and the nurse and her awareness of feelings. She presents nursing as a maturing educative force that uses the experiential learning method for both patient and nurse (Fig. 22-3).

LOGICAL FORM

The process Peplau uses is an inductive approach to theory building. Empirical generalizations are inductively established. "Induction is a type of relationship in which . . . one observes empirical events and generalizes from specific events to all similar events."[17:8] According to Peplau,[31:37] "Nursing situations provide a field of observations from which unique nursing concepts can be derived and used for the improvement of the professional's work." The selected concepts Peplau uses are organized into a

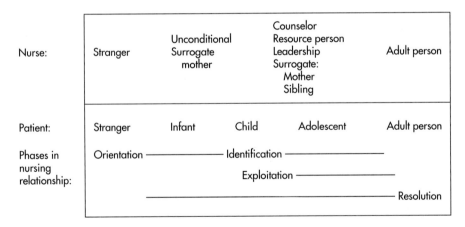

Fig. 22-3 **Phases and changing roles in nurse-patient relationships.** *From Peplau, H.E. (1952). Interpersonal relations in nursing (p. 54). New York: G.P. Putnam & Sons. Used with permission.*

larger component, forming relationships that are logical and complete. The relationships describe behaviors that occur in the nurse-patient interaction.

ACCEPTANCE BY THE NURSING COMMUNITY

Practice

Grace Sills[39:123] recalls Peplau brought "a new perspective, a new approach, a theoretically based foundation for nursing practice for therapeutic work with patients." She states, "Peplau's work is responsible for a second order change in the nursing culture."[39:123] Peplau's ideas provided a design for the practice of psychiatric nursing with explication of the design in usable form.

Some of Peplau's ideas were not accepted in the early years, such as the concept of experiential learning for the patient and students.[39] In a panel discussion on psychotherapeutic strategies, Mertz, Mereness, and Mellow disagreed with Peplau on the methodology of psychotherapeutic functions and the role of nurse as surrogate.[37] Later criticisms of Peplau's model indicate the lack of development of social systems that would broaden the knowledge base for understanding the patient's problems.

Peplau[27] used the interpersonal and intrapersonal theories of Sullivan and Freud as the theoretical base for her model and did not take into consideration interrelationships between man and society. These concepts were later developed in general systems theory by Ludwig von Bertalanffy[47] and included in the curriculum of the Rutgers graduate program in psychiatric nursing in which Peplau chaired. In 1968 Peplau began the first workshop on family therapy under a grant from NIMH to the University of New Mexico.

Today, Peplau's model continues to be used by clinicians. In her article "Peplau's Therapy: An Application to Short-Term Individual Therapy," Thompson[44] used Peplau's model to analyze short-term individual therapy. She stated, "In working with individuals with psychological problems, the development of the interpersonal process is of the utmost importance. Without the development of a therapeutic relationship, little work could be accomplished by the nurse-counselor."[44:32]

Forchuk and Brown[10] tested Peplau's conceptualization of the nurse-client relationship in their development of an instrument to measure the phases of the relationship. Further, Forchuk et al.[9] incorporated Peplau's theory into a case management model, which emphasized the importance of the interactive interpersonal relationship between client and practitioner.

Education

Peplau's book *Interpersonal Relations in Nursing* was written specifically as an aid to graduate nurses and nursing students. It was originally a hardback edition, but Macmillan printed it in paperback in 1988.

There are few early critiques of Peplau's model in the literature. Her model was designed and published in 1952, 1957, and 1962, with a particular emphasis in psychiatric nursing. The specialty journals in psychiatric nursing did not begin publication until 1963, 11 years after the model was first published. However, psychiatric nursing authors did write textbooks. Smoyak and Rouslin[40] state that after 1952, no psychiatric nursing text could ignore Peplau's work. Peplau's impact was reflected in books in the 1950s and 1960s, such as G. Burton's[5] *Personal, Impersonal, and Interpersonal Relations* (1958), Burd and Marshall's *Some Clinical Approaches to Psychiatric Nursing*[4] (1963), Hofling and Leininger's[16] *Basic Psychiatric Concepts in Nursing* (1960), and Orlando's *The Dynamic Nurse-Patient Relationship*[24] (1961), to name a few. Most comments on Peplau and her work were written 25 or more years after her published model. Anita O'Toole and Sheila Rouslin Welt have compiled Peplau's unpublished notes and lectures on the interpersonal theory. They have named the book *Interpersonal Theory in Nursing Practice: Selected Works of Hildegard E. Peplau.*[25] They state that "Peplau's theoretical ideas, particularly her definition of nursing and nursing process, elaboration of anxiety and learning, and her psychotherapeutic methods, have become a part of the collective culture of the discipline of nursing."[25:365]

Research

Sills[38] states that Peplau's work influenced the direction of clinical work and studies. Initial efforts to use research as a tool to develop a body of nursing knowledge were uneven in quality and quantity, and often did not explicitly recognize underlying assumptions. Early research followed the assumption that patient problems were within-the-person phenomena and were explored in nurse-patient relationship studies. This followed Peplau's conceptual model. Since the 1960s, research has shifted to "within-the-social-system" point of view, as studies have examined broader sets of relationships.

For more than 30 years Peplau's model has formed the basis for numerous applications of research methods. Thomas, Baker, and Estes[45] used Peplau's concept of anxiety as a means to constructively resolve angry feelings through experiential learning within the nurse-patient relationship. Hays[15] described a study teaching the concept of anxiety that is predominantly based on Peplau's concept of anxiety and used her conceptual model. Hays, a Rutgers graduate student in psychiatric nursing, was a student of Peplau's. This study is one example of Peplau's influence on new nursing leaders with graduate education in the field of psychiatric nursing. Topf and Dambacher[46] interpret the findings in their study using Peplau's role of the nurse as a stranger. Garrett, Manuel, and Vincent[13] cite Peplau's concept of anxiety for their operational definition of stress and its relationship to learning. Spring and Turk[41] developed a behavior scale using Peplau's conceptual framework and her assumption that therapeutic behavior in the nurse-patient relationship promotes experiential learning. The authors concluded that their behavior score was objective, reliable, and valid. Methven and Schlotfeldt,[22] who developed a tool to evaluate verbal responses, based their study on Peplau's assumption that therapeutic communication can be used to reduce or redirect anxiety.

Assumptions from Peplau's model continue to be used in current research. La Monica[19] devised an empathy instrument using Peplau's model (and work from other theorists) as a theoretical framework. She states, "The primary goal of nurses . . . is to provide services that assist in moving clients to their optimum health levels . . . and involves a helping relationship."[19:389]

Recent use of Peplau's theoretical model focused on the concept of pattern integrations. Beeber and Caldwell[2] piloted a program which consisted of a collaborative relationship between primary care providers, two psychiatric–mental health clinical nurse specialists, and young women suffering with the symptoms of depression. Particular emphasis was placed on creating a "learning laboratory out of everyday experiences." Peplau's model was ideal in this setting, offering a cost-effective alternative to more expensive treatment interventions. Interpersonal intervention structures were found to allow patients to achieve maximum quality of life by enlisting the support of others.

The impact and significance of Peplau's conceptual model may be best described by Suzanne Lego[20] in a thorough discussion of the history, trends, patterns, and assessment of published research that notes the direction of the one-to-one nurse-patient relationship. She states that ambiguity about the nurse-patient relationship abruptly ended in the literature as a result of Peplau's *Interpersonal Relations in Nursing* (1952).[27] As she would continue to do for the next 22 years, Peplau pulled together loose, ambiguous data and put them into systematic, scientific terms that could be tested, applied, and integrated into the practice of psychiatric nursing.[20:68]

Lego[20] states that most of the published literature describing the one-to-one nurse-patient relationship is based on theoretical concepts inspired principally by Peplau.

Peplau makes a significant contribution to the nursing community through the research done to evaluate, validate, and make more precise the Theory of Interpersonal Relations.

FURTHER DEVELOPMENT

As nursing broadens its scope, there appears to be a need for further development of Peplau's theory for use with the healthy patient, group, and community. Further development is also indicated for clients who are unable to use their communication skills effectively. Increased use of Peplau's theory in practice is needed. Continued research is needed to further refine the theory and to build on nursing's knowledge base.

Peplau herself continues to write[32,33] about the expansion and development needed to test her Theory of Interpersonal Relations and to offer explanations of such constructs as concepts, processes, patterns, problems, energy, and anxiety. Further, she suggests that the constructs of focal attention, dissociation, forbidding gestures, and personification deserve additional study.

CRITIQUE
Simplicity

The major focus of Peplau's theory, interpersonal relations between patient and nurse, is easily understood. The theory's basic assumptions and key concepts are defined. Of the assumptions Peplau listed, two are explicit and one is implicit. Peplau sequentially describes her four phases of the interpersonal process. The roles of the nurse and the four psychobiological experiences are clearly indicated. Her logic is based on inductive reasoning. Ideas are taken from observations of the specific and applied to the general. Peplau draws from other disciplines' theories. She is consistent with established theories and principles, such as those of Sullivan, Freud, and Maslow. Peplau deals with the relationships of the interpersonal process, nurse, patient, and psychobiological experiences. Each of these relationships is then developed, within the theory, in an understandable way. Thus Peplau's theory can be described as meeting the evaluative quality of simplicity.

Generality

In meeting the criteria of generality, Peplau[27] states, "While clinical situations are stressed, any nurse can apply principles that are presented in any other interpersonal relationship in any other area of living." The one drawback to the theory's generality is that an interpersonal relationship must exist. The theory is adaptable only to nursing settings where there can be communication between the patient and nurse. Its use is limited in working with the comatose, se-

nile, or newborn patient. In such situations, the nurse-patient relationship is often one-sided. The nurse and the patient cannot work together to become more knowledgeable, develop goals, and mature. Even Peplau[27:41] admits, "Understanding of the meaning of the experience to the patient is required in order for nursing to function as an educative, therapeutic, maturing force." Since Peplau's theory cannot be applied to all patients, the quality of generality is not met.

Empirical Precision

Peplau provides us with a theory based on reality. The relationship between the theory and empirical data allows for validation and verification of the theory by other scientists. The definitions described by Peplau are in a middle range on a connotative-denotative continuum. Peplau operationally defines the four phases of the interpersonal process, the nurse with regard to her roles, and the patient with regard to his state of dependence. According to Duffey and Mullencamp,[6:573] "Peplau relates behavior to theory by naming and categorizing, operationalizing definitions of behavior, thematic abstractions of interaction phenomena, and diagnosis of problems and principles guiding nursing interactions." Peplau's theory can be considered empirically precise. With further research and development, the degree of precision will increase.

Derivable Consequences

In historical perspective, Peplau is one of the first theorists since Nightingale to present a theory for nursing. Therefore her work can be considered pioneering in the nursing field. "She provided nursing with a meaningful method of self-directed practice at a time when medicine dominated the health care field."[8:44]

Peplau's work, thoughts, and ideas have touched many nurses, from students to practitioners. Although her book was published in 1952, four decades ago, it continues to provide direction for nursing practice, education, and research. Peplau's work has provided a significant contribution to nursing's knowledge base. The evaluative criteria of derivable consequences are unquestionably met.

CRITICAL THINKING *Activities*

1 Describe how the six subroles of the psychiatric nurse would be used during a therapeutic relationship with an acutely psychotic schizophrenic patient. For example, the nurturing needs of the patient when the patient is unable to carry out simple tasks would be met by the subrole of mother surrogate.

2 During the therapeutic relationship, patients may distort their perceptions of others. Therefore, they may relate to the nurse not on the basis of the nurse's realistic attributes, but wholly or chiefly on the basis of interpersonal relationships existing in their environment. With the above patient and nurse roles you have described, discuss how these distorted perceptions may affect the patient's care and the nurse-patient relationship.

3 Considering the above-created nurse-patient relationship, discuss the phases and changing roles that would be considered when working with this patient. Consider experiences in which you would and would not be able to accomplish the appropriate goals of each phase.

REFERENCES

1. Andreoli, R.G., & Thompson, C.E. (1977, June). The nature of science in nursing. *Image, 9*(2), 32-37.
2. Beeber, L., & Caldwell, C. (1996). Pattern integrations in young depressed women: Part II. *Archives of Psychiatric Nursing, 10*(3), 157-164.
3. Belcher, J.R., & Fish, L.J. (1980). Hildegard E. Peplau. In Nursing Theories Conference Group, J.B. George, Chairperson, *Nursing theories: The base for professional nursing practice.* Englewood Cliffs, NJ: Prentice Hall.
4. Burd, S.F. (1963). The development of an operational definition using the process of learning as a guide. In S.F. Burd & A. Marshall (Eds.), *Some clinical approaches to psychiatric nursing.* New York: Macmillan.
5. Burton, G. (1958). *Personal, impersonal, and interpersonal relations.* Cited by S.A. Smoyak & S. Rouslin (Eds.) (1982). *A collection of classics in psychiatric nursing literature.* Thorofare, NJ: Charles B. Slack.
6. Duffey, M., & Mullencamp, A.F. (1974, Sept.). A framework for theory analysis. *Nursing Outlook, 22,* 570-574.
7. Field, W.E., Jr. (Ed.). (1979). *The psychotherapy of Hildegard E. Peplau.* New Brunfels, TX: PSF Publications.
8. Fitzpatrick, J.J., & Whall, A.L. (1983). *Conceptual models of nursing, analysis, and application.* Bowie, MD: Robert J. Brady.
9. Forchuk, C., Beaton, S., Crawford, L., Ide, L., Voorberg, N., & Bethune, J. (1989). Incorporating Peplau's theory and case management. *Journal of Psychosocial Nursing, 27*(2), 35-38.
10. Forchuk, C., & Brown, B. (1989). Establishing a nurse-client relationship. *Journal of Psychosocial Nursing, 27*(2), 30-34.
11. Freud, S. (1936). The problem of anxiety. Cited by H.E. Peplau. (1952). *Interpersonal relations in nursing.* New York: G.P. Putnam's Sons.
12. Fromm, E. (1947). Man for himself. Cited by H.E. Peplau. (1952). *Interpersonal relations in nursing.* New York: G.P. Putnam's Sons.
13. Garrett, A., Manuel, D., & Vincent, C. (1976, Nov.). Stressful experiences identified by student nurses. *Journal of Nursing Education, 15*(6), 9-21.
14. Gregg, D.E. (1978). Hildegard E. Peplau: Her contributions. *Psychiatry Care, 16,* 118-121.
15. Hays, D. (1961, Spring). Teaching a concept of anxiety. *Nursing Research, 10*(2), 108-113.
16. Hofling, C.K., & Leininger, M.M. (1960). Basic psychiatric concepts in nursing. Cited by S.A. Smoyak & S. Rouslin (Eds.) (1982). *A collection of classics in psychiatric nursing literature.* Thorofare, NJ: Charles B. Slack.
17. Jacox, A. (1974, Jan.-Feb.). Theory construction in nursing: An overview. *Nursing Research 23,* 4-12.
18. Johnson, D.E. (1959). The nature of a science of nursing. *Nursing Outlook, 7,* 292.
19. La Monica, E. (1981). Construct validity of an empathy instrument. *Research in Nursing and Health, 4,* 389-400.
20. Lego, S. (1980). The one-to-one nurse-patient relationship. *Perspectives in Psychiatric Care, 18*(2), 67-89. (Reprinted from *Psychiatric nursing 1946-1974: A report on the state of the art.* American Journal of Nursing Co.)
21. Maslow, A.H., & Mittleman, B. (1941). *Principles in abnormal psychology.* New York: Harper & Brothers.
22. Methven, D., & Schlotfeldt, R.M. (1962, Spring). The social intervention inventory. *Nursing Research, 11*(2), 83-88.
23. Miller, N.E., & Dollard, J. (1941). *Social learning and initiation.* New Haven, CT: Yale University Press.
24. Orlando, I. (1961). *The dynamic nurse-patient relationship.* Cited by S.A. Smoyak & S. Rouslin (Eds.) (1982). *A collection of classics in psychiatric nursing literature.* Thorofare, NJ: Charles B. Slack.

25. O'Toole, A., & Welt, S. (1989). *Interpersonal theory in nursing practice: Selected works of Hildegard E. Peplau*. New York: Springer.

26. Pavlov, I. (1927). *Conditioned reflexes: An investigation of the physiological activity of the cerebral cortex*. London: Oxford University Press.

27. Peplau, H.E. (1952). *Interpersonal relations in nursing*. New York: G.P. Putnam's Sons. (English edition reissued as a paperback in 1988 by Macmillan Education Ltd., London.)

28. Peplau, H.E. (1957). Therapeutic concepts. In S.A. Smoyak & S. Rouslin (Eds.) (1982). *A collection of classics in psychiatric nursing literature*. Thorofare, NJ: Charles B. Slack. (Reprinted from *National League for Nursing League Exchange No. 26:* Aspects of psychiatric nursing.)

29. Peplau, H.E. (1962). Interpersonal techniques: The crux of psychiatric nursing. *American Journal of Nursing, 62,* 629-633.

30. Peplau, H.E. (1964). *Basic principles of patient counseling* (2nd ed.). Philadelphia: Smith, Kline, & French Laboratories.

31. Peplau, H.E. (1969). Theory: The professional dimension. In C. Norris (Ed.), *Proceedings of the first nursing theory conference* (March 21-28). University of Kansas Medical Center, Department of Nursing Education, Kansas City.

32. Peplau, H.E. (1989). Future directions in psychiatric nursing from the perspective of history. *Journal of Psychosocial Nursing, 27*(2), 18-28.

33. Peplau, H.E. (1992). Interpersonal relations: A theoretical framework for application in nursing practice. *Nursing Science Quarterly, 5*(1), 13-18.

34. Peplau, H.E. (1996, July). Personal correspondence.

35. Phillips, J.R. (1977, Feb.). Nursing systems and nursing models. *Image, 9*(1), 6.

36. Profile. (1974, Feb.). *Nursing 74, 4,* 13.

37. Psychotherapeutic strategies. (1968). Current concepts in psychiatric care: The implications for psychiatric nursing practice. Proceedings of the Institute on Psychiatric Nursing, cosponsored by Yale School of Nursing, Department of Psychiatric Nursing and the Community Mental Health Center Department of Nursing. In *Perspectives of Psychiatric Care, 6*(6), 271-289.

38. Sills, G.M. (1977, May-June). Research in the field of psychiatric nursing 1952-1977. *Nursing Research, 28*(3), 201-207.

39. Sills, G.M. (1978). Hildegard E. Peplau: Leader, practitioner, academician, scholar, and theorist. *Perspectives in Psychiatric Care, 16*(3), 122-128.

40. Smoyak, S.A., & Rouslin, S. (Eds.) (1982). Introduction. *A collection of classics in psychiatric nursing literature*. Thorofare, NJ: Charles B. Slack.

41. Spring, F.E., & Turk, H. (1962, Fall). A therapeutic behavior scale. *Nursing Research, 11*(4), 214-218.

42. Sullivan, H.S. (1947). Conceptions of modern psychiatry. Cited by H.E. Peplau. (1952). *Interpersonal relations in nursing*. New York: G.P. Putnam's Sons.

43. Symonds, P. (1946). *The dynamics of human adjustments*. New York: Appleton-Century-Crofts.

44. Thompson, L. (1986, Aug.). Peplau's therapy: An application to short-term individual therapy. *Journal of Psychosocial Nursing, 24*(8), 26-31.

45. Thomas, M.D., Baker, J.M. & Estes, N.J. (1970, Dec.). Anger: A tool for developing self-awareness. *American Journal of Nursing, 70*(12), 2586-2590.

46. Topf, M., & Dambacher, B. (1979). Predominant source of interpersonal influence in relationships between psychiatric patients and nursing staff. *Research in Nursing and Health, 2*(1), 35-43.

47. Von Bertalanffy, L. (1968). *General systems theory: Foundations, development, applications*. New York: G. Braziller.

BIBLIOGRAPHY

Primary sources

Books

Peplau, H.E. (1952). *Interpersonal relations in nursing*. New York: G.P. Putnam & Sons.

Peplau, H.E. (1964). *Basic principles of patient counseling* (2nd ed.). Philadelphia: Smith, Kline, & French Laboratories.

Book chapters

Peplau, H.E. (1969). Theory: The professional dimension. In C. Norris (Ed.), *Proceedings of the first nursing theory conference* (March 21-28). University of Kansas Medical Center, Department of Nursing Education, Kansas City.

Peplau, H.E. (1987). Nursing science: A historical perspective. In R. Parse, *Nursing science: Major paradigms, theories, critiques*. Philadelphia: W.B. Saunders.

Journal articles

Peplau, H.E. (1942, Oct.). Health program at Bennington College. *Public Health Nursing, 34*(10), 573-575, 581.

Peplau, H.E. (1947, May). Discussion: A democratic participation technique. *American Journal of Nursing, 47*(5), 334-336.

Peplau, H.E. (1951, Dec.). Toward new concepts in nursing and nursing education. *American Journal of Nursing, 52*(12), 722-724.

Peplau, H.E. (1952, Dec.). The psychiatric nurses' family group. *American Journal of Nursing, 52*(12), 1475-1477.

Peplau, H.E. (1953, Feb.). The nursing team in psychiatric facilities. *Nursing Outlook, 1*(2), 90-92.

Peplau, H.E. (1953, Oct.). Themes in nursing situations: Power. *American Journal of Nursing, 53*(10), 1221-1223.

Peplau, H.E. (1953, Nov.). Themes in nursing situations: Safety. *American Journal of Nursing, 53*(11), 1343-1346.

Peplau, H.E. (1955, Dec.). Loneliness. *American Journal of Nursing, 55*(12), 1476-1481.

Peplau, H.E. (1956). Discussion. The League Exchange No. 18: *Psychology and psychiatric nursing research*, pp. 20-22.

Peplau, H.E. (1956, Spring). Present day trends in psychiatric nursing. *Neuropsychiatry, 111*(4), 190-204.

Peplau, H.E. (1956, July 8). An undergraduate program in psychiatric nursing. *Nursing Outlook, 4*, 400-410.

Peplau, H.E. (1957, July). What is experiential teaching? *American Journal of Nursing, 57*(7), 884-886.

Peplau, H.E. (1958). Educating the nurse to function in psychiatric services. *Nursing Personnel for Mental Health Programs*, Southern Regional Educational Board, Atlanta, Ga., pp. 37-42.

Peplau, H.E. (1958, Sept.). Public health nurses promote mental health. *Public Health Reports, 73*(9), 828.

Peplau, H.E. (1960). Talking with patients. *American Journal of Nursing, 60*, 964-967.

Peplau, H.E. (1960, Jan). Must laboring together be called teamwork? Problems in team treatment of adults in state mental hospitals. *American Journal of Orthopsychiatry, 30*, 103-108.

Peplau, H.E. (1960, March). A personal responsibility: A discussion of anxiety in mental health. *Rutgers Alumni Monthly*, pp. 14-16.

Peplau, H.E. (1960, May). Anxiety in the mother-infant relationship. *Nursing World, 134*(5), 33-34.

Peplau, H.E. (1962). The crux of psychiatric nursing. *American Journal of Nursing, 62*, 50-54.

Peplau, H.E. (1963). An approach to research in psychiatric nursing. *Training for Clinical Research in Psychiatric-Mental Health Nursing*. The Catholic University of America, pp. 5-44.

Peplau, H.E. (1963, Oct.-Nov.). Interpersonal relations and the process of adaptations. *Nursing Science, 1*(4), 272-279.

Peplau, H.E. (1964). Psychiatric nursing skills and the general hospital patient. *Nursing Forum, 3*(2), 28-37.

Peplau, H.E. (1964, Nov.). Professional and social behavior: Some differences worth the notice of professional nurses. *Quarterly, 50*(4), 23-33. (Published by the Columbia University–Presbyterian Hospital School of Nursing Alumni Association, New York.)

Peplau, H.E. (1965). The 91st day: A challenge to professional nursing. *Perspectives in Psychiatric Care, 3*(2), 20-24.

Peplau, H.E. (1965, April). The heart of nursing: Interpersonal relations. *Canadian Nurse, 61*(4), 273-275.

Peplau, H.E. (1965, Aug.). Specialization in professional nursing. *Nursing Science, 3*(4), 268-287.

Peplau, H.E. (1965, Nov.). The nurse in the community mental health program. *Nursing Outlook, 13*(11), 68-70.

Peplau, H.E. (1966). Nurse-doctor relationships. *Nursing Forum, 5*(1), 60-75.

Peplau, H.E. (1966). Nursing's two routes to doctoral degrees. *Nursing Forum, 5*(2), 57-67.

Peplau, H.E. (1966, March-April). An interpretation of the ANA position. *NJSNA-News Letter, 22*(2), 6-10.

Peplau, H.E. (1966, May-June). Trends in nursing and nursing education. *NJSNA-News Letter, 22*(3), 17-27.

Peplau, H.E. (1967, Feb.). The work of psychiatric nurses. *Psychiatric Opinion, 4*(1), 5-11.

Peplau, H.E. (1967, Nov.). Interpersonal relations and the work of the industrial nurse. *Industrial Nurse Journal, 15*(10), 7-12.

Peplau, H.E. (1968). Psychotherapeutic strategies. *Perspectives in Psychiatric Care, 6*(6), 264-289.

Peplau, H.E. (1969). Professional closeness as a special kind of involvement with a patient, client, or family group. *Nursing Forum, 8*(4), 342-360.

Peplau, H.E. (1969, Fall). The American Nurses' Association and nursing education. *Utah Nurse, 20*(3), 6.

Peplau, H.E. (1970, Jan.). ANA's new executive director states her views. *American Journal of Nursing, 70*, 84-88.

Peplau, H.E. (1970, Summer). Professional closeness as a special kind of involvement with a patient, client or family group. *Comprehensive Nurse Quarterly, 5*(3), 66-81.

Peplau, H.E. (1970, Nov.-Dec.). Changed patterns of practice. *Washington State Journal of Nursing, 42*, 4-6.

Peplau, H.E. (1970, Nov.-Dec.). Keynote address at the 68th annual convention of the New Jersey State Nurses' Association. *New Jersey Nurse, 26*, 3-10.

Peplau, H.E. (1970, Dec.). ANA: Who needs it? *Nursing News, 43*, 5-8.

Peplau, H.E. (1970, Dec.). What it means to be a professional nurse today. *Alabama Nurse, 24*, 8-17.

Peplau, H.E. (1970, Dec.). The road ahead. *Maine Nurse, 1*(3), 3-8.

Peplau, H.E. (1971). Dilemmas of organizing nurses. *Image, 4*, 4-8.

Peplau, H.E. (1971, Jan.). ANA: Who needs it? *Nursing News, 44*(1), 12-14.

Peplau, H.E. (1971, Spring). In support of nursing research. *Journal of the New York State Nurses' Association, 2*, 5.

Peplau, H.E. (1971, Summer). Time of decision. *Nevada Nurses' Association Quarterly Newsletter*, pp. 1-3.

Peplau, H.E. (1971, July). Responsibility, authority, evaluation, and accountability of nursing in patient care. *Michigan Nurse, 44*, 5-7.

Peplau, H.E. (1971, Sept.). The task ahead. *American Journal of Nursing, 71*, 1800-1802.

Peplau, H.E. (1971, Nov.). The now nurse in nursing: Some problems of diversity. *Oklahoma Nurse, 46*, 1.

Peplau, H.E. (1971, Nov.). What it means to be a professional nurse in today's society. *Kansas Nurse, 46*, 1-3.

Peplau, H.E. (1971, Winter). Communication in crisis intervention. *Psychiatric Forum, 2*, 1-7.

Peplau, H.E. (1971, Winter). Where do we go from here? *Pelican News, 27*, 14-16.

Peplau, H.E. (1972, Spring). The nurse's role in health care delivery systems. *Pelican News, 28*, 12-14.

Peplau, H.E. (1972, May). The independence of nursing. *Imprint, 9*, 11.

Peplau, H.E. (1972, June). The president challenges nurses in address to delegates. *Kansas Nurse*, pp. 2-4.

Peplau, H.E. (1972, Nov.-Dec.). Some issues and developments that should be of concern to nurses. *New Jersey State Nurses' Association News, 2*, 14-16.

Peplau, H.E. (1973, July). Meeting the challenge. *Mississippi RN, 35*, 1-6.

Peplau, H.E. (1974). Creativity and commitment in nursing. *Image: Journal of Nursing Scholarship, 6*, 3-5.

Peplau, H.E. (1974). Is health care a right? Affirmative response. *Image: Journal of Nursing Scholarship, 7*, 4-10.

Peplau, H.E. (1974, Jan.). Nurses: Collaborate or isolate. *Pennsylvania Nurse, 29*, 2-5.

Peplau, H.E. (1974, Autumn). Talking with patients. *Comprehensive Nursing Quarterly, 9*(3), 30-39.

Peplau, H.E. (1975, March-April). An open letter to a new graduate. *Nursing Digest, 3*, 36-37.

Peplau, H.E. (1975, Oct.). Interview with Dr. Peplau: Future of nursing. *Japanese Journal of Nursing, 39*(10), 1046-1050.

Peplau, H.E. (1975, Oct.). Midlife crisis. *American Journal of Nursing, 75*, 1761-1765.

Peplau, H.E., & Reinkemeyer, A.G. (1976, Aug.). What future for nursing? *AORN, 24*, 217-235.

Peplau, H.E. (1977, March-April). The changing view of nursing. *International Nursing Review, 24*, 43-45.

Peplau, H.E. (1978, March-April). Psychiatric nursing: Role of nurses and psychiatric nurses. *International Nursing Review, 25*, 41-47.

Peplau, H.E. (1980, April). New statement defines scope of practice. *American Nurse, 12*(4), 1, 8, 24.

Peplau, H.E. (1980, May-June). The psychiatric nurses: Accountable? to whom? for what? *Perspectives in Psychiatric Care, 18*, 128-134.

Peplau, H.E. (1982, Aug.). Some reflections on earlier days in psychiatric nursing. *Journal of Psychosocial Nursing Mental Health Services, 20*, 17-24.

Peplau, H.E. (1984, Jan.-Feb.). Internal versus external regulation. *New Jersey Nurse, 14*, 12-14.

Peplau, H.E. (1985, Feb.). Is nursing self-regulatory power being eroded? *American Journal of Nursing, 85*(2), 140-143.

Peplau, H.E. (1987, Jan.). Tomorrow's world. *Nursing Times*, pp. 29-32.

Peplau, H.E. (1987, May). American Nurses Association social policy statement: Part I. *Archives of Psychiatric Nursing, 1*(5), 301-307.

Peplau, H.E. (1988, Feb.). The art and science of nursing: Similarities, differences, and relations. *Nursing Science Quarterly, 1*(1), 8-15.

Peplau, H.E. (1988, Spring). Peplau responds. *Pacesetter Newsletter of the American Nurses Association Council on Psychiatric and Mental Health Nursing, 15*(1), 1-4.

Peplau, H.E. (1989). Future direction in psychiatric nursing from the perspective of history. *Journal of Psychosocial Nursing, 27*(2), 18-28.

Peplau, H.E. (1992). Interpersonal relations: A theoretical framework for application in nursing practice. *Nursing Science Quarterly, 5*(1), 13-18.

Peplau, H.E. (1995). Hildegard Peplau in a conversation with Mark Welch. Part I. *Nursing Inquiry, 2*(1), 53-56.

Peplau, H.E. (1995). Hildegard Peplau in a conversation with Mark Welch. Part II. *Nursing Inquiry, 2*(2), 115-116.

Peplau, H.E. (1996). Commentary. *Archives of Psychiatry Nursing, 10*(1), 14-15.

Interviews

Peplau, H.E. (1985, May). Help the public maintain mental health. *Nursing Success Today, 2*(5), 30-34.

Peplau, H.E. (1985, Aug.). The power of the dissociative state. *Journal of Psychosocial Nursing, 23*(8), 31-33.

Chapters, pamphlets, proceedings, reports

Peplau, H.E. (1951). *Understanding ourselves.* Fifty-seventh annual report. New York: National League for Nursing Education.

Peplau, H.E. (1952). *The responsibility of professional nursing in psychiatry.* Fifty-eighth annual report. New York: National League for Nursing Education.

Peplau, H.E. (1954, Sept. 15). *Some problems of the psychiatric nursing team.* Second Annual Psychiatric Institute, New Jersey Neuropsychiatric Institute, Proceedings.

Peplau, H.E. (1956). *The yearbook of modern nursing.* New York: G.P. Putnam's Sons.

Peplau, H.E. (1958, June). Current concepts of psychiatric nursing care. *ANA Proceedings.*

Peplau, H.E. (1959). Principles of psychiatric nursing. In *American Handbook of Psychiatry* (Vol. 2). New York: Basic Books.

Peplau, H.E. (1960). Ward atmosphere: Cliche or task. In *Nursing papers.* Illinois State Psychiatric Institute.

Peplau, H.E. (1962). Will automation change the nurse, nursing, or both? *Technical innovations in health care: Nursing implications.* (Pamphlet 5). New York: American Nurses Association.

Peplau, H.E. (1963). Counseling in nursing practice. In E. Harms & P. Schreiber (Eds.), *Handbook of counseling techniques.* New York: Pergamon.

Peplau, H.E. (1963). Leadership responsibility in toleration of stress: The leader's role in helping staff to tolerate stress. In *Conferences on preparation for leadership in psychiatric nursing service.* Department of Nursing Education, Teachers College, Columbia University, New York.

Peplau, H.E. (1963, Dec. 2-3). A personal challenge for immediate action. In *AHA Conference Group in Psychiatric Nursing Practice*, National Institute Proceedings, Kansas City.

Peplau, H.E. (1967). Psychiatric nursing. In A.M. Freedman & A.I. Kaplan (Eds.). *Comprehensive textbook of psychiatry.* New York: Williams & Wilkins.

Peplau, H.E. (1968). Operational definitions and nursing practice. In L.T. Zderad & H.C. Belcher (Eds.), *Developing behavioral concepts in nursing.* Atlanta: Southern Regional Education Board (SREB).

Peplau, H.E., & Smoyak, S. (1968, Nov. 14-16). *Pattern perpetuation and intellectual competencies in schizophrenia.* Paper presented at Conference on Schizophrenia: Current concepts and research. Waldorf Astoria, New York.

Peplau, H.E. (1969, March 20-21). *Theory: The professional dimension.* Presented at the Nursing Theory Conference, University of Kansas Medical Center, Kansas City.

Peplau, H.E. (1969). Pattern perpetuation in schizophrenia. In D. Sankar, *Schizophrenia: Current concepts and research.* Hicksville, NY: PJD Publications.

Peplau, H.E. (1974). *Associate degree education for nursing: Current issues, 1974.* ANA and the professional nurse. Pub. No. 23-1539. National League for Nursing, Department of Associate Degree Programs.

Peplau, H.E. (1992). Notes on Nightingale. In F. Nightingale. *Notes on nursing: What it is, and what it is not.* Philadelphia: J.B. Lippincott.

Peplau, H.E. (1995). Another look at schizophrenia from a nursing standpoint. *Psychiatric Nursing 1946 to 1994: A report on the state of the art.* St. Louis: Mosby.

Peplau, H.E. (1995). Preface: Psychiatric nursing 1946 to 1974: A report on the state of the art. *Psychiatric nursing 1946 to 1994: A report on the state of the art.* St. Louis: Mosby.

Videotape

The nurse theorist: Portraits of excellence: Hildegard Peplau. (1988). Oakland, CA: Studio III. Video is available from Fuld Video Project, Studio III, 370 Hawthorne Avenue, Oakland, CA 94609.

Thesis

Peplau, H.E. (1953). *An exploration of some process elements which restrict or facilitate instructor-student interaction in a classroom, Type B.* Doctoral Project, Teachers College, Columbia University, New York.

Forewords

Peplau, H.E. (1963). In S. Armstrong & S. Rouslin, *Group psychotherapy in nursing practice.* New York: Macmillan.

Peplau, H.E. (1963). In S.F. Burd & M.A. Marshall (Eds.), *Some clinical approaches to psychiatric nursing.* New York: Macmillan.

Peplau, H.E. (1987). In P. Martin, *Psychiatric nursing: A therapeutic approach.* London: Macmillan Education Ltd.

Editorial statements, letters, reactions

Letter to Editor (1962, March). *American Journal of Nursing,* 62(3), 16, 25, 26.

Peplau, H.E. (1963, Sept.). Nursing has lost its way. *Journal RN,* 25(9), 103-105.

Peplau, H.E. (1963, Jan.-Feb.). On semantics. *Perspectives in Psychiatric Care, 1,* 10-11.

Reviews

Peplau, H.E. (1955, May). Review of *The psychiatric interview* by H.S. Sullivan. *American Journal of Nursing,* 55(5), 614.

Peplau, H.E. (1957, April). Review of *The foundation of human behavior* by T. Muller. *Mental Hygiene,* 41(2), 285-286.

Peplau, H.E. (1957, Oct.). Review of *Beyond laughter* by M. Grotjohn. *American Journal of Nursing,* 57(10), 1349-1450.

Peplau, H.E. (1963). Review of *The management of the anxious patient* by Ainslic Meares. *Perspectives in Psychiatric Care,* 2(1) [1964]: 46-47.

Peplau, H.E. (1964). Review of *More for the mind: A study of psychiatric services in Canada. Perspectives in Psychiatric Care,* 11(3), 39-42.

Peplau, H.E. (1964, Fall). Review of *Attitudes of nursing students toward direct patient care* by Sr. L.M. Vaugh. *Journal of Nursing Research,* 13(4), 348-349.

Correspondence

Peplau, H.E. (June, 1992). Personal correspondence.

Peplau, H.E. (July, 1996). Personal correspondence.

Secondary sources

American Nurses Association new executive director states her views. (1970, Jan.). *American Journal of Nursing,* 70(1), 84-88.

Armstrong, M., & Kelly, A. (1993). Enhancing staff nurses' interpersonal skills: Theory to practice. *Clinical Nurse Specialist,* 7(6), 313-317.

Armstrong, M., & Kelly, A. (1995). More than the sum of their parts: Martha Rogers and Hildegard Peplau. *Archives of Psychiatric Nursing,* 9(1), 40-44.

Barker, P. (1993). The Peplau legacy . . . Hildegard Peplau. *Nursing Times,* 89(11), 48-51.

Belcher, J.R., & Fish, L.J. (1980). Hildegard E. Peplau. In Nursing Theories Conference Group, J.B. George, Chairperson, *Nursing theories: The base for professional practice.* Englewood Cliffs, NJ: Prentice-Hall.

Burd, S.F. (1963). The development of an operational definition using the process of learning as a guide. In S.F. Burd & A. Marshall, *Some clinical approaches to psychiatric nursing.* New York: Macmillan.

Burton, G. (1958). Personal, impersonal, and interpersonal relations. Cited by S.A. Smoyak & S. Rouslin (Eds.). (1982). *A collection of classics in psychiatric nursing literature.* Thorofare, NJ: Charles B. Slack.

Chinn, P.L., & Jacobs, M.K. (1983). *Theory and nursing: A systematic approach.* St. Louis: Mosby.

Comley, A. (1994). A comparative analysis of Orem's self-care model and Peplau's interpersonal theory. *Journal of Advanced Nursing,* 20(4), 755-760.

Doncliff, B. (1994). Putting Peplau to work. *Nursing New Zealand, 2*(1), 20-22.

Field, W.E., Jr. (Ed.). (1979). *The psychotherapy of Hildegard E. Peplau.* New Brunfels, TX: PSF Publications.

Fitzpatrick, J.J., & Whall, A.L. (1983). *Conceptual models of nursing: Analysis and application:* Bowie, MD: Robert J. Brady.

Forchuk, C. (1994). The orientation phase of the nurse-client relationship: Testing Peplau's theory. *Journal of Advanced Nursing, 20*(3), 532-537.

Forchuk, C., & Dorsay, J. (1995). Hildegard Peplau meets family systems nursing: Innovation in theory-based practice. *Journal of Advanced Nursing, 21*(1), 110-115.

Fowler, J. (1994). A welcome focus on a key relationship: Using Peplau's model in palliative care. *Professional Nurse, 10*(3), 194-197.

Fowler, J. (1995). Taking theory into practice: Using Peplau's model in the care of patients. *Professional Nurse, 10*(4), 226-230.

Garrett, A., Manuel, D., & Vincent, C. (1976, Nov.). Stressful experiences identified by student nurses. *Journal of Nursing Education, 15*(6), 9-21.

Gregg, D.E. (1978, May-June). Hildegard E. Peplau: Her contributions. *Perspective Psychiatric Care, 16*(3), 118-121.

Hall, K. (1994). Peplau's model of nursing: Caring for a man with AIDS. *British Journal of Nursing, 3*(8), 418-422.

Hays, D. (1961, Spring). Teaching a concept of anxiety. *Nursing Research, 10*(2), 108-113.

Hofling, C.K., & Leininger, M.M. (1960). Basic psychiatric concepts in nursing. Cited by S.A. Smoyak & S. Rouslin (Eds.). (1982). *A collection of classics in psychiatric nursing literature.* Thorofare, NJ: Charles B. Slack

Iveson, J. (1982, Nov.). A two-way process ... theories in nursing practice ... Peplau's nursing model. *Nursing Mirror, 155*(18), 52.

Jones, A. (1995). Utilizing Peplau's psychodynamic theory for stroke patient care. *Journal of Clinical Nursing, 4*(1), 49-54.

Keda, A. (1970, Winter). From Henderson to Orlando to Wiedenback: Thoughts on completion of translation of *Basic principles of clinical nursing. Comprehensive Nursing Quarterly, 5*(1), 85-94.

LaMonica, E. (1981). Construct validity of an empathy instrument. *Research in Nursing and Health, 4,* 389-400.

Lego, S. (1980). The one-to-one nurse-patient relationship. *Perspectives in Psychiatric Care, 18*(2), 67-89. (Reprinted from *Psychiatric nursing 1946-1974: A report on the state of the art,* American Journal of Nursing Co.)

Marshall, J. (1963, March-April). Dr. Peplau's strong medicine for psychiatric nurses. *Smith, Kline & French Reporter, 7,* 11-14.

McCarter, P. (1980, April). New statement defines scope of practice discussion with Dr. Lane and Dr. Peplau. *American Nurse, 12*(4), 1, 8, 24.

Methven, D., & Schlotfeldt, R.M. (1962, Spring). The social interaction inventory. *Nursing Research, 11*(2), 83-88.

Miller, N.E., & Dollard, J. (1941). *Social learning and imitation.* New Haven, CT: Yale University Press.

Nursing Theories Conference Group, J.B. George, Chairperson. (1980). *Nursing theories: The base for professional nursing practice.* Englewood Cliffs, NJ: Prentice-Hall, pp. 73-89.

Orlando, I. (1961). The dynamic nurse-patient relationship. Cited by S.A. Smoyak & S. Rouslin (Eds.). (1982). *A collection of classics in psychiatric nursing literature.* Thorofare, NJ: Charles B. Slack.

Osborne, O. (1984, Nov.). Intellectual traditions in psychiatric nursing. *Journal of Psychosocial Nursing, 22*(1), 27-32.

Peden, A. (1993). Recovering in depressed women: Research with Peplau's theory. *Nursing Science Quarterly, 6*(3), 140-146.

Profile. (1974, Feb.). *Nursing 74, 4,* 13.

Psychotherapeutic strategies. (1968). Current concepts in psychiatric care: The implications for psychiatric nursing practice. Proceedings of the Institute on Psychiatric Nursing, cosponsored by Yale School of Nursing, Department of Psychiatric Nursing and the Community Mental Health Center Department of Nursing. In *Perspectives of Psychiatric Care, 6*(6), 271-289.

Sills, G.M. (1977, May-June). Research in the field of psychiatric nursing 1952-1977. *Nursing Research, 28*(3), 201-207.

Sills, G.M. (1978). Hildegard E. Peplau: Leader, practitioner, academician, scholar, and theorist. *Perspectives in Psychiatric Care, 16*(3), 122-128.

Smoyak, S.A., & Rouslin, S. (Eds.). (1982). Introduction. In *A collection of classics in psychiatric nursing literature.* Thorofare, NJ: Charles B. Slack.

Spring, F.E., & Turk, H. (1962, Fall). A therapeutic behavior scale. *Nursing Research, 11*(4), 214-218.

Thomas, M.D., Baker, J.M., & Estes, N.J. (1970, Dec.). Anger: A tool for developing self-awareness. *American Journal of Nursing, 70*(12), 2586-2590.

Topf, M., & Dambacher, B. (1979). Predominant source of interpersonal influence in relationships between psychiatric patients and nursing staff. *Research in Nursing and Health, 2*(1), 35-43.

Other sources

Andreoli, R.G., & Thompson, C.E. (1977, June). The nature of science in nursing. *Image: Journal of Nursing Scholarship, 9*(2), 32-37.

Arnold, W., & Nieswiadomy, R. (1993). Peplau's theory with an emphasis on anxiety. In S.M. Ziegler (Ed.), *Theory-directed nursing practice.* New York: Springer.

Duffey, M., & Mullencamp, A.F. (1974, Sept.). A framework for theory analysis. *Nursing Outlook, 22,* 570-574.

Forchuk, C. (1993). Hildegarde E. Peplau: Interpersonal nursing theory. Newbury Park, CA: Sage.

Freud, S. (1936). The problem of anxiety. Cited by H.E. Peplau. (1952). *Interpersonal relations in nursing.* New York: G.P. Putnam's Sons.

Fromm, E. (1947). Man for himself. Cited by H.E. Peplau. (1952). *Interpersonal relations in nursing.* New York: G.P. Putnam's Sons.

Jacox, A. (1974, Jan.-Feb.). Theory construction in nursing: An overview. *Nursing Research, 23,* 4-12.

Johnson, D.E. (1959). The nature of a science of nursing. *Nursing Outlook, 7,* 272.

Maslow, A.H. (1943, July). A theory of human motivation. *Psychological Review, 50,* 370-396.

Maslow, A.H., & Mittleman, B. (1941). *Principles in abnormal psychology.* New York: Harper & Brothers.

Miller, N.E., & Dollard, J. (1941). *Social learning and imitation.* New Haven, CT: Yale University Press.

Mullahy, P. (1948). *Oedipus: Myth and complex.* New York: Hermitage House.

Pavlov, I. (1927). *Conditioned reflexes: An investigation of the physiological activity of the cerebral cortex.* London: Oxford University Press.

Phillips, J.R. (1977, Feb.). Nursing systems and nursing models. *Image: Journal of Nursing Scholarship, 9*(1), 6.

Popper, K.R. (1963). *Conjectures and refutations: The growth of scientific knowledge.* New York: Basic Books.

Reynolds, P.D. (1971). *A primer in theory construction.* Indianapolis: Bobbs-Merrill.

Solomon, A.P. (1943). Rehabilitation of patients with psychologically protracted convalescence. *Archives of Physical Therapy, 24,* 270-273.

Sullivan, H.S. (1947). Concepts of modern psychiatry. Cited by H.E. Peplau. (1952). *Interpersonal relations in nursing.* New York: G.P. Putnam's Sons.

Sullivan, H.S. (1948). *The meaning of anxiety in psychiatry and in life.* Washington, DC: William Alanson White Psychiatric Foundation.

Symonds, P. (1946). *The dynamics of human adjustment.* New York: Appleton-Century-Crofts.

von Bertalanffy, L. (1968). *General systems theory: Foundations, development, applications.* New York: Braziller.

Wertheimer, M. (1945). *Productive thinking.* New York: Harper & Brothers.

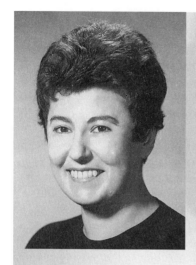

CHAPTER 23

Ida Jean Orlando (Pelletier)

Nursing Process Theory

Larry P. Schumacher, Susan Fisher, Ann Marriner Tomey, Deborah I. Mills, Marcia K. Sauter

CREDENTIALS AND BACKGROUND OF THE THEORIST

Ida Jean Orlando was born August 12, 1926. In 1947, she received a diploma in nursing from New York Medical College, Flower Fifth Avenue Hospital School of Nursing, in New York. She received a B.S. in Public Health Nursing from St. John's University in Brooklyn, New York, in 1951 and an M.A. in Mental Health Consultation from Columbia University Teachers College in New York in 1954. While pursuing her education, Orlando worked intermittently, and sometimes concurrently, as a staff nurse in obstetrical, medical, surgical, and emergency nursing services. She also worked as a supervisor in a general hospital. In addition, as an assistant director of nurses, she was responsible for a general hospital's nursing service and for teaching several courses in the hospital's nursing school.

After receiving her master's degree in 1954, Orlando attended the Yale School of Nursing in New Haven, Connecticut for 8 years. She was a research associate and principal investigator on a federal project grant entitled "Integration of Mental Health Concepts in a Basic Curriculum" until 1958. The project focused on identifying factors influencing the integration of mental health principles in a basic nursing curriculum. Orlando carried out this project by observing and participating in student experiences with patients, and medical, nursing, and instructional personnel throughout the basic curriculum. She recorded her observations for 3 years and spent a fourth year analyzing the accumulated data.

351

She reported her findings in 1958 in her first book, *The Dynamic Nurse-Patient Relationship: Function, Process and Principles of Professional Nursing Practice.*[23] Although written in 1958, this book was not published until 1961. Since then, five foreign language editions have been printed. The formulations in this book provided the foundation for Orlando's nursing theory.[25:243] During the next 4 years (1958 to 1961) as an associate professor and then as Director of the Graduate Program in Mental Health and Psychiatric Nursing, Orlando used her theory as the foundation of the program. She married Robert J. Pelletier and left Yale in 1961.

From 1962 through 1972, Orlando was Clinical Nursing Consultant at McLean Hospital in Belmont, Massachusetts. While in this position, she studied the interactions of nurses with patients, peers, and other staff members. She also studied how these interactions affected the processes used by the nurse to help patients. Orlando convinced the hospital director that a training program for nurses was needed. As a result, the nursing service of McLean hospital was reorganized and a training program based on her theory was implemented.[25:45] Orlando subsequently applied for and received federal funding to evaluate training in the nursing process discipline.

While at McLean Hospital, Orlando published "The Patient's Predicament and Nursing Function" in a 1967 issue of *Psychiatric Opinion.*[27] In 1972, she reported the 10 years of work at the hospital in her second book, *The Discipline and Teaching of Nursing Process: An Evaluative Study.*[24]

From 1972 to 1981, Orlando lectured, served as a consultant, and conducted about 60 workshops in her theory throughout the United States and Canada. She has served on the Board of the Harvard Community Health Plan in Boston, Massachusetts, from 1972 to 1984, and on the Hospital Committee of the Board from 1979 to 1985. She has since served in various capacities such as on the membership, program, and services committees.

In 1981, Orlando accepted a position as Nurse Educator for Metropolitan State Hospital in Waltham, Massachusetts. From 1984 until 1987, she held various administrative nursing positions there. In September 1987, Orlando became the Assistant Director

of Nursing for Education and Research at Metropolitan State Hospital.[28] In 1992 Orlando retired from nursing.[29]

In 1990, the National League for Nursing (NLN) reprinted Orlando's 1961 publication. In the preface to the NLN edition, Orlando states, "If I had been more courageous in 1961, when this book was first written, I would have proposed it as 'nursing process theory' instead of as a 'theory of effective nursing practice.'"[25:vii]

Orlando's nursing theory emphasizes the reciprocal relationship between patient and nurse. Both are affected by what the other says and does. She was one of the first nursing leaders to emphasize the elements of nursing process and the critical importance of the patient's participation during the nursing process. Orlando may have facilitated the development of nurses as logical thinkers, as well as conformers, in carrying out the medical orders of a physician.[22:133]

Orlando stated that her search for facts in observing nursing situations influenced her most before the development of her theory and that she derived her theory from the conceptualization of those facts.[28] Her overall goal was to find an organizing principle for professional nursing, that is, a distinct function.[23:viii]

Orlando has made a major contribution to nursing theory and practice. Her conceptualizations fulfill the criteria of theory because she presents interrelated concepts that present a systematic view of nursing phenomena; she specifies relationships among the concepts; she explains what happens during the nursing process and why; she prescribes how nursing phenomena can be controlled; and she explains how the control leads to prediction of outcome. Although nursing writers such as Fitzpatrick and Whall[14:15] do not believe any current nursing model meets a level of specificity, Orlando's theory has considerable merit in application to practice, education, and research.

THEORETICAL SOURCES

Orlando acknowledges no theoretical sources for the development of her theory. None of her publications include a bibliography.

MAJOR CONCEPTS & DEFINITIONS

Orlando describes her model as revolving around five major interrelated concepts: (1) the function of professional nursing, (2) the presenting behavior of the client, (3) the immediate or internal response of the nurse, (4) the nursing process discipline, and (5) improvement.[13:39]

Nurse's Responsibility "Whatever help the patient may require for his needs to be met (i.e., for his physical and mental comfort to be assured as far as possible while he is undergoing some form of medical treatment or supervision)."[25:5] It is the nurse's responsibility to see that "the patient's needs for help are met, either directly by her own activity or indirectly by calling in the help of others."[23:29]

Need "Situationally defined as a requirement of the patient which, if supplied, relieves or diminishes his immediate distressor and improves his immediate sense of adequacy or well-being."[25:6]

Presenting Behavior of Patient Any observable verbal or nonverbal behavior.[13:39]

Immediate Reactions Include both the nurse and patient's individual perceptions, thoughts, and feelings.[13:39]

Nursing Process Discipline Includes the nurse communicating to the client his/her own immediate reaction, clearly identifying that the item expressed belongs to the nurse, and then asking for validation or correction[13:39]; was called *deliberative nursing process* in Orlando's first book; also called *nursing process* and *process discipline*.

Improvement "Means to grow better, to turn to profit, to use to advantage."[25]

Purpose of Nursing "Supply the help a patient requires in order for his needs to be met."[25:9]

Automatic Nursing Action "Those nursing actions decided upon for reasons other than the patient's immediate need."[5:167]

Deliberative Nursing Action "Those actions decided upon after ascertaining a need and then meeting this need."[5:167]

USE OF EMPIRICAL EVIDENCE

Orlando synthesized facts from observations to develop her theory. She asserted that her theory was valid and applied it in her work with patients and nurses and the teaching of students. Orlando gathered a considerable amount of data before constructing her theory. She used a research process but did not follow research methodology for quantitative analysis.[11:59]

At McLean Hospital, Orlando implemented the nursing process theory that she had developed at Yale. During her last 3 years there, she received a research grant to do evaluative research of the training program to test what she thought had happened. She published the results in her second book.

MAJOR ASSUMPTIONS

Nearly all the assumptions in Orlando's theory are implicit. Meleis[21] thinks that one of the major problems with Orlando's assumptions is that it is not totally clear how they were derived. No documentation exists.[21]

Nursing

Orlando's major assumption about nursing is that it should be a distinct profession that functions autonomously. Although nursing has been historically aligned with medicine and continues to have a close relationship with medicine, nursing and the practice of medicine are clearly separate professions.[23:18,12] These assumptions are reflected in Orlando's definition of the function of professional nursing.

Orlando[24:20] states that "the function of professional nursing is conceptualized as finding out and meeting the patient's immediate need for help." It is the nurse's responsibility to see that "the patient's needs for help are met, either directly by her own activity or indirectly by calling in the help of others."[23:29] This may be more fully developed by Orlando's approach to nursing process discipline, which she proposes is composed of the following basic elements: "(1) the behavior of the patient, (2) the reaction of the nurse, and (3) the nursing actions which are designed for the patient's benefit. The interaction of these elements with each other is nursing process."[19:36]

Another assumption Orlando[24:19] makes is that nurses should help relieve physical or mental discomfort and should not add to the patient's distress. This assumption is evident in Orlando's concept of improvement in the patient's behavior as the intended outcome of nursing actions.

Orlando is concerned with providing direct assistance to individuals in whatever setting they are found for the purpose of avoiding, relieving, diminishing, or curing the person's sense of helplessness.[13]

Person

Orlando assumes that persons behave verbally and nonverbally. Evidence of this assumption is found in Orlando's emphasis on behavior. Orlando assumes that persons are sometimes able to meet their own needs for help in some situations but that persons become distressed when unable to do so. This is the basis for Orlando's assertion[23:22] that professional nurses should be concerned only with those persons who are unable to meet their need for help independently. She also stated that each patient is unique and individual in his or her response and that a professional nurse can recognize that the same behavior in different patients can signal quite different needs.[25:59]

Health

Orlando[30:9] does not define health but assumes that freedom from mental or physical discomfort and feelings of adequacy and well-being contribute to health.[23:9]

Environment

Orlando does not define environment. She assumes that a nursing situation occurs when there is a nurse-patient contact and that both nurse and patient perceive, think, feel, and act in the immediate situation. She does point out, however, that a patient may react with distress to any aspect of an environment that was designed for therapeutic and helpful purposes.[25:11]

THEORETICAL ASSERTIONS

Orlando[30:8] views the professional function of nursing as finding out and meeting the immediate needs for help of the patient. This function is fulfilled when the nurse ascertains and meets the patient's immediate needs for help. Consequently, Orlando's theory focuses on how to produce improvement in the patient's behavior.

A person becomes a patient requiring nursing care when he/she has unmet needs for help that cannot be met independently because of physical limitations, a negative reaction to an environment, or experiences preventing the patient from communicating needs for help.[23:11] Orlando[23:10] asserts that these limitations on the patient's ability to meet his needs are most likely to occur while the patient is receiving medical care or supervision. Thus the restrictions Orlando has frequently placed on the concept of patient can be seen as a function of the impediments that persons have in meeting their needs.

Patients experience distress or feelings of helplessness as a result of unmet needs for help.[23:61] Orlando[23:46-47] believes there is a positive correlation between the length of time the patient experiences the unmet needs and the degree of distress. Therefore immediacy is emphasized throughout her theory. In Orlando's view,[23:22] when persons are able to meet their own needs, they do not feel distress and do not require care from a professional nurse. For those persons who do have a need for help, it is essential the nurse obtain correction or verification of the nurse's perceptions, thoughts, and feelings to determine whether the patient is in need of help.[23:29]

Individuals in contact with each other go through an action process that involves observation of the other's behavior, the resulting thoughts and feelings about this observation, and an action chosen by each individual in response to the reaction.[24:25] When the nurse acts, an action process transpires. This action process by the nurse in the nurse-patient contact is called *nursing process*.[24:29] The nursing process may be automatic or deliberative. Any behavior of the patient observed by the nurse must be viewed as a possible signal of distress because it is possible for the patient to "react with distress to any aspect of an environment that was designed for therapeutic and helpful purposes."[23:17] Perception of patient behavior produces thoughts and feelings in the nurse. Orlando defines *immediate reaction* as including perception, a physical stimulation of any one of a person's five senses; thought, an idea that occurs in an individual's mind; and feeling, a state of mind inclining a person toward or against a perception, thought, or feeling.[23:25] The nurse's reaction precipitates nursing actions.[23:61]

The nurse's asking the patient about the nurse's perception of the patient's behavior is more effective and less time consuming because the physical stimulus for perception has objective validity. Nursing actions that are not deliberative are automatic.[23:60] Automatic nursing actions are those having nothing to do with finding out and meeting the patient's needs for help. Deliberative nursing actions are those designed to identify and meet the patient's immediate need for help and, therefore, to fulfill the professional nursing function. Deliberative nursing actions require that the nurse seek validation or correction of her thoughts and feelings with the patient before she and the patient can know what nursing action will meet the need for help.[23:41]

In her second book, Orlando renamed deliberative nursing action a *process discipline* with three specific requirements. Application of the nursing process discipline qualifies as a *disciplined professional response*.[24:29,31] Despite this change in terminology, Orlando provides a clear procedure for nurses to ascertain and meet a patient's needs for help. First, the nurse expresses to the patient any or all of the items contained in her reaction to the patient's behavior. Second, the nurse verbally states to the patient that the expressed item belongs to the nurse by use of the personal pronoun (an "I" message). Finally, the nurse asks about the item expressed, attempting to verify or correct her perceptions, thoughts, or feelings (reaction).[35:29-30]

The value of the nursing process discipline is in determining whether the patient feels distressed and ascertaining what help is required to relieve the distress.[20:29] Without the investigation required by the nursing process discipline, the nurse does not have a reliable database for action.[24:32] When the nurse responds automatically, the perceptions, thoughts, and feelings of each person are not available to the other. When the nurse uses the nursing process discipline, the perceptions, thoughts, and feelings of the nurse are available to the patient and vice versa.[24:25-27] This latter response is viewed by Orlando[23:67] as a form of "continuous reflection as the nurse tries to understand the meaning to the patient of the behavior she observed and what he needs from her in order to be helped." The nurse evaluates her actions by comparing the patient's verbal and nonverbal behavior at the end of the contact with the behavior that was present when the process started.[23:68]

LOGICAL FORM

Orlando's theory is inductive. Orlando collected records of her observations of nurse-patient situations during a 3-year period. In analyzing this material, Orlando looked for "good" versus "bad" outcomes. Good outcomes were defined as those that improved the patient's behavior. Bad outcomes were defined as absence of improvement. Orlando concluded that the nurse's use of the nursing process discipline was an effective means of achieving a good outcome. On this basis, Orlando synthesized her theory.[11:34]

If Walker and Avant's criteria[38:125-128] are used for theory analysis, Orlando's theory is logically adequate. Although inductive argument can produce false conclusions even when the premises are true, Orlando's conclusions seem reasonable. The structure of relationships is clear and sufficiently precise; and it is possible to represent the relationships schematically. The relationships progress from existence and conditional statements to prediction and control. The predictions Orlando makes are acceptable to the nursing profession, as improvement in patient care is always valuable. There are no logical fallacies within Orlando's theory because relationships are sufficiently developed.

ACCEPTANCE BY THE NURSING COMMUNITY

Orlando's theory is clearly applicable to nursing practice. However, there is little evidence of this application in the literature. Schmidt[33:72] reported using Orlando's theory as a basis for practice in 1972. Peitchinis[26] suggested that Orlando's nursing process discipline reflected the elements of the therapeutic relationship, which include expression of empathy, warmth, and genuineness. She proposed that nursing practice based on Orlando's theory would increase the therapeutic effectiveness of nursing.[26:146]

The use of Orlando's theory as a basis of practice in the Mid Missouri Mental Health Center and its use in a new psychiatric unit in a general hospital in Antigonish, Nova Scotia, are other examples of acceptance by the nursing community. Henderson[18:119] wrote in 1978 that Orlando's insistence on validation was an important contribution to the practice of nursing. More recently, Schmieding[34] reported the advantages of adopting Orlando's theory throughout a department of nursing. Implementation of Orlando's theory produced several benefits. They included increased effectiveness in meeting patient needs; improvement in decision-making skills among staff nurses, particularly in determining what constituted nursing versus nonnursing actions; more effective conflict resolution among staff nurses and between staff and physicians; and a greater sense of identity and unity among staff.[34:761]

Schmieding[35] also discussed "how specific types of actions facilitate or thwart problem identification" and, using Orlando's theory, analyzed managerial responses in face-to-face contacts. Boston's Beth Israel Hospital Division of Nursing Statement of Philosophy and Purpose represents their nursing service based on Henderson, Weidenback, and Orlando. Consequently, there is evidence that Orlando's theory is used at the patient care level, managerial level, and nursing division level.

Orlando's nursing process discipline is confined to every immediate nurse-patient contact. Observa-

tion of the patient's verbal and nonverbal behavior provides data for determining the patient's level of distress when the nursing process discipline is used. The nurse then takes actions to meet the patient's need for help. Finally, the nurse investigates her newer observations to learn whether the action actually relieved the distress (evaluation). If the distress is not relieved, the process begins again.

Education

Orlando's theory is a conceptual framework for the process by which professional nursing should be practiced. Orlando's process recording has made a significant contribution to nursing education. Orlando[24:32-33] found that "training" in the nursing process discipline was necessary for the nurse to be able to control the nursing process and achieve improvement in the patient's behavior. She therefore developed the process recording, a tool to facilitate self-evaluation of whether or not the nursing process discipline was used. This "systematic repetitious examination and study of the nursing process" was designed to help students learn how to express their immediate reactions to patients and to ask for correction or verification.[24:32-33] The process recording is an educational tool still used in nursing education.

Orlando[23:vii] wrote her first book "to offer the professional nursing student a theory of effective practice." Since 1961, numerous psychiatric nursing texts have included Orlando's theory. Orlando deserves credit for providing guidelines for the nurse to use in contacts with patients. Orlando's theory was instrumental in development of the interaction theory currently used in psychiatric nursing.[2:117]

Winder[39] identifies the need to provide a "facilitating environment and implementing the caring process" in the nursing curriculum. He suggests that Orlando's theory provides a model for such a training process in her book *The Discipline and Teaching of Nursing Process.*

Haggerty[16] analyzed nursing students' responses to distressed patients based on Orlando's nursing process concept. She found that "emphasis on communication and psychosocial foundations in BSN curriculums may not translate into more effective exploratory skills in these students." She recommends Orlando's model for teaching B.S.N. students to conceptualize the interactional process and its goals.

Research

Orlando's theory has enjoyed considerable acceptance in the area of nursing research and has been applied to a variety of research settings. Many of the studies have provided empirical evidence that Orlando's theoretical assertions are valid. These are discussed under Empirical Precision.

Dracup and Breu[6:213] used Orlando's definition of the concept *need for help* in their study of the needs of grieving spouses; Hampe[17:114] used the definition in a similar study. Orlando's *nursing process discipline* has been designated the *experimental approach* in several studies to examine its effects on a patient's distress during admission and before surgery. Anderson, Mertz, and Leonard[1:151] found that deliberative nursing actions promoted stress reduction during admission. Wolfer and Visintainer[40:248] demonstrated this same result with children and their parents. Dumas and Johnson[8:140] determined that preoperative exploration with patients to determine the real source of distress permitted the nurse to take appropriate action to relieve the distress and that lower distress before surgery correlated with fewer postoperative complications. Nursing process discipline was used as the experimental nursing action by Dumas and Leonard[9:12] in their study of postoperative vomiting.

As alluded to earlier, Haggerty[16] used Orlando's nursing process concept to conduct research on nursing students' responses to distressed patients. Princeton[32] tested the effects of using the nursing process discipline with breast-feeding mothers and their infants. These studies using the nursing process discipline can be considered both theory-testing and theory-generating. They have provided empirical support for Orlando's theory (theory-testing) and have produced new principles for practice, especially in the area of preoperative teaching (theory-generating).

In 1988 Schmieding[36] did a study on the use of Orlando's theory to investigate the action process of nurse administrators to realistic hypothetical situations presented to them by their staff. The findings indicated the administrators' first thought was seldom about their staff's reaction to the situation. Schmieding concludes that the quality of nursing is reflected in the quality of help nurses receive from their administrators in the problem-solving process. The results of this study indicate that the quality of this help may be less than optimal. Sheafor[37:30] in a review of this study concludes that Orlando's theory should be included in a graduate program for nursing administrators. They also suggested that the use of Orlando's theory in the graduate education of clinical specialists is important. In a study of adult cancer patients, Ponte[31] examined the relationships among empathy and Orlando's nursing process discipline. A positive relationship was found between empathy skills in the primary nurse and the use of nursing process discipline. Ponte encourages further research in the area of nurses' interpersonal skills and patient outcomes.

FURTHER DEVELOPMENT

The process discipline needs to be taught and then implemented in a variety of settings. Orlando's study could be replicated to validate that the process discipline is directly related to effectiveness of a nursing system.

CRITIQUE
Clarity

Orlando's first book, *The Dynamic Nurse-Patient Relationship*, presented concepts clearly. Her second book, *The Discipline and Teaching of Nursing Process*, redefined and renamed *deliberative nursing process* as *nursing process discipline*. Orlando's writing style involves defining concepts minimally at first and then developing them throughout the book. Because of the evolution of the theory the reader must be familiar with both books to evaluate her theory thoroughly.

Simplicity

As Orlando deals with relatively few concepts and their relationships with each other, her theory would be considered simple. Her theory may also be viewed as simplistic because she is able to make some predictive statements as opposed to just description and explanation. The simplicity of Orlando's theory has benefited research application.

Walker and Avant[38] use Orlando's theory as an example of grand nursing theory. They state that grand nursing theories have provided a global perspective, but by virtue of their generality and abstractness, most grand theories are untestable in their current form. Although Orlando's theory has undergone testing, its global perspective would support labeling this work as a grand theory. Orlando's theory has also been described as a practice theory. Practice theories provide a framework to specify when the guidelines should be applied, describe the means to be used, and specify the goals to be used for outcome evaluation.[13:40]

Generality

Orlando discussed and illustrated nurse-patient contacts in which the patient is conscious, able to communicate, and in need of help. Although she did not focus on unconscious patients and groups, application of her theory to unconscious patients or groups is feasible. Actually, any other person could make use of the nursing process discipline with any other group if educated properly. Therefore, although Orlando's theory focuses on a limited number of situations, it could be adapted to other nursing situations and other professional fields.

Empirical Precision

Two thirds of Orlando's second book is a report of a research project designed to test the validity of her nursing formulations. A training program based on her formulations had been in progress for 3 years before the project began.[24:44] Nurses were trained to use the nursing process discipline in nurse-patient contacts. Those nurses who became clinical nursing supervisors were trained to use the nursing process discipline in their supervisory contacts and other contacts as well. The following is a brief description of the research methodology.

The purpose of the project was to evaluate the effectiveness of the nursing process discipline in the nurse's contacts at work and the effectiveness of the training program. But these evaluations could not take place before hypothetical measures for the nursing process discipline and the effectiveness of the nursing process discipline were identified. A discipline variable was defined.[24:60] Effectiveness was determined by the presence or absence of a *helpful outcome*, as judged by two reliable outcome coders. The outcome coders compared the beginning behavior of the subject with the behavior at the end of the record.[24:76] Testing the relationship of the nursing process discipline (in use) with the presence or absence of a helpful outcome in patient, staff, and supervisee contacts was also done. Evaluation of the training program was done by testing whether nurses increased their use of the nursing process discipline after being trained.[24:63-66]

Two groups of nurses were included in the study. The control group consisted of "veterans"—previously trained supervisors and staff nurses. The experimental group consisted of "novices"—untrained supervisors and staff nurses. Transcripts were made of tape-recorded 10-minute periods (six for each subject) of novices' and veterans' contacts at work.

This report is extensive and detailed and may be difficult to read and interpret for those without a good understanding of statistics and research methodology. The study concludes that training in the nursing process discipline and its use achieves helpful outcomes in patient, supervisee, and staff contacts.

Although Orlando's work is difficult to understand, numerous studies by Orlando's first graduate students at Yale in the 1960s supported the validity of her theory.[1,3,4,7-12] Several that incorporated Orlando's nursing process discipline approach have already been mentioned in research application. Others, who specifically tested the usefulness of the nursing process discipline approach, included the following: Pienschke,[30:484-489] who found that nursing intervention was more effective under conditions of open disclosure because patients' needs were perceived more accurately; Bochnak,[3:191-192] who found that the nursing process discipline was more effective in relieving patients' pain; Dye,[10:194] who controlled for staff-patient ratios and amount of nursing time and still demonstrated that deliberative nursing actions met patient needs effectively; and Cameron,[4:192] who revealed that the nursing process discipline led to the most consistent effective results in verifying patient needs.

Orlando asserts that patient distress stems from reaction to the environment that the patient cannot control alone. Dye provided empirical evidence for this assertion in her study on clarifying patient needs. She found patients experienced distress more as a reaction to the hospital setting than to their illness.[11:59]

Orlando also asserts patient distress stems from misinterpretation by the nurse of the patient's experience or from the patient's initial inability to clearly communicate the need for help. Both necessitate use of the nursing process discipline.

Two studies, one down by Elder[12] and the other by Gowan and Morris,[15] provided support for this assertion. Both studies demonstrated that although patients frequently did not express their needs clearly, deliberative nursing actions alleviated the problem.[1,3,4,7-12]

Derivable Consequences

Orlando's theory is potentially beneficial in achieving valued outcomes. Identifying the patient's needs for help and the nurse's ability to meet these needs are very important to nursing practice.

Incorporating validation into the nursing process discipline, as Orlando suggests, allows for maximum participation by the patient in his/her care. Several researchers have also demonstrated that the use of disciplined professional response enables the nurse to ascertain and meet the patient's needs. The study of what nurses say and do in their practice and the resulting effect displayed by the patient is valuable content for nursing education. The nursing process discipline also allows nurses to view the patient from a nursing perspective, rather than from a medical disease orientation.

CRITICAL THINKING *Activities*

1 George is a 70-year-old client that has been assigned to you as a community-based nurse case manager. George has severe congestive heart failure, peripheral vascular disease, and no family or social support. George has had 15 admissions to the hospital and 35 visits to the emergency department this year due to noncompliance with his medication and diet regimen. He receives a monthly social security check, which he spends on food, gambling (primarily bingo), and medications, in that order.

   a. Describe your immediate reactions to George, who really is uncertain of the need for a nurse.

   b. Place yourself in George's shoes and describe the immediate reactions to yourself as a nurse.

   c. What would your first interaction with George be like; describe the dialogue.

   d. Define your automatic nursing actions in relation to George.

   e. Define deliberative nursing actions in relation to George.

2 Select two situations when a client would not require medical interventions that professional nursing would be necessary.

   a. List two deliberative nursing actions for each situation.

   b. List two automatic nursing actions for each situation.

3 Describe how Orlando's theory can be used in practice when the nurse-patient relationship is extremely short term, as in the extremely short lengths of stay experienced by hospitalized clients.

REFERENCES

1. Anderson, B., Mertz, H., & Leonard, R. (1965). Two experimental tests of a patient-centered admission process. *Nursing Research, 14,* 151-156.
2. Artinian, B. (1983). Implementation of the intersystem patient-care model in clinical practice. *Journal of Advanced Nursing, 8,* 117-124.
3. Bochnak, M. (1963). The effect of an automatic and deliberative process of nursing activity on the relief of patients' pain: A clinical experiment. *Abstract in Nursing Research, 12,* 191-192.
4. Cameron, J. (1963). An exploratory study of the verbal responses of the nurses in twenty nurse-patient interactions. *Abstract in Nursing Research, 12,* 292.
5. Crane, M. (1985). Ida Jean Orlando. In J.B. George (Ed.). *Nursing theories: The base for professional nursing practice* (pp.158-179). Englewood Cliffs, NJ: Prentice-Hall.
6. Dracup, K., & Breu, C. (1978). Using nursing research findings to meet the needs of grieving spouses. *Nursing Research, 27,* 212-216.
7. Dumas, R. (1963). Psychological preparation for surgery. *American Journal of Nursing, 63,* 52-55.
8. Dumas, R., & Johnson, B. (1972). Research in nursing practice: A review of five clinical experiments. *International Journal of Nursing Studies, 9,* 137-149.
9. Dumas, R., & Leonard, R. (1963). The effect of nursing on the incidence of postoperative vomiting. *Nursing Research, 12,* 12-15.
10. Dye, M. (1963). A descriptive study of conditions conducive to an effective process of nursing activity. *Abstract in Nursing Research, 12,* 194.
11. Dye, M. (1963). Clarifying patients' communications. *American Journal of Nursing, 63,* 56-59.
12. Elder, R. (1963). What is the patient saying? *Nursing Forum, 11,* 25-37.
13. Forchuk, C. (1991). A comparison of the works of Peplau and Orlando. *Archives of Psychiatric Nursing, 5*(1), 38-45.
14. Fitzpatrick, J., & Whall, A. (1983). *Conceptual models of nursing: Analysis and application.* Bowie, MD: Robert J. Brady.
15. Gowan, N., & Morris, M. (1964). Nurses' responses to expressed patient needs. *Nursing Research, 13,* 68-71.
16. Haggerty, L. (1987). An analysis of senior nursing students' immediate responses to distressed patients. *Journal of Advanced Nursing, 12,* 451-461.
17. Hampe, S. (1975). Needs of the grieving spouse in a hospital setting. *Nursing Research, 24,* 113-120.
18. Henderson, V. (1978). The concept of nursing. *Journal of Advanced Nursing, 3,* 113-130.
19. Larson, P., Sr. (1977). Nurse perceptions of patient characteristics. *Nursing Research, 26,* 416-421.
20. McCann-Flynn, J., & Heffron, B. (1984). *Nursing: From concept to practice.* Bowie, MD: Robert J. Brady.
21. Meleis, A.I. (1991). *Theoretical nursing: Development and progress* (2nd ed., pp. 338-348). New York: J.B. Lippincott.
22. Nursing Theories Conference Group, J.B. George, Chairperson. (1980). *Nursing theories: The base for professional practice.* Englewood Cliffs, NJ: Prentice-Hall.
23. Orlando, I. (1961). *The dynamic nurse-patient relationship: Function, process and principles of professional nursing practice.* New York: G.P. Putnam's Sons.
24. Orlando, I. (1972). *The discipline and teaching of nursing process: An evaluative study.* New York: G.P. Putnam's Sons.
25. Orlando, I.J. (1990). *The dynamic nurse-patient relationship* (Pub. No. 15-2341). New York: National League for Nursing.
26. Peitchinis, L. (1972). Therapeutic effectiveness of counseling by nursing personnel. *Nursing Research, 21,* 138-147.
27. Pelletier, I.O. (1967). The patient's predicament and nursing function. *Psychiatric Opinion, 4,* 25-30.
28. Pelletier, I.O. (1984). Personal correspondence.
29. Pelletier, I.O. (1996). Telephone interview.
30. Pienschke, D., Sr. (1973). Guardedness or openness on the cancer unit. *Nursing Research, 22,* 484-490.
31. Ponte, P.A.R. (1988). *The relationships among empathy and the use of Orlando's deliberative process by the primary nurse and the distress of the adult cancer patient.* Unpublished doctoral dissertation, Boston University, Boston.
32. Princeton, J. (1986). Incorporating a deliberative nursing care approach with breast-feeding mothers. *Health Care for Women International, 7,* 277-293.
33. Schmidt, J. (1972). Availability: A concept of nursing practice. *American Journal of Nursing, 72,* 1086-1089.
34. Schmieding, N. (1984). Putting Orlando's theory into practice. *American Journal of Nursing, 84,* 759-761.
35. Schmieding, N. (1987). Analyzing managerial responses in face-to-face contacts. *Journal of Advanced Nursing, 12,* 357-365.
36. Schmieding, N.J. (1988). Action process of nurse administrators to problematic situations based on Orlando's theory. *Journal of Advanced Nursing, 13,* 99-107.
37. Sheafor, M. (1991). Productive work groups in complex hospital units. *Journal of Nursing Administration, 21*(5), 25-30.
38. Walker, L., & Avant, K. (1983). *Strategies for theory construction in nursing.* Norwalk, CT: Appleton-Century-Crofts.
39. Winder, A. (1984). A mental health professional looks at nursing care. *Nursing Forum, 21,* 184-188.
40. Wolfer, J., & Visintainer, M. (1975). Pediatric surgical patients' and parents' stress responses and adjustment. *Nursing Research, 24,* 244-255.

BIBLIOGRAPHY

Primary sources

Books

Orlando, I. (1961). *The dynamic nurse-patient relationship.* New York: G.P. Putnam's Sons.

Orlando, I. (1972). *The discipline and teaching of nursing process.* New York: G.P. Putnam's Sons.

Orlando, I.J. (1990). *The dynamic nurse-patient relationship* (Pub. No. 15-2341). New York: National League for Nursing.

Book chapter

Orlando, I. (1962). Function, process and principle of professional nursing practice. In *Integration of mental health concepts in the human relations professions.* New York: Bank Street College of Education.

Journal articles

Orlando, I. (1987). Nursing in the 21st century: Alternate path. *Journal of Advanced Nursing, 12,* 405-412.

Orlando, I.J., & Dugan, A. (1989 Feb.). Independent and dependent paths: The fundamental issue for the nursing profession. *Nursing and Health Care, 2,* 77-80.

Pelletier, I.O. (1967). The patient's predicament and nursing function. *Psychiatric Opinion, 4,* 25-30.

Video

Pelletier, I.O. (1988). *The nurse theorist: Portraits of excellence. Ida Orlando Pelletier.* Athens, OH: Fuld Institute for Technology in Nursing Education.

Correspondence

Pelletier, I.O. (1984). Personal correspondence.
Pelletier, I.O. (1985). Personal correspondence.
Pelletier, I.O. (1988). Personal correspondence.

Interviews

Pelletier, I.O. (1984). Telephone interviews.
Pelletier, I.O. (1985). Telephone interviews.
Pelletier, I.O. (1988). Telephone interviews.
Pelletier, I.O. (1996). Telephone interviews.

Secondary sources

Book

Schmieding, N.J. (1993). *Ida Jean Orlando: A nursing process theory.* Newbury Park, CA: Sage.

Book reviews

Orlando, I. (1961). *The dynamic nurse-patient relationship.*
*AAINJ, 10,*41, March 1962.
Nursing Outlook, 10, 221, April 1962.
Catholic Nurse, 10, 54, June 1962.
Journal of Psychiatric Nursing, 1, 65, Jan. 1963.

Orlando, I. (1972). *The discipline and teaching of nursing process.*
Nursing Research, 22, 10, Jan.-Feb. 1973.
Supervisor Nurse, 4, 48-49, Feb. 1973.
American Journal of Nursing, 73, 926, May 1973.
Nursing Outlook, 21, 432, July 1973.

Journal of Nursing Administration, 4, 12, Jan.-Feb. 1974.

Dissertations

Ponte, P.A.R. (1988). *The relationships among empathy and the use of Orlando's deliberative process by the primary nurse and the distress of the adult cancer patient.* Unpublished doctoral dissertation. Boston University, Boston.

Schmieding, N. (1983). *A description and analysis of the directive process used by directors of nursing, supervisors, and head nurses in problematic situations based on Orlando's theory of nursing experience.* Unpublished doctoral dissertation, Boston University, Boston.

Sellers, S.C. (1991). *A philosophical analysis of conceptual models of nursing.* Unpublished doctoral dissertation, Iowa State University, Ames, Iowa.

Book chapters

Andrews, C. (1983). Ida Orlando's model of nursing. In J. Fitzpatrick & A. Whall, *Conceptual models of nursing: Analysis and application.* Bowie, MD: Robert J. Brady.

Crane, M.D. (1980). Ida Jean Orlando. In Nursing Theories Conference Group, J.B. George, Chairperson, *Nursing theories: The base for professional nursing practice.* Englewood Cliffs, NJ: Prentice-Hall.

Crane, M.D. (1985). Ida Jean Orlando. In Nursing Theories Conference Group, J.B. George, Chairperson, *Nursing theories: The base for professional nursing practice.* Englewood Cliffs, NJ: Prentice-Hall.

Fawcett, J. (1993). Orlando's theory of the deliberative nursing process. In *Analysis and evaluation of nursing theories.* Philadelphia: F.A. Davis.

Meleis, A.I. (1985). Ida Orlando. In Meleis, A.I., *Theoretical nursing: Development and progress.* Philadelphia: J.B. Lippincott.

Meleis, A.I. (1991). Ida Orlando. In Meleis, A.I., *Theoretical nursing: Development and progress.* Philadelphia: J.B. Lippincott.

Mertz, H. (1962). Nurse actions that reduce stress in patients. In *Emergency intervention by the nurse* (Monograph 1). New York: American Nurses Association.

Schmieding, N.J. (1983). An analysis of Orlando's theory based on Kuhn's theory of science. In P.L. Chinn, *Advances in nursing theory development.* Rockville, MD: Aspen.

Journal articles

Anderson, B., Mertz, H., & Leonard, R. (1965). Two experimental tests of a patient-centered admission process. *Nursing Research, 14,* 151-156.

Artinian, B. (1983). Implementation of the intersystem patient-care model in clinical practice. *Journal of Advanced Nursing, 8,* 117-124.

Beckstrand, J.A. (1980). A critique of several conceptions of practice model in nursing. *Research in Nursing and Health, 3,* 69-79.

de la Cuesta, C. (1983). The nursing process: From development to implementation. *Journal of Advanced Nursing, 8,* 365-371.

Diers, D. (1970). Faculty research development at Yale. *Nursing Research,* 19(1), 64-71.

Dixon, J., Dixon, J., & Spinner, J. (1989). Perceptions of life-pattern disintegrity as a link in the relationship between stress and illness. *Advances in Nursing Science,* 11(2), 1-11.

Dracup, K., & Breu, C. (1978). Using nursing research findings to meet the needs of grieving spouses. *Nursing Research, 27,* 212-216.

Dumas, R. (1963). Psychological preparation for surgery. *American Journal of Nursing, 63,* 52-55.

Dumas, R., & Johnson, B. (1972). Research in nursing practice: A review of five clinical experiments. *International Journal of Nursing Studies, 9,* 137-149.

Dumas, R., & Leonard, R. (1963). The effect of nursing on the incidence of postoperative vomiting. *Nursing Research, 12,* 12-15.

Dye, M. (1963). Clarifying patients' communications. *American Journal of Nursing, 63,* 56-59.

Eisler, J., Wolfer, J., & Diers, D. (1972). Relationship between need for social approval and postoperative recovery and welfare. *Nursing Research, 21,* 520-525.

Elder, R. (1963). What is the patient saying? *Nursing Forum, 11,* 25-37.

Elms, R., & Leonard, R. (1966). Effects of nursing approaches during admission. *Nursing Research, 15,* 39-48.

Forchuk, C. (1991). A comparison of the works of Peplau and Orlando. *Archives of Psychiatric Nursing,* 5(1), 38-45.

Gowan, N., & Morris, M. (1964). Nurses' responses to expressed patient needs. *Nursing Research, 13,* 68-71.

Haggerty, L. (1987). An analysis of senior nursing students' immediate response to distressed patients. *Journal of Advanced Nursing, 12,* 451-461.

Hampe, S. (1975). Needs of the grieving spouse in a hospital setting. *Nursing Research, 24,* 113-120.

Henderson, V. (1978). The concept of nursing. *Journal of Advanced Nursing, 3,* 113-130.

Huckabay, L. (1991). The role of conceptual frameworks in nursing practice, administration, education, and research. *Nursing Administration Quarterly,* 15(3), 17-28.

Larson, P., Sr. (1977). Nursing perceptions of patient characteristics. *Nursing Research, 26,* 416-421.

Lipson, J., & Meleis, A.I. (1983, Dec.). Issues in health care of Middle-Eastern patients. *The Western Journal of Medicine, 139,* 854-861.

Madden, B. (1990). The hybrid model for concept development: Its value for the study of therapeutic alliance. *Advances in Nursing Science,* 12(4), 75-86.

McKenna, H. (1989). The selection by ward managers of an appropriate nursing model for long-stay psychiatric patient care. *Journal of Advanced Nursing, 14,* 762-775.

Peitchinis, L. (1972). Therapeutic effectiveness of counseling by nursing personnel. *Nursing Research, 21,* 138-147.

Pienschke, D., Sr. (1973). Guardedness or openness on the cancer unit. *Nursing Research, 22,* 484-490.

Pillar, B., Jacox, A., & Redman, B. (1990). A classification of nursing technology. *Nursing Outlook,* 38(2), 81-85.

Powers, M., & Woldridge, P. (1982). Factors influencing knowledge, research, and compliance of hypertensive patients. *Research in Nursing and Health, 5,* 171-182.

Princeton, J. (1986). Incorporating a deliberative nursing approach with breast-feeding mothers. *Health Care for Women International, 7,* 277-293.

Rhymes, J. (1964). A description of nurse-patient interaction in effective nursing activity. *Nursing Research, 13,* 365.

Schmidt, J. (1972). Availability: A concept of nursing practice. *American Journal of Nursing, 72,* 1086-1089.

Schmieding, N. (1986). Evaluation of nurse administrators' actions. American Nurses Association Council of Nursing Administrators. *Nurse Facilitator, 10,* 4.

Schmieding, N. (1984). Putting Orlando's theory into practice. *American Journal of Nursing, 83,* 759-761.

Schmieding, N. (1987). Analyzing managerial responses in face-to-face contacts. *Journal of Advanced Nursing, 12,* 357-365.

Schmieding, N. (1987). Problematic situations in nursing: Analysis of Orlando's theory based on Dewey's theory of inquiry. *Journal of Advanced Nursing, 12,* 431-440.

Schmieding, N. (1988). Action process of nurse administrators to problematic situations based on Orlando's theory. *Journal of Advanced Nursing, 13,* 99-107.

Schmieding, N. (1990). A model for assessing nurse administrator's actions. *Western Journal of Nursing,* 12(3), 293-306.

Schmieding, N. (1990). An integrative nursing theoretical framework. *Journal of Advanced Nursing, 15,* 463-467.

Schmieding, N. (1990). Do head nurses include staff in problem solving? *Nursing Management,* 21(3), 58-60.

Schmieding, N. (1991). Relationship between head nurse responses to staff nurses and staff nurse responses to patients. *Western Journal of Nursing Research,* 13(6), 746-760.

Schmieding, N.J. (1993). Nurse empowerment through context, structure and process. *Journal of Professional Nursing,* 9(4), 239-245.

Schmieding, N.J. (1993). Successful superior-subordinate relationships require mutual management. *Health Care Supervisor,* 11(4), 52-63.

Sheafor, M. (1991). Productive work groups in complex hospital units. *Journal of Nursing Administration,* 21(5), 25-30.

Silva, M. (1979). Effects of orientation information on spouses' anxieties and attitudes toward hospitalization and surgery. *Research in Nursing and Health, 2,* 127-136.

Stevens, B. (1971). Analysis of structured forms used in nursing curricula. *Nursing Research, 20,* 388-397.

Thibaudeau, M., & Reidy, M. (1977). Nursing makes a difference: A comparative study of the health behavior of mothers in three primary care agencies. *International Journal of Nursing Studies, 14,* 97-107.

Tryon, P.A. (1963). An experiment of the effects of patients' participation in planning the administration of a nursing procedure. *Nursing Research, 12,* 262-265.

Tryon, P.A., & Leonard, R.C. (1964). The effect of patients' participation on the outcome of a nursing procedure. *Nursing Forum, 3*(2), 79-89.

Williamson, J. (1978). Methodologic dilemmas in tapping the concept of patient needs. *Nursing Research, 27,* 172-177.

Winder, A. (1984). A mental health professional looks at nursing care. *Nursing Forum, 21,* 184-188.

Wolfer, J., & Visintainer, M. (1975). Pediatric surgical patients' and parents' stress responses and adjustment. *Nursing Research, 24,* 244-255.

Books

Beck, C.M., Rawlins, R., & Williams, S. (1984). *Mental health: Psychiatric nursing.* St. Louis: Mosby.

Carter, F. (1981). *Psychosocial nursing.* New York: Macmillan.

Chaska, N. (1978). *The nursing profession: Views through the mist.* New York: McGraw-Hill.

Chinn, P.L., & Jacobs, M.K. (1983). *Theory and nursing: A systematic approach.* St. Louis: Mosby.

Chinn, P.L., & Kramer, M.K. (1991). *Theory and nursing: A systematic approach* (3rd ed., pp. 177-178). St. Louis: Mosby.

Fitzpatrick, J., & Whall, A. (1983). *Conceptual models of nursing practice: Analysis and application.* Bowie, MD: Robert J. Brady.

Joel, L., & Collins, D. (1978). *Psychiatric nursing: Model and application.* New York: McGraw-Hill.

McCann-Flynn, J., & Heffron, B. (1984). *Nursing: From concept to practice.* Bowie, MD: Robert J. Brady.

Meleis, A. (1985). *Theoretical nursing: Development and progress.* Philadelphia: J.B. Lippincott.

Meleis, A. (1991). *Theoretical nursing: Development and progress* (2nd ed., pp. 338-348). New York: J.B. Lippincott.

Murray, R., & Huelskoetter, M. (1983). *Psychiatric–mental health nursing: Giving emotional care.* Englewood Cliffs, NJ: Prentice-Hall.

Nursing Theories Conference Group, J.B. George, Chairperson (1980). *Nursing theories: The base for professional nursing practice.* Englewood Cliffs, NJ: Prentice-Hall.

Stuart, G., & Sundeen, S. (1983). *Principles and practice of psychiatric nursing.* St. Louis: Mosby.

Torres, G. (1986). *Theoretical foundations in nursing.* Norwalk, CT: Appleton-Century-Crofts.

Wilson, H., & Kneisel, C. (1983). *Psychiatric nursing.* Reading, MA: Addison Wesley.

Research abstracts

Barron, M.A. (1966). The effects varied nursing approaches have on patients' complaints of pain (Abstract). *Nursing Research, 15*(1), 90-91.

Bochnak, M. (1963). The effect of an automatic and deliberative process of nursing activity on the relief of patients' pain: A clinical experiment (Abstract). *Nursing Research, 12,* 191-192.

Cameron, J. (1963). An exploratory study of the verbal responses of the nurses in twenty nurse-patient interactions (Abstract). *Nursing Research, 12,* 192.

Diers, D.K. (1966). The nurse orientation system: A method for analyzing the nurse-patient interactions (Abstract). *Nursing Research, 15*(1), 91.

Dye, M. (1963). A descriptive study of conditions conducive to an effective process of nursing activity (Abstract). *Nursing Research, 12,* 194.

Faulkner, S. (1963). A descriptive study of needs communicated to the nurse by some mothers on a postpartum service (Abstract). *Nursing Research, 12,* 26.

Fichelis, M. (1963). An exploratory study of labels nurses attach to patient behavior and their effect on nursing activities (Abstract). *Nursing Research, 12,* 195.

Joyce Travelbee

Human-to-Human Relationship Model

Sheila Rangel, William H. Hobble, Theresa Lansinger,
Jude A. Magers, Nancy J. McKee

CREDENTIALS AND BACKGROUND OF THE THEORIST

Joyce Travelbee was a psychiatric nurse practitioner, educator, and writer. Born in 1926, she completed her basic nursing preparation in 1946 at Charity Hospital School of Nursing in New Orleans. She earned a B.S. degree in nursing education from Louisiana State University in 1956 and an M.S. degree in nursing from Yale in 1959. In the summer of 1973, Travelbee began a doctoral program in Florida but was unable to complete the program because of

The authors wish to express appreciation to Leigh DeNoon, Mary Ellen Doona, Joyce Lee, and Katharine Taylor for assistance with data collection. The authors have been unable to obtain a picture of Joyce Travelbee.

her untimely death later that year.[1,2,9] She died at the age of 47 after a brief illness, leaving no survivors.[5]

Travelbee began her career as a nursing educator in 1952, teaching psychiatric nursing at Depaul Hospital Affiliate School, New Orleans, while working on her baccalaureate degree. She also taught psychiatric nursing at Charity Hospital School of Nursing, at Louisiana State University, at New York University in New York City, and at the University of Mississippi in Jackson. In 1970, she was named Project Director at Hotel Dieu School of Nursing in New Orleans. At the time of her death, Travelbee was the director of graduate education at Louisiana State University School of Nursing.[1,2,9]

Travelbee began publishing articles in nursing journals in 1963. Her first book, *Interpersonal Aspects of Nursing,* was published in 1966 and 1971. A second book, *Intervention in Psychiatric Nursing,* was published in 1969.

THEORETICAL SOURCES

Travelbee's experiences in her basic nursing education and initial practice in Catholic charity institutions greatly influenced the development of her theory. Travelbee believed the nursing care given patients in these institutions lacked compassion.[9] She felt nursing needed "a humanistic revolution—a return to focus on the 'caring' function of the nurse—in the caring for (and) the caring about ill persons and predicted if this did not occur, consumers would demand the 'services of a new and different kind of health worker.'"[11:2]

Travelbee was probably also influenced by Ida Jean Orlando, who was one of her instructors during her graduate studies at Yale. Orlando's model possesses some similarities to the model Travelbee proposes. Orlando stated,[7:6] "The nurse is responsible for helping the patient avoid and alleviate the distress of unmet needs." Orlando[7:8] also stated that the nurse and patient interact with each other. The similarities between the two models are shown by Travelbee's assertion that the nurse and patient interact with each other and by her definition of the purpose of nursing. Travelbee stated[11:7] that the purpose of nursing is to assist "an individual, family, or community to prevent or cope with the experience of illness and suffering, and, if necessary, to find meaning in these experiences."

Travelbee also appears to have been influenced by Viktor Frankl, a survivor of Auschwitz and other Nazi concentration camps. As a result of his experiences, Frankl[3:153] proposed the theory of logotherapy, in which a patient "is actually confronted with and reoriented toward the meaning of his life." Travelbee[11:158] based the assumptions of her theory on the concepts of logotherapy.

USE OF EMPIRICAL EVIDENCE

Katharine Taylor,[9] a former student and colleague of Travelbee, remembers Travelbee as a prolific reader whose office was often crammed with files of bibliography cards. Apparently, Travelbee's theory is based on her cumulative nursing experiences and her readings rather than the evidence of a particular research study.

MAJOR CONCEPTS & DEFINITIONS

Human Being "A human being is defined as a unique irreplaceable individual—a one-time being in this world—like yet unlike any person who has ever lived or ever will live."[11-26]

Patient The term *patient* is a stereotype useful for communicative economy. "Actually there are no patients. There are only individual human beings in need of the care, services, and assistance of other human beings, whom, it is believed, can render the assistance that is needed."[11:32]

Nurse The nurse is also a human being. "The nurse possesses a body of specialized knowledge and the ability to use it for the purpose of assisting other human beings to prevent illness, regain health, find meaning in illness, or to maintain the highest maximal degree of health."[11:40]

Illness Illness is "a category and a classification."[11:49] Travelbee did not use the term *illness* as a definition of being unhealthy, but rather explored the human experience of illness. Travelbee defined illness by objective and subjective criteria. The objective criteria are determined by the outward effects of illness on the individual.[11:52] The subjective criteria refer to the way in which a human being perceives himself as ill.[11:52]

Suffering "Suffering is a feeling of displeasure which ranges from simple transitory mental, physical, or spiritual discomfort to extreme anguish, and to those phases beyond anguish, namely, the malignant phase of despairful 'not caring,' and the terminal phase of apathetic indifference."[11:62] Suf-

Continued

MAJOR CONCEPTS & DEFINITIONS—cont'd

fering can be placed on a continuum, which is illustrated in Fig. 24-1.

Pain "Pain itself is not observable—only its effects are noted."[11:72] Pain is a lonely experience that is difficult to communicate fully to another individual.[11:72] The experience of pain is unique to each individual.

Hope "Hope is a mental state characterized by the desire to gain an end or accomplish a goal combined with some degree of expectation that what is desired or sought is attainable."[11:77] Hope is related to dependence on others, choice, wishing, trust and perseverance, and courage and is future oriented.[11:78-80]

Hopelessness Hopelessness is being devoid of hope.[11:81]

Communication "Communication is a process which can enable the nurse to establish a human-to-human relationship and thereby fulfill the purpose of nursing, namely, to assist individuals and families to prevent and to cope with the experience of illness and suffering and, if necessary, to assist them to find meaning in these experiences."[11:93]

Interaction "The term *interaction* refers to any contact during which two individuals have reciprocal influence on each other and communicate verbally and/or nonverbally."[11:120]

Nurse-Patient Interaction "The term *nurse-patient interaction* refers to any contact between a nurse and an ill person and is characterized by the fact that both individuals perceive the other in a stereotyped manner."[11:120]

Nursing Need "A nursing need is any requirement of the ill person (or family) which can be met by the professional nurse practitioner and which lies within the scope of the legal definition of nursing practice."[11:125]

Therapeutic Use of Self "The therapeutic use of self is the ability to use one's personality consciously and in full awareness in an attempt to establish relatedness and to structure nursing intervention."[11:19] It "requires self-insight, self-understanding, an understanding of the dynamics of human behavior, ability to interpret one's own behavior as well as the behavior of others, and the ability to intervene effectively in nursing situations."[11:19]

Empathy "Empathy is a process wherein an individual is able to comprehend the psychological state of another."[11:143]

Sympathy Sympathy implies a desire to help an individual undergoing stress.[10:68-69]

Rapport "Rapport is a process, a happening, an experience, or series of experiences, undergone simultaneously by the nurse and the recipient of her care. It is composed of a cluster of interrelated thoughts and feelings, these thoughts, feelings and attitudes being transmitted, or communicated, by one human being to another."[11:150]

Human-to-Human Relationship "A human-to-human relationship is primarily an experience or series of experiences between a nurse and the recipient of her care. The major characteristic of these experiences is that the nursing needs of the individual (or family) are met."[11:123] "The human-to-human relationship, in nursing situations, is the means through which the purpose of nursing is accomplished."[11:119] The human-to-human relationship is established when the nurse and the recipient of her care attained a rapport after having progressed through the stages of the original encounter, emerging identities, empathy, and sympathy[11:119-120] (see Fig. 24-2).

Transitory feeling of displeasure	Extreme anguish	Malignant phase of despairful not caring	Terminal phase of apathetic indifference

Fig. **24-1 Continuum of suffering.** *Conceptualized by Theresa Lansinger based on Joyce Travelbee's definition.*

MAJOR ASSUMPTIONS

Nursing

Travelbee[11:7] defined nursing as an "interpersonal process whereby the professional nurse practitioner assists an individual, family, or community to prevent or cope with the experience of illness and suffering and, if necessary, to find meaning in these experiences." Nursing is an interpersonal process because it is an experience that occurs between the nurse and an individual or group of individuals.[10:8]

Person

The term *person* is defined as a human being. Both the nurse and the patient are human beings. A human being is a unique, irreplaceable individual who is in the continuous process of becoming, evolving, and changing.[11:26-27]

Health

Travelbee defined health by the criteria of subjective and objective health. A person's subjective health status is an individually defined state of well-being in accord with self-appraisal of physical-emotional-spiritual status.[11:9] Objective health is "an absence of discernible disease, disability, or defect as measured by physical examination, laboratory tests, assessment by a spiritual director, or psychological counselor."[11:10]

Environment

Travelbee does not explicitly define environment in the theory. She does define the human condition and life experiences encountered by all human beings as suffering, hope, pain, and illness. These conditions can be equated to the environment.

THEORETICAL ASSERTIONS

1. "The purpose of nursing is achieved through the establishment of a human-to-human relationship."[11:16]
2. The human condition is shared by all human beings and is dichotomous in nature.[11:29]
3. Most people, at one time or another and in varying degrees, will experience joy, contentment, happiness, and love.[11:29]
4. "All persons, at some time in their lives, will be confronted by illness and pain (mental, physical, or spiritual suffering), and eventually they will encounter death."[11:29]
5. The quality and quantity of nursing care delivered to an ill human being is greatly influenced by the nurse's perception of the patient.[11:32]
6. The terms *patient* and *nurse* are stereotypes and only useful for communicative economy.
7. The roles of the nurse and patient must be transcended to establish a human-to-human relatedness.[11:33]
8. Illness and suffering "are spiritual encounters as well as emotional-physical experiences."[11:61]
9. The communication process enables "the nurse to establish a human-to-human relationship and thereby fulfill the purpose of nursing."[11:93]
10. "Individuals can be assisted to find meaning in the experience of illness and suffering. The meanings can enable the individual to cope with the problems engendered by these experiences."[11:158]
11. "The spiritual and ethical values of the nurse, or her philosophical beliefs about illness and suffering, will determine the extent to which she will be able to assist individuals and families to find meaning (or no meaning) in these difficult experiences."[11:158]
12. "It is the responsibility of the professional nurse

practitioner to assist individuals and families to find meaning in illness and suffering (if this be necessary)."[11:158]

Human-to-Human Relationship

The human-to-human relationship model, shown in Fig. 24-2, represents the interaction between the nurse and patient. The half circles at the point of the original encounter indicate the possibility of and need for developing the encounter into a therapeutic relationship. As the interaction process progresses toward rapport, the circles join into one full circle, representing that the potential for a therapeutic relationship has been attained.

Original encounter. The original encounter is characterized by first impressions by the nurse of the ill person and by the ill person of the nurse. The nurse and ill person perceive each other in stereotyped roles.[11:131]

Emerging identities. The emerging identities phase is characterized by the nurse and ill person perceiving each other as unique individuals. The bond of a relationship is beginning to form.[11:132]

Empathy. The empathy phase is characterized by the ability to share in the other person's experience. The result of the empathic process is the ability to predict the behavior of the individual with whom one has empathized.[11:137] Travelbee believed two qualities that enhanced the empathy process were similarities of experience and the desire to understand another person.[11:138]

Sympathy. Sympathy goes beyond empathy and occurs when the nurse desires to alleviate the cause

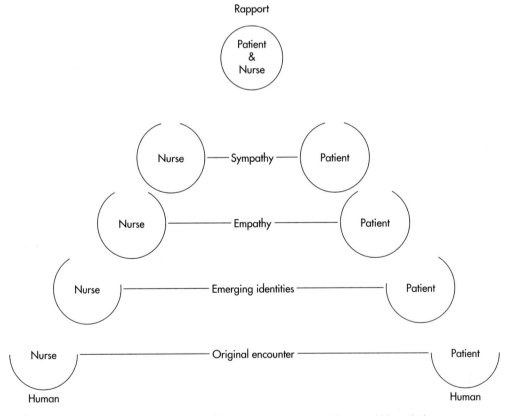

Fig. **24-2 Human-to-human relationship.** *Conceptualized by William Hobble and Theresa Lansinger based on Joyce Travelbee's writings.*

of the patient's illness or suffering. "When one sympathizes, one is involved but not incapacitated by the involvement."[11:142] The nurse is to create helpful nursing action as a result of reaching the phase of sympathy. "This helpful nursing action requires a combination of the disciplined intellectual approach combined with the therapeutic use of self."[11:149]

Rapport. Rapport is characterized by nursing actions that alleviate an ill person's distress. The nurse and ill person are relating as human being to human being. The ill person exhibits both trust and confidence in the nurse. "A nurse is able to establish rapport because she possesses the necessary knowledge and skills required to assist ill persons, and because she is able to perceive, respond to, and appreciate the uniqueness of the ill human being."[11:155]

LOGICAL FORM

Travelbee's theory is inductive. She has used specific nursing situations to create general ideas. Travelbee appears to follow a logical form by first defining the labels in her theory, then listing the assumptions, and finally establishing specific nursing goals.

ACCEPTANCE BY THE NURSING COMMUNITY
Practice

Travelbee believed the condition of an individual exhibiting apathetic indifference is just as critical as that of an individual who is hemorrhaging. She believed that both people need emergency resuscitative measures. But an examination of patient care given by nurses today indicates the patient's physical needs still hold top priority. The acceptance and use of nursing diagnosis does appear to focus nursing care more on the total needs of the patient as compared with 25 years ago when Travelbee published her theory. However, nursing has not yet reached the humanistic revolution Travelbee proposed.

Hospice is the one area of nursing practice where the philosophy closely adheres to the tenets of Travelbee's theory. The hospice nurse attempts to develop a rapport with the patient and significant others. Most hospice nurses agree with Elisabeth Kübler-Ross[4:2]

"that death does not have to be a catastrophic, destructive thing; indeed, it can be viewed as one of the most constructive, positive, and creative elements of culture and life." Travelbee[11:162] asserted that finding meaning in illness and suffering enables the ill individual not only to accept the illness but also to use it as a self-actualizing life experience. An ill individual's perception of meaninglessness in his illness and suffering leads to nonacceptance of his illness and a feeling of hopelessness. One hospice nurse believes the dying person must find meaning in his death before he can ever begin to accept the actuality of his death, just as his loved ones must find meaning in his death before they can complete the grieving process.[8]

Education

Nursing education appears to have identified the need to prepare nurses to address the emotional and spiritual needs of patients. The focus of nursing education has changed from the disease entity approach—that is, signs, symptoms, and nursing interventions—to a more holistic care approach. However, basic nursing programs do not seem to prepare nurses adequately to help individuals find meaning in illness and suffering as Travelbee proposed. Travelbee's second book, *Intervention in Psychiatric Nursing: Process in the One-to-One Relationship*, has been used in various nursing programs. However, this book alone does not adequately prepare nurses to help individuals find meaning in illness and suffering. Nursing programs need to offer a much broader background in communication techniques, values clarification, and thanatology. Courses in philosophy and religion would also be helpful in preparing nurses adequately to fulfill the purpose of nursing as stated in Travelbee's theory.

Research

Some aspects of the one-to-one relationship proposed by Travelbee have been cited by several sources in research studies. One study by O'Connor, Wicker, and Germino,[6] which is closely related to some of Travelbee's ideas, explored how individuals who were recently diagnosed with cancer described their personal search for meaning. Six major themes, which were (1) seeking an understanding of the personal significance of the cancer diagnosis, (2) looking at the consequences of the cancer diagnosis, (3) review of life, (4) change in outlook toward self, life, others, (5) living with cancer, and (6) hope, were identified, and two major sources of support were found—faith and social support. The findings of this study revealed that the search for meaning seems to be both a spiritual and psychosocial process. Nursing interventions that would support this process were identified. No other major research studies generated by Travelbee's specific theory, which could stimulate further development, were found.

FURTHER DEVELOPMENT

The advent of diagnostic-related groups (DRGs) has created the need to produce the highest quality nursing care by the most economical method. Tools such as patient acuity systems have been devised to determine nursing staffing patterns in accordance with the nursing needs of patients. Although this type of tool can account for the emotional needs of patients, emotional needs are not weighed as heavily as patients' physical needs. DRGs may shift the nursing focus back to meeting only the patient's physical needs. If nurses are to prevent this shift, they must prove to health care administrators and health care consumers that the time taken by the nurse to meet a patient's emotional and spiritual needs is a valuable investment. Travelbee's theory could be used to provide the research data to justify this time investment. However, Travelbee's theory does not currently contain the empirical precision to support such research data. To be more readily accepted, the theory's major assumptions must be assigned operational definitions. Then the theory could perhaps generate the data needed to facilitate further acceptance.

CRITIQUE

Clarity

All concepts are defined in the Travelbee theory, but definitions are not consistent with regard to origin and explicitness. Some are the author's own defini-

tions, whereas others were adopted from Webster's dictionary. Some of the definitions are explicitly presented, but others are derived from contextual usage. None of the concepts is operationally defined. Travelbee also uses different terms for the same definition. The terms *rapport, human-to-human relationship*, and *human-to-human relatedness* all had the same definition.

The goal or purpose of nursing, as stated in Travelbee's definition of nursing, is inconsistent with the emphasis of her presentation. Travelbee focused on adult individuals who are ill and the nurse's role in assisting them in finding meaning in their illness and suffering. She addressed families and their needs minimally, and communities were not included at all.

Simplicity

Travelbee's theory does not possess simplicity because there are many variables. The theory is designed to help nurses appreciate not only the patient's humanness but also the nurse's humanness. To be human is to be unique; so the variables present in each phase of the human-to-human relationship will be numerous.

Generality

Travelbee's theory has a wide scope of application. It was primarily generated as a result of Travelbee's experience with psychiatric patients but is not limited to use in this setting. It is applicable whenever the nurse encounters ill persons in distress. It would seem to be most useful when working with those who are chronically ill, those who are undergoing long-term rehabilitation, or those who are terminally ill.

Empirical Precision

Travelbee's theory appears to have a low degree of empirical validity. Most of the lack of empirical validity can be traced to the lack of simplicity in the theory. Concepts have been theoretically defined, but they have not been operationally defined. Because the model has not been tested, there is no empirical support.

Derivable Consequences

The usefulness of a theory is related to its ability to describe, explain, predict, and control phenomena. Travelbee's theory does describe some variables that may affect the establishment of a therapeutic relationship between nurse and patient. However, the lack of empirical precision also creates a lack of derivable consequences. Travelbee's theory focuses on the development of the attribute of caring. In this respect, the theory can be useful, because caring is a major characteristic of the nursing profession.

CRITICAL THINKING *Activities*

1 Review a clinical experience in which you as a nurse observed or provided clinical care to an individual. Identify the opportunities and/or potential topics for client education (either client or family) during routine care.

2 Conduct a comprehensive nursing assessment of an individual in a health care setting, and do the following:

 a. Identify actual and potential client needs.

 b. Categorize each need according to Maslow's hierarchy and rank the needs according to priorities.

 c. Describe conditions creating barriers to the client's successful attainment of needs.

 d. Describe nursing actions to assist the client to meet his/her individual needs.

3 Describe a parable or some type of story that might assist an individual to cope with a difficult diagnosis.

4 Design a nursing care plan for an individual, paying special attention to the spiritual needs of the individual client.

REFERENCES

1. Doona, M.E. (1984, Oct.). Personal interview. (Nursing instructor, Boston College.)
2. Doona, M.E. (1984, Oct.). Telephone interview.
3. Frankl, V. (1963). *Man's search for meaning: An introduction to logotherapy.* New York: Washington Square Press.
4. Kübler-Ross, E. (1975). *Death: The final stage of growth.* Englewood Cliffs, NJ: Prentice-Hall.
5. Obituary for Joyce Travelbee. (1973, Sept.). *New Orleans Times-Picayune,* Section 1, p. 22.
6. O'Connor, A.P., Wicker, C.A., & Germino, B.B. (1990). Understanding the cancer patient's search for meaning. *Cancer Nursing, 13*(3), 167-175.
7. Orlando, I.J. (1961). *The dynamic nurse-patient relationship.* New York: G.P. Putnam.
8. Schoon, F. (1984, Oct.). Personal interview. (Hospice nurse.)
9. Taylor, K. (1984, Oct.). Telephone interview. (Former student and colleague of Joyce Travelbee.)
10. Travelbee, J. (1964, Jan.). What's wrong with sympathy? *American Journal of Nursing, 64,* 68-71.
11. Travelbee, J. (1971). *Interpersonal aspects of nursing.* Philadelphia: F.A. Davis.

BIBLIOGRAPHY

Primary sources

Books

Travelbee, J. (1966). *Interpersonal aspects of nursing.* Philadelphia: F.A. Davis.
Travelbee, J. (1969). *Intervention in psychiatric nursing: Process in the one-to-one relationship.* Philadelphia: F.A. Davis.
Travelbee, J. (1971). *Interpersonal aspects of nursing* (2nd ed.). Philadelphia: F.A. Davis.
Travelbee, J., & Doona, M.E. (1979). *Travelbee's intervention in psychiatric nursing* (2nd ed.). Philadelphia: F.A. Davis.

Journal articles

Travelbee, J. (1963, Feb.). Humor survives the test of time. *Nursing Outlook, 11,* 128.
Travelbee, J. (1963, Feb.). What do we mean by rapport? *American Journal of Nursing, 63,* 70-72.
Travelbee, J. (1964, Jan.). What's wrong with sympathy? *American Journal of Nursing, 64,* 68-71.

Secondary sources

Book reviews

Travelbee, J. (1966). *Interpersonal aspects of nursing.*
 Nursing Outlook, 14, 77, June 1966.
 American Journal of Nursing, 66, 1504, July 1966.
 Nursing Mirror, 122, 438, Aug. 5, 1966.
 Supervisor Nurse, 2, 44, Dec. 1971.
 Nursing Outlook, 20, 278, April 1972.
 Journal of Nursing Administration, 3, 14-15, Jan.-Feb. 1973.
Travelbee, J. (1969). *Intervention in psychiatric nursing: Process in the one-to-one relationship.*
 American Journal of Nursing, 70, 101-102, Jan. 1970.
 Nursing Outlook, 18, 16, Aug. 1970.
 Nursing Mirror, 131, 31, Sept. 18, 1970.

Book chapters

Chinn, R. (1974). The utility of system models and development models for practitioners. In J. Riehl & C. Roy (Eds.), *Conceptual models for nursing practice* (pp. 46-53). New York: Appleton-Century-Crofts.

Meleis, A.I. (1985). Joyce Travelbee. In A.I. Meleis, *Theoretical nursing: Development and progress* (pp. 254-262). Philadelphia: J.B. Lippincott.

Roy, C. (1974). Travelbee's developmental approach. In J.P. Riehl & C. Roy (Eds.), *Conceptual models for nursing practice* (pp. 267-268). New York: Appleton-Century-Crofts.

Thibodeau, J.A. (1983). An interaction model: The Travelbee model. In *Nursing models: Analysis and evaluation* (pp. 89-104). Belmont, CA: Wadsworth.

Journal articles

Aggleton, P., & Chalmers, H. (1987). Models of nursing, nursing practice and nurse education. *Journal of Advanced Nursing, 12*(5), 573-581.

Arnold, H.M. (1976). Working with schizophrenic patients: Guide to one-to-one relationships. *American Journal of Nursing, 76,* 941-943.

Axelsson, K., Norbert, A., & Asplund, K. (1986). Relearning to eat late after a stroke by systematic nursing intervention: A case report. *Journal of Advanced Nursing, 11,* 553-559.

Barker, P.J. (1989). The nursing care of people experiencing affective disorder: A review of the literature. *Journal of Advanced Nursing, 14*(8), 618-629.

Barker, P.J. & Reynolds, B. (1994). A critique: *Watson's caring ideology:* The proper focus of psychiatric nursing? *Journal of Psychosocial Nursing, 32*(5), 17-22.

Barker, P.J., Reynolds, W., & Ward, T. (1995). The proper focus of nursing: A critique of the "caring" ideology. *International Journal of Nursing Studies, 32*(4), 386-397.

Belcher, A.E., Dettmore, D., & Holzemer, S.P. (1989). Spirituality and sense of well-being in persons with AIDS. *Holistic Nursing Practice, 3*(4), 16-25.

Brumbach, A.E. (1994). What gives nurses hope? *Journal of Christian Nursing, 11*(4), 30-35.

Bullough, V.L., & Seidl, A. (1987). Attitudes on sexuality in nursing texts today and yesterday. *Holistic Nursing Practice, 1*(4), 84-92.

Carson, V., Soeken, K.L., & Grimm, P.M. (1988). Hope and its relationship to spiritual well-being. *Journal of Psychology and Theology, 16*(2), 159-167.

Cohen, M.Z. (1987). A historical overview of the phenomenologic movement. *Image, 19*(1), 31-34.

Comp, H.D.R. (1995). Satisfying a hunger: A personal journey of self-discovery through further nursing education. *Nursing practice in New Zealand, 10*(1), 12-21.

Criddle, L. (1993). Healing from surgery: A phenomenological study. *Image, 25*(3), 208-213.

DiSalvo, V.S., Larsen, J.K., & Backus, D.K. (1986). The health care communicator: An identification of skills and problems. *Communication Education, 35*(3), 231-242.

Dobson, S.M. (1989). Conceptualizing for transcultural health visiting: The concept of transcultural reciprocity. *Journal of Advanced Nursing, 14*(2), 97-102.

Fenton, M.V. (1987). Development of the scale of humanistic nursing behaviors. *Nursing Research, 36,* 82-93.

Flaskerud, J.H. (1986). On "Toward a theory of nursing action: Skills and competency in nurse-patient interaction." *Nursing Research, 35,* 250-252.

Forbes, S.B. (1994). Hope: An essential human need in the elderly. *Journal of Gerontological Nursing, 20*(6), 5-10.

Forchuk, C. (1994). The orientation phase of the nurse-client relationship: Testing Peplau's theory. *Journal of Advanced Nursing, 20*(3), 532-537.

Freihofer, P., & Felton, G. (1976). Nursing behaviors in bereavement. *Nursing Research, 25,* 332-337.

Gould, D. (1990). Empathy: A review of the literature with suggestions for an alternative research strategy. *Journal of Advanced Nursing, 15*(10), 1167-1174.

Hagland, M.R. (1995). Nurse-patient communication in intensive care: A low priority? *Intensive Critical Care Nursing, 11*(2), 111-115.

Hall, J.M., & Stevens, P.E. (1991). Rigor in feminist research. *Advances in Nursing Science, 13*(3), 16-29.

Henault, M. (1985). Un obstacle de plus pour l'enfant qui eprouve des problemes psychosociaux. *Nursing Quebec, 5*(7), 24-27.

Herth, K. (1990). Fostering hope in terminally-ill people. *Journal of Advanced Nursing, 15*(11), 1250-1259.

Hinds, P.S. (1984). Introducing a definition of hope through the use of grounded theory methodology. *Journal of Advanced Nursing, 9,* 357-362.

Hinds, P.S. (1988). Adolescent hopefulness in illness and health. *Advances in Nursing Science, 10*(3), 79-88.

Holmes, C.A. (1990). Alternatives to natural-science foundations for nursing. *International Journal of Nursing Studies, 27*(3), 187-198.

Johnson, J. (1994). The communication training needs of registered nurses. *Journal of Continuing Education, 25*(5), 213-218.

Kasch, C.R. (1986). Skills and competency in nurse-patient interaction. *Nursing Research, 35,* 226-229.

Koshi, P.T. (1976). Cultural diversity in nursing curricula. *Journal of Nursing Education, 15,* 14-21.

Laine, L., Shulman, R.J., Bartholomew, K., Gardner, P., Reed, T., & Cole, S. (1989). An educational booklet diminishes anxiety in parents whose children receive total parenteral nutrition. *American Journal of Diseases of Children, 143*(3), 374-377.

Larson, P.A. (1977). Nurse perceptions of patient characteristics. *Nursing Research, 26,* 416-421.

Limandri, B.J., & Boyle, D.W. (1978). Instilling hope. *American Journal of Nursing, 78,* 78-80.

Marshall, C. (1994). The concept of advocacy. *British Journal of Theater Nursing, 4*(2), 11-13.

McBride, A.B. (1986). Theory and research: Present issues and future perspectives of psychosocial nursing. *Journal of Psychosocial Nursing, 24*(9), 29-32.

McKenna, H.P. (1989). The selection by ward managers of an appropriate nursing model for long-stay psychiatric patient care. *Journal of Advanced Nursing, 14*(9), 762-775.

McMahon, R. (1988). The 24-hour reality orientation type of approach to the confused elderly: A minimum standard for care. *Journal of Advanced Nursing, 13*(6), 693-700.

Mickley, J.R., Soeken, K., & Belcher, A. (1992). Spiritual well-being, religiousness and hope among women with breast cancer. *Image, 24*(4), 267-272.

Moch, S.D. (1989). Health within illness: Conceptual evolution and practice possibilities. *Advances in Nursing Science, 11*(4), 23-31.

Moch, S.D. (1990). Health within the experience of breast cancer. *Journal of Advanced Nursing, 15*(12), 1426-1435.

Morse, B.W., & Vandenberg, E. (1978). Interpersonal relationships in nursing practice, interdisciplinary approach. *Communication Education, 27*, 158-163.

Morse, J.M., et al. (1992). Exploring empathy: A conceptual fit for nursing practice? *Image, 24*(4), 273-280.

Muxlow, J. (1995). The relationship between nurse and patient. *Professional Nurse, 11*(1), 63-65.

Narayanasamy, A. (1993). Nurses' awareness and educational preparation in meeting their patients' spiritual needs. *Nurse Education Today, 13*, 196-201.

Nix, J., & Dillon, K. (1986). Short-term nursing therapy: A conceptual model for inpatient psychiatric care. *Hospital and Community Psychiatry, 37*(5), 493-496.

Norberg, A., & Athlin, E. (1989). Eating problems in severely demented patients: Issues and ethical dilemmas. *Nursing Clinics of North America, 24*(3), 781-789.

Nowotny, M.L. (1989). Assessment of hope in patients with cancer: Development of an instrument. *Oncology Nursing Forum, 16*(1), 57-61.

Owen, D.C. (1989). Nurses' perspectives on the meaning of hope in patients with cancer: A qualitative study. *Oncology Nursing Forum, 16*(1), 75-79.

Paul, D., Hagan, L., & Lambert, J. (1985). Au-dela du malade. *Nursing Quebec, 5*(7), 18-23.

Peterson, E.A., & Nelson, K. (1987). How to meet your clients' spiritual needs. *Journal of Psychosocial Nursing, 25*(5), 34-39.

Pinch, W.J., & Spielman, M.L. (1989). Ethical decision-making for high-risk infants: The parents' perspective. *Nursing Clinics of North America, 24*(4), 1017-1023.

Podrasky, D.L., & Sexton, D.L. (1988). Nurses' reactions to difficult patients. *Image, 20*(1), 16-21.

Ramos, M.C. (1992). The nurse-patient relationship: Theme and variations. *Journal of Advanced Nursing, 17*(4), 496-506.

Sarter, B. (1987). Evolutionary idealism. *Advanced Nursing Science, 9*(2), 1-9.

Schweer, S.F., & Dayani, E.C. (1973). Extended role of professional nursing: Patient education. *International Nursing Review, 20*, 174.

Shelly, J., & Fish, S. (1995). Praying with patients: Why, when, and how. *Journal of Christian Nursing, 12*(1), 9-13.

Sodestrom, K.E., & Martinson, I.M. (1987). Patients' spiritual coping strategies: A study of nurse and patient perspectives. *Oncology Nursing Forum, 14*(2), 41-44.

Sorgen, L.M. (1979). Student learning following an educational experience at an alcohol rehabilitation center in Saskatoon, Saskatchewan, Canada. *International Journal of Nursing Studies, 16*, 41-50.

Spratlen, L.P. (1976). Introducing ethnic-cultural factors in models of nursing: Some mental health applications. *Journal of Nursing Education, 15*, 23-29.

Stephenson, C. (1991). The concept of hope revisited for nursing. *Journal of Advanced Nursing, 16*(12), 1456-1461.

Stetler, C.B. (1977). Relationship of perceived empathy to nurses' communication. *Nursing Research, 26*, 432-438.

Stoll, R.I. (1979). Guidelines for spiritual assessment. *American Journal of Nursing, 79*, 1574-1577.

Stuart, E.M., Deckro, J.P., & Mandle, C.L. (1989). Spirituality in health and healing: A clinical program. *Holistic Nursing Practice, 3*(3), 35-44.

Swanson, K.M. (1993). Nursing as informed caring for the well-being of others. *Image, 25*(4), 352-357.

Sweeting, H.N., & Gilhooly, M.L.M. (1992). Doctor, am I dead: A review of social death in modern societies. *Omega: Journal of Death and Dying, 24*(4), 251-269.

Wallston, K.A., & Wallston, B.S. (1975). Role-playing simulation approach toward studying nurses' decisions to listen to patients. *Nursing Research, 24*, 16-22.

Wallston, K.A., Wallston, B.S., & Devellis, B.M. (1976). Effect of a negative stereotype on nurse's attitudes toward an alcoholic patient. *Journal of Studies on Alcohol, 37*, 659-665.

Webb, C., & Hope, K. (1994). What kind of nurses do patients want? *Journal of Clinical Nursing, 4*, 101-108.

Wesley, R.L., & McHugh, M.K. (1992). Appendix B: Additional nursing theorists and the nursing metaparadigm. In *Nursing Theories and Models.* Springhouse, PA: Springhouse, p. 132.

Young, J.C. (1988). Rationale for clinician self-disclosure and research agenda. *Image, 20*(4), 196-199.

Correspondence

Doona, M.E. (1984, Oct. 19). Personal communication.

Interviews

Doona, M.E. (1984, Oct.). Telephone interview.

Taylor, K. (1984, Oct.). Telephone interview.

Other sources

Barrett-Lennard, G.T. (1962). Dimensions of therapist responses as causal factors in therapeutic change. *Psychological Monographs, 76*, 43 (Whole No. 562).

Cartwright, R.D., & Lerner, B. (1963). Empathy, need to change, and improvement with psychotherapy. *Journal of Consulting Psychology, 27,* 138-144.

Chinsky, J.M., & Rappaport, J. (1970). Brief critique of the meaning and reliability of "accurate empathy" ratings. *Psychological Bulletin, 73,* 379-382.

Frankl, V. (1963). *Man's search for meaning: An introduction to logotherapy.* New York: Washington Square Press.

Kurtz, R.R., & Grummon, D.L. (1972). Different approaches to the measurement of therapist empathy and their relationship to therapy outcomes. *Journal of Consulting and Clinical Psychology, 30,* 106-115.

May, R. (1953). *Man's search for himself.* New York: W.W. Norton.

McBride, M.A. (1967). Nursing approach, pain, and relief: An exploratory experiment. *Nursing Research, 16*(4), 337-341.

Critical thinking activities references

Books

Bandman, E., & Bandman, B. (1995). *Critical thinking in nursing.* Norwalk, CT: Appleton-Lange.

Hoover, K.G. (1993). *Study guide to accompany fundamentals of nursing.* St. Louis: Mosby.

LeFevre, R.A. (1995). *Critical thinking in nursing.* Philadelphia: W.B. Saunders.

Journal articles

Adams, M.H., et al. (1996). Critical thinking as an educational outcome: An evaluation of current tools of measurement. *Nurse Educator, 21*(3), 23-32.

Heiney, S.P. (1995). The healing power of story. *Oncology Nursing Forum, 22*(6), 899-903.

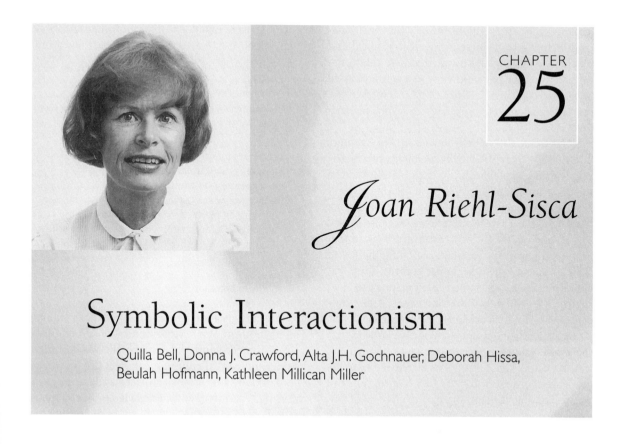

CHAPTER

25

Joan Riehl-Sisca

Symbolic Interactionism

Quilla Bell, Donna J. Crawford, Alta J.H. Gochnauer, Deborah Hissa,
Beulah Hofmann, Kathleen Millican Miller

CREDENTIALS AND BACKGROUND OF THE THEORIST

Although Joan Riehl was born in Davenport, Iowa, she spent most of her childhood and young adult life in a Chicago suburb. She attended the University of Illinois in Urbana and Chicago, where she obtained her B.S.N. After graduation, she worked as a clinical instructor, a supervisor, and an in-service director in Texas and in California before returning to college for her master's degree in nursing. After receiving her M.S.N. from the University of California, Los Angeles (UCLA), Riehl taught pediatric nursing at California State University for 3 years before joining the

faculty at UCLA. There she began teaching theoretical concepts and their application. Two major professional events resulted from this instruction. First, she began writing nursing textbooks on conceptual models to use for teaching graduate students, and she began to identify her own theoretical framework. Her interest resulted in doctoral study at UCLA in sociology, which afforded her the opportunity to pursue the knowledge base needed to develop the particulars of her model. Symbolic interactionism is the foundation on which this model is built. Role theory and self-concept are components of the theory. They constituted her dissertational investigation for her Ph.D., which she received in 1980.

Like many nurses who attend graduate school, Riehl worked part-time to maintain her clinical and

The authors wish to express appreciation to Dr. Joan Riehl-Sisca for critiquing the original chapter.

research skills. The positions she held during this period included staff nurse in medical-surgical and psychiatric nursing and in the intensive care unit–cardiac care unit and supervisor in a gerontological hospital in southern California. She also worked as a research assistant and coordinator in several research projects at UCLA.

After graduation, Riehl moved to San Antonio, Texas. While there she taught sociology, psychiatric nursing, and mental health concepts as a lecturer in the Department of Social Science at the University of Texas and as an associate professor in the Division of Nursing at Incarnate Word College. She also served as a research evaluator on a government grant that examined numerous variables regarding the RN to B.S.N. student. When the 3-year grant in Texas was completed, Riehl was named chairperson of the Department of Nursing at the Harrisburg Area Community College in Harrisburg, Pennsylvania.

In 1985, Riehl became an associate professor at the graduate level in the Department of Nursing at Indiana University of Pennsylvania. She served as the graduate coordinator for the M.S.N. program and was responsible for teaching master's-prepared students theoretical foundations; research; curriculum theory and practice; ethical, legal and political dimensions of health care; family theory and practice; and administration theory and practicum. Riehl is currently residing in California and working on a state-supported research project to determine whether it is possible to reduce hospitalization of the mentally ill and in what manner the reduction can be accomplished. She is writing a paper about one part of the project. Riehl continues to receive national and international recognition as a pioneer and leader for publishing in the field of nursing theory.

Riehl has been a member of numerous professional organizations. They include the National League for Nursing, American Nurses' Association, the ANA Council of Nurse Researchers, Sigma Theta Tau, the American Sociological Association, and the American Association for the Advancement of Science. We were unable to obtain information about Joan Riehl-Sisca's activities for the past few years.

THEORETICAL SOURCES

Riehl's theory is derived from symbolic interactionism (SI). In SI Theory,

> interaction occurs between human beings who interpret or define each others' actions instead of merely reacting to them. The response is based on the meaning which the individual attaches to the action. Human interaction is mediated by the use of symbols, by interpretation, or by ascertaining the meaning of one another's action. This mediation is equivalent to inserting a process of interpretation between the stimulus and the response in the case of human behavior.[4:8]

"Communication is a key component of symbolic interactionism. While verbal communication is usually the major source of exchange between human beings, nonverbal communication is often considered equally important. This certainly applies in nursing."[11] Consequently, Riehl claims several theoretical sources from sociology and social psychology, including George Mead, Herbert Blumer, Arnold Rose, L. Edward Wells, Gerald Marwell, and Robert E.L. Faris.

USE OF EMPIRICAL EVIDENCE

During the past 50 years, the SI Theory has been supported by numerous empirical studies. Many theoretical sources, including those mentioned earlier, have illustrated the utility of this theory and have contributed to further refinement and clarification of its components. Blumer[1:viii] eloquently states, "It is my conviction that an empirical science necessarily has to respect the nature of the empirical world that is its object of study. In my judgment symbolic interactionism shows that respect for the nature of human group life and conduct."

MAJOR CONCEPTS & DEFINITIONS

Riehl's theory and model adapt four key concepts from the SI Theory described by Blumer.[1:50] In addition, Riehl uses the "me" and "I" concepts developed by Mead. Finally, she identifies role reversal and sick role as examples of the concept.

People "People, individually and collectively, are prepared to act on the basis of the meaning of the objects that comprise their world."[1:50] In the Riehl model, the term *people* includes the patient, the nurse, other health care professionals, and the patient's family and friends. Riehl and Roy[5:17] describe the nurse as one who knows her capabilities, is self-directed, and assumes more than one role in a given period.

Association "The association of people is necessarily in the form of a process in which they are making indications to one another and interpreting each other's indications."[1:50] Riehl summarizes this as the defining process of role taking, a social-psychological concept instituted by Mead. Role taking occurs when an individual cognitively internalizes another person's perceptions of reality in varied situations.[5:352] Hence, the formative meanings of actions arise from this reciprocal interaction. The nurse-patient interface is an example of this interaction.

Social Acts "Social acts, whether individual or collective, are constructed through a process in which the actors note, interpret, and assess the situations confronting them."[1:50] Riehl[4:46] states, "Their interpretation of these situations influence their social acts toward each other." She expounds on the interpretive phase as described by Faris, in which a delayed response promotes clear thought, reduced frustration, and prospective learning.[5:354] This concept correlates to Riehl's method of process recordings, which allows the nurse to as-

sess and respond more appropriately to a patient's behavior.

Interlinkages "The complex interlinkages of acts that comprise organizations, institutions, division of labor, and networks of interdependency are moving and not static affairs."[1:50] From this concept Riehl derives that patient assessment is a dynamic process that often necessitates the use of several resources in meeting patients' needs, particularly in long-term care.

Me Riehl defines *me* synonymously with a role taker in a given situation. In other words, the me learns and assumes the attitudes of others. This is a concept used in the development of one's behavior as well as a method of understanding another's actions.

I (Self-Concept) Riehl defines *I*, or *self-concept*, as the individual's total behavioral perceptions, reflecting the summation of roles. She states, "The self-concept refers to a global, relatively constant self-perception that an individual holds and it changes only gradually."[4:64]

Role Reversal Role reversal is an example of a potential consequence resulting during the interaction between nurse and patient. Riehl[5:355] defines role reversal as an inadvertent situation in which "the patient assumes the therapeutic role while the nurse becomes the recipient of the care." Rectification of this situation may require assistance from a third person.

Sick Role Riehl defines the *sick role* "as the position one assumes when one perceives himself as ill."[10] There may be a problem "when a patient is reluctant to part with the sick role."[5:355] As with role reversal, this situation suggests the need of additional resources for the patient's rehabilitation.

MAJOR ASSUMPTIONS

Riehl relates Arnold Rose's genetic and analytical assumptions to nursing and uses them in her derived theory. Rose divides his assumptions into two categories. The first, genetic assumptions, deals with only the child. The second is the analytic assumptions, which focus on all ages of man other than the child.

Genetic Assumptions

Rose cites the following four genetic assumptions applicable to the SI theory:
1. "Society—a network of interacting individuals—with its culture—the related meanings and values by means of which individuals interact—precedes any existing individual."[5:353]
2. "The process by which socialization takes place can be thought of as occurring in three stages."[5:353] These stages are:
   a. "The infant is habituated to a certain sequence of behaviors and events through a psychogenic process such as trial and error."[5:353]
   b. "When the habit is blocked, the image of the incomplete act arises in the infant's mind and he thus learns to differentiate the object . . . in that act by a symbol."[5:353]
   c. "As the infant acquires a number of meanings he uses them to designate to others, and to himself, what he is thinking."[5:353]
3. "The individual is socialized into the general culture and also into various subcultures."[5:353]
4. "While some groups and personal meanings and values may be dropped and become lower on the reference-relationship scale, they are not lost or forgotten."[5:353]

Analytical Assumptions

The five analytical assumptions pertaining to the SI Theory according to Rose follow.
1. "Man lives in a symbolic as well as in a physical environment and can be stimulated to act by symbols as well as by physical stimuli."[5:351]
2. "Through symbols, man has the capacity to stimulate others in ways other than those in which he himself is stimulated."[5:351] Rihel[5:351] states that role taking, a concept included under this assumption, is important in nursing.
3. "Through communication of symbols, man can learn huge numbers of meanings and values—and hence ways of acting—from other men."[5:351] Riehl summarizes that as a result of this assumption man's behavior is not learned through trial and error or through conditioning, but rather through symbolic communication.[5:351] "According to the SI theory, an individual's perception of how others evaluate him is more important in forming his self-concept than the actual evaluation that others hold."[4:12] Riehl[5:351] explains that it can be deduced from this assumption that "through the learning of a culture, or subculture, men are able to predict each other's behavior and gauge their own behavior accordingly."
4. "The symbols—and the meanings and values to which they refer—do not occur in isolated bits, but in large and complex clusters."[5:351] This assumption refers to man's role. As defined in the discussion of concepts, the "me" is the role-taker and the "I," or self-concept, is the perception of a person as a whole. "Since the 'me' is made up of the attitudes of others, these others can take this role and predict an individual's behavior in a given capacity."[4:351] Consequently, a person is able to gain insight into another's problem by taking the other's role, anticipating how he will act, and implementing a plan of action to help him accomplish his goal.[5:352]
5. "Thinking is the process by which possible symbolic solutions and other future courses of action are examined, assessed for their relative advantages and disadvantages in terms of the values of the individual, and chosen for action or rejected."[5:352] Riehl discusses two major points involving this assumption. First, the assumption encompasses the four steps of the nursing process: "nursing assessment, diagnosis, planned intervention, and evaluation of action."[5:352] Second, she points out, "Since meaning arises in the process of interaction between

two persons, and individuals differ, even the most carefully thought out plan may go awry."[5:352]

THEORETICAL ASSERTIONS

Riehl has identified several theoretical assertions in her model. These include:

1. "The premise that social action is built up by the acting unit through the process of noting, interpreting, etc., implies how social action should be studied."[5:354] Riehl identifies the acting unit as the individual.

2. "According to Blumer (1969), in order to treat and analyze social action, one must observe the process by which it is constructed." Riehl[5:354] identifies "one" as the nurse, who must view the social action as the individual sees it.

3. "Since the self-concept is an integral part of this model, the nurse must continue to develop self-insight through self-evaluation regarding his/her own actions to understand end results of interactions with others."[6,8]

4. "The goal of action is to guide the patient in maintaining and regaining a higher level of wellness to improve the quality of life and to gain insight during life's journey regardless of the health problem."[10] "The goal of action is based on a key factor of SI, which is taking the role of the others."[5:354] Riehl[5:354] identifies three methodological approaches the nurse uses to achieve this goal. The first approach, role taking, allows the nurse to understand why the patient does what he does. The second method entails interpretation of these actions. The third involves the use of process recordings. Riehl does not advocate recording all interactions, but she does recommend that recordings be used until the nurse is able to respond effectively during on-the-spot interactions.

5. "It must be realized that it is not completely possible to take the role of the other, but genuine attempts to do so convey understanding of the other's position."[8,9]

6. "Three additional elements must be included to meet the requirements of an effective con-

ceptual model for nursing, namely, the source of difficulty, the intervention, and the consequences."[5:354] Riehl[6,7] equates the source of difficulty with the nursing diagnosis and the intervention with the plan of care arrived at after role taking, interpretation, and process recordings.

7. The eclipse shown in her model (Fig. 25-1), "should never be complete, however, because maintaining a certain distance is essential for the preservation of the individuality of each person."[5:356] As the nurse and patient gain knowledge and insight from their interactions, the circles in the model move toward each other and form an ecliptical image. However, Riehl[5,6] emphasizes that if the circles form a complete eclipse, objectivity and independence will be lost.

LOGICAL FORM

Riehl's theory uses deductive and inductive logic. It is deductive because Riehl draws relationships between nursing and the SI Theory. Her statements are consistent with Mead's concepts of role taking and self-concept. Her theoretical assertions deduced from Rose's assumptions demonstrate further consistency. This allows for each identification of the interrelationships between the theoretical components and thus enhances the generation of hypotheses for empirical testing. It is inductive because Riehl uses SI as a foundation on which to build and develop her concepts into a nursing theory.[10]

ACCEPTANCE BY THE NURSING COMMUNITY

Practice

Riehl's theory is becoming more widely accepted in the United States and it is used fairly extensively in Canada, England, Japan, and the Middle East.[10] It has been considered a middle-range theory in nursing.[2:13] The middle range constitutes a relatively broad scope of phenomena. However, Riehl's theory and model have been found applicable to all age groups and in a variety of clinical settings.[3]

As Fig. 25-1 illustrates, Riehl views the nurse-therapist and the patient as actively exchanging information and gleaning knowledge. This is accomplished through mutual role taking in conjunction with the nurse selecting and using known theoretical approaches. The unshaded areas of the model indicate active processes in the relationship, whereas the arrows represent the complex interdependencies of these elements, allowing for continual reassessment and evaluation.

Riehl's model provides a realistic approach for nursing practice in any situation where the focus is on role interaction in the nurse-patient relationship. Preisner demonstrates the applicability of Riehl's model in the psychiatric setting.[5:362-371] The nurse selects from multiple theories, therapies, and allied health disciplines in planning and implementing effective nursing interventions.

Wood demonstrates the use of role taking in a patient's hospital admission.[5:357-361] The nurse interprets

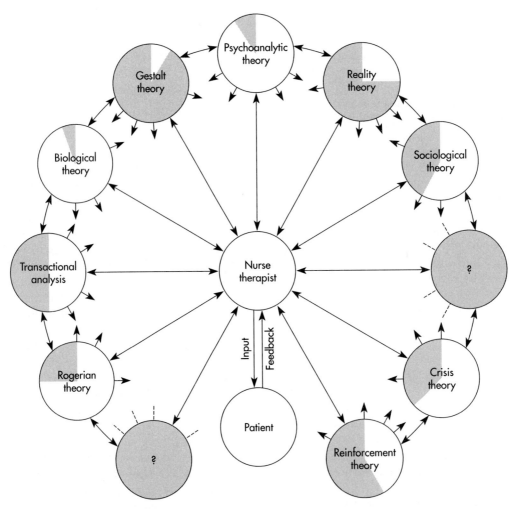

Fig. **25-1** **Schematic representation of model.** *From Preisner, J.M. (1980). A proposed model for the nurse therapist. In J.P. Riehl and C. Roy (Eds.),* Conceptual models for nursing practice. *New York: Appleton-Century-Crofts, p. 363. Used with permission.*

the patient's response to the new environment and thereby helps the patient acquire the necessary perceptual changes or new roles in the health care system.

The nursing implications are evident yet not restrictive to the interaction between the nurse and patient. The role interaction framework may also be effective in nurse-nurse relationships (nursing management, for example), nurse-physician dyads, nurse-patient-family triads, and other interactive situations. However, the model's emphasis is on the nurse-patient-family relationships.

Education

The SI Theory has long been prevalent among schools of sociology and psychology. The Riehl Interaction Model was introduced to the nursing discipline in 1980. The number of educational institutions that have incorporated it into their nursing curriculum is uncertain. The Riehl Interaction Model was considered as part of the organizing framework of the curriculum at both Harrisburg Area Community College and Indiana University of Pennsylvania.

In addition, interaction models as a group are moderately employed in B.S.N. programs.[5:396-398] Nursing is presently concerned with developing a distinct body of knowledge and delineating its professional role. Riehl's model, which focuses on the therapeutic processes in the nurse-patient and nurse-patient-family relationships, continues to contribute to these goals.

Research

The earliest research relevant to Riehl's theory can be found in her own doctoral dissertation. This study examines autistic children's ability to role take compared with that of their "normal" siblings. It implicates a positive correlation between the level of development of self-concept and the ability to role take.

The generation of implications for further research is inherent in empirical studies. Riehl makes several suggestions for further testing dealing specifically with autistic children, such as investigating their perceptions of their parent's treatment of them

and simply increasing the sample size to study more variables in this population. Examples of other recommendations include applying this study to other handicapped children and developing more tools for measuring self-conception.

Research on Riehl's theory and model supports their applicability to a wide variety of patients and clinical settings. These studies include use of the model with pregnant women, with adults in a medical clinic and the concept of personal space, with diabetic children and their self-esteem, with patients being transported by helicopter to acute-care settings, and with a woman with postpartum psychosis.[3] Continued research is needed for Riehl's theory to gain credibility, acceptance, and future application.

FURTHER DEVELOPMENT

In operationalizing her model, Riehl has developed an assessment tool in the form of a matrix with the *mnemonic* FANCAP down the left side and the parameters physiological, psychological, sociological, cultural, and environmental across the top. With this approach, each factor intersects with each parameter and is therefore addressed (Fig. 25-2). After analyzing the collected data and making a diagnosis, a plan of care is made with the patient and/or family. The diagnosis and plan of care are prioritized (nurse with patient and/or family) and evaluated after implementation. This tool has been tested and Riehl indicates that it is valid and reliable.[3]

Riehl has introduced an interesting and valuable model of SI to nursing. She has included further development of her theory in her third edition of *Conceptual Models for Nursing Practice*.

More explicit definitions of many concepts in the current model, including *I, me, process recordings,* and *SI* itself, are needed for in-depth descriptions in regard to the relationship statements between Blumer's concepts and nursing and between Rose's assumptions and nursing. Furthermore, the theoretical assertions require refinement for lucidity and depth.

As a therapeutic nursing approach, Riehl's theory merits the involvement of the profession for progress

	Physiological	Psychological	Sociological	Cultural	Environmental
Fluids					
Aeration					
Nutrition					
Communication					
Activity					
Pain					

Fig. **25-2** Riehl Interaction Model assessment tool. *(Drawn by Deborah Hissa from a description given by Riehl.)*

in its development, understanding, and validation. Abundant potential for both nursing research and subsequent contributions to the theory seems to lie particularly in the psychiatric nurse setting. This testing may also generate new information. "Theory development is important to the growth of any discipline" and should be pursued.[5:3]

Riehl continued to work with the theory. A book written in England compiles information from various sources about the use of the theory. Development of a consortium is being planned to add clarifications to the concepts as they apply to various nursing situations.

CRITIQUE
Complexity

The Riehl Interaction Model contains several key concepts and theoretical relationships; thus, it is complex. The future development of concepts and relationships will increase the level of complexity.

Generality

Riehl's interaction model is generalizable to the broad scope of nursing. With a nonresponsive comatose patient, however, the model may be applied by using nonverbal forms of communication. The exact interpretations may vary from patient to patient and nurse

to nurse. A team approach is important and the help of family and friends is invaluable.[11,12]

Empirical Precision

The derived concepts from Blumer and Mead have been defined explicitly and grounded in observable reality within their parent discipline. Riehl does not clarify all her concepts with denotative definitions. "Peripheral nuances exist. Slight variations on the theme can be adjusted to the individual situation without changing the basic theory."[11,12] The means for accurate testability and the degree of empirical precision will remain with the individual researcher.

Derivable Consequences

Riehl's Interaction Model uses the nursing process in implementing nursing care. Emphasis is on the nurse assessing and interpreting the patient's actions and then making predictions about the patient's behavior to plan interventions with the patient and his family. Furthermore, the evaluation phase in the theory presents important nursing implications regarding potential patient problems. The theory's usefulness is evident not only in the delivery of nursing care but also in delineating the nurse's professional role.

SUMMARY

Riehl continued the development of her nursing theory, which is derived from SI. SI, as defined by Blumer, involves the interaction that transpires between people who "interpret or define each other's actions instead of just relating to them."[5:350] Riehl uses Rose's genetic and analytic assumptions as her own. She identifies Blumer's concepts, the I and me concepts of Mead, and the role reversal and sick role concepts in describing her model.

With use of these assumptions and concepts, Riehl relates nursing to the SI Theory. She believes that the nurse must view the actions of the individual as he perceives them. By role playing, explicitly or implicitly the nurse is able to understand why the patient does what he does and is thus better able to identify the source of difficulty, or nursing diagnosis. Then, having interpreted the patient's action and studied the process recordings, the nurse is able to intervene with a plan of care. The plan of care involves helping the patient and/or family assume roles they have used in the past, or are currently using, to cope with the present illness. The evaluation process is then used to determine the success of this role taking. Riehl views this dynamic process as one that changes daily, requiring continuous assessment by both the nurse and the patient.

Although testing of Riehl's theory within the science of nursing has occurred only since 1985, its contribution to nursing is apparent.

CRITICAL THINKING *Activities*

1 Discuss the major assumptions of SI Theory.

2 After reviewing the concepts and definitions of SI Theory, use the assessment tool (Fig. 25-2) to develop a plan of care from a scenario you create.

3 Apply SI Theory in an analysis of the following:

   a. A curriculum framework

   b. A process recording

4 Use SI Theory to design a research study.

5 Use summative and formative evaluative processes to analyze a clinical setting with use of SI Theory.

REFERENCES

1. Blumer, H. (1969). *Symbolic interactionism: Perspective and method*. Englewood Cliffs, NJ: Prentice-Hall.
2. Kim, H.S. (1983). *The nature of theoretical thinking in nursing*. Norwalk, CT: Appleton-Century-Crofts.
3. Riehl, J. (Ed.). (1989). *Conceptual models for nursing practice* (3rd ed.). Norwalk, CT: Appleton & Lange.
4. Riehl, J.P. (1980). *The self-conception and role relationships of autistic children: A symbolic interactionist perspective*. Doctoral dissertation, University of California, Los Angeles, Department of Sociology.
5. Riehl, J.P., & Roy, C. (Eds.). (1980). *Conceptual models for nursing practice* (2nd ed.). New York: Appleton-Century-Crofts.
6. Riehl-Sisca, J. (1984). Personal correspondence.
7. Riehl-Sisca, J. (1984). Telephone interviews.
8. Riehl-Sisca, J. (1985). Personal correspondence.
9. Riehl-Sisca, J. (1985). Telephone interviews.
10. Riehl-Sisca, J. (1988). Personal correspondence.
11. Riehl-Sisca, J. (1992). Personal correspondence.
12. Riehl-Sisca, J. (1992). Telephone interviews.

BIBLIOGRAPHY

Primary sources

Books

Riehl, J. (Ed.). (1989). *Conceptual models for nursing practice* (3rd ed.). Norwalk, CT: Appleton & Lange.
Riehl, J.P., & McVay, J.W. (Eds.). (1973). *The clinical nurse specialist: Interpretations*. New York: Appleton-Century-Crofts.
Riehl, J.P., & Roy, C. (Eds.). (1974). *Conceptual models for nursing practice*. New York: Appleton-Century-Crofts.
Riehl, J.P., & Roy, C. (Eds.). (1980). *Conceptual models for nursing practice* (2nd ed.). New York: Appleton-Century Crofts.
Riehl-Sisca, J, (Ed.). (1985). *The science and art of self-care*. East Norwalk, CT: Appleton-Century-Crofts.

Book chapters

Chrisman, M., & Riehl, J.P. (1974). The systems-developmental stress model. In J.P. Riehl & C. Roy (Eds.), *Conceptual models for nursing practice*. New York: Appleton-Century-Crofts.
McVay, J.W., Riehl, J.P., & Chen, S. (1973). The clinical nurse specialist as perceived by the deans of baccalaureate and higher degree programs. In J.P. Riehl & J.W. McVay (Eds.), *The clinical nurse specialist: Interpretations*. New York: Appleton-Century-Crofts.

Riehl, J.P. (1973). Role change and resistance: The baccalaureate student as practitioner. In J.P. Riehl & J.W. McVay (Eds.), *The clinical nurse specialist: Interpretations.* New York: Appleton-Century-Crofts.

Riehl, J.P. (1974). Application of interaction theory. In J.P. Riehl & C. Roy (Eds.). *Conceptual models for nursing practice.* New York: Appleton-Century-Crofts.

Riehl, J.P. (1980). Nursing models in current use. In J.P. Riehl & C. Roy (Eds.), *Conceptual models for nursing practice* (2nd ed.). New York: Appleton-Century-Crofts.

Riehl, J.P. (1980). The Riehl interaction model. In J.P. Riehl & C. Roy (Eds.), *Conceptual models for nursing practice* (2nd ed.). New York: Appleton-Century-Crofts.

Riehl, J. (1989). Preface and introductions to each unit. In J. Riehl (Ed.), *Conceptual models for nursing practice* (3rd ed.). East Norwalk, CT: Appleton & Lange.

Riehl, J. (1989). Prologue and epilogue chapters. In J. Riehl (Ed.), *Conceptual models for nursing practice* (3rd ed.). East Norwalk, CT: Appleton & Lange.

Riehl, J. (1989). The Riehl interaction model. In J. Riehl (Ed.), *Conceptual models for nursing practice* (3rd ed.). East Norwalk, CT: Appleton & Lange.

Riehl, J.P., & Roy, C. (1974). Conceptual models in nursing: Use of nursing models in education, research, and service. In J.P. Riehl & C. Roy (Eds.), *Conceptual models for nursing practice.* New York: Appleton-Century-Crofts.

Riehl, J.P., & Roy, C. (1974). Discussion of a unified nursing model. In J.P. Riehl & C. Roy (Eds.), *Conceptual models for nursing practice.* New York: Appleton-Century-Crofts.

Riehl, J.P., & Roy, C. (1974). The nature and history of models: Models related to theory: Use of models in other fields; and history of nursing models. In J.P. Riehl & C. Roy (Eds.), *Conceptual models for nursing practice.* New York: Appleton-Century-Crofts.

Riehl, J.P., & Roy, C. (1974). Toward a unified nursing model. In J.P. Riehl & C. Roy (Eds.), *Conceptual models for nursing practice.* New York: Appleton-Century-Crofts.

Riehl, J.P., & Roy, C. (1980). The nature of nursing models. In J.P. Riehl & C. Roy (Eds.), *Conceptual models for nursing practice* (2nd ed.). New York: Appleton-Century-Crofts.

Riehl, J.P., & Roy, C. (1980). A unified model of nursing. In J.P. Riehl & C. Roy (Eds.), *Conceptual models for nursing practice* (2nd ed.). New York: Appleton-Century-Crofts.

Riehl-Sisca, J. (1985). Determining criteria for graduate and undergraduate self-care curriculums. In J. Riehl-Sisca (Ed.), *The science and art of self-care.* East Norwalk, CT: Appleton-Century-Crofts.

Riehl-Sisca, J. (1985). Epilogue: Future implications for the science and art of self-care. In J. Riehl-Sisca (Ed.), *The science and art of self-care.* East Norwalk, CT: Appleton-Century-Crofts.

Riehl-Sisca, J. (1985). Orem's general theory of nursing: An interpretation. In J. Riehl-Sisca (Ed.), *The science and art of self-care.* East Norwalk, CT: Appleton-Century-Crofts.

Skolny, M.A., & Riehl, J.P. (1974). Hope: Solving patient and family problems by using a theoretical framework. In J.P. Riehl & C. Roy (Eds.), *Conceptual models for nursing practice.* New York: Appleton-Century-Crofts.

Journal articles

Riehl, J.P. (1965). The effect of naturally occurring pain on the galvanic skin response and heart rate: A clinical study. *American Nurses' Association Regional Clinical Conference, 3,* 16-23

Riehl, J.P., & Chambers, J. (1976, July). Better salvage for the stroke victim. *Nursing, 6,* 24-31.

Riehl-Sisca, J. (1981, Aug.). Preparing to take the state board exams. *California Nurse, 77,* 5.

Riehl-Sisca, J. (1982). Nontraditional RN-BSN programs for ethnic minority students: A research paradigm. *Journal of Nursing Education, 21*(8), 75.

Riehl-Sisca, J., & Kerr, J. (1984). Passing the state board examination. *Journal of Nursing Education, 23*(8), 358-360.

Professional papers

Riehl, J.P. (1965). *The effect of naturally occurring pain on the galvanic skin response and heart rate: A clinical study.* Master's thesis, University of California, Los Angeles, Department of Nursing.

Riehl, J.P. (1980). *The self-conception and role relationships of autistic children: A symbolic interactionist perspective.* Doctoral dissertation, University of California, Los Angeles, Department of Sociology.

Secondary sources

Book reviews

Riehl, J.P., & McVay, J.W. (Eds.). (1973). *The clinical nurse specialist: Interpretations.*
  Canadian Nurse, 69, 38, Nov. 1973.
  Nursing Outlook, 21, 689-690, Nov. 1973.
  Nursing Research, 23, 76-77, Jan.-Feb. 1974.
  American Journal of Nursing, 74, 960, May 1974.
  Hospitals, 48, 36, May 16, 1974.
  Nursing Mirror, 141, 72, Oct. 2, 1975.

Riehl, J.P., & Roy, C. (Eds.). (1974). *Conceptual models for nursing practice.*
  Canadian Nurse, 76, 48, Dec. 1980.
  Nursing Times, 77, 825, May 7, 1981.
  Nursing Research, 30, 379, Nov.-Dec. 1981.
  American Journal of Nursing, 82, 696, April 1982.
  Nursing Clinics of North America, 21, 461-471, Sept. 1986.

Riehl, J.P., & Roy, C. (Eds.). (1980). *Conceptual models for nursing practice.*
  Journal of Advanced Nursing, 11, 197-202, Nov. 1986.

Books

Chinn, P.L., & Jacobs, M.K. (1983). *Theory and nursing: A systematic approach.* St. Louis: Mosby.

Kim, H.S. (1983). *The nature of theoretical thinking in nursing.* Norwalk, CT: Appleton-Century-Crofts.

Marriner, A. (Ed.). (1986). *Nursing theorists and their work.* St. Louis: Mosby.

Meleis, A.J. (1985). *Theoretical development and progress.* Philadelphia: JB Lippincott.

Nicoll, L.H. (Ed.). (1986). *Perspectives on nursing theory.* Boston: Little, Brown.

Walker, L.O., & Avant, K. (1983). *Strategies for theory construction in nursing.* Norwalk, CT: Appleton-Century-Crofts.

Book chapters

Preisner, J.M. (1980). A proposed model for the nurse therapist. In J.P. Riehl & C. Roy (Eds.), *Conceptual models for nursing practice* (2nd ed.) (pp. 362-371). New York: Appleton-Century-Crofts.

Wood, M.J. (1980). Implementing the Riehl interaction model in nursing administration. In J.P. Riehl & C. Roy (Eds.), *Conceptual models for nursing practice* (2nd ed.) (pp. 357-361). New York: Appleton-Century-Crofts.

Correspondence

Riehl-Sisca, J. (1984, Nov.). Curriculum vitae, revised.

Riehl-Sisca, J. (1984, Nov. 2). Personal correspondence.

Riehl-Sisca, J. (1985). Personal correspondence.

Riehl-Sisca, J. (1987). Curriculum vitae, revised.

Riehl-Sisca, J. (1988, April). Personal correspondence.

Riehl-Sisca, J. (1992, June 5, 30). Personal correspondence.

Interviews

Riehl-Sisca, J. (1984, Oct. 10). Telephone interview.

Riehl-Sisca, J. (1984, Oct. 17). Telephone interview.

Riehl-Sisca, J. (1984, Nov. 30). Telephone interview.

Riehl-Sisca, J. (1985). Telephone interview.

Riehl-Sisca, J. (1992, July, Aug.). Telephone interviews.

Other sources

Blumer, H. (1969). *Symbolic interactionism: Perspective and method.* Englewood Cliffs, NJ: Prentice-Hall.

Faris, R.E.L. (1964). *Handbook of modern sociology.* Chicago: Rand McNally.

Mead, G.H. (1934). *Mind, self, and society* (C.V. Morris, Ed.). Chicago: University of Chicago.

Rose, A.M. (1962). *Human behavior and social processes.* Boston: Houghton Mifflin.

Wells, L.E., & Marwell, G. (1976). *Self-esteem: Its conceptualization and measurement.* Beverly Hills, CA: Sage.

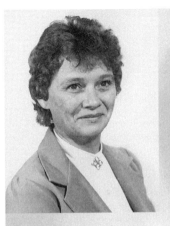

*H*elen C. Erickson

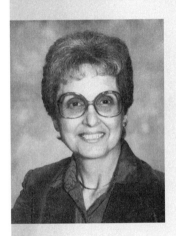

*E*velyn M. Tomlin

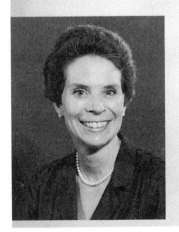

*M*ary Ann P. Swain

Modeling and Role-Modeling

Margaret E. Erickson, Jane A. Caldwell-Gwin, Lisa A. Carr,
Brenda Kay Harmon, Karen Hartman, Connie Rae Jarlsberg,
Judy McCormick, Kathryn W. Noone

CREDENTIALS AND BACKGROUND OF THE THEORISTS

Helen C. Erickson

Helen C. Erickson received a diploma from Saginaw General Hospital, Saginaw, Michigan, in 1957. Her degrees include a Bachelor of Science in Nursing in 1974, a Master of Science in Psychiatric Nursing in 1976, and a Doctor of Educational Psychology in 1984, all from the University of Michigan.

Erickson's professional experience began in the emergency room of the Midland Community Hospital in Midland, Texas, where she was the head nurse for 2 years. She then worked in Mt. Pleasant, Michigan, as night supervisor of nursing in the State Home for the Handicapped. She was then Director of Health Services at the Inter-American University in San German, Puerto Rico, from 1960 to 1964. On her return to the United States, she worked as a staff nurse at both St. Joseph's and University Hospitals in Ann Arbor, Michigan. Erickson later served as a psychiatric nurse consultant to the Pediatric Nurse Practitioner Program at the University of Michigan and the University of Michigan Hospitals–Adult Care. Her academic career began as a teaching assistant in the RN Studies Program at the University of Michi-

gan School of Nursing, where she later served as chairperson of the undergraduate program and Dean for Undergraduate Studies.

Erickson was an assistant professor of nursing at the University of Michigan from 1978 to 1986. In 1986, Erickson left Michigan to go to the University of South Carolina College of Nursing. Initially, she served as associate professor and assistant dean for academic programs; later she held the position of Associate Dean for Academic Affairs. Since 1988, Dr. Erickson has been a professor of nursing at the University of Texas at Austin and Chair of Adult Health. She currently holds the additional title of Special Assistant to the Dean, Graduate Programs. Erickson has maintained an independent nursing practice since 1976.

Erickson is a member of the American Nurses Association, American Nurses' Foundation, the Charter Club, American Holistic Nurses' Association, Texas Nurses' Association, Sigma Theta Tau, and the Institute for the Advancement of Health. In addition, she has served as president of the Society for the Advancement of Modeling and Role-Modeling from 1986 to 1990. She was the chairperson of the First National Symposium on Modeling and Role-Modeling (1986) and served on the planning committee for the Second, Third, Fourth, Fifth, and Sixth National Conferences in 1988, 1990, 1992, 1994, and 1996, respectively.

The authors wish to express appreciation to Helen C. Erickson, Evelyn M. Tomlin, and Mary Ann P. Swain for critiquing the chapter.

Erickson has been listed in *Who's Who Among University Students* and is a member of Phi Kappa Phi. She received the Sigma Theta Tau Rho Chapter Award of Excellence in Nursing in 1980, the Amoco Foundation Good Teaching Award in 1982, and was accepted into ADARA, a University of Michigan honor society, in 1982. In 1990 she received the Faculty Teaching Award, University of Texas at Austin, School of Nursing.[25] She was nominated for the Sigma Theta Tau International Honor Society in Nursing, Excellence in Education Award by the Epsilon Theta Chapter in 1993, received the Graduate Faculty Teaching Award, University of Texas at Austin School of Nursing in 1995, and was accepted as a Fellow in the American Academy in 1996.[22]

Erickson is actively researching the Modeling and Role-Modeling Theory and has presented numerous seminars and papers on various aspects of the theory both nationally and internationally. She has served as a consultant in the implementation of the theory into clinical practice at the University of Michigan Medical Center in the surgical area, at Brigham and Women's Hospital, Boston, and at the University of Pittsburgh Hospitals. She has consulted with faculty in various schools of nursing and service agencies that have adopted the theory into their curriculum and practice. Humboldt University School of Nursing, in Arcata, California, is the first school to be accredited by the National League for Nursing using the Modeling and Role-Modeling Theory as its conceptual base. Metropolitan State University at St. Paul, Minnesota, has adopted the Modeling and Role-Modeling Theory for its RN/B.S.N. and M.S.N. programs. The University of Texas at Galveston has adopted concepts in the theory as the basis for the academic/service model at the University of Texas Medical Branch-Galveston.[22,23,25,26,29]

Erickson has been an invited speaker at multiple national and international conferences and has participated in numerous workshops, including the Third and Fourth International Congresses on Ericksonian Approaches to Hypnosis sponsored by the Erickson Foundation and the Seventh and Eighth International Psychology of Health, Immunity and Disease Conferences sponsored by the National Institute for the Clinical Application of Behavioral Medicine in 1995 and 1996. Erickson has also been involved in activities sponsored by the American Association for Holistic Nursing. She served as a content expert for certification curricula and will be included in a forthcoming book featuring nurse healers.[26]

Evelyn M. Tomlin

Evelyn M. Tomlin's nursing education began in Southern California. She attended Pasadena City College, Los Angeles County General Hospital School of Nursing, and the University of Southern California, where she received her Bachelor of Science in Nursing. She received a Master of Science in Psychiatric Nursing from the University of Michigan in 1976.

Tomlin's professional experiences are varied, beginning when she was a clinical instructor at Los Angeles County General Hospital School of Nursing in surgical nursing and maternal and premature infant nursing. She later lived in Kabul, Afghanistan, where she taught English at the Afghan Institute of Technology. In addition, she also served as school nurse and practiced family nursing in the overseas American and European communities with which she was associated, a role that included attending more than 40 home deliveries with a certified nurse-midwife. After the establishment of medical services at the United States Embassy Hospital, Tomlin functioned as relief staff nurse. When she returned to the United States, she was employed by the Visiting Nurse Association as a staff nurse in Ann Arbor, Michigan. She was then the coordinator and clinical instructor for student practical nurses. She was a staff nurse in a coronary care unit for 5 years, worked in the respiratory intensive care unit, and was also the head nurse of the emergency department at St. Joseph's Mercy Hospital in Ann Arbor. She was also an assistant professor in the RN Studies Program at the University of Michigan School of Nursing. She served as the mental health consultant to the pediatric nurse-practitioner program at the University of Michigan. For 8 years she was an assistant professor of nursing in the fundamentals at the University of Michigan.

Tomlin was among the first 14 nurses in the United States to be certified by the American Association of Critical Care Nurses. With several colleagues, she opened one of the first offices for independent nursing practice in Michigan. She continued her independent practice until 1993.

Tomlin is a member of Sigma Theta Tau Rho Chapter, the California Scholarship Federation, and the Philathian Society. She has presented programs incorporating a variety of nursing topics based on the Modeling and Role-Modeling Theory and paradigm, with an emphasis on clinical applications.

In late 1985, Tomlin moved with her husband to Big Rock, Illinois, where she enjoyed teaching small community and nursing groups and working with a community shelter serving the women and children of Fox Valley. Later she moved to Geneva, Illinois, where she currently resides with her husband. Tomlin has had inquiries from staff nurses for help in integrating the framework into practice. Tomlin states that "elements of the theory and paradigm can be introduced easily in many settings and can be very valuable" for practicing nurses. Tomlin was first editor for the newsletter of the Society for the Advancement of Modeling and Role-Modeling.[57-61]

Tomlin currently identifies herself as a Christian in retirement from nursing for pay, but not from nursing practice. She is pursing her interest in the practice of healing prayer, stating that she has always been interested in the interface of the Modeling and Role-Modeling Theory and Judeo-Christian principles. She is on the Board of Directors and works as a volunteer at Wayside Cross Ministries in Aurora, Illinois, where she teaches and counsels homeless women, most of whom are single mothers. She stated that her goal is to help them develop skills necessary to live healthier, happier lives.[57-61]

Mary Ann P. Swain

Mary Ann P. Swain's educational background is in psychology. She received her Bachelor of Arts in psychology from DePauw University in Greencastle, Indiana, and her Master of Science and doctoral degrees from the University of Michigan, both in the field of psychology.

Swain has taught psychology research methods and statistics as a teaching assistant at DePauw University and later as a lecturer and an associate professor of psychology in nursing at the University of Michigan. She became the director of the Doctoral Program in Nursing in 1975 and served in that capacity for 1 year. She was chairperson of nursing research from 1977 to 1982 and is currently professor of nursing research at the University of Michigan. In 1983, Swain became Associate Vice President for Academic Affairs at the University of Michigan.[49]

Swain is a member of the American Psychological Association and an associate member of the Michigan Nurses' Association. She has developed and taught classes of psychology, research, and nursing research methods. She has collaborated with nurse researchers on various projects, including health promotion among diabetics and influencing compliance among hypertensive patients, and has worked with Erickson to develop a model for assessing potential adaptation to stress, which is significant to the Modeling and Role-Modeling Theory.

Swain received the Alpha Lambda Delta, Psi Chi, Mortar Board, and Phi Beta Kappa awards while at DePauw University. In 1981, she was recognized by the Rho Chapter of Sigma Theta Tau for Contributions to Nursing and in 1983 became an honorary member of Sigma Theta Tau.

Swain currently holds the position of Provost for the New York State University System and resides in Appalachia, New York with her husband.

THEORETICAL SOURCES

The theory and paradigm were developed by a retroductive process. The original model was derived inductively from the primary author's clinical and personal life experiences. The works of Abraham Maslow, Erik Erikson, Jean Piaget, George Engle, Hans Seyle, and Milton H. Erickson were then integrated and synthesized into the original model to label, further articulate, and refine a holistic theory and paradigm for nursing. Erickson[19] argued that people have mind-body relations and have an identifiable resource potential that predicts their ability to contend with stress. She also articulated a relationship between needs status and developmental processes, satisfaction with needs and attachment objects, loss and illness, and health and need satisfaction. Tomlin and Swain validated and affirmed Erickson's practice model and helped to expand and articulate labeled phenomena, concepts, and theoretical relationships.

Maslow's Theory of Human Needs was used to label and articulate the authors' personal observations "all people want to be the best that they can possibly be; unmet basic needs interfere with holistic growth whereas satisfied needs promote growth."[30:45] The authors further integrated the model to say that unmet basic needs create need deficits, which can lead to initiation or aggravation of physical or mental distress or illness. At the same time, need satisfaction creates assets that provide resources needed to contend with stress and promote health, growth, and development.

Piaget's Theory of Cognitive Development provides a framework for understanding the development of thinking. On the other hand, integration of Erikson's work on the stages of psychosocial development through the life span provides a theoretical basis for understanding the psychosocial evolution of the individual. Each of his eight stages represent developmental tasks. As an individual resolves each task, strengths are gained that contribute to character and health. Furthermore, as an outcome of each stage, people develop a sense of their own worth and therefore a projection of themselves into the future. "The utility of Erikson's theory is the freedom we may take to view aspects of people's problems as uncompleted tasks. This perspective provides a hopeful expectation for the individual's future since it connotes something still in progress."[30:62-63]

The works of Winnicott, Klein, Mahler, and Bowlby on object attachment were integrated with the original model to develop and articulate the concept of affiliated-individuation (AI). Object relations theory proposes that an infant initially forms an attachment to his or her caregiver after having repeated positive contacts. As the child grows and begins to move toward a more separate and individuated state, a sense of autonomy develops. During this time he or she usually transfers some attachment to an inanimate object such as a cuddly blanket or a teddy bear.

Later, the child may attach to a favorite baseball glove, doll, or pet and finally onto more abstract things in adulthood, such as an educational degree, professional role, or relationship. On the basis of the work of these individuals, a theoretical relationship was identified between object attachment and need satisfaction. According to the theorists, when an object repeatedly meets an individual's basic needs, attachment or connectedness to that object occurs. After further synthesis of these theoretical linkages and research findings, the authors identified a new concept, AI. They defined AI as the inherent need to be connected with significant others at the same time that there is a sense of separateness from them that enhances the uniqueness. AI runs across the life span from birth to death. Research supports that AI, as well as object attachment, is essential to need satisfaction, adaptive coping, and healthy growth and development.

The authors further stated that "object loss results in basic need deficits."[30:88] Loss is real, threatened, or perceived; can be a normal part of the developmental process; or can be situational. Loss always results in grief; normal grief is resolved in approximately 1 year. When there are inadequate or inappropriate objects available to meet needs, morbid grief results. Morbid grief interferes with the individual's ability to grow and develop to maximum potential. The work of Selye and Engle provides additional conceptual basis for the beliefs the theorists hold regarding loss and an individual's stress response to that loss or losses. Seyle's theory pertains to an individual's biophysical responses to stress, whereas Engle's work explores the psychosocial responses to stressors.

The synthesis of these theories, along with the integration of the primary author's clinical observations and lived experiences, resulted in the development of the Adaptive Potential Assessment Model (APAM). The focus of the APAM is the ability of the individual to mobilize resources when confronted with stressors rather than the adaptation process. This model was first developed by Erickson[19] and published by Erickson and Swain in 1982.[29]

Finally, Erickson credits Milton H. Erickson with influencing her clinical practice and providing inspiration and direction in the development of this theory. Initially, the formulation of modeling and role-modeling was articulated by Erickson when he urged her to "model the client's world, understand it as they do, then role-model the picture the client has drawn—building a healthy world for them."[20]

USE OF EMPIRICAL EVIDENCE

Several studies have provided initial evidence for philosophical premises and theoretical linkages implied in the original book by Erickson, Tomlin, and Swain[30] and later specified by Erickson.[18] The APAM (Figs. 26-1 and 26-2) has been tested as a classification model,[4,19,44] as a predictor for health status,[5] and

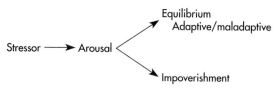

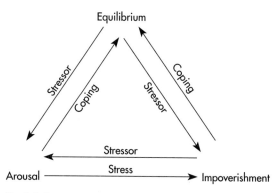

Fig. **26-1** Adaptive Potential Assessment Model. *From Erickson, H.C., Tomlin, E.M., & Swain, M.A.P. (1983).* Modeling and role-modeling: A theory and paradigm for nursing. *Englewood Cliffs, NJ: Prentice Hall, p. 81. Reprinted with permission.*

Fig. **26-2** Dynamic relationship among the states of the Adaptive Potential Assessment Model. *From Erickson, H.C., Tomlin, E.M., & Swain, M.A.P. (1983).* Modeling and role-modeling: A theory and paradigm for nursing. *Englewood Cliffs, NJ: Prentice Hall, p. 82. Reprinted with permission.*

length of hospital stay,[29] and as it relates to basic need status.[6] Findings provide beginning evidence for the proposed three-state model across populations, a relationship between health and ability to mobilize resources, and ability to mobilize resources and needs status. Two other studies have shown relationships between stressors (measured as life events) and propensity for accidents[3] and resource state and ability to take in and use new information.[12]

Relationships among self-care knowledge, resources, and activities have been demonstrated in several studies.[1,37,39,49] The self-care knowledge construct, first studied by Erickson,[16,22,25] was replicated and found to be significantly associated with perceived control.[8] Self-directedness, need for harmony (affiliation), and need for autonomy (individuation) were found when multidimensional scaling was used to explore relationships among self-care knowledge, resources, and actions. The author concluded that a positive attitude was a major factor when health-directed self-care actions were assessed.[53] Physical activity in post–myocardial infarction patients was shown to be affected by life satisfaction (not physical condition); life satisfaction was predicted by availability of self-care resources and resources needed. Furthermore, resources needed served as a suppresser for resources available.[2] In a sample of caregivers, social support predicted for stress level and self-worth and had an indirect effect on hope through self-worth,[37] whereas persons with diabetes with spiritual well-being were better able to cope.[46]

When the Theory of Modeling and Role-Modeling was used as a guideline, interviews were used to determine the client's model of the world and seven themes emerged: the cause of the problem, which was unique to the individual; related factors (also unique to the individual); expectations for the future; types of perceived control; affiliation (or lack of); and trust in the caregiver.[18] Each model was unique and each warranted individualized interventions. Other qualitative studies on self-care knowledge showed that postcardiac patients perceived monitoring, caring, presence, touch, and voice tones as comforting[41]; healthy adults sought need satisfaction from the nurse-practitioner in primary care[7]; and hospice patients benefited from nurse empathy.[51]

Studies also showed relationships between or among mistrust and length of stay in hospitalized subjects,[33] perceived support, control, and well-being in the elderly,[10] and loss, morbid grief, and onset of symptoms of Alzheimer's disease.[27]

Other studies addressed linkages between role-modeled interventions and outcomes. Nursing students who perceived that they were supported were more able to attain their goals for advanced education[55]; the elderly who felt supported reported higher need satisfaction and were better able to cope[40]; those with a strong social network reported better health[15]; and persons convicted of sexual offenses and then provided with support to "remodel" their worlds were able to develop new behaviors and "move on" with their lives.[54] Families and post–myocardial infarction patients who were able to participate in planning their own care through contracting had less anxiety and more perceived control and perceived support,[36] and caregivers of adults with dementia who experienced theory-based nursing using the Modeling and Role-Modeling Theory perceived that their needs were met and that they were healthier.[39] They also reported feeling that they were encouraged, which helped them accept the situation and transcend the experience of caregiving.[39]

Self-care resources, measured as needs, have been found to be related to perceived support and coping in women with breast cancer,[40] physical well-being in persons with chronic obstructive pulmonary disease,[45] and anxiety in hospitalized cardiac patients and their families.[36] When affiliated individuation was tested as a buffer between stress and well-being, a mediation effect was found.

Other studies operationalizing self-care resources by measuring developmental residuals have shown that identity resolution in facially disfigured adolescents can be predicted by previous developmental residual[50]; trust predicts for adolescent clients' involvement in the prescribed medical regimen[34]; perceived support and adaptation are related to developmental residual in families with newborn infants[14]; mistrust predicts for hospital stay; and positive residual serves as a buffer.[32] Positive residual in the intimacy stage of healthy adults predicts for health behaviors[47]; developmental residual predicts for hope; trust-mistrust residual predicts for generalized hope; autonomy-shame/doubt residual predicts for particularized hope in the elderly[13]; and negative residual is related to speed/impatience behaviors in a healthy sample of military personnel.[43] Case study methods have been used to show relationships among needs, attachment, and developmental residual[42] and needs and coping,[39] and two other unpublished studies have shown relationships between healthy adults and need status.[28]

Tools that have been developed to test the Modeling and Role-Modeling Theory include the Basic Needs Satisfaction Inventory,[45] the Erikson Psychosocial Stage Inventory,[14] the Perceived Enactment of Autonomy tool designed to measure a prerequisite to self-care actions,[35] the Self-Care Resource Inventory,[2] the Robinson Self-Appraisal Inventory designed to measure denial (the first stage in the grief process) in post–myocardial infarction patients,[52] and the Erickson Maternal Bonding-Attachment Tool designed to measure self-care knowledge as motivational style (i.e., deficit or being motivation) and self-care resources.[31]

MAJOR CONCEPTS & DEFINITIONS

The theory and paradigm modeling and role-modeling contains multiple concepts.

Modeling "The act of Modeling, then, is the process the nurse uses as she develops an image and understanding of the client's world—an image and understanding developed within the client's framework and from the client's perspective. . . . The art of Modeling is the development of a mirror image of the situation from the client's perspective. . . . The science of Modeling is the scientific aggregation and analysis of data collected about the client's model."[30:95]

MAJOR CONCEPTS & DEFINITIONS—cont'd

"Modeling occurs as the nurse accepts and understands her client."[30:96]

Role-Modeling "The art of Role-Modeling occurs when the nurse plans and implements interventions that are unique for the client. The science of Role-Modeling occurs as the nurse plans interventions with respect to her theoretical base for the practice of nursing. . . . Role-Modeling is . . . the essence of nurturance. . . . Role-Modeling requires an unconditional acceptance of the person as the person is while gently encouraging the facilitating growth and development at the person's own pace and within the person's own model."[30:95]

"Role-Modeling starts the second the nurse moves from the analysis phase of the nursing process to the planning of nursing interventions."[30:95]

Nursing "Nursing is the holistic helping of persons with their self-care activities in relation to their health. This is an interactive, interpersonal process that nurtures strengths to enable development, release, and channeling of resources for coping with one's circumstances and environment. The goal is to achieve a state of perceived optimum health and contentment."[30:49]

Nurturance "Nurturance fuses and integrates cognitive, physiological and affective processes, with the aim of assisting a client to move toward holistic health. Nurturance implies that the nurse seeks to know and understand the client's personal model of his or her world and to appreciate its value and significance for that client from the client's perspective."[30:48]

Unconditional Acceptance "Being accepted as a unique, worthwhile, important individual—with no strings attached—is imperative if the individual is to be facilitated in developing his or her own potential. The nurse's use of empathy helps the individual learn that the nurse accepts and respects him or her as is. The acceptance will facilitate the mobilization of resources needed as this individual strives for adaptive equilibrium."[30:49]

Person People are alike because of their holism, lifetime growth and development, and their need for affiliated-individuation. They are different because of their inherent endowment, adaptation, and self-care knowledge.

How People Are Alike

Holism "Human beings are holistic persons who have multiple interacting subsystems. Permeating all subsystems are the inherent bases. These include genetic makeup and spiritual drive. Body, mind, emotion, and spirit are a total unit and they act together. They affect and control one another interactively. The interaction of the multiple subsystems and the inherent bases creates holism: Holism implies that the whole is greater than the sum of the parts."[30:44-45]

Basic needs "All human beings have basic needs that can be satisfied, but only from within the framework of the individual."[31:58] "Basic needs are only met when the individual perceives that they are met."[30:57]

Lifetime development Lifetime develoment evolves through psychological and cognitive stages.

PSYCHOLOGICAL STAGES "Each stage represents a developmental task or decisive encounter resulting in a turning point, a moment of decision between alternative basic attitudes (for example, trust versus mistrust or autonomy versus shame and doubt). As a maturing individual negotiates or resolves each age-specific crisis or task, the individual gains enduring strengths and attitudes that contribute to the character and health of the individual's personality in his or her culture."[30:61]

COGNITIVE STAGES "Consider how thinking develops rather than what happens in psychosocial or affective development. . . . Piaget believed that cognitive learning develops in a sequential manner and he has identified several periods in this process. Essentially, there are four periods: sensorimotor, preoperational, concrete operations, and formal operations."[30:63-64]

Continued

MAJOR CONCEPTS & DEFINITIONS—cont'd

Affiliated-individuation "Individuals have an instinctual need for affiliated-individuation. They need to be able to be dependent on support systems while simultaneously maintaining independence from these support systems. They need to feel a deep sense of both the 'I' and the 'we' states of being and to perceive freedom and acceptance in both states."[30:47]

How People Are Different

Inherent endowment "Each individual is born with a set of genes that will to some extent predetermine appearance, growth, development, and responses to life events. . . . Clearly, both genetic makeup and inherited characteristics influence growth and development. They might influence how one perceives oneself and one's world. They make individuals different from one another, each unique in his or her own way."[30:74-75]

Adaptation Adaptation occurs as the individual responds to external and internal stressors in a health- and growth-directed manner. Adaptation involves mobilizing internal and external coping resources. No subsystem is left in jeopardy when adaptation occurs.[30:47]

The individual's ability to mobilize resources is depicted by APAM. The APAM identifies three different coping potential states: arousal, equilibrium (adaptive and maladaptive), and impoverishment. Each of these states represents a different potential to mobilize self-care resources.[30:80] "Movement among the states is influenced by one's ability to cope [with ongoing stressors] and the presence of new stressors."[30:80-81] Nurses can use this model to predict an individual's potential to mobilize self-care resources in response to stress.

Mind-body relationships "We are all biophysical, psychosocial beings who want to develop our potential, this is, to be the best we can be."[30:70]

Self-care Self-care involves the use of knowledge, resources, and action.

SELF-CARE KNOWLEDGE "At some level a person knows what has made him or her sick, lessened his or her effectiveness, or interfered with his or her growth. The person also knows what will make him or her well, optimize his or her effectiveness or fulfillment (given circumstances), or promote his or her growth."[30:48]

"The person also knows what will make him or her well, optimize his or her effectiveness or fulfillment (given circumstances), or promote his or her growth."[30:48]

SELF-CARE RESOURCES Self-care resources are "the internal resources, as well as additional resources, mobilized through self-care action that help gain, maintain, and promote an optimum level of holistic health."[30:254-255]

SELF-CARE ACTION Self-care action is "the development and utilization of self-care knowledge and self-care resources."[30:254]

MAJOR ASSUMPTIONS

Nursing

"The nurse is a facilitator, not an effector. Our nurse-client relationship is an interactive, interpersonal process that aids the individual to identify, mobilize, and develop his or her own strengths."[30:48]

Person

A differentiation is made between patients and clients in this theory. A patient is given treatment and instruction; a client participates in his own care. "Our goal is for nurses to work with clients."[30:21] "A client is one who is considered to be a legitimate member of the decision-making team, who always has some control over the planned regimen, and who is incorporated into the planning and implementation of his or her own care as much as possible."[30:20]

Health

"Health is a state of physical, mental, and social well-being, not merely the absence of disease or infirmity. It connotes a state of dynamic equilibrium among the various subsystems [of a holistic person]."[30:46]

Environment

"Environment is not identified in the theory as an entity of its own. The theorists see environment in the social subsystems as the interaction between self and others both cultural and individual. Biophysical stressors are seen as part of the environment."[24]

THEORETICAL ASSERTIONS

The theoretical assertions of the Modeling and Role-Modeling Theory are based on the linkages between completion of developmental tasks and basic need satisfaction; among basic need satisfaction, object attachment and loss, and developmental tasks; and between the ability to mobilize coping resources and need satisfaction. Three generic theoretical assertions that constitute a number of theoretical linkages implied in the theory but less specifically delineated are as follows:

1. "The degree to which developmental tasks are resolved is dependent on the degree to which human needs are satisfied."[30:87]
2. "The degree to which needs are satisfied by object attachment depends on the availability of those objects and the degree to which they provide comfort and security as opposed to threat and anxiety."[30:90]
3. "An individual's potential for mobilizing resources—the person's state of coping according to the APAM [Adaptive Potential Assessment Model]—is directly associated with the person's need satisfaction level."[30:91]

LOGICAL FORM

The Modeling and Role-Modeling Theory is formulated by the use of retroductive thinking. The theorists go through all four levels of theory development and then recycle from inductive to deductive to inductive to deductive.[24] The theoretical sources were used to validate clinical observations. Clinical observations were tested in light of the theoretical bases. These sources were synthesized with their observations, which enabled Erickson, Tomlin, and Swain to develop a "multi-dimensional new theory and paradigm—Modeling and Role-Modeling."[21]

The theorists label Modeling and Role-Modeling as a theory and a paradigm. The Modeling and Role-Modeling Theory meets the five functions of a paradigm as identified by Merton,[48:70] who said paradigms "provide a compact arrangement of central concepts and their interrelations that are utilized for description and analysis." First, the theorists provide a clear presentation of their central concepts and build on the relationships as they described them. Second, "paradigms lessen the likelihood of inadvertently introducing hidden assumptions and concepts, for each new assumption and concept must be either logically derived from previous components or explicitly introduced into it."[32:71] Erickson, Tomlin, and Swain build on previous components as their paradigm is developed, each component being logically derived from clinical observations or based in theory. "Third, paradigms advance the cumulation of theoretical interpretation."[32:71] The assumptions and concepts allow for interpretation in multiple clinical and research situations in which the concepts may be applied, thereby expanding the theory base of nursing. Fourth, "paradigms promote analysis rather than descriptions of concrete details."[32:71] The Modeling and Role-Modeling Theory promotes analysis of significant concepts. The interrelationships among the concepts can be empirically examined because they have broad applicability, and lend themselves to multiple research questions. "Fifth, paradigms make for codification of qualitative analysis in a way that approximates the logic if not the empirical rigor of quantitative analysis."[32:71] Erickson states that a qualitative approach has been used to form concepts. On the basis of that approach, scales were built with deductive logic to test those concepts.[21] The methods used will become available for replication of studies as they are published.

ACCEPTANCE BY THE NURSING COMMUNITY

Practice

Publication of the book *Modeling and Role-Modeling: A Theory and Paradigm for Nursing* and a chapter on self-care on *Introduction to Person-Centered Nursing*, as well as publication of research studies based on the theory, have exposed practicing nurses to this theory. Nurses on surgical units at the University of Michigan Medical Center are using an assessment tool based on the Modeling and Role-Modeling Theory. The tool is used to gather information to identify the client's need assets, deficits, developmental residual, attachment-loss and grief status, and potential therapeutic interventions (see Appendix at end of this chapter).[9,22]

The theorists have spoken on their theory and have held one-to-one consultations that exposed nurses from various practice and educational backgrounds to the theory. Nurses in critical care, adult health, mental health, and hospices are using the theory. Erickson[21] has noted that what seemed to be a revolutionary idea as recently as 11 to 12 years ago—calling for the client to be head of the health care team—is rapidly gaining acceptance, as is the notion that nurses can practice nursing independently. According to Erickson,[21] negative responses to the theory came from individuals who cannot accept the idea of listening to the client first or who do not take the concept of holism seriously.

Brigham and Women's Hospital in Boston has used the Modeling and Role-Modeling Theory as a theoretical basis for their professional practice model in the institution for the past several years. The nurses use the theory as a framework to structure care planning and conduct case conferences. Jenny James,[38] prior vice president for nursing, states that "consistency of language, the way care is talked about and planned" is one of the major advantages of using this theoretical basis. The basic fundamentals of the theory are easy to apply in practice, and with a small amount of knowledge an individual can begin to apply the theory. Nurses at Brigham and Women's Hospital use an adaptation of the assessment tool developed at University of Michigan Medical Center. At the Fourth National Conference on Modeling and Role-Modeling held in Boston in October 1992, information on the implementation of the professional practice model at Brigham and Women's Hospital, as well as case studies, were presented by staff nurses.[38]

Nurses at the University of Pittsburgh Medical Center in Pittsburgh Pennsylvania, as well as other hospitals and state agencies across the country, have also adopted modeling and role-modeling as a theoretical foundation for their professional practice model.

Education

The theory is introduced into the curriculum in the sophomore year at the University of Michigan School of Nursing and is required for returning RN students as well. Faculty members at several nursing schools have contacted Erickson regarding the use of the theory in their curricula. Humboldt State University at Arcata, California, has selected modeling and role-modeling as a conceptual framework for their curriculum and has been accredited by the National League for Nursing.[26] Other nursing programs that use modeling and role-modeling as a basis for curriculum include the University at St. Paul, Minnesota. Finally, Foo Yin College of Nursing and Medical Technology is developing a baccalaureate program based on this theory and will translate the book into Chinese.

Introduction to Person-Centered Nursing, with a chapter on self-care by Tomlin, is being used as a text in various schools of nursing and is expanding exposure to the theory concepts.[57]

Research

Erickson and Swain continue to research the Modeling and Role-Modeling Theory. One study completed was entitled "Modeling and Role-Modeling: Testing Nursing Theory." Research activity continues to support and validate the self-care knowledge construct and the importance of support and control.[19,23] The initial study provided evidence that psychosocial factors are significantly related to physical health problems. A follow-up study (1988) supported these findings, and subsequent research has provided for expansion and enrichment of the concepts. Key concepts include perceived support, perceived control, hope for the future, and satisfaction with daily life. The 1988 study was authored by Erickson, S. Lock, and Swain.[22]

The theorists identify several other research projects that are tests of the theory. Several doctoral students at the University of Michigan School of Nursing, the University of Texas at Austin, and other universities are pursuing various research questions based on the theory. A research study was conducted at the University of Michigan Medical Center by three nurses who hypothesized that length of hospital stay correlated with stages of development. A nursing assessment tool was adapted from the assessment model proposed by the theorists D. Finch, J. Campbell, and M. Hunt and was used to measure a patient's psychosocial development and to relate developmental status to the length of hospitalization and the number of health problems identified during hospitalization. Results indicate that the balance of trust-mistrust accounts for a large percentage of the variance in the length of hospitalization. There was no significant relationship between psychosocial coping skills and number of health problems identified.[9]

Erickson was the principal investigator of a research project, Modeling and Role-Modeling with Alzheimer's Patients, funded by the National Institutes of Health, National Center for Nursing Research. This research project included 10 other investigators. Results supported the constructs of self-care knowledge and affiliated individuation.[26]

Numerous graduate students have also used the Theory of Modeling and Role-Modeling as a basis for their theses and dissertations. In addition, extensive work has been published that substantiates many of the major constructs and theoretical linkages of the theory.[17] Finally, an integrative review of all research using modeling and role-modeling (through 1992) as a theoretical basis was conducted by Baas and Hertz.[35] Empirical evidence has provided bases for validation, refinement, and revision of the theory. It is expected that research will continue to expand the Modeling and Role-Modeling Theory.

FURTHER DEVELOPMENT

This theory is in its infancy; therefore, there is much potential for further development. Currently, the theory is gaining national and international attention. One reason for this increased attention is the founding of the Society for the Advancement of Modeling and Role-Modeling. The society was formed to develop a network of colleagues who could advance the development and application of the Modeling and Role-Modeling Theory. One of the goals is to promote continued research related to the theory. The society held its first national symposium in 1986 and has met biennially thereafter. At the 1988 conference, held at Hilton Head, South Carolina, the membership chair announced that society members came from 12 different states.[22] By the time of the 1990 conference in Austin, members represented more than 30 states.[26] These conferences are a forum for researchers, educators, and practitioners to disseminate knowledge pertaining to the Modeling and Role-Modeling Theory and paradigm.[22]

The Fourth National Conference on Modeling and Role-Modeling Theory and Paradigm for Professionals, held in Boston in October 1992, demonstrated the breadth and depth of the current use and research for the Modeling and Role-Modeling Theory. Presentations included studies based in critical care units and community-based practice, multiple types of educational settings, and across the age span.

The biennial conferences continue to provide an opportunity for nurses to discuss interrelationships among nursing practice, theory, research, and education.

Much of the research data related to the theory is yet to be published. Erickson[20] states, "Every part of it [the theory] needs further development. . . . There are a thousand research questions in that book. . . . You can take any one statement we make and ask a research question about it. . . . Modeling and Role Modeling has only begun."

CRITIQUE

Clarity

Erickson, Tomlin, and Swain present their theory clearly. Definitions in the theory are denotative, with the concepts explicitly defined. They use everyday language and offer many examples to illustrate their meaning. Their definitions and assumptions are consistent, and there is a logical progression from assumptions to assertions.

Simplicity

The theory appears simple at first. On closer inspection, however, it becomes complex. It is based on biological and psychological theories and several of the theorists' own assumptions. The interactions among the major concepts, assumptions, and assertions add depth to the theory and increase its complexity.

Generality

Because major assumptions that deal with developmental tasks, basic needs satisfaction, object attachment and loss, and adaptive potential are broad enough to be applicable in multiple diverse nursing situations, the theory is generalizable to all nursing and client situations. The theorists cite many examples of the applicability of their concepts, both in clinical practice and research. Although it may be argued that the theory lacks applicability in the pediatric or comatose population, the theorists believe the theory is also applicable in these situations, although it may take some creativity by the clinician to achieve. The Modeling and Role-Modeling Theory is generalizable to all aspects of professional nursing practice.

Empirical Precision

Empirical precision is increased if the theory has operationally defined concepts, identifiable subconcepts, and denotative definitions. The major concepts, modeling and role-modeling, are reality-based, which makes them more empirical than general. Definitions in the theory are denotative, making it

possible to test empirically the concepts identified. The theorists provide an outline for collecting, analyzing, and synthesizing data and guidelines for implementing their theory based on the client's model. These explicit guidelines increase the empirical precision of the theory by allowing any practitioner to test the theory using these tools.

Chinn and Jacobs state,[11:42] "Empirical precision is necessarily increased with research testing." Data reflecting research testing of the theory is not currently readily available; however, as has been stated, studies are ongoing. We believe the Theory of Modeling and Role-Modeling will gain empirical precision when data become available for critical analysis. The theorists recognize the need for further research of their theory and encourage practicing nurses to do it.[8]

Derivable Consequences

One of the many challenges facing the profession of nursing is the development of a unique, scientific knowledge base. One aid in this process is the use of nursing theory as a basis for professional practice. Erickson, Tomlin, and Swain's Theory of Modeling and Role-Modeling can provide the stimulus to accomplish this goal.

Although this theory is relatively new, it is gaining recognition in the nursing community. As interest grows, additional research supporting its theoretical statements will be generated. Many nurses are engaged in research based on this theory. Publication of the findings will lend credence to the theoretical propositions.

Chinn and Jacobs[11] state that a theory should be evaluated in terms of its derivable consequences. The derivable consequences can be determined by examining whether the theory guides research, directs practice, generates new ideas, and differentiates the focus of nursing from other professions.[11:42] In terms of these criteria, this theory does appear to possess inherent value, although the scope is undeterminable at this time. As the theory matures, the extent of its merit and worth will become evident; however, one thing can undoubtedly be said. Erickson, Tomlin, and Swain's Theory of Modeling and Role-Modeling encourages, as well as challenges, nurses to practice theory-based nursing.

CRITICAL THINKING *Activities*

1 Interview a client and use the theory to interpret the data. Identify nursing diagnoses based on the interpretations.

2 Given the findings, propose a nursing plan of care. Identify what predictions can be made if the care is not given.

3 Assuming that the goal is to promote the client's health and development, predict the outcome on the basis of the proposed nursing plan of care.

4 Assess the client from primary, secondary, and tertiary sources. Compare for congruency among the three types of sources.

REFERENCES

1. Acton, G. (1993). *Relationships among stressors, stress, affiliated-individuation, burden, and well-being in care-givers of adults with dementia: A test of the theory and par-adigm for nursing, modeling and role-modeling.* Doctoral dissertation, University of Texas, Austin.
2. Baas, L.S. (1992). *The relationships among self-care knowl-edge, self-care resources, activity level and life satisfaction in persons three to six months after a myocardial infarction.* Doctoral dissertation, University of Texas, Austin. *Dissertation Abstracts International, 53,* 1780B.
3. Babcock, M., & Mueller, P. (1980). *Accidents and life stress.* Unpublished master's thesis, University of Michigan.
4. Barnfather, J.S. (1987). Mobilizing coping resources related to basic need status in healthy, young adults. *Dissertation Abstracts International, 49/02-B,* 0360.
5. Barnfather, J.S. (1990). Mobilizing coping resources related to basic need status. In Kinney, C., & Erickson, H. (Eds.), *Modeling and role-modeling: Theory, practice and research* (Vol. 1) (pp. 156-169). Society for Advancement of Modeling and Role-Modeling.
6. Barnfather, J. (1993). Testing a theoretical proposition for modeling and role-modeling: A basic need and adaptive potential status. *Issues in Mental Health Nursing, 13,* 1-18.
7. Boodley, C.A. (1990). The experience of having a healthy examination. In H. Erickson & C. Kinney (Eds.), *Modeling and role-modeling: Theory, practice and research* (Vol. 1) (pp. 1170-1177). Society for Advancement of Modeling and Role-Modeling.
8. Cain, E., & Perzynski, K. (1986). *Utilization of the self care knowledge model with wife caregivers.* Unpublished master's thesis, University of Michigan.
9. Campbell, J., Finch, D., Allport, C., Erickson, H.C., & Swain, M.A. (1985). A theoretical approach to nursing assessment. *Journal of Advanced Nursing, 10,* 111-115.
10. Chen, Y. (1996). *Relationships among health control orien-tation, self-efficacy, self-care, and subjective well-being in the elderly with hypertension.* Doctoral dissertation, University of Texas, Austin.
11. Chinn, P.L., & Jacobs, M.K. (1983). Theory and nursing: A systematic approach. St. Louis: Mosby.
12. Clementino, D., & Lapinske, M. (1980). *The effects of dif-ferent preparatory messages on distress from a bronchoscopy.* Unpublished master's thesis, University of Michigan.
13. Curl, E.D. (1992). *Hope in the elderly: Exploring the rela-tionship between psychosocial developmental residual and hope.* Doctoral dissertation, University of Texas, Austin. *Dissertation Abstracts International, 47,* 992B.
14. Darling-Fisher, C., & Leidy, N. (1988). Measuring Erik-sonian development of the adult: The modified Erikson psychosocial stage inventory. *Psychological Reports, 62,* 747-754.
15. Doornbos, M. (1983). *The relationship of the social net-work to emotional health in the aged.* Unpublished master's thesis, University of Michigan.
16. Erickson, H. (1985). Self-care knowledge: Relations among the concepts support, hope, control, satisfaction with life, and physical health. In *Social support and health: New directions for theory development and research* (pp. 208-212). University of Rochester.
17. Erickson, H. (1990). Modeling and role-modeling with psychophysiological problems. In J.K. Zeig & S. Gilligan (Eds.), *Brief therapy: Myths, methods, and metaphors* (pp. 473-491). New York: Brunner/Mazel.
18. Erickson, H. (1990). Theory based nursing. In C. Kinney & H. Erickson (Eds.), *Modeling and role-modeling: Theory, practice and research* (Vol. 1) (pp. 1-27). Society for Advancement of Modeling and Role-Modeling.
19. Erickson, H.C. (1976). *Identification of states of coping uti-lization physiological and psychological data.* Unpublished Master's thesis, University of Michigan.
20. Erickson, H.C. (1984, Nov. 5). Telephone interview.
21. Erickson, H.C. (1984, Nov. 7). Telephone interview.
22. Erickson, H.C. (1988). Personal correspondence.
23. Erickson, H.C. (1988, Feb.). Curriculum vitae.
24. Erickson, H.C. (1988, March 30). Telephone interview.
25. Erickson, H.C. (1992, July). Curriculum vitae.
26. Erickson, H.C. (1992, July 1). Personal correspondence.
27. Erickson, H.C., Kinney, C., Becker, H., Acton, G., Irvin, B., Hopkins, R., & Jensen, B. (1994). *Modeling and role-modeling with Alzheimer's patients.* (National Institutes of Health funded grant). University of Texas, Austin. Un-published manuscript.

28. Erickson, H.C., Kinney, C., Stone, D., & Acton, G. (1990). *Self-care activities, knowledge, and resources related to physical health.* Unpublished manuscript, University of Texas, Austin.

29. Erickson, H.C., & Swain, M.A. (1982). A model for assessing potential adaptation to stress. *Research in Nursing and Health, 5,* 93-101.

30. Erickson, H.C., Tomlin, E.M., & Swain, M.A. (1983). *Modeling and role-modeling: A theory and paradigm for nursing.* Englewood Cliffs, NJ: Prentice-Hall.

31. Erickson, M. (1996). *Relationships among support, needs satisfaction, and maternal attachment in the adolescent mother.* Doctoral dissertation, University of Texas, Austin.

32. Finch, D. (1987). *Testing a theoretically based nursing assessment.* Doctoral dissertation, University of Michigan.

33. Finch, D.A. (1990). Testing a theoretically based nursing assessment. In C. Kinney & H. Erickson (Eds.), *Modeling and role-modeling: Theory, practice and research* (Vol. 1) (pp. 203-213). Society for Advancement of Modeling and Role-Modeling.

34. Hannan, J., & McLaughlin, K. (1983). *Relationship between interpersonal trust and compliance in the adolescent with diabetes.* Unpublished master's thesis, University of Michigan.

35. Hertz, J.E.G. (1991). *The perceived enactment of autonomy scale: Measuring the potential for self-care action in the elderly.* Doctoral dissertation, University of Texas, Austin. *Dissertation Abstracts International, 52,* 1953B.

36. Holl, R.M. (1992). *The effect of role-modeled visiting in comparison to restricted visiting on the well-being of clients who had open heart surgery and their significant family members in the critical care unit.* Doctoral dissertation, University of Texas, Austin. *Dissertation Abstracts International, 53,* 4030B.

37. Irvin, B.L. (1993). *Social support, self-worth and hope as self-care resources for coping with caregiver stress.* Doctoral dissertation, University of Texas, Austin. *Dissertation Abstracts International, 54* (06), B2995.

38. James, J. (1992, July 6). Telephone interview.

39. Jensen, B. (1995). *Caregiver responses to a theoretically based intervention program: Case study analysis.* Doctoral dissertation, University of Texas, Austin.

40. Keck, V.E. (1989). *Perceived social support, basic needs satisfaction, and coping strategies of the chronically ill.* Doctoral dissertation, University of Michigan. *Dissertation Abstracts International, 50,* 3921B.

41. Kennedy, G.T. (1991). *A nursing investigation of comfort and comforting care of the acutely ill patient.* Doctoral dissertation, University of Texas, Austin. *Dissertation Abstracts International, 52,* 6318B.

42. Kinney, C.K. (1990). Facilitating growth and development: A paradigm case for modeling and role-modeling. *Issues in Mental Health Nursing, 11,* 375-395.

43. Kinney, C. (1992). Psychosocial developmental correlates of coronary prone behavior in healthy adults. Manuscript submitted for publication.

44. Kleinbeck, S. (1977). *Coping states of stress.* Unpublished master's thesis, University of Michigan.

45. Kline, N.W. (1988). *Psychophysiological processes of stress in people with a chronic physical illness.* Doctoral dissertation, University of Michigan. *Dissertation Abstracts International, 49,* 2129B.

46. Landis, B.J. (1991). *Uncertainty, spiritual well-being, and psychosocial adjustment to chronic illness.* Doctoral dissertation, University of Texas, Austin. *Dissertation Abstracts International, 52,* 4124B.

47. MacLean, T.T. (1987). *Erikson's development and stressors as factors in healthy lifestyle.* Doctoral dissertation, University of Michigan. *Dissertation Abstracts International, 48,* 1710A.

48. Merton, R.K. (1968). Social theory and social structure. New York: The Free Press.

49. Miller, E.W. (1994). *The meaning of encouragement and its connection to the inner-spirit as perceived by caregivers of the cognitively impaired.* Doctoral dissertation, University of Texas, Austin.

50. Miller, S.H. (1986). *The relationship between psychosocial development and coping ability among disabled teenagers.* Doctoral dissertation, University of Michigan. *Dissertation Abstracts International, 47,* 4113B.

51. Raudonis, B. (1991). *A nursing study of empathy from the hospice patient's perspective.* Doctoral dissertation, University of Texas, Austin.

52. Robinson, K.R. (1992). *Developing a scale to measure responses of clients with actual or potential myocardial infarctions.* Doctoral dissertation, University of Texas, Austin. *Dissertation Abstracts International, 53,* 6226B.

53. Rosenow, D.J. (1991). *Multidimensional scaling analysis of self-care actions for reintegrating holistic health after a myocardial infarction: Implications for nursing.* Doctoral dissertation, University of Texas, Austin. *Dissertation Abstracts International, 53,* 1789B.

54. Scheela, R. (1991). *The remodeling process: A grounded study of adult male incest offenders' perceptions of the treatment process.* Doctoral dissertation, University of Texas, Austin.

55. Smith, K. (1980). *Relationship between social support and goal attainment.* Unpublished master's thesis, University of Michigan.

56. Swain, M.A.P. (1988, Feb.). Curriculum vitae.

57. Tomlin, E.M. (1984, Oct.). Curriculum vitae.

58. Tomlin, E.M. (1988, Feb.). Curriculum vitae.

59. Tomlin, E.M. (1992, July). Curriculum vitae.

60. Tomlin, E.M. (1992, July). Telephone interview.

61. Tomlin, E.M. (1996, July 10). Telephone interview.

BIBLIOGRAPHY
Primary sources
Books

Erickson, H., & Kinney, C. (Eds.), (1990). *Modeling and role-modeling: Theory, practice and research.* Austin, TX: Society for Advancement of Modeling and Role-Modeling.

Erickson, H.C., Tomlin, E.M., & Swain, M.A. (1990). *Modeling and role-modeling: A theory and paradigm for nursing.* Austin, TX: EST. Original publication Englewood Cliffs, NJ: Prentice-Hall (1983).

Book chapters

Barnfather, J. (1990). An overview of the ability to mobilize coping resources related to basic needs. In H. Erickson & C. Kinney (Eds.), *Modeling and role-modeling: Theory, practice and research* (Vol. 1) (pp. 156-169). Austin, TX: Society for Advancement of Modeling and Role-Modeling.

Boodley, C.A. (1990). The experience of having a healthy examination. In H. Erickson & C. Kinney (Eds.), *Modeling and role-modeling: Theory, practice and research* (Vol. 1) (pp. 1170-1177). Austin, TX: Society for Advancement of Modeling and Role-Modeling.

Erickson, H. (1977). Communication in nursing. In *Professional nursing matrix: A workbook* (pp. 1-150). Ann Arbor, MI: Media Library, University of Michigan.

Erickson, H. (1985). Modeling and role modeling: Ericksonian approaches with physiological problems. In J. Zeig & S. Langton (Eds.), *Ericksonian psychotherapy: The state of the art.* New York: Brunner/Mazel.

Erickson, H. (1990). Modeling and role-modeling with psychophysiological problems. In J.K. Zeig & Gilligan, S., (Eds.), *Brief therapy: Myths, methods, and metaphors* (pp. 473-491). New York: Brunner/Mazel.

Erickson, H. (1990). Self-care knowledge: An exploratory study. In C. Kinney & H. Erickson (Eds.), *Modeling and role-modeling: Theory, practice and research* (Vol. 1) (pp. 178-202). Austin, TX: Society for Advancement of Modeling and Role-Modeling.

Erickson, H. (1990). Theory based nursing. In C. Kinney & H. Erickson (Eds.), *Modeling and role-modeling: Theory, practice and research* (Vol. 1) (pp. 1-27). Austin, TX: Society for Advancement of Modeling and Role-Modeling.

Finch, D.A. (1990). Testing a theoretically based nursing assessment. In C. Kinney & H. Erickson (Eds.), *Modeling and role-modeling: Theory, practice and research* (Vol. 1) (pp. 203-213). Austin, TX: Society for Advancement of Modeling and Role-Modeling.

MacLean, T. (1990). Health behaviors, developmental residual and stressors. In C. Kinney & H. Erickson (Eds.), *Modeling and role-modeling: Theory, practice and research* (Vol. 1) (pp. 147-155). Austin, TX: Society for Advancement of Modeling and Role-Modeling.

Tomlin, E.M. (1983). Self-care. In J. Lindberg, M. Hunter, & A. Kruszewski (Eds.), *Introduction to person-centered nursing* (pp. 51-60). Philadelphia: JB Lippincott.

Journal articles

Acton, G., & Miller, E. (1996). Affiliated-individuation in caregivers of adults with dementia. *Issues in Mental Health Nursing, 17,* 245-260.

Barnfather, J. (1993). Testing a theoretical proposition for modeling and role-modeling: A basic need and adaptive potential status. *Issues in Mental Health Nursing, 13,* 1-18.

Barnfather, J., Swain, M.A., Erickson, H. (1989). Construct validity of an aspect of the coping process: Potential adaptation to stress. *Issues in Mental Health Nursing, 10,* 23-40.

Barnfather, J., Swain, M.A., & Erickson, H. (1989). Evaluation of two assessment techniques. *Nursing Science Quarterly, 4,* 172-182.

Beery, T., & Baas, L. (1996). Medical devices and attachment: Holistic healing in the age of invasive technology. *Issues in Mental Health Nursing, 17,* 233-243.

Campbell, J., Finch, D., Allport, C., Erickson, H., & Swain, M. (1985). A theoretical approach to nursing assessment. *Journal of Advanced Nursing, 10,* 111-115.

Darling-Fisher, C., & Leidy, N. (1988). Measuring Eriksonian development of the adult: The modified Erikson psychosocial stage inventory. *Psychological Reports, 62,* 747-754.

Erickson, H. (1983, March). Coping with new systems. *Journal of Nursing Education,* 132-136.

Erickson, H. (1991). Erickson, H. Modeling y role-modeling con psychophysiological problemas. *Rapport. Journal of Instituto de Hipnoterapia Ericksoniana.* Buenes Aires, Argentina.

Erickson, H., & Swain, M.A. (1982). A model for assessing potential adaptation to stress. *Research in Nursing and Health, 5,* 93-101.

Erickson, H., & Swain, M.A. (1990). Mobilizing self-care resources: A nursing intervention for hypertension. *Issues in Mental Health Nursing, 11,* 217-236.

Erickson, M. (1996). Factors that influence the mother-infant dyad relationships and infant well-being. *Issues in Mental Health Nursing, 17,* 185-200.

Hertz, J. (1996). Conceptualization of perceived enactment of autonomy in the elderly. *Issues in Mental Health Nursing, 17,* 261-273.

Irvin, B., & Acton, G. (1996). Stress mediation in caregivers of cognitively impaired adults: Theoretical model testing. *Nursing Research, 45*(3), 160-166.

Irvin, B., & Acton, G. Stress, hope and well-being of women caring for family members with Alzheimer's disease. *Holistic Nursing Practice.* In press.

Kinney, C. (1996). Transcending breast cancer: Reconstructing one's self. *Issues in Mental Health Nursing, 17,* 201-216.

Kinney, C., & Erickson, H. (1990). Modeling the client's world: A way to holistic care. *Issues in Mental Health Nursing, 11,* 93-108.

Kinney, C.K. (1990). Facilitating growth and development: A paradigm case for modeling and role-modeling. *Issues in Mental Health Nursing, 11,* 375-395.

Landis, B.J. (1996). Uncertainty, spiritual well-being, and psychosocial adjustment to chronic illness. *Issues in Mental Health Nursing, 17,* 217-231.

Leidy, N. (1990). A structural model of stress, psychosocial resources and symptomatic experience in chronic physical illness. *Nursing Research, 39,* 230-236.

Leidy, N. (1994). Operationalizing Maslow's theory: Development and testing of the Basic Needs Satisfaction Inventory. *Issues in Mental Health Nursing, 15,* 277-295.

Leidy, N.K. (1989). A physiological analysis of stress and chronic illness. *Journal of Advanced Nursing, 14,* 868-876.

Leidy, N.K., & Traver, G.A. (1995). Psychophysiological factors contribution to functional performance in people with COPD: Are there gender differences? *Research in Nursing and Health, 18,* 535-546.

MacLean, T. (1992). Influence of psychosocial development and life events on the health practices of adults. *Issues in Mental Health Nursing, 13,* 403-414.

Miller, E.W. (1995). Encouraging Alzheimer's caregivers. *Journal of Christian Nursing, 12*(4), 7-12.

Ozbolt, J. (1987). Developing decision support systems for nursing—theoretical bases for advanced computer systems. *Computers in Nursing, 5,* 105-111.

Robinson, K.R. (1994). Developing a scale to measure denial levels of clients with actual or potential myocardial infarctions. *Heart and Lung, 23,* 36-44.

Rogers, S. (1990). Facilitative affiliation: Nurse-client interactions that enhance healing. *Issues in Mental Health Nursing, 17,* 171-184.

Sappington, J., & Kelley, J.H. (1996). Modeling and role-modeling theory: A case study of holistic care. *Journal of Holistic Nursing, 14*(2), 130-141.

Walsh, K.K., Vanden Bosch, T.M., & Boehm, S. (1989). Modeling and role-modeling: Integrating nursing theory into practice. *Journal of Advanced Nursing, 14,* 775-761.

Abstracts

Erickson, H. (1985). Self-care knowledge: Relations among the concepts support, hope, control, satisfaction with life, and physical health. *Social Support and Health: New Directions for Theory Development and Research* (pp. 208-212). University of Rochester.

Erickson, H. (1989). Mind-body relationships as a factor in the care of people with diabetes. *Third Annual Conference of the Southern Nursing Research Society* (p. 47).

Erickson, H. (1989). Study of the self-care knowledge construct. *Third Annual Conference of the Southern Nursing Research Society* (p. 10).

Erickson, H. (1990). The McKennell model: using qualitative methods to guide instrument development. *Fourth Annual Conference of the Southern Nursing Research Society* (p. 115).

Erickson, H. (1991). The relationships among self-care knowledge, self-care resources and physical health. *Proceedings of the Fifth Annual Conference of the Southern Nursing Research Society.*

Erickson, H. (1993). Intervention research with cognitively impaired persons and their caregivers. *Nursing's Challenge: Leadership in Changing Times.* STTI 32nd Biennial Convention. Indianapolis, IN.

Erickson, H. (1995). Caring, comforting and healing. Conference Proceedings. *Sixth National AJN Conference on Medical-Surgical and Geriatric Nursing.*

Erickson, H., Acton, G., Baas, L., Robinson, K., & Rossi, L. (1992). Strategies to humanize care in the ICU. *Proceedings: Celebrating Patnerships.* AACN NTI. New Orleans, LA.

Erickson, H., & Kennedy, G. (1992). Viewing the world through the patient's eyes. *Proceedings: Celebrating Partnerships.* AACN NTI. New Orleans, LA.

Erickson, H., Kinney, C., Acton, G., Becker, H., Irvin, B., Jensen, B., & Miller, E. (1994). An intervention study: Persons with Alzheimer's disease and their caregivers. Conference Proceedings. *The Fifth National Conference for the Theory of Modeling and Role-Modeling.*

Erickson, H., Lock, S., & Swain, M. (1989). Continuation of the study of the self-care knowledge construct in the modeling and role-modeling theory. *Advances in International Nursing Scholarship. Sigma Theta Tau International Research Congress* (p. 84). Taipei, Taiwan: Sigma Theta Tau International Honor Society.

Erickson, H.C., & Swain, M.A. (1977). The utilization of a nursing care model for treatment of essential hypertension. *Circulation* 56 (Suppl III), 145.

Theses

Babcock, M., & Mueller, P. (1980). *Accidents and life stress.* Unpublished master's thesis, University of Michigan.

Cain, E., & Perzynski, K. (1986). *Utilization of the self care knowledge model with wife caregivers.* Unpublished master's thesis, University of Michigan.

Calvin, A. (1991). *Personal control: Conceptual analysis and its role in the nursing theory of modeling and role-modeling.* Unpublished master's thesis, University of Texas, Austin.

Cehaich, K., & Nalski, J. (1984). *Life change events, self-concept, and the injury rate of female high school basketball players.* Unpublished master's thesis, University of Michigan.

Clementino, D., & Lapinske, M. (1980). *The effects of different preparatory messages on distress from a bronchoscopy.* Unpublished master's thesis, University of Michigan.

Doornbos, M. (1983). *The relationship of the social network to emotional health in the aged.* Unpublished master's thesis, University of Michigan.

Finch, D. (1987). *Testing a theoretically based nursing assessment.* Unpublished master's thesis, University of Michigan.

Hannan, J., & McLaughlin, K. (1983). *Relationship between interpersonal trust and compliance in the adolescent with diabetes.* Unpublished master's thesis, University of Michigan.

Kirk, L. (1996). *A descriptive study of level of hope in cancer patients.* Unpublished master's thesis, University of Texas, San Antonio.

Kleinbeck, S. (1977). *Coping states of stress.* Unpublished master's thesis, University of Michigan.

Merritt, J., & Swender, K. (1984). *Marital status and social support in elderly women.* Unpublished master's thesis, University of Michigan.

Smith, K. (1980). *Relationship between social support and goal attainment.* Unpublished master's thesis, University of Michigan.

Stein, K. (1986). *Beyond self-esteem: New dimensions in the relationship between the self concept and coping.* Unpublished preliminary examination, University of Michigan.

Walker, M. (1990). *Modeling and role-modeling and quantum physics.* Unpublished master's thesis, University of Texas, Austin.

Dissertations

Acton, G. (1993). *Relationships among stressors, stress, affiliated-individuation, burden, and well-being in caregivers of adults with dementia: A test of the theory and paradigm for nursing, Modeling and Role-modeling.* Doctoral dissertation, University of Texas, Ausin.

Baas, L.S. (1992). *The relationships among self-care knowledge, self-care resources, activity level and life satisfaction in persons three to six months after a myocadial infarction.* Doctoral dissertation, University of Texas, Austin. *Dissertation Abstracts International, 53,* 1780B.

Barnfather, J.S. (1987). *Mobilizing coping resources related to basic need status in healthy, young adults.* Doctoral dissertation, University of Michigan. *Dissertation Abstracts International, 49,* 360B.

Boodley, C.A. (1986). *A nursing study of the experience of having a health examination.* Doctoral dissertation, University of Michigan. *Dissertation Abstracts International, 47,* 992B.

Chen, Y. (1996). *Relationships among health control orientation, self-efficacy, self-care, and subjective well-being in the elderly with hypertension.* Doctoral dissertation, University of Texas, Austin.

Curl, E.D. (1992). *Hope in the elderly: Exploring the relationship between psychosocial developmental residual and hope.* Doctoral dissertation, University of Texas, Austin. *Dissertation Abstracts International, 47,* 992B.

Daniels, R. (1994). *Exploring the self-care variables that explains a wellness lifestyle in spinal cord injured wheelchair basketball athletes.* Doctoral dissertation, University of Texas, Austin.

Darling-Fisher, C.S. (1987). *The relationship between mothers' and fathers' Eriksonian psychosocial attributes, perceptions of family support, and adaptation to parenthood.* Doctoral dissertation, University of Michigan. *Dissertation Abstracts International, 48,* 1640B.

Erickson, M. (1996). *Relationships among support, needs satisfaction, and maternal attachment in the adolescent mother.* Doctoral dissertation, University of Texas, Austin.

Hertz, J.E.G. (1991). *The perceived enactment of autonomy scale: Measuring the potential for self-care action in the elderly.* Doctoral dissertation. University of Texas, Austin. *Dissertation Abstracts International, 52,* 1953B.

Holl, R.M. (1992). *The effect of role-modeled visiting in comparison to restricted visiting on the well-being of clients who had open heart surgery and their significant family members in the critical care unit.* Doctoral dissertation, University of Texas, Austin. *Dissertation Abstracts International, 53,* 4030B.

Hopkins, B. (1994). *Assessment of adaptive potential.* Doctoral dissertation, University of Texas, Austin.

Irvin, B.L. (1993). *Social support, self-worth and hope as self-care resources for coping with caregiver stress.* Doctoral dissertation, University of Texas, Austin. *Dissertation Abstracts International, 54*(06), B2995.

Jensen, B. (1995). *Caregiver responses to a theoretically based intervention program: Case study analysis.* Doctoral dissertation, University of Texas, Austin.

Kennedy, G.T. (1991). *A nursing investigation of comfort and comforting care of the acutely ill patient.* Doctoral dissertation, University of Texas, Austin. *Dissertation Abstracts International, 52,* 6318B.

Kline, N.W. (1988). *Psychophysiological processes of stress in people with a chronic physical illness.* Doctoral dissertation, University of Michigan. *Dissertation Abstracts International, 49,* 2129B.

Landis, B.J. (1991). *Uncertainty, spiritual well-being, and psychosocial adjustment to chronic illness.* Doctoral dissertation, University of Texas, Austin. *Dissertation Abstracts International, 52,* 4124B.

MacLean, T.T. (1987). *Erikson's development and stressors as factors in healthy lifestyle.* Doctoral dissertation, University of Michigan. *Dissertation Abstracts International, 48,* 1710A.

Miller, E.W. (1994). *The meaning of encouragement and its connection to the inner-spirit as perceived by caregivers of the cognitively impaired.* Doctoral dissertation, University of Texas, Austin.

Miller, S.H. (1986). *The relationship between psychosocial development and coping ability among disabled teenagers.* Doctoral dissertation, University of Michigan. *Dissertation Abstracts International, 47,* 4113B.

Raudonis, B. (1991). *A nursing study of empathy from the hospice patient's perspective.* Doctoral dissertation, University of Texas, Austin.

Robinson, K.R. (1992). *Developing a scale to measure responses of client with actual or potential myocardial infarctions.* Doctoral dissertation, University of Texas, Austin. *Dissertation Abstracts International, 53,* 6226B.

Rosenow, D.J. (1991). *Multidimensional scaling analysis of self-care actions for reintegrating holistic health after a myocardial infarction: Implications for nursing.* Doctoral dissertation, University of Texas, Austin. *Dissertation Abstracts International, 53,* 1789B.

Scheela, R. (1991). *The remodeling process: A grounded study of adult male incest offenders' perceptions of the treatment process.* Doctoral dissertation, University of Texas, Austin.

Sofhauser, C. (1996). *The relationships among self-esteem, psychosocial residual, self-concept, and hostility in persons with coronary heart disease.* Doctoral dissertation, University of Texas, Austin.

Straub, H. (1993). *The relationship among intellectual, psychosocial, and ego development of nursing students in associate, baccalaureate, and baccalaureate-completion programs.* Doctoral dissertation, University of Texas, Austin.

Weber, G. (1995). *Employed mothers with pre-school aged children: An exploration of their lived experiences and the nature of their well-being.* Doctoral dissertation, University of Texas, Austin.

Correspondence

Erickson, H.C. (1984, Oct.). Curriculum vitae.

Erickson, H.C. (1988). Personal correspondence.

Erickson, H.C. (1988, Feb.). Curriculum vitae.

Erickson, H.C. (1992, July). Curriculum vitae.

James, J. (1992, July). Curriculum vitae.

Swain, M.A. (1984, Oct.). Curriculum vitae.

Swain, M.A.P. (1988. Feb.). Curriculum vitae.

Tomlin, E.M. (1984, Oct.). Curriculum vitae.

Tomlin, E.M. (1988, Feb.). Curriculum vitae.

Tomlin, E.M. (1992, July). Curriculum vitae.

Interviews

Erickson, H. (1984, Nov. 5). Telephone interview.

Erickson, H. (1984, Nov. 7). Telephone interview.

Erickson, H.C. (1988, March 30). Telephone interview.

Erickson, H.C. (1992, July 1). Personal correspondence.

James, J. (1992, July 6). Telephone interview.

Tomlin, E.M. (1992, July 6). Telephone interview.

Erickson, H.C. (1996, July 9). Personal interview.

Tomlin, E.M. (1996, July 10). Telephone interview.

Secondary sources

Book reviews

Erickson, H.C., Tomlin, E.M., & Swain, M.A. (1983). *Modeling and role-modeling: A theory and paradigm for nursing.* Englewood Cliffs, NJ: Prentice-Hall.
American Journal of Nursing, 83, 1355, Sept. 1983.
Nursing and Health Care, 4, 413, Sept. 1983.
Nursing Outlook, 32, 116, Feb. 1984.

Correspondence

Barnfather, J.S. (1988, March). Personal correspondence.

Finch, D. (1988, March). Personal correspondence.

Other sources

Adamson, J., & Schmale, A. (1965). Object loss, giving up, and the onset of psychiatric disease. *Psychosomatic Medicine, 27,*(6), 557-576.

Bartholomew, K. (1990). Avoidance of intimacy: An attachment perspective. *Journal of Social and Personal Relationships, 7,* 147-178.

Bowlby, J. (1958). The nature of the child's tie to his mother. *International Journal of Psychoanalysis, 39,* 89-97.

Bowlby, J. (1960). Child care and the growth of love. In M. Haimowitz & N. Haimowitz, *Human development* (2nd ed.) (pp. 155-166). New York: Thomas Y. Crowell.

Bowlby, J. (1961). Childhood mourning and its explications for psychiatry. *American Journal of Psychiatry, 118,* 481-498.

Bowlby, J. (1961). Process of mourning. *International Journal of Psychoanalysis, 42,* 317-340.

Bowlby, J. (1969). *Attachment.* New York: Basic Books.

Bowlby, J. (1973). *Separation.* New York: Basic Books.

Bowlby, J. (1980). *Loss.* New York: Basic Books.

Bowlby, J., Robertson, J., & Rosenbluth, D. (1952). A two-year-old goes to the hospital. *Psychoanalytic Study of the Child, 7,* 89-94.

Chinn, P.L., & Kramer, M.K. (1994). *Theory and nursing: A systematic approach* (3rd ed.). St. Louis: Mosby.

Engel G. (1968). A life setting conducive to illness: The giving-up: Given-up complex. *Annuals of Internal Medicine, 69,*(2), 293-300.

Engel, G.S. (1962). *Psychological development in health and disease.* Philadelphia: WB Saunders.

Erikson, E. (1960). The case of Peter. In M. Haimowitz & N. Haimowitz, *Human development.* (2nd ed.) (pp. 355-359). New York: Thomas Y. Crowell.

Erikson, E. (1960). Identity versus self-diffusion. In M. Haimowitz & N. Haimowitz, *Human development* (2nd ed.) (pp. 766-770). New York: Thomas Y. Crowell.

Erikson, E. (1963). *Childhood and society.* New York: WW Norton.

Erickson, H. (1986). Synthesizing clinical experiences: A step in theory development. Ann Arbor, MI: Biomedical Communications.

Haley, J. (1973). *Uncommon therapy: The psychiatric techniques of Milton H. Erickson, M.D.* New York: WW Norton.

Hassan, A., & Hassan, B.M. (1987). Interpersonal development across the life span: Communion and its interaction with agency in psychosocial development. In L.A. Meachem (Ed.), *Contributions to human development* (Vol. 18) (pp. 102-127). Basel: Werner Druck AG.

Klein, M. (1952). Some theoretical conclusions regarding the emotional life of the infant. In J. Riviere, *Developments in psycho-analysis* (pp. 198-236). London: Hogarth Press.

Mahler, M.S. (1967). On human symbiosis and the vicissitudes of individuation. *Journal of the American Psychoanalytic Association, 15,* 740-763.

Mahler, M.S., & Furer, M. (1968). *On human symbiosis and the vicissitudes of individuation* (Vol. I). *Infantile psychosis.* New York: International Universities Press.

Maslow, A.H. (1936). The need to know and the fear of knowing. *Journal of General Psychology, 68,* 111-125.

Maslow, A.H. (1968). *Toward a psychology of being* (2nd ed.). New York: D. Von Nostrand.

Maslow, A.H. (1970). *Motivation and personality* (2nd ed.). New York: Harper & Row.

Merton, R.K. (1968). *Social theory and social structure.* New York: The Free Press.

Montgomery, C., & Webster, D. (1993). Caring and nursing's metaparadigm: Can they survive the era of managed care? *Perspectives in Psychiatric Care, 29*(4), 5-12.

Piaget, J. (1952). *The origins of intelligence in children.* New York: International Universities Press.

Piaget, J. (1974). The pathway between subjects' recent life changes and their near-future illness reports: Representative results and methodological issues. In B.S. Dohrenwend & B.P. Dohrenwend, *Stressful life events: Their nature and effects* (pp. 73-86). New York: John Wiley & Sons.

Piaget, J., & Inhelder, B. (1969). *The psychology of the child.* New York: Basic Books.

Rossi, E. (1986). *The psychobiology of mind-body healing.* New York: WW Norton.

Selye, H. (1974). *Stress without distress.* Philadelphia: JB Lippincott.

Selye, H. (1976). *The stress of life* (2nd ed.). New York: McGraw-Hill.

Selye, H. (1979). Further thoughts on stress without distress. *Resident and Staff Physician, 25,* 125-134.

Stoddard, J., & Stoddard, H.J. (1985). Affectional bonding and the impact of bereavement. *Advances: Institute for the Advancement of Health, 2*(2), 19-28.

Winnicott, D.W. (1953). Transitional objects and transitional phenomena: A study of the first not-me possession. *International Journal of Psychoanalysis, 34,* 89-97.

Winnicott, D.W. (1965). The theory of the parent-infant relationship. In D.W. Winnicott, *The maturational processes and the facilitating environment.* London: Hogarth Press.

APPENDIX

ASSESSMENT TOOL BASED ON MODELING AND ROLE-MODELING*

1. Description of the situation
   a. Overview of the situation
   b. Etiology
      (1) Eustressors
      (2) Stressors
      (3) Distressors
   c. Therapeutic needs
2. Expectations
   a. Immediately
   b. Long-term
3. Resource potential
   a. External
      (1) Social network
      (2) Support system
      (3) Health care system
   b. Internal
      (1) Strengths
      (2) Adaptive potential
      (a) Feeling states
      (b) Physiological parameters
4. Goals and life tasks
   a. Current
   b. Future

DATA INTERPRETATION TOOL BASED ON MODELING AND ROLE-MODELING†

1. Interpret data for ability to mobilize resources (APAM)
2. Interpret data for needs status (assets, deficits related to type of need), attachment objects, loss, grief (normal or morbid), life tasks (developmental: actual and chronological)

DATA ANALYSIS TOOL BASED ON MODELING AND ROLE-MODELING‡

1. Step one
   a. Articulate relationships between stressors and needs status

*Interview questions and thoughts that guide critical thinking are suggested in Erickson, et al., *Modeling and Role-Modeling: A Theory and Paradigm for Practice.* Chapters 9-10, pp. 116-168. Suggestions for interviewing techniques can be found in Erickson, Self-care Knowledge. In Erickson & Kinney (1990), *Modeling and Role-Modeling: Theory, Practice and Research.*
†Critical thinking guidelines for data interpretation are suggested in Erickson, et al., Chapter 10, pp. 148-166, and Erickson, Theory based nursing. In Erickson & Kinney (1990), *Modeling and Role-Modeling: Theory, Practice and Research.*
‡Critical thinking guidelines for data analysis are suggested in Erickson, et al., Chapter 10, p. 148-166, and Erickson, Theory based nursing. In Erickson & Kinney (1990), *Modeling and Role-Modeling: Theory, Practice and Research.* *Continued*

APPENDIX—cont'd

b. Articulate relationships between needs status and ability to mobilize resources

c. Articulate relationships between needs status and loss of attachment

d. Articulate relationships between loss and type of grief response

e. Articulate relationships between type of need assets and deficits and developmental residual

f. Articulate relationships between chronological developmental task and developmental residual

2. Step two

a. Articulate relationships among stressors, resource potential, needs status, loss, grief status, developmental residual, chronological task, and attachment potential

b. Articulate relationships among needs, status, potential resources, developmental residual, and personal goals

PLANNING TOOL BASED ON MODELING AND ROLE-MODELING§

1. Aims of interventions

a. Build trust

b. Promote positive orientation

c. Promote client control

d. Promote strengths

e. Set health-directed goals

2. Intervention goals

a. Develop a trusting and functional relationship between yourself and your client

b. Facilitate a self-projection that is futuristic and positive

c. Promote affiliated-individuation with the minimum degree of ambivalence possible

d. Promote a dynamic, adaptive, and holistic state of health

e. Promote and nurture coping mechanism that satisfies basic needs and permits growth-need satisfaction

f. Facilitate congruent actual and chronological developmental stages

§Critical thinking guidelines are suggested in Erickson, et al., Chapter 11, pp. 169-220, and Erickson, Theory based nursing. In Erickson & Kinney (1990), *Modeling and Role-Modeling: Theory, Practice and Research.*

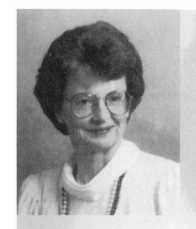

$\mathcal{R}$amona T. Mercer

Maternal Role Attainment

Mary M. Meighan, Alberta M. Bee, Denise Legge, Stephanie Oetting

CREDENTIALS AND BACKGROUND OF THE THEORIST

Ramona T. Mercer began her nursing career in 1950, when she was graduated from St. Margaret's School of Nursing, Montgomery, Alabama. She was graduated with the L.L. Hill Award for Highest Scholastic Standing. In the 10 years that followed, she worked as a nurse, head nurse, and instructor in the areas of pediatrics, obstetrics, and contagious diseases before returning to school in 1960. She completed a Bachelor of Science in Nursing degree in 1962, graduating with distinction from the University of New Mexico, Albuquerque. She went on to earn an M.S.N. in maternal child health nursing from Emory University in 1964 and a Ph.D. in maternity nursing from the University of Pittsburgh in 1973.

The authors wish to express appreciation to Ramona T. Mercer for critiquing the original chapter.

From 1961 to 1963, while pursuing studies in nursing, Mercer worked as a clinical instructor. In 1964 she was awarded the Department of Health, Education, and Welfare Public Health Service Nurse Trainee Award and was inducted into Sigma Theta Tau. From 1964 to 1971, she was an assistant professor of maternal child health nursing at Emory University. During this time she was again awarded a Department of Health, Education, and Welfare Public Health Service Nurse Trainee Award and also the Bixler Scholarship for Nursing Education and Research, Southern Regional Board.

Mercer moved to California in 1973 and accepted the position of assistant professor, Department of Family Health Care Nursing, at the University of California, San Francisco. She held that position until 1977, when she was promoted to associate professor. In 1983 she accepted a position as a professor in the same department and remained in that role until her retirement in 1987. Currently Dr. Mercer is professor emeritus in family health nursing at the University of California, San Francisco. She remains active in writing, speaking engagements, and consultations.[20]

In early research efforts, Mercer focused on the behaviors and needs of breast-feeding mothers, mothers with postpartum illness, and mothers bearing infants with defects. The results were published in several articles and led to the writing of *Nursing Care for Parents at Risk*, which was published in 1977 and received an *American Journal of Nursing* Book of the Year Award in 1978. This prior research led Mercer to study mothers of various ages, family relationships, and antepartal stress as related to familial relationships and the maternal role. A portion of that work, concerning teenage mothers over the first year of motherhood, resulted in the book *Perspectives on Adolescent Health Care*, which in 1980 also received an *American Journal of Nursing* Book of the Year Award. In 1986, Mercer's work on mothers at various ages was drawn together in *First-time Motherhood: Experiences From Teens to Forties*.

Mercer's fifth book, *Parents at Risk*, published in 1990, also received an *American Journal of Nursing* Book of the Year Award. *Parents at Risk* focuses on strategies for facilitating early parent-infant interactions and promoting parental competence in relation to specific risk situations.[18]

In 1995, *Becoming a Mother: Research on Maternal Role Identity Since Rubin*, Mercer's sixth book, was published by Springer Publishing Company of New York. Since her first publication in 1968, she has published numerous articles for both nursing and nonnursing journals, six books, six book chapters, many abstracts, forewords, editorials, commentaries, and book reviews.

Mercer has maintained membership in seven professional organizations, including the American Nurses Association and the American Academy of Nursing and has been an active member on many national committees. From 1983 to 1990 she was the associate editor of *Health Care for Women International*. She has served on the review panel for *Nursing Research* and *Western Journal of Nursing Research* and was on the executive advisory board of *California Nursing* and *Nurseweek*. She has also served as a re-

viewer for numerous grant proposals. Additionally, she has been actively involved with regional, national, and international scientific and professional meetings and workshops.

Other honors and awards she has received include Maternal Child Health Nurse of the Year Award by the National Foundation March of Dimes and American Nurses Association, Division of Maternal Child Health Practice in 1983; Fourth Annual Helen Nahm Lecturer, University of California, San Francisco, School of Nursing in 1984; ASPO/Lamaze National Research Award in 1987; in 1988 the Distinguished Research Lectureship Award, Western Institute of Nursing, Western Society for Research in Nursing; and in 1990 the American Nurses Foundation's Distinguished Contribution to Nursing Science Award.[16,19,21]

THEORETICAL SOURCES

Reva Rubin, who is well known for her work in maternal role identity, was Mercer's professor and mentor at the University of Pittsburgh, where Mercer earned her Ph.D. Rubin's research not only served as a stimulus, but became the foundation for Mercer's research on variables that affect the attainment of the maternal role.

Both role and developmental theories provide the overall framework for Mercer's Theory of Maternal Role Attainment.[6,14] She relied heavily on an interactionist approach to role theory, using Mead's theory on role enactment and Turner's theory on the "core self."[14] At the same time, Thornton's and Nardi's role acquisition process also helped shape Mercer's theory, as did the work of Burr, Leigh, Day, and Constantine.[6,14] Werner's and Erikson's developmental process theories contributed as well.[14] Mercer's work is also based on Ludwig von Bertalanffy's general system theory. This is apparent by her description of family as a dynamic system that includes subsystems, both individual and dyads.

The complexity of her research interest led Mercer to rely on many other theoretical sources to identify and study variables that affect maternal role attainment. Although much of her work was based on Rubin's theories, she also looked to Gottlieb's research on attachment and caretaking roles, as well as the most current research on maternal-infant relationships.[7] In her work with high-risk families she examined the Life Span Developmental Models of Baltes, Reese, and Lipsitt and research on families by Rankin and Weekes.[17] Gloger-Tippelt's Process Model for the Course of Pregnancy also influenced Mercer to examine maternal role attainment as a process.[14] On that basis, she established five intervals for data collection in her study: early postpartum, 1 month, 4 months, 8 months, and 1 year.

Mercer selected both maternal and infant variables for her research on the basis of her extensive review of the literature and findings of many researchers. Maternal variables included age at first birth, birth experience, early separation from the infant, social stress, social support, personality traits, self-concept, child-rearing attitudes, and health. Infant temperament and health status were also included.

Mercer used many measurement tools to test the variables under investigation in her maternal role research. To measure early postpartum and the first-month attachment, she used E.R. Broussard and Hartner's prediction of neonatal outcomes and perceptions work, and later she used the Degree of Bothersome Inventory to measure stress related to infant behavior. Samko and Schoenfeld's measurement tool was adapted by Mercer and Marut to a 29-item questionnaire to assess the effect of the perception of the birth experience. Leifer's How I Feel About My Baby questionnaire was used to measure attachment at 1, 4, 8, and 12 months. She also used Leifer's Child-Trait Checklist at 1 month because of its representation of the claiming behaviors described by Gottlieb (1978), Robson and Moss (1970), and Rubin (1961, 1972).[13:342] Gratification of the maternal role was measured by adaptation of Russell's (1974) Gratification Checklist. Maternal behavior was measured by Disbrow and associates (1977, 1982). Ways Parents Handle Irritating Behavior Scale was originally used for discriminating between abusive and nonabusive parents. Maternal behavior in Mercer's studies, as observed by the raters, was measured by an adaptation from Blank's (1974) scale.

To measure social stress, Mercer used the Life Experience Survey constructed by Sarason, Johnson

and Siegel (1978). She also used the Checklist of Bothersome Factors to reflect infant stress in the transition to parenthood developed by Hobbs (1965), who revised it for a replicated study (Hobbs and Cole, 1976). A seven-item subscale derived from the Hobbs Checklist relating to change in the mate relationship was used during the 8-month test periods. An adaptation of Burr and associates' (1979) Scale of Role Strain was used as a reflection of stress in the role of parenting at 4, 8, and 12 months. Mercer also used a 12-item empathy scale from Stotland's 96-item scale by Disbrow's Child Abuse Prediction Project.

To measure maternal rigidity, she used a 15-item scale constructed by Larsen (1966). Maternal temperament was measured by using Thomas, Mittelman, and Chess's (1982) 140-item Early Adult Life Temperament Questionnaire. This questionnaire was chosen because of "its high isomorphism with the Carey Infant Temperament Questionnaire that was used to measure infant temperament" (Carey 1970, Carey and McDevitt, 1978).[13:350] The Tennessee Self Concept Scale was selected by Mercer to measure maternal self-concept, personality integration, and personality disorders in her research subjects. Two measures, the Parent Child-Rearing Attitude Scales developed by Disbrow and associates (1977) and the Maternal Attitude Scale (MAS) developed by Cohler and associates (1970), were used for those variables.

In her research on the effects of antepartum stress on mothers' and fathers' health status, mate relationships, attachment to their infants, and family functioning, a family developmental approach was used to study changes from pregnancy over 8 months postpartum within the family system and subsystems. Measures used in this study were Feetham's Family Function Scale[12:270]; Locke and Wallace's Marital Adjustment Test [28:87]; Cranley's Fetal Attachment Scale[23:272]; Leifer's How I Feel About My Baby Scale[23:271]; Davies and Ware's General Health Index[12:270]; Revisions of Hobel's Pregnancy, Intrapartal, and Newborn Risk Scores[23:271]; Norbeck's revision of the Life Experiences Survey[12:270]; Rosenburg's Self-Esteem Scale[12:270]; Barerra's Inventory of Socially Supportive Behaviors (received support)[12:270]; McMillan and Wandersman's Feelings of Support (perceived support)[12:270]; Checklist of Supportive Persons (network support)[12:270]; Pearlin's Sense of Mastery[12:270]; Spielberger and associates; Trait and State Anxiety Scales[12:271]; Radloff's Center for Epidemiologic Studies Depression Scale[12:271]; and Gibaud-Wallston and Wandersman's Parental Sense of Competence Scale.[23:270]

USE OF EMPIRICAL EVIDENCE

Mercer's theory is based on the evidence of her extensive research. Although the work of Reva Rubin on maternal role attainment stimulated Mercer's initial interest, the focus of her work has gone beyond that of her predecessor to encompass adolescents, older mothers, ill mothers, mothers with defective children, families experiencing antepartal stress, parents at high risk, mothers who had cesarean deliveries, paternal-infant attachment, and paternal role competence.

While Rubin dealt with role attainment from the point of acceptance of the pregnancy to 1-month postpartum, Mercer has looked beyond that period to 12 months postpartum.

MAJOR CONCEPTS & DEFINITIONS

Mercer bases her theory for Maternal Role Attainment on the following factors.

Maternal Role Attainment An interactional and developmental process occurring over a period of time during which the mother becomes attached to her infant, acquires competence in the caretaking tasks involved in the role, and expresses pleasure and gratification in the role.[13:2-6] "The movement to the personal state in which the mother experiences a sense of harmony, confidence, and competence in how she performs the role is the end point of maternal role attainment—maternal identity."[7:74]

Maternal Age Chronological and developmental.[14:25]

Perception of Birth Experience A woman's perception of her performance during labor and birth.[18:202]

Early Maternal-Infant Separation Separation from the mother after birth due to illness and/or prematurity.[18:202]

Self-Esteem "An individual's perception of how others view one and self-acceptance of the perceptions."[30:341]

Self-Concept (Self-Regard) "The overall perception of self that includes self-satisfaction, self-acceptance, self-esteem, and congruence or discrepancy between self and ideal self."[13:18]

Flexibility Roles are not rigidly fixed; therefore, who fills the roles is not important.[18:21]

"Flexibility of childrearing attitudes increases with increased development. . . . Older mothers have the potential to respond less rigidly to their infants and to view each situation in respect to the unique nuances."[13:43;18:12]

Childrearing Attitudes Maternal attitudes or beliefs about childrearing.[13:19]

Health Status "The mother's and father's perception of their prior health, current health, health outlook, resistance-susceptibility to illness, health worry concern, sickness orientation, and rejection of the sick role."[30:342]

Anxiety "A trait in which there is specific proneness to perceive stressful situations as dangerous or threatening, and as situation-specific state."[30:342]

Depression "Having a group of depressive symptoms, and in particular the affective component of the depressed mood."[30:342]

Role Strain The conflict and difficulty felt by the woman in fulfilling the maternal role obligation.[11:199]

Gratification "The satisfaction, enjoyment, reward, or pleasure that a woman experiences in interacting with her infant, and in fulfilling the usual tasks inherent in mothering."[12:296]

MAJOR CONCEPTS & DEFINITIONS—cont'd

Attachment A component of the parental role and identity. Attachment is viewed as a process in which an enduring affectional and emotional commitment to an individual is formed.[18:19]

Infant Temperament An easy versus a difficult temperament, it is related to whether the infant sends hard-to-read cues, leading to feelings of incompetence and frustration in the mother.[13:76]

Infant Health Status Illness causing maternal-infant separation, interfering with the attachment process.[13:76]

Infant Characteristics Temperament, appearance, and health status.[7:74,76]

Family "A dynamic system which includes subsystems—individuals (mother, father, fetus/infant) and dyads (mother-father, mother-fetus/infant, and father-fetus/infant) within the overall family system."[30:339]

Family Functioning The individual's view of the activities and relationships between the family and its subsystems and broader social units.[27:270]

Stress Positively and negatively perceived life events and environmental variables[18:15]

Social Support "The amount of help actually received, satisfaction with that help, and the persons (network) providing that help."[30:341]

Four areas of social support are the following.

Emotional support "Feeling loved, cared for, trusted, and understood."[13:14]

Informational support "Helps the individual help herself by providing information that is useful in dealing with the problem and/or situation."[13:14]

Physical support A direct kind of help.[29:251]

Appraisal support "A support that tells the role taker how she is performing in the role; it enables the individual to evaluate herself in relationship to others' performance in the role."[13:14]

Mother-Father Relationship Perception of the mate relationship that includes intended and actual values, goals, and agreements between the two.[7:343]

MAJOR ASSUMPTIONS

For maternal role attainment, Mercer stated the following assumptions[13:24-25]:

1. A relatively stable "core self," acquired through lifelong socialization, determines how a mother defines and perceives events; her perceptions of her infant's and others' responses to her mothering, along with her life situation, are the real world to which she responds.

2. In addition to the mother socialization, her developmental level and innate personality characteristics also influence her behavioral responses.

3. The mother's role partner, her infant, will reflect the mother's competence in the mothering role through growth and development.

4. The infant is considered an active partner in the maternal role-taking process, affecting and being affected by the role enactment.[7:74]

5. Maternal identity develops along with maternal attachment and each depends on the other (Rubin, 1977).[20]

Nursing

Mercer does not define *nursing* but refers to nursing as a science emerging from a "turbulent adolescence to adulthood."[8] Nurses are the health professionals having the most "sustained and intense interaction with women in the maternity cycle."[8] Nurses are responsible for "promoting the health" of families and children; nurses are "pioneers" in developing and sharing assessment strategies for these clients.[6]

Obstetrical nursing, according to Mercer, is the diagnosis and treatment of women's and men's responses to actual or potential health problems during pregnancy, childbirth, and the postpartum period.[10:29]

Person

Mercer does not specifically define *person* but refers to the "self" or "core self."[11:198] She views the self as separate from the roles that are played. Through maternal individuation, a woman may regain her own "personhood" as she extrapolates her "self" from the mother-infant dyad.[13:295] The core self evolves from a culture context and determines how situations are defined and shaped.[11:198]

Health

In her theory, Mercer defines *health status* as the mother's and father's perception of their prior health, current health, health outlook, resistance-susceptibility to illness, health worry or concern, sickness orientation, and rejection of the sick role. Health status of the newborn is the extent of disease present and infant health status by parental rating of overall health.[13:342] The health status of a family is negatively affected by antepartum stress. Health status is an important indirect influence on satisfaction with relationships in childbearing families.

Environment

Mercer does not define *environment*. She does, however, address the individual's culture, mate, family and/or support network and size of that network as it relates to maternal role attainment.[13:50] A mate's love, support, and nurturance were important factors in enabling a woman to mother her child. The responses of mates, parents, other relatives, and friends are closely evaluated by the role taker. Supportive responses provided sanction for their mothering role and seemed to communicate confidence in their ability to mother. The mate, parents, family, and friends were also identified as sources of coping and help for the new mother.[13:50]

THEORETICAL ASSERTIONS

Mercer's Model of Maternal Role Attainment is placed within Bronfenbrenner's (1979) nested circles of the microsystem, exosystem, and macrosystem[21] (Fig. 27-1).

1. The immediate environment in which the maternal role attainment occurs is the microsystem, which includes the family, and factors such as family functioning, mother-father relationships, social support, and stress. The variables contained within the microsystem interact with one or more of the other variables in affecting maternal role. The infant as an individual is embedded within the family system. The family is viewed as a semiclosed system maintaining boundaries and control over interchange between the family system and other social systems.[18:19]

2. The exosystem encompasses, influences, and delimits the microsystem. The mother-infant unit is not contained within the exosystem, but the exosystem may determine in part what happens to the developing maternal role and the child.

3. The macrosystem refers to the general prototypes existing in a particular culture or transmitted cultural consistencies.

Maternal role attainment is a process that follows four stages of role acquisition (adapted from Thornton and Nardi, 1975)[18:26-37]:

1. Anticipatory—Begins social and psychological adjustment to the role by learning the expectations of the role. The mother fantasizes about the role, relates to the fetus in utero, and begins role play.

2. Formal—Begins with assumption of the role at birth; role behaviors are guided by formal, consensual expectations of others in the mother's social system.

3. Informal—Begins as mother develops unique ways of dealing with the role not conveyed by the social system.

4. Personal—The mother experiences a sense of harmony, confidence, and competence in the way she performs the role; maternal role is achieved.

LOGICAL FORM

Mercer used both deductive and inductive logic in developing the theoretical framework for studying

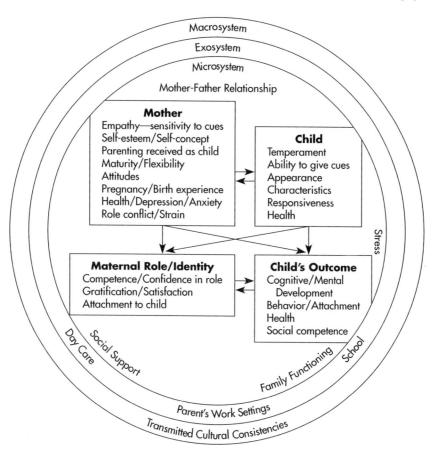

Fig. **27-1** **Proposed model of Maternal Role Attainment.** *Paper presented by Ramona T. Mercer at symposium, "Maternal Role: Models and Consequences," at the International Research Conference sponsored by the Council of Nurse Researchers and the American Nurses Association. Los Angeles, CA. Copyright © 1991 by Ramona T. Mercer. Reprinted with permission.*

factors that influence maternal role attainment in the first year of motherhood.

Deductive logic is demonstrated in Mercer's use of works from other researchers and disciplines. Both role and developmental theories and the work of R. Rubin on maternal role attainment provided a base for the framework.

Mercer also used inductive logic in the development of her Maternal Role Attainment Theory. Through practice and research, she observed adaptation to motherhood from a variety of circumstances. She noted that differences existed in adaptation to motherhood when maternal illness complicated the postpartum period, when a child with a defect was born, and when a teenager became a mother. These observations directed the research about those situations and subsequently the development of her theoretical framework.

ACCEPTANCE BY THE NURSING COMMUNITY
Practice

Mercer's theory is highly practice oriented. The concepts in her theory have been cited in many obstetrical textbooks and have been used in practice by nurses and those in other disciplines. Both the theory and the proposed model are capable of serving as a framework for assessment, planning, implementing, and evaluating nursing care of new mothers and their infants.

Concepts in the research conducted by Neeson, Patterson, Mercer, and May, "Pregnancy Outcomes for Adolescents Receiving Prenatal Care by Nurse Practitioners in Extended Roles," were used in setting up a clinical practice. In her book *First-Time Motherhood: Experiences From Teens to Forties*, Mercer links her research findings with nursing practice at each time interval from birth through the first year. Her summaries and implications are extremely useful to practicing nurses across many maternal-child settings.

Education

As previously stated, Mercer's work has appeared extensively in nursing texts, but not just as it relates to maternal role attainment; rather, each individual piece of research is used and valued.

Mercer's theory and model help to simplify a complex process, thus enhancing understanding and making Mercer's contribution extremely valuable to nursing education.

Research

Mercer has advocated the involvement of students in faculty research. During her tenure at the University of California, San Francisco, she chaired committees and was a committee member for numerous graduate theses and/or dissertations. Her work has been used as the basis for several graduate students' topics of research.[15,16] Collaborative research with a graduate student and junior faculty member in 1977 and 1978 led to the development of a highly reliable, valid instrument to measure mothers' attitudes about the labor and delivery experience.[16] Numerous researchers have requested permission to use the instrument.

Mercer's work has served as a springboard for future research. The theoretical framework for the correlational study exploring differences between three

age groups for first-time mothers (ages 15-19, 20-29, and 30-42 years) has been tested in part by others, including Lorraine Walker and associates, University of Texas, Austin, and reported in *Nursing Research*. Angela B. McBride wrote, "Maternal role attainment has been a fundamental concern of nursing since the pioneering work of Mercer's mentor, Rubin, almost two decades ago. It is now becoming the research-based, theoretically sound construct that nurse researchers have been searching for in their analysis of the experience of new mothers."[5:72]

FURTHER DEVELOPMENT

In her book *First-Time Motherhood: Experiences From Teens to Forties*, Mercer presents a model of four phases occurring in the process of maternal role attainment during the first year of motherhood. The four phases are labeled as follows: the physical recovery phase, occurring from birth to 1 month; the achievement phase from 2 to 4 or 5 months; the disruptions phase, occurring from 6 to 8 months; and finally the reorganization phase, from after the eighth month and still in process at 1 year.[13:299-314] Additionally, adaptation to the maternal role is proposed to occur at three levels—biological, psychological, and social—which are interacting and interdependent throughout the phases. These phases and levels of adaptation are briefly described and applied to her research on maternal role attainment. This model appears logical and useful but is in need of further explanation, exposure, and development.

Mercer used her initial research, which led to her Theory of Maternal Role Attainment, as a building block for other studies. In later research, Mercer aimed at identifying predictors of maternal-infant attachment on the basis of maternal experience with childbirth and maternal risk status. She also examined paternal competence on the basis of experience with childbirth and pregnancy risk status. In another study, she developed and tested a causal model to predict partner relationships in high- and low-risk pregnancy.

According to Mercer, there are several areas in need of further research. More testing and revision of the proposed causal model developed to predict partner relationships are needed.[26] In addition, more information is needed about the antecedents and mediators of partner relationships when pregnancy is at high risk.[24,25] Mercer also emphasized the need for more research into sources of stress and anxiety that potentially interfere with maternal-infant attachment and role competence.[2-4]

In paternal-infant attachment and paternal role competence studies, Mercer noted higher rates of depression among inexperienced fathers. She stresses the need for further research to develop interventions for depression among first-time fathers during the first year.[3] Continued testing of the application of Mercer's framework in a variety of perinatal situations, including multiple gestation, would be useful, and investigation of theory beyond the first year is also warranted.

CRITIQUE
Clarity

The concepts, variables, and relationships are not always explicitly defined but rather are described and implied. They are, however, theoretically defined and operationalized. The operational and theoretical definitions are consistent. Some interchanging of terms and labels used to identify concepts (e.g., adaptation and attainment, social support and support network) can create some confusion for the reader. Additionally, *maternal role attainment* is not consistently defined and thus obstructs clarity. Overall, the concepts, assumptions, and goals are organized into a logical and coherent whole, and understanding the interrelationships among the concepts is relatively easy.

Simplicity

In spite of numerous concepts and relationships, the theoretical framework for maternal role attainment organizes a rather complex phenomenon into an easily understood and useful form. The theory is predictive in nature and thus readily lends itself to guide practice.[1:142] Concepts are not specific to time and place, and so are abstract, but are described and operationalized to the extent that meanings are not eas-

ily misinterpreted. It should be noted, however, that the research completed to define and support the theoretical relationships was very complex, largely due to the great number of concepts.

Generality

Maternal role attainment is a theory specific to parent-child nursing. The theory can be generalized to all women during pregnancy through the first year after birth, regardless of age, parity, or environment. Mercer has also respecified her theory to study and predict parental attachment, including the pregnant woman's partner.[23]

Mercer's work has done much to broaden the range of application of previously existing theories on maternal role attainment because her studies have spanned various developmental levels and situational contexts, a quality that other studies do not share.

Empirical Precision

Mercer's work was derived from extensive research efforts. The concepts, assumptions, and relationships are grounded predominantly in empirical observations and are congruent. The degree of concreteness and the completeness of operational definitions further increase the empirical precision.[1:144] The theoretical framework for exploring differences between age groups of first-time mothers lends itself well to further testing and is being used by others, as previously discussed in the acceptance section of this chapter.

Derivable Consequences

The theoretical framework for maternal role attainment in the first year has proved to be useful, practical, and valuable to nursing. Mercer's work is repeatedly used in research, practice, and education. The framework is also readily applicable to any discipline that works with mothers and children in the first year of motherhood. McBride wrote, "Dr. Mercer is the one who developed the most complete theoretical framework for studying one aspect of parental experience, namely, the factors that influence the attainment of the maternal role in the first year of motherhood."[5:72]

According to Chinn and Jacobs, nursing theory should "differentiate the focus of nursing from other service professions."[1:145] By combining the social, psychological, and biological sciences, Mercer achieves this criterion.

Throughout her career, Mercer has consistently linked research to practice. Implications for nursing and/or nursing interventions are addressed and provide the bond between research and practice in most of her works. She believes that nursing research is the "bridge to excellence" in nursing practice.[9]

CRITICAL THINKING *Activities*

1 In your own practice, consider Mercer's Theory and Model of Maternal Role Attainment as a guide. In what ways is it useful?

2 High-risk families often continue to experience problems for years after the birth of a child with a congenital problem. Can Mercer's framework and proposed model be adapted to help in assessment and intervention for these mothers and their families beyond the first year? What areas need further research and development?

3 Consider the current health care environment. Does the model proposed by Mercer adequately address current changes in health care delivery and the impact on the family? What changes in the proposed model, if any, would you suggest?

4 In the following high-risk perinatal case, Mercer's framework should be useful for nursing assessment and intervention to facilitate maternal role attainment. How would you use it as a guide in planning care for Susan?

Susan B., a 19-year-old woman, was prematurely delivered of her first infant 5 days ago. Although her postpartum course has been relatively uneventful, the infant has had difficulty and must remain hospitalized. Susan and her young husband visit the nursery every afternoon to be with the baby, but they ask very few questions. In talking with the couple, the nurse learns that the only living grandparents of the baby live a great distance away. Susan will not have any family or friends to turn to when she takes the baby home.

REFERENCES

1. Chinn, P.I., & Jacobs, M.K. (1987). *Theory and nursing: A systematic approach*. St. Louis: Mosby.
2. Ferketich, S.L., & Mercer, R.T. (1995). Paternal-infant attachment of experienced and inexperienced fathers during infancy. *Nursing Research, 44*, 31-37.
3. Ferketich, S.L., & Mercer, R.T. (1995). Predictors of paternal role competence by risk status. *Nursing Research, 43*, 80-85.
4. Ferketich, S.L., & Mercer, R.T. (1995). Predictors of role competence for experienced and inexperienced fathers. *Nursing Research, 44*, 89-95.
5. McBride, A.B. (1984). The experience of being a parent. *Annual Review of Nursing Research, 2*, 63-81.
6. Mercer, R.T. (1981). Foreword. In C. Kehoe (Ed.), *The cesarean experience*. New York: Appleton-Century-Crofts.
7. Mercer, R.T. (1981). A theoretical framework for studying factors that impact on the maternal role. *Nursing Research, 30*, 73-77.
8. Mercer, R.T. (1982). Foreword. In S. Hummenick (Ed.), *Assessment evaluation: A clinical and technical review of selected assessment strategies for use in the health care of families in pregnancy and early parenting years*. New York: Appleton-Century-Crofts.
9. Mercer, R.T. (1984). Nursing research: The bridge to excellence in practice. *Image: The Journal of Nursing Scholarship, 16*(2), 47-51.
10. Mercer, R.T. (1985). Obstetric nursing research: Past, present and future. *Birth Defects: Original Article Series, 21*(3), 29-70.
11. Mercer, R.T. (1985). The process of maternal role attainment over the first years. *Nursing Research, 34*, 198-204.
12. Mercer, R.T. (1985). The relationship of age and other variables to gratification in mothering. *Health Care for Women International, 6*, 295-308.
13. Mercer, R.T. (1986). *First-time motherhood: Experiences from teens to forties*. New York: Springer.
14. Mercer, R.T. (1986). The relationship of developmental variables to maternal behavior. *Research in Nursing & Health, 9*, 25-33.
15. Mercer, R.T. (1987, Feb.). Curriculum vitae.
16. Mercer, R.T. (1988). Curriculum vitae.
17. Mercer, R.T. (1989). Response to "Life-span development: A review of theory and practice for families with chronically ill members." *Scholarly Inquiry for Nursing Practice, 3*, 23-26.
18. Mercer, R.T. (1990). *Parents at risk*. New York: Springer.
19. Mercer, R.T. (1992). Curriculum vitae.

20. Mercer, R.T. (1992, Feb.). Personal correspondence.
21. Mercer, R.T. (1992, March). Personal correspondence.
22. Mercer, R.T., & Ferketich, S.L. (1990). Predictors of family functioning eight months following birth. *Nursing Research, 39,* 76-82.
23. Mercer, R.T., & Ferketich, S.L. (1990). Predictors of parental attachment during early parenthood. *Journal of Advanced Nursing, 15,* 268-280.
24. Mercer, R.T., & Ferketich, S.L. (1994). Maternal-infant attachment of experienced and inexperienced mothers during infancy. *Nursing Research, 43,* 344-350.
25. Mercer, R.T., & Ferketich, S.L. (1995). Experienced and inexperienced mothers' maternal competence during infancy. *Research in Nursing & Health, 18,* 333, 343.
26. Mercer, R.T., Ferketich, S.L., & DeJoseph, J.F. (1993). Predictors of partner relationships during pregnancy and infancy. *Research in Nursing & Health, 16,* 45-56.
27. Mercer, R.T., Ferketich, S.L., DeJoseph, J., May, K.A., & Sollid, D. (1988). Effects of stress on family functioning during pregnancy. *Nursing Research 37,* 268-275.
28. Mercer, R.T., Ferketich, S., May, K., DeJoseph, J., & Sollid, D. (1988). Further exploration of maternal and paternal fetal attachment. *Research in Nursing & Health, 11,* 83-95.
29. Mercer, R.T., Hackley, K.C., & Bostrom, A. (1984). Social support of teenage mothers. *Birth Defects: Original Article Series, 20*(5), 245-290.
30. Mercer, R.T., May, K.A., Ferketich, S., & DeJoseph, J. (1986). Theoretical models for studying the effect of antepartum stress on the family. *Nursing Research, 35,* 339-346.

BIBLIOGRAPHY
Primary sources
Books

Mercer, R.T. (1977). *Nursing care for parents at risk.* Thorofare, NJ: Charles B. Slack.
Mercer, R.T. (1979). *Perspectives on adolescent health care.* Philadelphia: JB Lippincott.
Mercer, R.T. (1986). *First-time motherhood: Experiences from teens to forties.* New York: Springer.
Mercer, R.T. (1990). *Parents at risk.* New York: Springer Publishers.
Mercer, R.T. (1995). *Becoming a mother: Research on maternal role identity since Rubin.* New York: Springer.
Mercer, R.T., Nichols, E.G., & Doyle, G. (1989). *Transitions in a woman's life: Major life events in developmental context.* New York: Springer.

Journal articles

Ferketich, S.L., & Mercer, R.T. (1989). Men's health status during pregnancy and early fatherhood. *Research in Nursing & Health, 12,* 137-148.

Ferketich, S.L., & Mercer, R.T. (1990). Effects of antepartal stress on health status during early motherhood. *Scholarly Inquiry for Nursing Practice: An International Journal, 4*(2), 127-149.
Ferketich, S.L., & Mercer, R.T. (1992). Focus on psychometrics: Aggregating family data. *Research in Nursing & Health, 15,* 313-317.
Ferketich, S.L., & Mercer, R.T. (1995). Paternal-infant attachment of experienced and inexperienced fathers during infancy. *Nursing Research, 44,* 31-37.
Ferketich, S.L., & Mercer, R.T. (1995). Predictors of paternal role competence by risk status. *Nursing Research, 43,* 80-85.
Ferketich, S.L., & Mercer, R.T. (1995). Predictors of role competence for experienced and inexperienced fathers. *Nursing Research, 44,* 89-95.
Highley, B.L., & Mercer, R.T. (1978). Safeguarding the laboring woman's sense of control. *MCN, The American Journal of Maternal-Child Nursing, 4,* 39-41.
Marut, J.S., & Mercer, R.T. (1979, Sept.-Oct.). A comparison of primiparas' perception of vaginal and cesarean birth. *Nursing Research, 28,* 260-266.
Marut, J.S., & Mercer, R.T. (1981). The cesarean birth experience: Implications for nursing. *Birth Defects: Original Article Series, 17,* 129-152.
Mercer, R.T. (1973, Spring). One mother's use of negative feedback in coping with her infant with a defect. *Maternal-Child Nursing Journal, 2,* 29-37.
Mercer, R.T. (1974). A focus on field methodology as a method of research in nursing practice. *Occasional Papers in Nursing Research, University of California, San Francisco, 2,* 14-17.
Mercer, R.T. (1974). Two fathers' early responses to the birth of a daughter with a defect. *Maternal-Child Nursing Journal, 3,* 77-86.
Mercer, R.T. (1974, March-April). Mothers' responses to their infants with defects. *Nursing Research, 23,* 133-137.
Mercer, R.T. (1975). Responses of mothers to the birth of an infant with a defect. *ANA Clinical Sessions* (pp. 340-349). New York: Appleton-Century-Crofts.
Mercer, R.T. (1976). Mothering at sixteen. *MCN, The American Journal of Maternal-Child Nursing, 1,* 44-52.
Mercer, R.T. (1977, July). Postpartum illness and the acquaintance-attachment process. *American Journal of Nursing, 77,* 1174-1178.
Mercer, R.T. (1977, Nov.). Crisis: A baby is born with a defect. *Nursing 77, 7,* 45-47.
Mercer, R.T. (1978). Internal and external constraints on teenage mothering. *Research in Education, 13*(8).
Mercer, R.T. (1979, Sept.-Oct.). She's a multip: She knows the ropes. *MCN, The American Journal of Maternal-Child Nursing, 4,* 301-304.
Mercer, R.T. (1980). Commentary on maternal identification and infant care: A theoretical perspective. *Western Journal of Nursing Research, 2,* 700-702.

Mercer, R.T. (1980, Jan.-Feb.). Teenage motherhood: The first year. Part I, The teenage mothers' views and responses. Part II, How their infants fared. *Journal of Obstetric, Gynecologic, and Neonatal Nursing, 9*, 16-27.

Mercer, R.T. (1981). Factors impacting on the maternal role the first year. *Birth Defects: Original Article Series, 17*, 233-252.

Mercer, R.T. (1981, March-April). A theoretical framework for studying factors that impact on the maternal role. *Nursing Research, 30*, 73-77.

Mercer, R.T. (1981, Sept.-Oct.). The nurse and maternal tasks of early postpartum. *MCN, The American Journal of Maternal-Child Nursing, 6*, 341-345.

Mercer, R.T. (1983, June). Assessing and counseling teenage mothers during the perinatal period. *Nursing Clinics of North America, 8*, 293-301.

Mercer, R.T. (1984). Commentary on subject mortality: Is it inevitable? *Western Journal of Nursing Research, 6*, 336-337.

Mercer, R.T. (1984). Health of the children of adolescents. *Adolescent Family, Report of Fifteenth Ross Roundtable on Critical Approaches to Common Pediatric Problems* (pp. 60-66). Columbus, OH: Ross Laboratories.

Mercer, R.T. (1984). Student involvement in faculty research: A mentor's view. *Western Journal of Nursing Research, 6*(4), 433-437.

Mercer, R.T. (1984, June). Challenges during the first year of motherhood. *The Fourth Helen Nahm Lecture*. San Francisco: University of California, School of Nursing.

Mercer, R.T. (1985). Obstetrical nursing: Past, present, and future. *Birth Defects: Original Article Series, 21*(3), 29-70.

Mercer, R.T. (1985). The relationship of age and other variables to gratification in mothering. *Health Care for Women International, 6*, 295-308.

Mercer, R.T. (1985). Teenage pregnancy as a community problem. *Annual Review of Nursing Research, 3*, 49-76.

Mercer, R.T. (1985, July-Aug.). The process of maternal role attainment over the first year. *Nursing Research, 34*(4), 198-204.

Mercer, R.T. (1985, July-Aug.). The relationship of the birth experience to later mothering behavior. *Journal of Nurse Midwifery, 30*(4), 204-211.

Mercer, R.T. (1986). Predictors of maternal role attainment at one year post-birth. *Western Journal of Nursing Research, 8*(1), 9-32.

Mercer, R.T. (1986). The relationship of developmental variables to maternal behavior. *Research in Nursing & Health, 9*, 25-33.

Mercer, R.T. (1987). The mentor and research outcomes. *Search: Improved Nursing Care Through Research, 11*(2), 1-2.

Mercer, R.T. (Spring, 1988). P's and Q's of monitoring and maintaining a research career. *Community Nursing Research*, Vol. 21. *Nursing: A socially responsible profession* (pp. 21-31). Boulder, CO: Western Institute of Nursing.

Mercer, R.T. (1989). Responses to life-span development: A review of theory and practice for families with chronically ill members. *Scholarly Inquiry for Nursing Practice: An International Journal, 3*, 23-26.

Mercer, R.T. (1990). After surgery, patients and families still face difficulties. *California Nursing Review, 12*(4), 14.

Mercer, R.T. (1990). Allocating scarce resources. *California Nursing Review, 12*(4), 17-18.

Mercer, R.T. (1990). Caring for patients of infants with birth defects. *Nurseweek, 3*(18), 12-13.

Mercer, R.T. (1990). Caring for pregnant teens. *Nurseweek, 3*(21), 8-10.

Mercer, R.T. (1990). Commentary by Mercer (Predicting paternal role enactment). *Western Journal of Nursing Research, 12*(2), 156-158.

Mercer, R.T. (1990). Fathers are parents, too! *Nurseweek, 3*(25), 810.

Mercer, R.T. (1990). Single-mother families require special care. *Nurseweek, 3*(14), 8-9.

Mercer, R.T. (1991). Caring for parents who have an infant in the NICU. *Nurseweek, 4*(8), 9-10.

Mercer, R.T. (1991). Commentary by Mercer (Mother's Perceptions of Problem-Solving Competence for Infant Care). *Western Journal of Nursing Research, 13*(2), 176-178.

Mercer, R.T. (1991). Family adjustment after a child's death. *Nurseweek, 4*(25), 10-11,14.

Mercer, R.T. (1991). Family adjustment to a chronically ill child. *Nurseweek, 4*(29), 8-9,11.

Mercer, R.T. (1991). Helping parents handle a cesarean birth. *Nurseweek, 4*(5), 8-9,19.

Mercer, R.T. (1991). Introduction. Adolescent Pregnancy: Nursing Perspectives on Prevention. *March of Dimes Birth Defects Foundation Birth Defects: Original Article Series, 27*(1), 1-8.

Mercer, R.T. (1991). Postpartum depression. *Nurseweek, 4*(21), 10-11,13.

Mercer, R.T. (1991). Summary and challenge to nursing. *March of Dimes Birth Defects Foundation Birth Defects: Original Article Series, 27*(1), 271-275.

Mercer, R.T. (1991). Second births: The myths and realities. *Nurseweek, 4*(8), 12-13,11.

Mercer, R.T. (1991). Unexpected hospitalization during pregnancy. *Nurseweek, 4*(8), 11,12-13.

Mercer, R.T. (1991). When parents suffer perinatal loss. *Nurseweek, 4*(20), 10-11,13.

Mercer, R.T. (1992). Facilitating parent-infant interaction. *Nurseweek, 5*(2), 10-12.

(Mercer) Evans, R.T. (1968). Needs identified among breastfeeding mothers. *ANA Clinical Sessions* (pp. 162-171). New York: Appleton-Century-Crofts.

Mercer, R.T. (1994). The evolution of maternity care: Driven by research or social change? *AWHONN Womens Health Nursing Scan, 8*, 1-2.

Mercer, R.T. (1995). A tribute to Reva Rubin. *MCN, 20*, 184.

Mercer, R.T., & Ferketich, S.L. (1988). Stress and social support as predictors of anxiety and depression during pregnancy. *Advances in Nursing Science, 10*(2), 26-39.

Mercer, R.T., & Ferketich, S.L. (1990). Predictors of family functioning eight months following birth. *Nursing Research, 29,* 76-82.

Mercer, R.T., & Ferketich, S.L. (1990). Predictors of parental attachment during early parenthood. *Journal of Advanced Nursing, 15,* 268-280.

Mercer, R.T., & Ferketich, S.L. (1990). Predictors of parental attachment during early parenthood. *Journal of Advanced Nursing, 15,* 268-280.

Mercer, R.T., & Ferketich, S.L. (1994). Maternal-infant attachment of experienced and inexperienced mothers during infancy. *Nursing Research, 43,* 344-350.

Mercer, R.T., & Ferketich, S.L. (1994). Predictors of maternal role competency by risk status. *Nursing Research, 43,* 38-43.

Mercer, R.T., & Ferketich, S.L. (1995). Experienced and inexperienced mothers' maternal competence during infancy. *Research in Nursing & Health, 18,* 333-343.

Mercer, R.T., Ferketich, S.L., & DeJoseph, J.F. (1993). Predictors of partner relationships during pregnancy and infancy. *Research in Nursing & Health, 16,* 45-56.

Mercer, R.T., Ferketich, S.L., DeJoseph, J., & Sollid, D. (1988, Sept.-Oct.). Effect of stress on family functioning during pregnancy. *Nursing Research, 37*(5), 268-275. Also in J. Fawcett & A. Whall (Eds.) (1991), *Family theory development in nursing: State of the science and art* (pp. 121-138). Philadelphia: F.A. Davis.

Mercer, R.T., Hackley, K.C., & Bostrom, A.G. (1983, July-Aug.). Relationship of psychosocial and perinatal variables to perception of childbirth. *Nursing Research, 32,* 202-207. Reprinted (1984) in *Taiwan Nursing Digest, 106*(21), 100-104.

Mercer, R.T., Hackley, K.C., & Bostrom, A.G. (1984). Adolescent motherhood: Comparisons of outcome with older mothers. *Journal of Adolescent Health Care, 4,* 7-13.

Mercer, R.T. Hackley, K.C., & Bostrom, A. (1984). Social support of teenage mothers. *Birth Defects: Original Article Series, 20*(5), 245-290.

Mercer, R.T., Highley, B.L. (1978). Maternity specialization: Where are the challenges? In M.R. Spaulding (Ed.), *Report of Conference on Crisis in Maternal-Child Nursing Leadership* (pp. 63-75). Richmond, VA: Medical College of Virginia, School of Nursing.

Mercer, R.T., Ferketich, S.L., May, K., DeJoseph, J., & Sollid, D. (1988). Further exploration of maternal and paternal fetal attachment. *Research in Nursing & Health, 11,* 83-95.

Mercer, R.T., May, K.A., Ferketich, S., & DeJoseph, J. (1986, Nov.-Dec.). Theoretical models for studying the effect of antepartum stress on the family. *Nursing Research, 35*(6), 339-346.

Mercer, R.T., Nichols, E., & Doyle, G. (1988). Transitions over the life cycle: A comparison of mothers and nonmothers. *Nursing Research, 37,* 144-151.

Mercer, R.T., & Stainton, M.C. (1984). Perceptions of the birth experience: A cross-cultural comparison. *Health Care for Women International 5,* 28-27.

(Mercer) Evans, R.T., Thigpen, L., & Hamrick, M. (1969, Jan.-Feb.). Exploration of factors involved in maternal physiological adaptation to breastfeeding. *Nursing Research, 18*(1), 28-33.

Neeson, J.D., Patterson, K.A., Mercer, R.T., & May, K.A. (1983, June). Pregnancy outcome for adolescents receiving prenatal care by nurse practitioners in extended roles. *Journal of Adolescent Health Care, 4,* 94-99.

Slavazza, K.L., Mercer, R.T., Marut, J.S., & Shnider, S.M. (1985, July-Aug.). Differences in maternal perceptions of anesthesia, analgesia for vaginal childbirth. *Journal of Obstetric, Gynecologic, and Neonatal Nursing, 14*(4), 321-329.

Correspondence

Mercer, R.T. (1988, Jan.). Curriculum vitae.

Mercer, R.T. (1988, Feb.). Revised curriculum vitae.

Mercer, R.T. (1992). Curriculum vitae.

Mercer, R.T. (1992, Feb.). Personal correspondence.

Mercer, R.T. (1992, March). Personal correspondence.

Grant reports

Mercer, R.T., Ferketich, S.L, May, K.A., DeJoseph, J., & Sollid, D. Antepartum stress: Effects on family health and functioning. Grant No. R01-NR-01064. National Center for Nursing Research, National Institutes of Health, San Francisco: Department of Family Health Care Nursing, University of California, San Francisco (1987).

Mercer, R.T., Hackley, K.C., & Bostrom, A. Factors having an impact on maternal role attainment the first year of motherhood. Grant No. MC-R-05-060435. Maternal and Child Health (Social Security Act, Title V), San Francisco: Department of Family Health Care Nursing, University of California, San Francisco (1982).

Mercer, R.T., & Virden, S. (1978). *Selected materials from a review of the literature to identify instruments to measure maternal role attainment and related factors.* Nursing Graduate Research Support Grant.

Book chapters

Mercer, R.T. (1981). Potential effects of anesthesia and analgesia on mother-infant attachment process of cesarean mothers. In C. Kehoe (Ed.), *The cesarean experience.* New York: Appleton-Century-Crofts.

Mercer, R.T. (1981). Reaction of parents following cesarean delivery. In S. Rosno (Ed.), *A humanistic approach to cesarean childbirth.* San Jose, CA: Cesarean Birth Control International, Inc.

Mercer, R.T. (1983). Parent-infant attachment. In L.J. Sontegard, K.M. Kowalski, & B. Jennings (Eds.), *Women's health:* Vol. II, *Childbearing.* New York: Grune & Stratton.

Mercer, R.T. (1987). Adolescent pregnancy. In L.J. Sontegard, K.M. Kowalski, & B. Jennings (Eds.), *Women's health*: Vol. III, *Crisis and illness in childbearing*. Orlando, FL: Grune & Stratton.

Mercer, R.T. (1988). Theoretical perspectives on the family. In B. Gilliss, B. Highley, B. Roberts, & I. Martinson (Eds.), *Toward a science of family nursing*. Menlo Park, CA: Addison-Wesley.

Mercer, R.T., & Marut, J.S. (1981). Comparative viewpoints: Cesarean versus vaginal birth. In D.D. Affonso (Ed.), *Impact of cesarean childbirth*. Philadelphia: FA Davis.

Abstracts

Hackley, K., & Mercer, R.T. (1981). Variables correlating with the mother's perception of her neonate early postpartum and at one month. *Proceedings Nurses' Association of American College of Obstetrics and Gynecologists, Third National Meeting, San Francisco, March 29-April 4, 1981*. Libertyville, IL: Hollister.

Hackley, K.C., Mercer, R.T., & Bostrom, A. (1982). Motherhood in the 30s: A preview of their experiences. *Western Journal of Nursing Research, 4*(3), 61. Also in *Communicating Nursing Research, 15*, 61.

Mercer, R.T. (1986). Needs identified among breastfeeding mothers. *American Journal of Nursing, 68*, 1274-1275.

Mercer, R.T. (1974). Responses of five multigravidae to the event of the birth of an infant with a defect. *Dissertation Abstracts International, 34*(10).

Mercer, R.T. (1979). Internal and external constraints on teenage mothering. Resources in Women's Educational Equity, *ERIC Documents*.

Mercer, R.T., Hackley, K., & Bostrom, A. (1980). Maternal age and role attainment at one month postpartum. *Nursing Research Advancing Clinical Practice for the 80's*. San Francisco: Department of Nursing Service, Stanford University Hospital, and Symposia Medicus.

Mercer, R.T. (1980). Teenage mothering. *Perinatal Press, 4*(5), 71.

Mercer, R.T., & Hackley, K. (1981). Factors correlated with the primipara's perception of her labor and delivery experience. *Proceedings Nurses' Association of American College of Obstetrics and Gynecologists, Third National Meeting, San Francisco, March 29-April 4, 1981*. Libertyville, IL: Hollister, Inc.

Mercer, R.T. (1982). The changing family. *Proceedings Seventh Annual March of Dimes Perinatal Nursing Conference, March 22 & 23, 1982*. Mead Johnson Nutritional Division.

Mercer, R.T., & Hackley, K. (1982). Factors correlating with maternal age early postpartum. *Nursing Research, 31*, 188.

Mercer, R.T. (1982). The early postpartum days: Expectations versus realities. *Pediatric Nursing Currents, 29*(1), 1-2.

Mercer, R.T., Hackley, K.C., & Bostrom, A., (1982). Adolescent mothers: Their assets and deficits. *Western Journal of Nursing Research, 4*, 59. Also in *Communicating Nursing Research, 15*, 59.

Mercer, R.T., Hackley, K.C., & Bostrom, A. (1983). Impact on motherhood after thirty. *Communicating Nursing Research, 16*, 51-52.

Mercer, R.T., Hackley, K.C., & Bostrom, A. (1983, April). Comparison of mothering behaviors. *Maternal and Child Health Technical Information Series,*, 8-9.

Mercer, R.T. (1983). Predictors of gratification for mothers 30 and older. *Proceedings Council on Nurse Researchers Conference, Minneapolis, September 21-23*. American Nurses' Association.

Mercer, R.T. (1983). The relationship of attitudes toward the birth experience and mothering behaviors. *Journal of Adolescent Health Care, 4*, 212.

Mercer, R.T. (1984). Predictors of maternal role attainment at one year post birth. *Western Journal of Nursing Research, 6*,(3), 62.

Mercer, R.T., & Hackley, K.C. (1984). A comparison of employed and unemployed mothers' responses and attitudes. *Western Journal of Nursing Research, 6*(3), 61.

Mercer, R.T., Ferketich, S., May, K., & DeJoseph, J. (1987). A comparison of maternal and paternal responses during pregnancy. *Proceedings Council of Nurse Researchers Conference, Arlington, Va., October 13-16*. American Nurses' Association.

Mercer, R.T., Nichols, E.G., & Doyle, G. (1987). Transitions in the life cycle of women: Mothers and nonmothers. *Proceedings Sigma Theta Tau International Biennial Conference, San Francisco, November 10*, Sigma Theta Tau International.

Mercer, R.T., Ferketich, S., May, K., DeJoseph, J., & Sollid, D. (1987). Maternal and paternal responses in high- and low-risk pregnancies. Symposium. *Proceedings Sigma Theta Tau International Biennial Conference, San Francisco, November 10*, Sigma Theta Tau International.

Mercer, R.T. (1991). Parenting models: Where are we? Where are we going? Symposium, Maternal role: Models and consequences. *1991 International Nursing Research Conference Abstracts, Nursing Research: Global Health Perspectives*, American Nurses' Association, Council of Nurse Researchers, p. 502.

Audiovisual

Beland, J.W., & Mercer, R.T. (1975). The crisis of loss, TIO, Psychiatric-Mental-Health Nursing. *American Journal of Nursing* Company, Educational Services Division.

Forewords

Foreword. (1981). In C. Kehoe (Ed.), *Nursing management in cesarean births*. New York: Appleton-Century-Crofts.

Foreword. (1982). In S. Hummenick (Ed.), *Assessment evaluation: A clinical and technical review of selected assessment strategies for use in the health care of families in pregnancy and early parenting years*. New York: Appleton-Century-Crofts.

Foreword. (1986). In J.D. Neeson & K.A. May (Eds.), *Comprehensive maternity nursing*. Philadelphia: JB Lippincott.

Foreword. (1990). In K.A. May & L.R. Mahlmeister (Eds.), *Comprehensive maternity nursing: Nursing process and the childbearing family* (2nd ed.). Hagerstown, MD: JB Lippincott.

Letters to editor

Mercer, R.T. (1976). Preparation of the breast for breastfeeding. *Nursing Research*, 25, 222.

Mercer, R.T. (1977). Moving out of the nursing ghetto. *MCN, American Journal of Nursing*, 2, 65.

Mercer, R.T. (1984). Eight stages of a doctoral dissertation. *Nursing Research*, 23, 435-436.

Book reviews

Mercer, R.T. (1983). *Parenting reassessed: A nursing perspective. American Journal of Nursing*, 83, 963.

Mercer, R.T. (1985). *Maternal identity and the maternal experience. American Journal of Nursing*, 85, 103-104.

Mercer, R.T. (1988). Gay and lesbian parents. *Image: Journal of Nursing Scholarship*, 20(4), 234-235.

Secondary sources

Journal articles

Barnard, K.E., & Neal, M.V., Maternal child nursing research: Review of the past and strategies for the future. *Nursing Research*, 26, 193-200.

Brouse, A.J. (1988). Easing the transition to the maternal role. *Journal of Advanced Nursing*, 13(2), 167-172.

Cranley, M.S., Hedahl, K.J., & Pegg, S.H. (1983). Women's perceptions of vaginal and cesarean deliveries. *Nursing Research*, 32(1), 10-15.

Crawford, G. (1982). A theoretical model of support network conflict experienced by new mothers. *Nursing Research*, 34, 100-102.

Curry, M.A. (1982). Maternal attachment behavior and the mother's self-concept: The effect of early skin-to-skin contact. *Nursing Research*, 32(2), 73-78.

Dunnington, R.M., & Glazer, G. (1991). Maternal identity and early mothering behavior in previously infertile and never infertile women. *Journal of Obstetric, Gynecologic and Neonatal Nursing*, 20(4), 309-318.

Gift, A.G., & Palmer, M.H. (1987). Planning clinical nursing research with a geriatric population. *Clinical Nurse Specialist*, 1(2), 56, 87.

Hawkins, J.W. (1986). Did we do all we could? *American Journal of Nursing*, 86, 158.

Lederman, R.P., Weingarten, C.T., & Lederman, E. (1981). Postpartum self-evaluation questionnaire: Measures of maternal adaptation. *Birth Defects: Original Article Series*, 17(6), 201-231.

Lin, R.C. (1986). A project for facilitating maternal adaptation with Chinese adolescent mothers in Taiwan. *Health Care For Women International* 7(4), 311-327.

Lipson, J.G., & Tilden, V.P. (1980). Psychological integration of the cesarean birth experience. *American Journal of Orthopsychiatry*, 50(4), 598-609.

Majewski, J.L, (1986). Conflicts, satisfactions, and attitudes during transition to the maternal role. *Nursing Research*, 35(1), 10-14.

Pridham, K.F., Lytton, D., Chang, A.S., & Rutledge, D. (1991). Early postpartum transition: Progress in maternal identity and role attainment. *Research in Nursing & Health*, 14(1), 21-31.

Proctor, S.E. (1986). A developmental approach to pregnancy prevention with early adolescent females. *Journal of School Health*, 56(8), 313-321.

Sadler, L.S., & Catrone, C. (1983). The adolescent parent: A dual developmental crisis. *Journal of Adolescent Health Care*, 4(2), 100-105.

Sims-Jones, N. (1986). Back to the theories: Another way to view mothers of prematures. *MCN, The Journal of Maternal-Child Nursing* 11(6), 394-397.

Slager-Ernest, S.E., Hoffman, S.J., & Beckman, C.J.A. (1987). Effects of a specialized prenatal adolescent program on maternal and infant outcomes. *Journal of Obstetric, Gynecologic and Neonatal Nursing*, 16(6), 422-429.

Spivak, H., & Weitzman, M. (1987). Social barriers faced by adolescent parents and their children. *Journal of Adolescent Health Care*, 258, 1500-1504.

Walker, L.O. (1989). A longitudinal analysis of stress process among mothers of infants. *Nursing Research*, 38(6), 339-343.

Walker, L.O. (1989). Stress process among mothers of infants: Preliminary model testing. *Nursing Research*, 38(1), 10-16.

Walker, L.O., & Best, M.A. (1991). Well-being of mothers with infant children: A preliminary comparison of employed women and homemakers. *Women & Health*, 17(1), 71-89.

Walker, L.O., Crain, H., & Thompson, E. (1986). Maternal role attainment and identity in the postpartum period: Stability and change. *Nursing Research*, 35(2), 68-71.

Walker, L.O., Crain, H., & Thompson, E. (1986). Mothering behavior and maternal role attainment during the postpartum period. *Nursing Research*, 35(6), 322-355.

Wassermun, G.A., & Rhiasom, A. (1985). Maternal withdrawal from handicapped toddlers. *Journal of Child Psychology and Psychiatry and Allied Disciplines*, 26, 381-387.

White, M., & Dawson, C. (1981). Impact of the at-risk infant on family solidarity. *Birth Defects*, 17, 253-284.

Yonger, J.B. (1991). A model of parenting stress. *Research in Nursing & Health*, 14(3), 197-204.

Yoos, L. (1987). Perspectives on adolescent parenting: Effect of adolescent egocentrism on the maternal-child interaction. *Journal of Pediatric Nursing*, 2(3), 193-200.

Zahr, L.K. (1991). The relationship between maternal confidence and mother-infant behaviors in premature infants. *Research in Nursing & Health, 14*(4), 279-286.

Zuskar, D.M. (1987). The psychological impact of prenatal diagnosis of fetal abnormality: Strategies for investigation and intervention. *Women's Health, 12,* 91-103.

Other sources

Baltes, P.B., Reese, H.W., & Lipsitt, L.P. (1980). Life-span developmental psychology. *Annual Review of Psychology, 31,* 65-110.

Bronfenbrenner, U. (1979). *The ecology of human development: Experiment by nature and design.* Cambridge, MA: Harvard University Press.

Burr, W.R., Leigh, G.K., Day, R.D. & Constantine, J. (1979). Symbolic interaction and the family. In W.R. Burr, R. Hill, F.I. Nye, & I.L. Reiss (Eds.), *Contemporary theories about the family* (Vol. 2) (pp. 42-111). New York: Free Press.

Erikson, E.H. (1959). Identity and the life cycle. *Psychological Issues* (Monograph), 1(1), 1-171.

Gloger-Tippelt, G. (1983). A process model of the pregnancy course. *Human Development, 26,* 134-138.

Gottlieb, L. (1978). Maternal attachment in primipara. *JOGN Nursing, 7,* 39-44.

Mead, G.H. (1934). *Mind, self and society.* Chicago: University of Chicago Press.

Rowe, G.P. (1966). The developmental conceptual framework to the study of the family. In F.I. Nye & F.M. Berardo (Eds.), *Emerging conceptual frameworks in family analysis* (pp. 198-222). New York: Macmillan.

Rubin, R. (1967). Attainment of the maternal role: Part I. Processes. *Nursing Research, 16,* 237-245.

Rubin, R. (1967). Attainment of the maternal role: Part II. Models and referrants. *Nursing Research, 16,* 342-346.

Rubin, R. (1977). Binding in the postpartum period. *Maternal-Child Nursing Journal, 6,* 67-75.

Rubin, R. (1984). *Maternal identity and the maternal experience.* New York: Springer.

Thorton, R., & Nardi, P.M. (1975). The dynamics of role acquisition. *American Journal of Sociology, 80,* 870-885.

Turner, J.H. (1978). *The structure of sociological theory.* (rev. ed.). Homewood, IL: Dorsey Press.

Von Bertalanffy, L. (1968). *General system theory.* New York: George Braziller.

Werner, H. (1957). The concept of development from a comparative and organismic point of view. In D.H. Harris (Ed.), *The concept of development* (pp. 125-148). Minneapolis: University of Minnesota.

CHAPTER
28

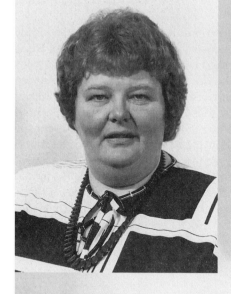

Kathryn E. Barnard

Parent-Child
Interaction Model

Julia M.B. Fine, Jill K. Baker, Debra A. Borchers, Debra Trnka Cochran,
Karla G. Kaltofen, Nancy Orcutt, Jean A. Peacock,
Elizabeth Godfrey Terry, Cynthia A. Wesolowski, Lorraine A. Yeager

CREDENTIALS AND BACKGROUND OF THE THEORIST

Kathryn E. Barnard was born April 16, 1938, in Omaha, Nebraska. In 1956 she enrolled in a prenursing program at the University of Nebraska and graduated with a Bachelor of Science in Nursing in June 1960. On graduation, she continued at the University of Nebraska in part-time graduate studies. That

The authors wish to thank Dr. Kathryn Barnard for her critique of the original chapter.

summer she accepted an acting head nurse position and in the fall became an assistant instructor in pediatric nursing.[8] In 1961 Barnard moved to Boston, Massachusetts, where she enrolled in a Master's program at Boston University. She also worked as a private duty nurse. After earning her Master of Science in Nursing in June 1962 and a certificate of Advanced Graduate Specialization in Nursing Education, she accepted a position as an instructor in maternal and child nursing at the University of Washington in Seattle. In 1965 she was named assistant professor.

She began consulting in the area of mental retardation and coordinated training projects for nurses in child development and the care of children with mental retardation and handicaps. Barnard became the project director for a research study to develop a method for nursing child assessment in 1971. The following year she earned a Ph.D. in the ecology of early childhood development from the University of Washington.[10:1]

In 1972 Barnard accepted a position at the University of Washington as a professor in parent-child nursing. Since 1985 she has also served as adjunct professor of psychology at the University of Washington and served as Associate Dean for Academic Affairs for the School of Nursing from 1987 to 1992.[10:2-3] Barnard has served as the project director or principal investigator for more than 20 research grants and projects since 1971 and from 1979 to the present has served as the principal researcher and advisor for the Nursing Child Assessment Satellite Training Project (NCAST)[10:1-3]

In addition to these research efforts, Barnard has provided consultation, presented lectures internationally, and served on multiple advisory boards. She has published articles in both nursing and nonnursing journals since 1966. Her books include a four-part series on child health assessment, two editions related to teaching the mentally retarded and developmentally delayed child, and work focusing on families of vulnerable infants.[7:2-14] Her most recent publications focus on school-age follow-up of children born preterm, affect regulation by adult and adolescent mothers with high and low social risk, and efficacy of hospital and home visit interventions for improving interaction between mothers and their preterm infants.[10:11-14]

Barnard[2:4] is a member of the American Nurses Association (ANA), where she has served on the Executive Committee for the Division of Maternal and Child Health Nursing. She is also an active member of nine other national organizations, including the Society for Research in Child Development, Sigma Theta Tau, American Public Health Association, and the World Association of Infant Mental Health.[10:6] She has served on numerous advisory boards and committees of these and other professional groups.[10:3-6]

In 1969 Barnard was presented with the Lucille Perry Leone Award by the National League for Nursing for her outstanding contribution to nursing education.[18] She was elected a Fellow of the American Academy of Nursing in 1975 and of the Institute of Medicine in 1985.[10:6] The ANA honored Barnard with the Maternal and Child Health Nurse of the Year Award in 1984[20:242] and named her the Nurse Scientist of the Year in 1987. She was the recipient of two research awards from Sigma Theta Tau in that same year.[7:9] In May 1990, Barnard received an honorary Doctor of Science Degree from the University of Nebraska Medical Center. In May 1992, the American Association for Care of Children's Health presented her with the T.B. Brazelton Lectureship Award.[10:6]

THEORETICAL SOURCES

Although Barnard cites various nursing theorists, such as Florence Nightingale, Virginia Henderson, and Martha Rogers, their direct influence on her research and theory development is uncertain.[3:208; 15:193-194]

Barnard refers to the Neal Nursing Construct, which has four expressions of health and illness: cognition, sensation, motion, and affiliation. Neal worked on a construct for practice, and Barnard and her associates developed measures related to the period of infancy. Barnard later stated, "In reviewing both the Maryland construct and the Washington research, we were impressed with how the design and results of the Nursing Child Assessment Project (NCAP) fit into the [Neal] construct."[15:195-196]

Barnard credits Florence Blake for the beliefs and values making up the foundation of current nursing practice. She describes Blake as:

a great pediatric nursing clinician and educator [who] turned our minds toward an orientation on the patient rather than the procedure. Blake saw the principal function of parenthood and nursing to be the capacity to establish and maintain constructive and satisfying relationships with others. She amplified for nursing important acts such as mother-infant attachment, maternal care, and separation of child from parents. She helped nursing understand the importance of the family.[15:194]

Many of Dr. Barnard's publications were coauthored by writers such as D. King and A.W. Pattullo, indicating a variety of influences. Barnard also coauthored the book, *Teaching the Mentally Retarded Child: A Family Care Approach,* with Marcene L. Powell. Four years later the authors developed a second edition, *Teaching Children with Developmental Problems: A Family Care Approach.* Of greater influence were the coinvestigators and consultants of the Nursing Child Assessment Project, including Sandra Eyres, Charlene Snyder, and Helen Bee Douglas.[14:iv] Barnard and her colleagues[15] state that they were influenced by child development theorists such as J. Piaget, J.S. Brunner, L. Sander, and T.B. Brazelton, in addition to nursing theorists.

USE OF EMPIRICAL EVIDENCE

Barnard used findings of many researchers, such as T. Berry Brazelton, Bettye Caldwell, H. Als, M.F. Waldrup, J.D. Goering, and L.M.S. Dubowitz, in the evolution of her model of parent-child interaction and adaptation.[15:6] The research findings contributed valuable knowledge for the task of developing tools to assess and measure interaction between a caregiver and a child.

In addition to tapping others' research, Barnard conducted her own. She began her research in 1968 by studying mentally and physically handicapped children and adults. In the early 1970s, she studied the activities of the well child and later expanded her study to include methods of evaluating growth and development of children. She also initiated a 10-year series of research projects to examine the effects of stimulation on sleep states in premature infants.

The majority of these research studies were funded by grants from the U.S. Department of Health, Education, and Welfare and later the Department of Health and Human Services.[8:2-3]

From 1976 to 1979, Barnard and colleagues from the University of Washington initiated work to determine how research results could be communicated to practicing nurses across the nation.[3] This led to the evolution of the Nursing Child Assessment Satellite Training Project. In 1977 Barnard began researching methods for disseminating information about newborns and young children to parents. Projects have been funded by the National Foundation of the March of Dimes and Johnson & Johnson, manufacturer of baby products. Barnard recently participated in a publication for parents entitled, "The Many Facets of Touch," which was also funded by Johnson & Johnson.

Barnard continued to study the mother-infant relationship, examining the nurse's role in relation to high-risk mothers and infants.[12:6] The Nursing Child Assessment Project (NCAP) formed the basis for Barnard's Child Health Assessment Interaction Theory. This was a longitudinal study "to identify poor [child development] outcomes before they occur and to examine the variability of the screening and assessment measures over time."[12:16] The study population included 193 infants and their parents. With use of various assessment scales and interviewing tools, the child and his or her parental relationships were assessed at six stages: prenatally, postnatally, and at 1 month, 4 months, 8 months, and 1 year of age. Additional funds were obtained to continue the project by reassessing the child and parent at 2 years of age, and again when the children were in the second grade.[12:16]

Researchers have used the NCAST instruments for both research and as a basis for public health nursing intervention for families with problems. Ruff[22] used the tools to assess the interaction between unmarried teenage mothers and their infants. The NCAST instruments were used as an outcome measure to evaluate differences between mothers and high-risk infants who participated in a monitoring program and those who did not. Farel and colleagues[17] conducted a research study to examine the usefulness of the NCAST instruments for assessing the interaction between high-risk infants and their mothers to determine the need for intervention and the focus for such services. The findings suggest that the NCAST instruments may be useful in screening for dysfunctional interactions between high-risk infants and their mothers and for directing more specialized intervention services in the high-risk infant population.[17]

The NCAST instruments have been standardized and normed for several different ethnic groups, including Caucasian, Hispanic, and African American.[24] More recently, the instruments were also used to assess urban Native Americans by Seideman and other researchers[23,24] and Alaskan Eskimos by MacDonald-Clark and Boffman.[21] These researchers found that, although both groups were less verbal than the ethnic groups on which the instruments were originally normed, the instruments were useful for both research and clinical use because of the universality of the conceptual framework.[24]

MAJOR CONCEPTS & DEFINITIONS

A major focus of Barnard's work was developing assessment tools to evaluate child health, growth, and development while viewing the parent and child as an interactive system. Barnard stated that the parent-infant system was influenced by individual characteristics of each member and that the individual characteristics were also modified to meet the needs of the system. She defines modification as adaptive behavior. The interaction between parent and child is diagrammed in the Barnard model in Fig. 28-1.

Barnard[15:9-12] has defined the terms in the diagram as follows:

Infant's clarity of cues

To participate in a synchronous relationship, the infant must send cues to his/her caregiver. The skill and clarity with which these cues are sent will make it either easy or difficult for the parent to "read" the cues and make the appropriate modification of his/her own behavior. Infants send cues of many kinds: sleepiness, fussiness, alertness, hunger and satiation, and changes in body activity, to name a few. Ambiguous or confusing cues sent by an infant can interrupt a caregiver's adaptive abilities.

Infant's responsiveness to the caregiver

Just as the infant must "send" cues so that the parent can modify his/her behavior, the infant must also "read" cues so that he/she can modify his/her behavior in return. Obviously, if the infant is unresponsive to the behavioral cues of his/her caregivers, adaptation is not possible.

Parent's sensitivity to the child's cues

Parents, like infants, must be able to accurately read the cues given by the infant if they are to appropriately modify their behavior. . . . There are also other influences on the parents' sensitivity. Parents who are greatly concerned about other aspects of their lives, such as occupational or financial problems, emotional problems, or marital stress, may be unable to be as sensitive as they would be otherwise. Only when these stresses are reduced are some parents able to "read" the cues of their young children.

Parent's ability to alleviate the infant's distress

Some cues sent by the infant signal that assistance from the parent is needed. . . . The effectiveness of parents in alleviating the distress of their infants depends upon several factors. First, they must recognize that distress is occurring. . . . Second, they must know (or figure out) the appropriate action which will alleviate distress. . . . Finally, they must be available to put this knowledge to work.

Parent's social and emotional growth-fostering activities

The ability to initiate social and emotional growth-fostering activities depends upon more global parent adaptation. The parent needs to be able to play affectionately with the child, engage in social interactions such as those associated with eating, and to provide appropriate social reinforcement of desirable behaviors. To do these things the parent must be aware of the child's level of development and be able to adjust his/her be-

MAJOR CONCEPTS & DEFINITIONS—cont'd

havior accordingly. . . . This depends as much upon the parent's available energy as on his/her knowledge and skill.

Parent's cognitive growth-fostering activities

It has been shown in a number of studies that cognitive growth is facilitated by providing stimulation which is just above the child's level of understanding. To do this, the parent must have a good grasp of the child's present level of understanding. . . . and the parent also [must] have the energy available to use these skills.

As the NCAP continued, Barnard's model became the foundation for her Child Health Assessment Interaction Theory. Three major concepts form the basis of this theory.

Child In describing the child, Barnard[15:16] used the characteristics of "newborn behavior, feeding

and sleeping patterns, physical appearance, temperament and the child's ability to adapt to his/her caregiver and environment."

Mother *Mother* refers to the child's mother or caregiver and his or her important characteristics. The mother's characteristics include her "psychosocial assets, her concerns about her child, her own health, the amount of life change she experienced, her expectations for her child, and most important, her parenting style and her adaptional skills."[15:17]

Environment The environment represents the environment of both child and mother. Characteristics of the environment include "aspects of the physical environment of the family, the father's involvement and the degree of parent mutuality in regard to child rearing."[15:17]

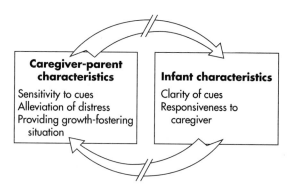

Fig. **28-1** Barnard model. *From Barnard, K.E., et al. (1977). The nursing child assessment training guide: Program learning manual, p. 8. Used with permission.*

MAJOR ASSUMPTIONS

Nursing

Except for nursing, Barnard does not define her major assumptions. In 1966 she defined *nursing* as "a process by which the patient is assisted in maintenance and promotion of his independence. This process may be educational, therapeutic, or restora-

tive: it involves facilitation of change, most probably a change in the environment."[1:629] Fifteen years later, in a 1981 keynote address to the first International Nursing Research Conference, she defined nursing as "the diagnosis and treatment of human responses to health problems."[4:2]

Person

When Barnard describes a person or human being, she speaks of the ability "to take in auditory, visual, and tactile stimuli but also to make meaningful associations from what he takes in."[15:15] This term includes infants, children, and adults.

Health

Although Barnard does not define health, she describes the family "as the basic unit of health care."[3:210] In *The Nursing Child Assessment Satellite Training Study Guide*, she states, "In health care, the ultimate goal is primary prevention."[15:2] Barnard emphasizes the importance of striving to reach one's maximum potential. She believes, "We must promote new values in American society, which up to now has valued not health, but the absence of disease."[4:9] She wrote the definition for the scope of practice on maternal child health.

Environment

Environment is an essential aspect of Dr. Barnard's theory. In *Child Health Assessment, Part II: The First Year of Life*, she states, "In essence, the environment includes all experiences encountered by the child: people, objects, places, sounds, visual and tactile sensations."[12:53] She distinguishes the animate from the inanimate environment. "The inanimate environment refers to the objects available to the child for exploration and manipulation. The animate environment includes the activities of the caretaker used in arousing and directing the young child to the external world."[12:53]

THEORETICAL ASSERTIONS

Barnard's Child Health Assessment Interaction Theory is based on the following 10 theoretical assertions[15:6-7]:

1. In child health assessment the *ultimate* goal is to identify problems at a point before they develop and when intervention would be most effective.
2. Environmental factors, as typified by the process of parent-child interaction, are important for determining child health outcomes.
3. The caregiver-infant interaction provides information that reflects the nature of the child's ongoing environment.
4. The caregiver brings a basic style and level of skills that are enduring characteristics; the caregiver's adaptive capacity is more readily influenced by responses of the infant and her environmental support.
5. In the adaptive parent-child interaction, there is a process of mutual modification in that the parent's behavior influences the infant or child and in turn the child influences the parent so that both are changed.
6. The adaptive process is more modifiable than the mother's or infant's basic characteristics;

therefore, in intervention the nurse should lend support to the mother's sensitivity and response to her infant's cues rather than trying to change her characteristics or styles.
7. An important quality of promoting the child's learning is in permitting child-initiated behaviors and in reinforcing the child's attempt at a task.
8. A major issue for the nursing profession is support of the child's caregiver during the first year of life.
9. Interactive assessment is important in any comprehensive child health care model.
10. Assessment of the child's environment is important in any child health assessment model.

The Child Health Assessment Interaction Model was developed to illustrate Barnard's theory (Fig. 28-2). "The smallest circle represents the child and his/her important characteristics. . . . The next largest circle represents the mother or caregiver and his/her important characteristics. . . . The largest circle represents the environment of both the child and mother."[15:16-17]

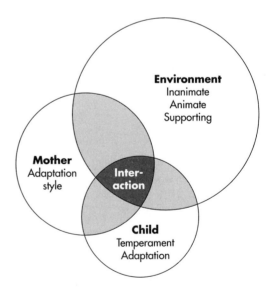

Fig. **28-2 Child Health Assessment Interaction Model.** *From Barnard, K.E., et al. (1977). The nursing child assessment training guide: Program learning manual, p. 19. Used with permission.*

Those portions of the model where two circles overlap represent interaction between the two concepts. The dark center area represents interaction among all three concepts. Barnard's theory focuses on this crucial mother-child-environment interactive process. The NCAP used this as the theoretical basis for the study of potential screening and assessment methods to be used with young children.[15:17]

LOGICAL FORM

According to Chinn and Jacobs,[16:61] "In inductive logic the reasoning method relies on observing particular instances and then combining those particulars into a larger whole." Inductive logic is the form Barnard used in developing her Child Health Assessment Interaction Theory. This theory was an outcome of the investigation and findings of the NCAP. Barnard concluded the most important aspect of child health assessment was the interaction and adaptation that occurs between parent and child.

ACCEPTANCE BY THE NURSING COMMUNITY

Practice

The NCAST has prepared more than 6000 nurses to use a series of standardized assessment tests over a period of more than 20 years. The scales are used to screen and to plan individualized interventions with families. The scales also give measurable outcomes for both the caregiver and the child and thus form an ongoing assessment and basis for evaluation. Trained nurses use these tools throughout the United States and in other countries for both research and daily clinical use.

Education

The nursing satellite training project initially used satellite communications and later videotaped classes to teach nurses how to use a series of standard assessment instruments. Interrater reliability of more than 85% has encouraged nurses to share their knowledge and observations with coworkers. The ex-

plicitness of the observations has made the task of educating others easier.

Research

One of the outcomes of the contract to develop accurate assessment tools was the creation of a research project. The purpose of the satellite training program was to quickly disseminate current research findings. Barnard has continued to refine the assessment scales and continues to receive funds for research. She is well recognized for her work, having been cited in the Citation Indices at least 35 times between 1976 and 1984. She has received awards recognizing her work from several organizations, including the American Medical Association, the American Public Health Association, and the Association of Women's Health, Obstetric, and Neonatal Nurses (formerly known as NAACOG). The NCAST scales have been used in numerous research studies both in the United States and in other countries.

FURTHER DEVELOPMENT

Barnard stated she has a model of interaction. She does not believe that her model fulfills the criteria set forth for evaluation of a theory.[9] If Barnard's model is critiqued by theoretical criteria, the greatest deficit is a lack of semantic clarity. Barnard does not explicitly define her major assumptions about nursing, person, health, and environment. Although the identification of major concepts is implied through the Nursing Child Health Assessment Interaction Model, Barnard fails to clearly define these concepts. This is an area requiring further development.

In the Child Health Assessment Interaction Theory, the mother is identified as a major concept, and the father is included in the description of the environment. Although this classification may describe the father's role in many families of the 1970s, a problem exists when the father or another relative or even a babysitter assumes the role of primary or part-time caregiver. In these instances, Barnard's model must be modified.

Barnard says her future endeavors will focus on further investigation of the child, the parents, and the environment. She plans to continue work in the area of teaching parents how to improve interaction skills with their children. From 1982 to 1988 she conducted research involving the high-risk infant. In 1987 she began a study to develop a nursing model for preterm infant follow-up and continues to research and refine nursing assessment and interventions for high-risk families.[10] Although Barnard's theory is a micro theory, she does not intend to broaden her scope. Rather, she will be looking more closely at individual variables and how these affect a child's development.[13]

CRITIQUE

Clarity

"Clarity in general refers to the lucidness and consistency of the theory. . . . An extremely important aspect of semantic clarity is that of definition of concepts."[16:137] Barnard does not identify or define her theoretical concepts. Rather, she describes and implies the definitions of these concepts. "In a theory with structural clarity, concepts are interconnected and organized into a coherent whole."[16:139] By using Barnard's Child Health Assessment Interaction Model, it is relatively easy for the reader to understand the interrelationships of her theoretical concepts. Barnard is consistent in the use of an inductive form of logic.

Simplicity

The Child Health Assessment Interaction Model is a simple way of communicating the main focus of Barnard's work as it relates to the parent-child interaction and the development of accurate assessment tools. However, there are several identified characteristics for both concepts and assertions, and consequently the complexity is great. It must also be noted that the research necessary to define and support the assertions is complex.

Generality

The original work involved interactions between parent and child during the child's first 12 months of life. Subsequent work lengthened the time period of the child assessment to 36 months. However, one can currently only generalize to parent-child interactions in the first 3 years of life. The parent-child interaction model approaches midrange theory as defined by Chinn and Jacobs.[16] Despite the narrow scope, Barnard's theory is applicable not only to nursing but also to other disciplines that deal with the parent-child relationship.

Empirical Precision

Much research was included in Barnard's original work. The scales were tested for reliability and established as reliable by studies of internal consistency and through test-retest procedures. Factorial and criterion-related validity have also been addressed.[15] By requiring certified NCAST training for clinicians or researchers to use the scales, Barnard and her colleagues have ensured a high degree of precision and reliability in the many research studies using the scales.

Derivable Consequences

More than 6000 nurses have been trained to use the NCAST assessment scales with greater than 85% interrater reliability. Nurses in the United States and in other countries use the observational skills in daily clinical practice.[11]

Throughout her writings, Barnard emphasizes the need for strong links among nursing research, theory, and practice. She indicates, "There has been no more exciting time in nursing than now. We have the clinical, research, scholarship, administrative, and educational expertise so carefully developed over the past years."[6:252]

In discussing research, she states, "We simply must attempt to be in closer alignment with practice from the beginning."[20:169] In the Nursing Child Assessment Satellite Training Project, she identifies her goal as the dissemination of research findings and the application of these findings to practice. This goal is a prime example of Barnard's efforts to link research, theory, and practice.

CRITICAL THINKING *Activities*

1 Picture youself as a public health nurse in Alaska. You provide health services to a number of traditional Yup'ik Eskimo villages. The state Division of Public Health Nursing has urged use of the NCAST scales for assessment because of a recent statewide increase in child abuse and the need for early identification and intervention to prevent problems. You must gain the permission of the village councils to assess the village families. State the points you would cover and how you would explain Barnard's Child Health Assessment Interaction Model, the NCAST scales, and nursing interventions to the village councils.

2 Do you think it would be possible to adapt Barnard's Child Health Assessment Interaction Model to other caregiver/care receiver situations, such as a wife caring for her husband with Alzheimer's disease? What changes in the concepts and definitions, assumptions, and theoretical assertions would be necessary?

REFERENCES

1. Barnard, K.E. (1966, Dec.). Symposium on mental retardation. *Nursing Clinics of North America, 1,* 629-630.
2. Barnard, K.E. (1979, Sept. 20). Child advocates must help parents, too. *American Nurse, 11,* 4.
3. Barnard, K.E. (1980, July). Knowledge for practice: Directions for the future. *Nursing Research, 29,* 208-212.
4. Barnard, K.E. (1982, Summer). The research cycle: Nursing, the profession, the discipline. *Western Journal of Nursing Research, 4,* 1-12.
5. Barnard, K.E. (1984). Curriculum vitae.
6. Barnard, K.E. (1985). Rituals that integrate nursing practice, education, and research. In K.E. Barnard & G.R. Smith (Eds.), *The second annual symposium in nursing faculty practice.* American Academy of Nursing.
7. Barnard, K.E. (1987, Oct.). Curriculum vitae.
8. Barnard, K.E. (1992, June). Curriculum vitae.
9. Barnard, K.E. (1992, June). Personal communication.
10. Barnard, K.E. (1994, May). Curriculum vitae.
11. Barnard, K.E. (1996, July). Personal communication.
12. Barnard, K.E., & Eyres, S.J. (Eds.). (1979). *Child health assessment, part II: The first year of life.* Hyattsville, MD: U.S. Department of Health, Education, and Welfare.

13. Barnard, K.E., & Neal, M.V. (1977, May-June). Maternal-child nursing research: Review of the past and strategies for the future. *Nursing Research, 26,* 193-200.
14. Barnard, K.E., & Powell, M.L. (1972). *Teaching the mentally retarded child: A family care approach.* St. Louis: Mosby.
15. Barnard, K.E., Spietz, A.L., Snyder, C., Douglas, H.B., Eyres, S.J., & Hill, V. (1977). *The nursing child assessment satellite training study guide.* Unpublished program learning manual.
16. Chinn, P., & Jacobs, M. (1987). *Theory and nursing: A systematic approach.* St. Louis: Mosby.
17. Farel, A.M., Freeman, V.A., Keenan, N.L., & Huber, C.J. (1991). Interaction between high-risk infants and their mothers: The NCAST as an assessment tool. *Research in Nursing and Health, 14,* 109-118.
18. Kathryn E. Barnard presented with the Lucille Petry Leone Award at NLN annual convention. (1969). *Washington State Journal of Nursing, 41,* 9.
19. Kathryn E. Barnard presented with the Maternal and Child Health Nurse of the Year Award, 1983, at ANA annual convention. (1984). *Nursing Outlook, 32,* 242.
20. King, D., Barnard, K.E., & Hoehn, R. (1981, March). Disseminating the results of nursing research. *Nursing Outlook, 29,* 164-169.
21. MacDonald-Clark, N.J., & Boffman, J.L. (1995). Mother-child interaction among the Alaskan Eskimos. *JOGNN, 24,* 450-457.
22. Ruff, C.C. (1987). How well do adolescents mother? *Maternal and Child Nursing, 12,* 249-253.
23. Seideman, R.Y., Haase, J., Primeaux, M., & Burns, P. (1992). Using NCAST instruments with urban American Indians. *Western Journal of Nursing Research, 14,* 308-321.
24. Seideman, R.Y., Williams, R., Burns, T., Jacobson, S., Weatherby, R., & Primeaux, M. (1994). Culture sensitivity in assessing urban Native American parenting. *Public Health Nursing, 11,* 98-103.

BIBLIOGRAPHY

Primary sources

Books

Barnard, K.E. (Ed.). (1983). *Structure to outcome: Making it work.* Kansas City, MO: American Academy of Nursing.
Barnard, K.E. (1984). *Social support and families of vulnerable infants.* White Plains, NY: March of Dimes Birth Defects Foundation.
Barnard, K.E. (Ed.). (1987). *Nursing child assessment satellite training: Learning resource manual.* Seattle, WA: Nursing Child Assessment Satellite Training Publications.
Barnard, K.E., & Brazelton, T.B. (Chairpersons). (1984). *The many facets of touch.* Somerville, NJ: Johnson & Johnson.
Barnard, K.E., & Brazelton, T.B. (Eds.). (1990). *Touch: The foundation of experience.* Clinical Infant Reports Series of the National Center for Clinical Infant Programs, 4, International Universities Press, Inc.

Barnard, K.E., & Douglas, H.B. (Eds.). (1974). *Child health assessment, part I: A literature review.* Bethesda, MD: U.S. Department of Health, Education, and Welfare.

Barnard, K.E., & Erickson, M.L. (1976). *Teaching children with developmental problems: A family care approach* (2nd ed.). St. Louis: Mosby.

Barnard, K.E., & Eyres, S.J. (Eds.). (1979). *Child health assessment, part II: The first year of life.* Hyattsville, MD: U.S. Department of Health, Education, and Welfare.

Barnard, K.E., & Powell, M.L. (1972). *Teaching the mentally retarded child: A family care approach.* St. Louis: Mosby.

Book chapters

Barnard, Kennell, Lubchenco, Parmelee: Panel discussion. (1980). In E.J. Sell (Ed.), *Follow-up of the high risk newborn: A practical approach* (pp. 187-195). Springfield, IL: Charles C Thomas.

Barnard, K.E. (1973). Nursing. In J. Wortis (Ed.), *Mental retardation and developmental disabilities: An annual review.* New York: Brunner-Mazel.

Barnard, K.E. (1975). Infant programming. In R. Koch (Ed.), *Proceedings of confidence on Down's syndrome.* New York: Brunner-Mazel.

Barnard, K.E. (1976). The state of the art: Nursing and early intervention with handicapped infants. In T. Tjossem (Ed.), *Proceedings of 1974 President's Committee on Mental Retardation Meeting on Infant Intervention.* Baltimore, MD: University Park Press.

Barnard, K.E. (1978). Introduction to parent-infant interaction studies. In G.P. Sackett (Ed.), *Observing behavior* (Vol. I): *Theory and application in mental retardation.* Baltimore, MD: University Park Press.

Barnard, K.E. (1979). How focusing on the family changes the health care system. In T.B. Brazelton & V.C. Vaughan (Eds.), *The family: Setting priorities.* New York: Science & Medicine.

Barnard, K.E. (1980). How nursing care may influence prevention of development delay. In E.J. Sell (Ed.), *Follow-up of the high risk newborn: A practical approach.* Springfield, IL: Charles C Thomas.

Barnard, K.E. (1980). Sleep organization and motor development in prematures. In E.J. Sell (Ed.), *Follow-up of the high risk newborn: A practical approach.* Springfield, IL: Charles C Thomas.

Barnard, K.E. (1981). An ecological approach to parent-child relations. In C.C. Brown (Ed.), *Infants at risk: Assessment and intervention.* Johnson & Johnson Pediatric Round Table.

Barnard, K.E. (1981). General issues in parent-infant interaction during the first years of life. In D.L. Yeung (Ed.), *Essays of pediatric nutrition.* Ontario, Canada: The Canadian Science Committee on Food and Nutrition, Canadian Public Health Association.

Barnard, K.E. (1981). The nursing role in the promotion of child development. In M. Tudor (Ed.), *Child development.* New York: McGraw-Hill.

Barnard, K.E. (1981). A program of temporarily patterned movement and sound stimulation for premature infants. In V.L. Smeriglio (Ed.), *Newborns and parents: Parent-infant contact and newborn sensory stimulation* (pp. 31-48). Hillsdale, NJ: Lawrence Erlbaum Associates.

Barnard, K.E. (1984). Nursing research in relation to infants and young children. In H. Werley & J. Fitzpatrick (Eds.), *Annual review of nursing research* (Vol. 1) (pp. 3-25). New York: Springer.

Barnard, K.E. (1985). Rituals that integrate nursing practice, education and research. In K.E. Barnard & G.R. Smith (Eds.), *The second annual symposium in nursing faculty practice.* American Academy of Nursing.

Barnard, K. (1986). Major issues in program evaluation. In *Program evaluation: Issues, strategies and models.* Washington, DC: National Center for Clinical Infant Programs.

Barnard, K.E. (1987). Paradigms for intervention: Infant state modulation. In N. Gunzenhauser (Ed.), *Infant stimulation: For whom, what kind, when, and how much?* (pp. 129-136). Skillman, NJ: Johnson & Johnson Baby Products Company.

Barnard, K.E., Bee, H.L., & Hammond, M.A. (1984). Home environment and cognitive development in a health, low-risk sample: The Seattle study. In A. Gottfried (Ed.), *Home environment and early cognitive development.* New York: Academic Press.

Barnard, K.E., Booth, C.L., Mitchell, S.K., & Telzow, R.W. (1988). Newborn nursing models: A test of early intervention to high-risk infants and families. In E. Hibbs (Ed.), *Children and families: Studies in prevention and intervention* (pp. 63-81). New York: International Universities Press.

Barnard, K.E., & Brazelton, T.B. (Eds.). (1987). Touch: The foundation of experience. National Center for Clinical Infant Programs, Monograph No. 4.

Barnard, K.E., Eyres, S.J., Lobo, M., & Snyder, C. (1983). An ecological paradigm for assessment and intervention. In T.B. Brazelton & B. Lester (Eds.), *New Approaches to developmental screening of infants.* New York: Elsevier.

Barnard, K.E., Hammond, M.A., Booth, C.L., Bee, H.L., Mitchell, S.K., & Spieker, S.J. (1989). Measurement and meaning of parent-child interaction. In F.J. Morrison, C.E. Lord, & D.P. Keating (Eds.). *Applied developmental psychology* (Vol. III). New York: Academic Press.

Barnard, K.E., Hammond, M.A., Mitchell, S.K., Booth, C.L., Spietz, A., Snyder, C., & Elsas, T. (1985). Caring for high-risk infants and their families. In M. Green (Ed.), *The psychological aspects of the family.* Lexington, MA: Lexington Books.

Barnard, K., & Hoehn, R.E. (Dec. 1978). Nursing child assessment satellite training. In R.A. Duncan (Ed.), *Biomedical communications experiments.* Lister Hill National Center for Biomedical Communications, Department of U.S. Health, Education, and Welfare, Public Health Service.

Barnard, K.E., & Kelly, J.F. (1988). Children with special needs—Early intervention. In H.M. Wallace, G. Ryan, & A.C. Oglesby (Eds.), *Maternal and child health practices* (3rd ed.). Oakland, CA: Third Party Publishing.

Barnard, K.E., & Kelly, J.F. (1990). Assessment of parent-child interaction. In S.J. Meisels, & J.P. Shonkoff (Eds.), *Handbook of early childhood intervention* (pp. 278-302). New York: Cambridge University Press.

Barnard, K.E., & Magyary, D.L. (1987). Early identification. In H. Wallace, A. Oglesky, R. Biehl, & L. Taft (Eds.), *Handicapped children and youth: A comprehensive community and clinical approach* (pp. 99-110). New York: Human Science Press.

Barnard, K.E., Magyary, D.L., Booth, C.L., & Eyres, S.J. (1987). Longitudinal design: Considerations and application to nursing research. In M. Cahoon (Ed.), *Recent advances in nursing: Research methodology*. Edinburgh: Churchill Livingstone.

Barnard, K.E., & Martell, L.K. (1995). Mothering. In M.H. Bornstein (Ed.), *Handbook of parenting*, Vol. 3: *Status and social conditions of parenting* (pp. 3-26). Hillsdale, NJ: Lawrence Erlbaum Associates.

Barnard, K.E., & Morisset, C.E. (1995). Preventive health and developmental care for children: Relationships as a primary factor in service delivery with at risk populations. In H.E. Fitzgerald, B.M. Lester, & B.S. Zuckerman (Eds.), *Children of poverty: Research, health, and policy issues. Reference books on family issues*, Vol. 23; *Garland reference library of social science*, Vol. 968 (pp. 167-195). New York: Garland Publishing.

Barnard, K.E., Morisset, C.E., & Spiker, S. (1993). Preventive interventions: Enhancing parent-infant relationships. In C.H. Zeanah (Ed.), *Handbook of infant mental health* (pp. 386-401). New York: Guilford Press.

Barnard, K.E., & Sumner, G.A. (June 1981). The health of women with fertility-related needs. In L.V. Klerman (Ed.), *Research priorities in maternal and child health: Report of a conference* (pp. 49-102). Waltham, MA: Brandeis University.

Barnard, K.E., Wenner, W., Weber, B., Gray, C., & Peterson, A. (1977). Premature infant refocus. In Mittler, P. (Ed.), *Research to practice in mental retardation: Biomedical aspects*, Vol. 3. I.A.S.S.M.D.

Booth, C.L., Spiker, S.J., Barnard, K.E., & Morisset, C.E. (1992). Infants at risk: The role of preventive intervention in deflecting a maladaptive developmental trajectory. In J. McCord & R.E. Tremblay, (Eds.), *Preventing antisocial behavior: Interventions from birth through adolescence* (pp. 21-42). New York: Guilford Press.

Kang, R., & Barnard, K. (1979). Using the Neonatal Behavioral Assessment Scale to evaluate premature infants. In *Birth defects: Original article series, XV* (7) 119-144. National Foundation. New York: Alan R. Liss.

Magyary, D., Barnard, K., & Brandt, P. (1988). Biophysical considerations in the assessment of young children with a developmental disability. In T.D. Wachs & R. Sheehan (Eds.), *Assessment of young developmentally disabled children: Perspectives in developmental psychology* (pp. 347-370). New York: Plenum Press.

Magyary, D., Brandt, P., Barnard, K.E., Hammond, M. (1992). School age follow-up of the development of preterm infants: Infant and family predictors. In M. Sigman (Ed.), *Advances in applied developmental psychology series: Low birth-weight children*. New York: Ablex Press.

Mitchell, S.K., Barnard, K.E., Booth, C., Magyary, D., and Spieker, S. (1985). Prediction of school problems and behavior problems in children followed from birth to age eight. In W.K. Frankenburg, R.N. Emde, & J. Sullivan (Eds.), *Early identification of children at risk: An international perspective*. New York: Plenum Press.

Mitchell, S.K., Magyary, D.A., Barnard, K.E., Summer, G.A., & Booth, C.L. (1988). A comparison of home-based prevention programs for families of newborns. In L.A. Bond & B. Wagner (Eds.), *Families in transition: Primary prevention programs that work*. Beverly Hills, CA: Sage.

Journal articles

Barnard, K., Boothe, C., Johnson, C., & Crowley, N. (1985). Infant massage and exercise: Worth the effort? *Maternal-Child Nursing, 10*(3), 184-189.

Barnard, K.E. (1966, April-May). New four-part training project is developed. *Children Limited, 15,* 2.

Barnard, K.E. (1966, Dec.). Symposium on mental retardation. *Nursing Clinics of North America, 1,* 629-630.

Barnard, K.E. (1968, Feb.). Teaching the mentally retarded child is a family affair. *American Journal of Nursing, 68,* 305-311.

Barnard, K.E. (1969, Oct.). Are professionals educable? *Alabama Journal of Medical Sciences, 6,* 388-391.

Barnard, K.E. (1973, Dec.). The effect of stimulation on the sleep behavior of the premature infant. *Communicating Nursing Research, 6,* 12-33.

Barnard, K.E. (1975, Oct.). Trends in the care and prevention of developmental disabilities. *American Journal of Nursing, 75,* 1700-1704.

Barnard, K.E. (1976, Oct.). Predictive nursing: The baby and parents. *Health Care Dimensions, 3,* 185-202.

Barnard, K.E. (1977, Aug. 15). A challenge for nursing care. *American Nurse, 9,* 4.

Barnard, K.E. (1978, March-April). The family and you. *American Journal of Maternal Child Nursing, 3,* 82-83.

Barnard, K.E. (1979, Sept. 20). Child advocates must help parents, too. *American Nurse, 11,* 4.

Barnard, K.E. (1980, July). Knowledge for practice: Directions for the future. *Nursing Research, 29,* 208-212.

Barnard, K.E. (1981, May-June). The research question. *American Journal of Maternal Child Nursing, 6,* 211.

Barnard, K.E. (1981, July-Aug.). Breast-feeding is best for U.S. babies, too. *American Nurse, 13,* 44.

Barnard, K.E. (1981, July, Aug.). Research designs: Descriptive method. *American Journal of Maternal Child Nursing, 6,* 243.

Barnard, K.E. (1981, Sept-Oct.). Research designs: Experimental method. *American Journal of Maternal Child Nursing, 6,* 321.

Barnard, K.E. (1981, Nov.-Dec.). Research designs: The historical method. *American Journal of Maternal Child Nursing, 6,* 391.

Barnard, K.E. (1982, Jan.-Feb.). Research designs: Sampling. *American Journal of Maternal Child Nursing, 7,* 15.

Barnard, K.E. (1982, March-April). Measurements: Reliability. *American Journal of Maternal Child Nursing, 7,* 101.

Barnard, K.E. (1982, May-June). Measurement: Validity. *American Journal of Maternal Child Nursing, 7,* 165.

Barnard, K.E. (1982, Summer). The research cycle: Nursing, the profession, the discipline. *Communicating Nursing Research, 15,* 1-12.

Barnard, K.E. (1982, Summer). The research cycle: Nursing, the profession, the discipline. *Western Journal of Nursing Research, 4,* 1-12.

Barnard, K.E. (1982, July-Aug.). Measurement descriptive statistics. *American Journal of Maternal Child Nursing, 7,* 235.

Barnard, K.E. (1982, Sept.-Oct.). Determining the focus of nursing research. *American Journal of Maternal Child Nursing, 7,* 299.

Barnard, K.E. (1982, Nov.-Dec.). Determining the role of nursing. *American Journal of Maternal Child Nursing, 7,* 36.

Barnard, K.E. (1983, Jan.). Social policy statement can move nursing ahead. *American Nurse, 15,* 4, 14.

Barnard, K.E. (1983, Jan.-Feb.). The case study method: A research tool. *American Journal of Maternal Child Nursing, 8,* 36.

Barnard, K.E. (1983, March-April). Identifying potential nursing research areas. *American Journal of Maternal Child Nursing, 8,* 117.

Barnard, K.E. (1983, May-June). Nursing diagnosis: A descriptive method. *American Journal of Maternal Child Nursing, 8,* 223.

Barnard, K.E. (1983, July-Aug.). Formulation of hypotheses. *American Journal of Maternal Child Nursing, 8,* 263.

Barnard, K.E. (1983, Aug.). Our concern for child health. NCAP follow-up at age two. *NCAST National News, 1,* 1.

Barnard, K.E. (1983, Sept.-Oct.). Informed consent. *American Journal of Maternal Child Nursing, 8,* 327.

Barnard, K.E. (1983, Nov.). Child health screening indicators. *NCAST National News, 1,* 2.

Barnard, K.E. (1983, Nov.-Dec.). Control groups. *Maternal Child Nursing, 8,* 431.

Barnard, K.E. (1984). Nursing research related to infants and young children. *Annual Review of Nursing Research, 1,* 3-25.

Barnard, K.E. (1984, Jan.-Feb.). The family as a unit of measurement. *American Journal of Maternal Child Nursing, 9,* 21.

Barnard, K.E. (1984, Feb.). Home based intervention projects described. Newborn nursing models program study 1980-1983. Clinical nursing models study 1982-1987. *NCAST National News, 1,* 3.

Barnard, K.E. (1984, March-April). Children: Our greatest national resource. *Public Health Currents, 24,* 8-10.

Barnard, K.E. (1984, March-April). Commonly understood outcomes. *American Journal of Maternal Child Nursing, 9,* 99.

Barnard, K.E. (1984, May-June). Knowledge development. *American Journal of Maternal Child Nursing, 9,* 175.

Barnard, K.E. (1984, July-Aug.). Planning experiments. *American Journal of Maternal Child Nursing, 9,* 247.

Barnard, K.E. (1984, Sept.-Oct.). Determining relationships. *American Journal of Maternal Child Nursing, 9,* 345.

Barnard, K.E. (1984, Dec.). Sleep behavior of infants—is it important? *NCAST National News, 1,* 6.

Barnard, K. (1985). Blending the art and science of nursing. *Maternal-Child Nursing, 10*(1), 63.

Barnard, K.E. (1985). Nursing systems toward effective parenting-premature. *NCAST National News, 1,* 9.

Barnard, K. (1985). Planning the analysis. *Maternal-Child Nursing, 10*(2), 139.

Barnard, K. (1985). Retention of research sample. *Maternal-Child Nursing, 10*(3), 214.

Barnard, K. (1985). Seeking approval of conducting research. *Maternal-Child Nursing, 10*(4), 292.

Barnard, K. (1985). Seeking funds for research. *Maternal-Child Nursing, 10*(6), 424.

Barnard, K. (1985). Studying patterns of behavior. *Maternal-Child Nursing, 10*(5), 358.

Barnard, K. (1985). Supportive measures for high-risk infants and families. *Birth Defects, 20*(5), 291-329.

Barnard, K.E. (1986). Research utilization: The clinician's role. *Maternal-Child Nursing, 11*(3), 224.

Barnard, K.E. (1986). Research utilization: The researcher's responsibilities. *Maternal-Child Nursing, 11*(2), 150.

Barnard, K.E. (1986). Writing a research proposal. *Maternal-Child Nursing, 11*(1), 76.

Barnard, K.E. (1986, April). Child health screening indicators. *NCAST National News, 22,* 2.

Barnard, K.E. (1986, Oct.). Parenting alterations. *NCAST National News, 2,* 4.

Barnard, K.E. (1987, Jan.). Systematic use of the NCAST scales. *NCAST National News, 3,* 1.

Barnard, K.E. (1987, Oct.). Clinical nursing models. *NCAST National News, 3,* 4.

Barnard, K.E. (1991, April). A construct for assessing families. *NCAST National News, 7,* 2.

Barnard, K.E. (1991, July). Family boundaries. *NCAST National News, 7,* 3.

Barnard, K.E. (1991, Oct.). Family communications. *NCAST National News, 7,* 4.

Barnard, K.E., & Bee, H.L. (1983). The impact of temporarily patterned stimulation on the development of preterm infants. *Child Development, 54,* 1156-1167.

Barnard, K.E., & Bee, H.L. (1984). Developmental changes in maternal interactions with term and preterm infants. *Infant Behavior and Development, 7,* 101-113.

Barnard, K.E., Bee, J.L., & Hammond, M.A. (1984). Developmental changes in maternal interactions with term and preterm infants. *Infant Behavior and Development, 1,* 101-113.

Barnard, K.E., & Blackburn, S. (1985). Making a case for studying the ecologic niche of the newborn. *Birth Defects, 21*(3), 71-88.

Barnard, K.E., & Collar, B.S. (1973, Feb.). Early diagnosis, interpretation and intervention: A commentary on the nurse's role. *Annals of the New York Academy of Science, 205,* 373-382.

Barnard, K.E., Collar, B.S., Spietz, A., Snyder, C., & Kang, R. (1976). Predictive nursing: The baby and parents. *Health Care Dimensions, 31*(1), 185-202.

Barnard, K.E., Hammond, M.A., Sumner, G.A., Kang, R., Johnson-Crowley, N., Snyder, C., Spietz, A., Blackburn, S., Brandt, P., & Magyary, D. (1987). Helping parents with preterm infants: Field test of a protocol. *Early Child Development and Care, 27*(2), 56-290.

Barnard, K.E., Magyary, D., Sumner, G., Booth, C.L., Mitchell, S.K., & Spieker, S. (1988). Prevention of parenting alternations for women with low social support. *Psychiatry, 51,* 248-253.

Barnard, K.E., & Neal, M.V. (1977, May-June). Maternal-child nursing research: Review of the past and strategies for the future. *Nursing Research, 26,* 193-200.

Barnard, K.E., Snyder, C., & Spietz, A. (1984). Supportive measures for high-risk infants and families. In K.E. Barnard, P.A. Brandt, B.S. Raff, & P. Carroll. (Eds.), *Social support and families of vulnerable infants. Birth Defects: Original Article Series, 20*(5). White Plains, NY: March of Dimes Birth Defects Foundation.

Bee, H.L., Barnard, K.E., Eyres, S.J., Gray, C.A., Hammond, M.A., Spitz, A.L., Snyder, C., & Clark, B. (1982). Prediction of IQ and language skill from perinatal status, child performance, family characteristics, and mother-infant interaction. *Child Development, 53,* 1134-1156.

Bee, H.L., Hammond, M.A., Eyres, J.J., Barnard, K.E., & Snyder, C. (1986). The impact of parental life change in the early development of children. *Research in Nursing and Health, 9*(1), 64-74.

Bee, H.L., Mitchell, S.K., Barnard, K.E., Eyres, S.J., & Hammond, M.A. (1984). Predicting intellectual outcomes: Sex differences in response to early environmental stimulation. *Sex Roles, 10.*

Booth, C.L., Barnard, K.E., Mitchell, S.K., & Spieker, S.J. (1987). Successful intervention with multi-problem mothers: Effects on the mother-infant relationship. *Infant Mental Health Journal, 9,* 288-306.

Booth, C.L., Lyons, N.B., & Barnard, K.E. (1984). Synchrony in mother-infant interaction: a comparison of measurement methods. *Child Study Journal, 14,* 95-114.

Booth, C.L., Mitchell, S.K., Barnard, K.E., & Spieker, S.J. (1989). Development of maternal social skills in multi-problem families: Effects on the mother-child relationship. *Developmental Psychology, 25*(3), 403-412.

Brandt, P., Magyary, D., Hammond, M., & Barnard, K. (1992). Learning and behavioral-emotional problems of children born preterm at second grade. *Journal of Pediatric Psychology, 17,* 291-311.

Hammer, S.L., & Barnard, K.E. (1966, Nov.). The mentally retarded adolescent: A review of the characteristics and problems of 44 non-institutionalized adolescent retardates. *Pediatrics, 38,* 845-857.

Hann, D.M., Osofsky, J.D., Barnard, K.E., & Leonard, G. (1994). Dyadic affect regulation in three caregiving environments. *American Journal of Orthopsychiatry, 64,* 263-269.

Houck, G.M., Booth, C.L., & Barnard, K.E. (1991). Maternal depression and locus of control orientation as predictors of dyadic play behavior. *Infant Mental Health Journal, 12,* 347-360.

Jacox, A., Lang, N., & Barnard, K.E. (1982, Oct.). Four nurses describe "dramatic" changes in education. *American Nurse, 9,* 8.

Kang, R., & Barnard, K. (1979). Using the neonatal behavioral assessment scale to evaluate premature infants. *Birth Defects: Original Article Series, 15*(7), 119-144. National Foundation. New York: Alan R. Liss.

Kang, R., Barnard, K., & Oshio, S. (1994). Description of the clinical practice of advanced practice nurses in family-centered early intervention in two rural settings. *Public Health Nursing, 11,* 376-384.

King, D., Barnard, K.E., & Hoehn, R. (1981, March). Disseminating the results of nursing research. *Nursing Outlook, 29,* 164-169.

Mitchell, S.K., Barnard, K.E., Booth, C.L., Magyary, D., & Spieker, S. (1986). The natural alliance of psychology and nursing: Substance as well as practice (commentary). *American Psychologist, 41*(10), 1170.

Morriset, C.E., Barnard, K.E., Greenberg, M.T., Booth, C.L., & Spieler, S.J. (1990). Environmental influences on early language development: The context of social risk. *Development and Psychopathology, 2,* 127-149.

Murray, B.L., & Barnard, K.E. (1966, Dec.). The nursing specialist in mental retardation. *Nursing Clinics of North America, 1,* 631-640.

Patteson, D.M., & Barnard, K.E. (1990). Parenting of low birth weight infants: A review of issues and interventions. *Infant Mental Health Journal, 11,* 37-56.

Pattullo, A.W., & Barnard, K.E. (1968, Dec.). Teaching menstrual hygiene to the mentally retarded. *American Journal of Nursing, 12,* 2572-2575.

Snyder, C., Eyres, S.J., & Barnard, K.E. (1979, Nov.-Dec.). New findings about mothers' antenatal expectations and their relationship to infant development. *American Journal of Maternal Child Nursing, 4,* 354-357.

Whitney, L., & Barnard, K.E. (1966, June). Implications of operant learning theory for nursing care of the mentally retarded. *Mental Retardation, 4,* 3.

Unpublished papers

Barnard, K.E. (1967, April). Nursing and mental retardation: A problem solving paper. U.S. Public Health Service, Mental Retardation Division, pp. 1-70.

Barnard, K.E. (1967, April). Planning for learning experiences in university affiliated centers. Proceedings of the 4th National Workshop for Nurses in Mental Retardation, U.S. Children's Bureau.

Barnard, K.E. (1975). Predictive nursing care. In *Proceedings of perinatal nursing conference,* sponsored by University of Washington School of Nursing and Maternal and Child Health Services, HSMHA, Seattle, WA.

Barnard, K.E. (1976, Feb.). A perspective on where we are in early intervention programs. Adapted from a Keynote Address at a conference on "The Nursing Role in Early Intervention Programs for Developing Disabled Children," sponsored by the University of Utah College of Nursing Division of Continuing Education and Utah State Division of Health, Denver, CO.

Barnard, K.E. (1977). Nursing child assessment satellite training fact sheet.

Barnard, K.E. (1981). Critical issues: Support of the caregiver. Maternal Child Nursing in the 80s: Nursing Perspective. A Forum in Honor of Katherine Kendall. School of Nursing, University of Maryland.

Barnard, K.E., Principal Investigator. Clinical nursing model for infants and their families. National Institute of Mental Health, Alcohol, Drug Abuse, and Mental Health Administration, Public Health Service, Department of Health and Human Services. Grant submitted May 1981.

Barnard, K.E., Principal Investigator. Premature infant refocus. Grant No. MC-R-530348. Maternal and Child Health and Crippled Children's Services, Bureau of Community Health Services, Health Services Administration, Public Health Service, Department of Health and Human Resources, Sept. 1, 1974-April 30, 1981.

Barnard, K.E., Principal Investigator. Models of newborn nursing services. Grant No. NU-00719. Division of Nursing, Bureau of Health Professions, Health Resources Administration, Public Health Service, Department of Health and Human Services, July 7, 1979-June 30, 1982.

Barnard, K.E. (Ed.) (1983). *Structure to outcome—making it work.* Papers of the First Faculty Practice Symposium, American Academy of Nursing. Kansas City: American Nurses' Association.

Barnard, K.E., & Bee, H.L. The assessment of parent-infant interaction by observation of feeding and teaching.

Barnard, K.E., & Bee, H.L. (1981, Sept.). Premature infant refocus. Final report on Grant No. MC-R-530348. Prepared for the Maternal and Child Health and Crippled Children's Services Research Grants Program, Bureau of Community Health Services, Health Services Administration, Public Health Service, Department of Health and Human Services.

Barnard, K.E., Booth, C.L., Mitchell, S.K., & Telzrow, R.W. (1983). *Newborn nursing models.* Final report on Grant No. R01-NU-00719. Prepared for the Division of Nursing, Bureau of Health Manpower, Health Resources Administration, Department of Health and Human Services.

Barnard, K.E., & Hoehn, R.E. (1978, Dec.). Nursing child assessment satellite training. In R.A. Duncan (Ed.), *Biomedical communications experiments.* Lister Hill National Center for Biomedical Communications, Department of Health, Education, and Welfare, Public Health Service.

Barnard, K.E., & Kelly, J.F. (1980, May). Infant intervention: Parental consideration. State of art paper. Guidelines for Early Intervention Programs. Based on a conference Health Issues in Early Intervention Programs, Washington, DC. Sponsored by College of Nursing, University of Utah, and School of Public Health, University of Hawaii. Office for Maternal and Child Health, Department of Health and Human Services.

Barnard, K.E., Lendzion, A., & Moser, J. (1974). Final report on the measuring interactions project, technical report No. 3, The first three years: Programming for atypical infants and their families. New York: United Cerebral Palsy Association.

Barnard, K.E., & Powell, M. (1967, April). Planning for learning experiences in university affiliated centers. Proceedings of the 4th National Workshop for Nurses in Mental Retardation, U.S. Children's Bureau.

Barnard, K.E., & Powell, M. (Revised 1969). *Washington guide to promoting development in the young child.* University of Washington, School of Nursing, mimeographed.

Barnard, K.E., Spietz, A.L., Snyder, C., Douglas, H.B., Eyres, S.J., & Hill, V. (1977). *The nursing child assessment satellite training study guide.* Unpublished program learning manual. University of Washington, Seattle, WA.

Barnard, K.E., Spietz, A.L., Snyder, C., Douglas, H.B., Eyres, S.J., & Hill, V. (1977). The nursing child assessment satellite training study guide. Program learning manual.

Barnard, K.E., & Summer, G.A. (1981, June). The health of women with fertility-related needs. In L.V. Klerman (Ed.), Research priorities in maternal and child health: Report of a conference, Brandeis University, Waltham, MA.

Bee, H.L., et al. (1981, April). Parent-child interaction during teaching in abusing and nonabusing families. Paper presented at the biennial meetings of the Society for Research in Child Development, Boston, MA.

Eyres, S.J., Barnard, K.E., & Gray, C.A. Child health assessment, part III: 2-4 years.

Hammond, M.A., et al. (1983, July). Child health assessment, part IV: Follow-up at second grade. Final report of Grant No. R01-NU-00816 prepared for Division of Nursing, Bureau of Health Professions, Health Resources and Services Administration, U.S. Public Health Service.

Interview

Barnard, K.E.(1984, Nov.). Cassette tape interview.

Correspondence

Barnard, K.E. (1984, Sept.). Curriculum vitae.
Barnard, K.E. (1987, Oct.). Curriculum vitae.
Barnard, K.E. (1992, June). Curriculum vitae.

Videotapes

Barnard, K.E. (1990). *Keys to caregiving: Self-instructional video series.* Nursing Child Assessment Satellite Training. University of Washington, Seattle, WA 98195, 206-543-8528.
Videotape (1984, July 27). NAACOG Invitational Research Conference, Indianapolis, Indiana.
Videotape Services, Nursing Child Assessment Satellite Training.

Secondary sources

Book chapters

Disbrow, M.A. (1983). Conducting interdisciplinary reseearch: Gratifications and frustrations. In N.L. Chaska (Ed)., *The nursing profession: A time to speak.* New York: McGraw-Hill.
Menke, E.M. (1983). Critical analysis of theory development in nursing. In N.L. Chaska (Ed)., *The nursing profession: A time to speak.* New York: McGraw-Hill.

Book reviews

Barnard, K.E., & Douglas, H.B. (Eds.). (1974). *Child health assessment, part I: A literature review.*
   Journal of Continuing Education in Nursing, 6, 52, Nov.-Dec. 1975.
   Nursing Mirror, 141, 71, Oct. 2, 1975.
   RN, 38, 122, Sept. 1975.
Barnard, K.E., & Erickson, M.L. (1976). *Teaching children with developmental problems: A family care approach* (2nd ed.).
   American Journal of Nursing, 77, 499, March 1977.
   Canadian Nurse, 73, 46, July 1977.
Barnard, K.E., & Powell, M.L. (1972). *Teaching the mentally retarded child: A family care approach.*
   American Journal of Nursing, 73, 729, April 1973.
   Canadian Nurse, 69, 54, March 1973.

Research abstract

Barnard, K.E. (1972, Oct.). The effect of stimulation on the duration and amount of sleep and wakefulness in the premature infant. *Dissertation Abstracts International, 33,* 2167-2168.

News releases

Kathryn E. Barnard named in *Directory of Nurses with Doctoral Degrees* (1984). St. Louis: American Nurses Association.
Kathryn E. Barnard named in *National Nursing Directory* (1982). Rockville, MD: Aspen Systems.
Kathryn E. Barnard named in *Sigma Theta Tau Directory of Nurse Researchers* (1983). Indianapolis: Sigma Theta Tau.

Kathryn E. Barnard presented with the Lucille Petry Leone Award at NLN annual convention (1969, May-June). *Washington State Journal of Nursing, 41,* 9.
Kathryn E. Barnard presented with the Maternal and Child Health Nurse of the Year Award for 1983 at ANA annual convention. (1984). *Nursing Outlook, 32,* 242.
Kathryn Elaine Barnard presented with the 1983 Martha May Eliot Award of the American Public Health Association, Maternal and Child Health Section (1984, March-April). *Public Health Currents, 24,* 7-8.

Other sources

(More than 122 articles document Barnard's work.)
Als, H. (1976, May). Personal communication.
Brazelton, T.B. (1973). *The neonatal behavioral assessment scale.* London: William Heinemann; Philadelphia: JB Lippincott.
Brunner, J.S. (1956). *A study of thinking.* New York: John Wiley & Sons.
Brunner, J.S. (1966). *Studies in cognitive growth.* New York: John Wiley & Sons.
Caldwell, B.M. (1965). *Daily program II: A manual for teachers.* Washington, DC: Office of Economic Opportunity.
Caldwell, B.M. (1967). What is the optimal learning environment for the young child? *American Journal of Orthopsychiatry, 37,* 8-21.
Caldwell, B.M. (1968). On designing supplementary environments for early child development. *BAEYC Reporter 10,* 1-11.
Caldwell, B.M. (1970). *Instruction manual inventory for infants* (Home Observation for Measurement of the Environment). Little Rock, AR.
Caldwell, B.M. (1970). The rationale for early intervention. *Exceptional Children, 36,* 717-726.
Caldwell, B.M. (1971). Impact of interest in early cognitive stimulation. In H. Rie (Ed.), *Perspectives in psychopathology.* Chicago: Aldine-Atherton.
Caldwell, B.M. (1971, Feb. 20). A timid giant grows bolder. *Saturday Review,* pp. 47-66.
Caldwell, B.M. (1972). Infant day care: Fads, facts, and fancies. In R. Elardo & B. Pagan (Eds.), *Perspectives on infant day care.* Orangeburg, SC: Southern Association on Children Under Six.
Caldwell, B.M. (1972). Kramer school: Something for everybody. In S.J. Braun & E.P. Wards (Eds.), *History and theory of early childhood education.* Worthington, OH: Charles A. Jones.
Caldwell, B.M. (1973). Do young children have a quality life in day care? *Young Children, 28,* 197-208.
Caldwell, B.M., & Elardo, R. (1972). Innovative opportunities for school psychologists in early childhood education. *School Psychology Digest, 1,* 8-16.
Caldwell, B.M., Hersher, L., Lipton, E., Richmond, J.B., Stern, G.A., Eddy, E., Drachman, R., & Rothman, A. (1963). Mother-infant interaction in monomatric and polymatric families. *American Journal of Orthopsychiatry, 33,* 653-664.

Caldwell, B.M., & Richmond, J.B. (1968). The children's center in Syracuse, NY. In L.L. Dittman (Ed.), *Early child care: The new perspectives.* New York: Atherton.

Caldwell, B.M., & Smith, L.E. (1970). Day care for the very young: Prime opportunity for primary prevention. *American Journal of Public Health, 60,* 690-697.

Caldwell, B.M., Wright, C.M., Honig, A.S., & Tannenbaum, B.S. (1970). Infant day care and attachment. *American Journal of Orthopsychiatry, 40,* 397-412.

Dubowitz, L.M.S., Dubowitz, L.M.S., Dubowitz, V., & Goldberg, C. Clinical assessment of gestational age in the newborn infant. *Pediatrics, 77,* 1-10.

Piaget, J. (1962). *Judgment and reasoning in the child.* New York: Humanities. (Reproduction of 1928 ed.)

Piaget, J. (1976). *The group of consciousness: Action and concept in young children.* Cambridge, MA: Harvard University Press.

Piaget, J. (1983). *The child's perception of physical causality.* New York: Adren Lib. (Reproduction of 1930 ed.)

Waldrop, M.F., & Goering, J.D. (1971). Hyperactivity and minor physical anomalies in elementary school children. *American Journal of Orthopsychiatry, 41*(4), 602-607.

Wesolowski, C. (1994, October). Using keys to caregiving in hospital-based nursing practice. *NCAST National News, 10*(4), 1-3. Available from NCAST National News, NCAST, WJ-10, University of Washington, Seattle, WA 98195.

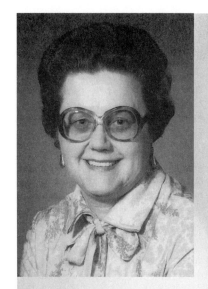

*M*adeleine Leininger

Culture Care: Diversity and Universality Theory

Alice Z. Welch, Sr. Judith E. Alexander, Carolyn J. Beagle, Pam Butler, Deborah A. Dougherty, Karen D. Andrews Robards, Kathleen C. Solotkin, Catherine Velotta

CREDENTIALS AND BACKGROUND OF THE THEORIST

Madeleine M. Leininger is the founder of transcultural nursing and a leader in transcultural nursing and human care theory. She is the first professional nurse with graduate preparation in nursing to hold a Ph.D. in cultural and social anthropology. She was born in Sutton, Nebraska, and began her nursing career after graduating from a diploma program at St. Anthony's School of

The authors wish to express appreciation to Madeleine Leininger for critiquing the chapter.

Nursing in Denver. She was a Cadet Corps nurse while pursuing the basic nursing program. In 1950 she obtained a B.S. degree in biological science from Benedictine College, Atchison, Kansas, with a minor in philosophy and humanistic studies. After graduation she served as an instructor, staff nurse, and head nurse on a medical-surgical unit and opened a new psychiatric unit as director of the nursing service at St. Joseph's Hospital in Omaha. During this time she did advanced study in nursing, nursing administration, teaching and curriculum in nursing, and tests and measurements at Creighton University in Omaha.[21,25]

In 1954 Leininger obtained an M.S.N. in psychiatric nursing from the Catholic University of America in Washington, D.C. She was then employed at the College of Health at the University of Cincinnati, where she began the first graduate clinical specialist program (M.S.N.) in child psychiatric nursing in the world. She also initiated and directed the first graduate nursing program in psychiatric nursing at the University of Cincinnati and the Therapeutic Psychiatric Nursing Center at the University Hospital. During this time she wrote one of the first basic psychiatric nursing texts with C. Hofling, entitled *Basic Psychiatric Nursing Concepts* (1960), which was published in 11 languages and used worldwide.[22]

While working at the child guidance home in the mid-1950s in Cincinnati, Leininger discovered the staff lacked understanding of cultural factors influencing the behavior of children. Among these children of diverse cultural backgrounds, she observed differences that deeply concerned her in the care and psychiatric treatments of the children. Psychoanalytical theories and therapy strategies did not seem to reach children who were of different cultural backgrounds and needs. She became increasingly concerned that her nursing decisions and actions, as well as with those of other staff, did not appear to adequately help these children. Leininger posed many questions to herself and the staff about cultural differences among children and therapy outcomes. She found few staff members were interested or knowledgeable about cultural factors in diagnosis and treatment of clients. A short time later, Margaret Mead became a visiting professor in the Department of Psychiatry, University of Cincinnati, and Leininger discussed with Mead the potential interrelationships between nursing and anthropology. Although she did not get any direct help, encouragement, or solutions from Mead, Leininger decided to pursue her interests with doctoral (Ph.D.) focus on cultural, social, and psychological anthropology at the University of Washington (Seattle).

As a doctoral student, Leininger studied many cultures and found anthropology fascinating and an area that should be of interest to all nurses. She then focused on the Gadsup people of the Eastern Highlands of New Guinea, where she lived alone with the indigenous people for nearly 2 years and undertook an ethnographic and ethnonursing study of two villages.[21,23] She was able to observe not only unique features of the culture but also a number of marked differences between Western and non-Western cultures related to caring health and well-being practices. From her in-depth study and first-hand experiences with the Gadsup, she continued to develop her Theory of Culture Care and the ethnonursing method.[3,4,15,21] Her research and theory has since helped nursing students to understand cultural differences in human care, health, and illness. She has been the major nurse leader who has encouraged many students and faculty to pursue graduate foundational studies in anthropology and to relate this knowledge to transcultural nursing education and practice. Her enthusiasm and deep interests in developing this field of transcultural nursing with a human care focus has sustained her for four decades.

During the 1950s and 1960s, Leininger identified several common areas of knowledge and theoretical research interests between nursing and anthropology, formulating transcultural nursing concepts, theory, principles and practices.[2,3] The book *Nursing and Anthropology: Two Worlds to Blend*, which was the first beginning book in transcultural nursing, laid the foundation for developing the field of transcultural nursing, her theory, and culturally based health care. Her next book, *Transcultural Nursing: Concepts, Theories, Research, and Practice* (1978), identified major concepts, theoretical ideas, and practices in transcultural nursing and was the first definitive publication on transcultural nursing in practice.[3] In her writings she has shown that transcultural nursing and anthropology are complementary to each other but different. Her theory and the conceptual framework for Culture Care Diversity and Universality were laid in this book. During the past 45 years, Leininger has established, explicated, and used the Theory of Culture Care to study many cultures within and outside the United States. She developed the ethnonursing qualitative research method to fit the theory, but especially to grasp the insider (emic) view of cultures.[15,21] The ethnonursing research method was the first nursing research method developed in nursing for nurses to examine complex care and cultural phenomena. In the past four decades, approximately 40 doctoral nurses, as well as many master's and baccalaureate students, have been prepared in transcultural nursing and have used the Leininger Theory of Culture Care. [11,15,26]

The first course offered in transcultural nursing was 1966 at the University of Colorado, where Leininger was a professor of nursing and anthropology. This marked the first joint appointment of a professor of nursing and another discipline in the United States. She also initiated and served as the director of the first nurse-scientist (Ph.D.) program in the United States. In 1969 Leininger was appointed Dean and Professor of Nursing and Lecturer in Anthropology at the University of Washington (Seattle). There she established the first academic nursing department on comparative nursing care systems to support master's and doctoral programs in transcultural nursing. Under her leadership, the Research Facilitation Office was established in 1968 and 1969. She initiated several transcultural nursing courses and guided the first nurses in a special Ph.D. program in transcultural nursing. During this time, she initiated the Committee on Nursing and Anthropology in 1968 with the American Anthropological Association. [3]

In 1974, Leininger was appointed Dean and Professor of Nursing at the College of Nursing and Adjunct Professor of Anthropology at the University of Utah in Salt Lake City. At this institution she initiated the first master's and doctoral programs in transcultural nursing[3] and established the first doctoral program offerings at this institution. The transcultural nursing courses were the first in the world with substantive courses and research focused specifically on transcultural nursing. She also initiated and was director of a new research facilitation office at the University of Utah.

In 1981 Leininger was recruited to Wayne State University, Detroit, where she was Professor of Nursing and Adjunct Professor of Anthropology and Director of Transcultural Nursing Offerings until her semiretirement in 1995. She was also Director of the Center for Health Research at this university for 5 years. While at Wayne State she again developed several courses and seminars in transcultural nursing, caring, and qualitative research methods for baccalaureate, master, doctoral, and postdoctoral students. Currently, this doctoral program has the largest number of master's and doctoral students studying transcultural nursing in the world.[3] In addition to directing the transcultural offerings at Wayne State University, Leininger taught and mentored many students and nurses in field research in transcultural nursing. As one of the first nurse leaders to use qualitative research methods in the early 1960s she has continued to teach these methods at different universities within and outside the United States. To date, she has studied 14 cultures and continues to be a consultant to many research projects and institutions, especially those that are using her Theory of Culture Care.

With the growing interest in transcultural nursing and health care, Leininger[22] has annually delivered keynote addresses and conducted workshops and conferences nationally and internationally since 1965. Her academic vitae records nearly 600 such conferences, keynote addresses, workshops, and consultant services in the United States, Canada, Europe, Pacific Islands, Asia, Africa, Australia, and the Scandinavian countries. She has been an invited guest specialist in most cultures and countries in the world. Educational and service settings continue to request her consultation to focus on transcultural nursing, humanistic caring, ethnonursing research, and her Theory of Culture Care, as well as futuristic trends in health care worldwide.

As the first professional nurse to complete a doctoral degree in anthropology and to initiate several master's and doctoral nursing education programs, Leininger has many areas of expertise and interests. She has studied 14 major cultures in depth and has had experience with many different additional cultures. Besides transcultural nursing with care as a central focus, her other areas of interest are comparative education and administration, nursing theories, politics, ethical dilemmas of nursing and health care, qualitative research methods, the future of nursing and health care, and nursing leadership. Her Theory of Culture Care is now used worldwide and is growing in relevance and importance to obtain grounded cultural data from diverse cultures.

In 1974 she initiated the National Transcultural Nursing Society organization and has been an active leader in this society since its inception. She also initiated the National Research Care Conference in 1978 to help nurses focus specifically on the study of human care phenomena.[4,5,7,11,15,26] She initiated the *Journal of Transcultural Nursing* in 1989 and served as its editor. The *Journal of Transcultural Nursing* remains the only publication focusing primarily on transcultural nursing phenomena.

Leininger has gained international recognition in nursing and in related fields by her transcultural nursing and care writings, theory, research, consultation, courses, and dynamic addresses. She has enthusiastically worked to persuade nurse educators and practitioners to incorporate transcultural nursing and culture-specific care concepts with research findings into nursing curricula and clinical practice as the new and futuristic direction of all aspects of nursing.[15,21,26] She also has found time to give lectures to anthropologists, physicians, social workers, pharmacists, and educators and to do research with other colleagues. She is one of the few nurses who has kept active in two disciplines and to contribute to both fields in national and international transcultural conferences and association meeting. Currently, Leininger resides in Omaha, Nebraska, and is semiretired but still active in worldwide consulting, writing, and lecturing. Her present interest is to establish transcultural nursing institutes to educate and do research on transcultural nursing and health phenomena.

Leininger has authored or edited more than 27 books. Examples of her books include *Nursing and Anthropology: Two Worlds to Blend* (1970); *Transcultural Nursing: Concepts, Theories and Practices* (1978); *Caring: An Essential Human Need* (1981); *Care: The Essence of Nursing and Health* (1984); *Qualitative Research Methods in Nursing* (1985); *Care: Clinical and Community Uses of Care* (1988); *Ethical and Moral Dimensions of Care* (1990); *The Caring Imperative in Education* (1990); *Culture Care Diversity and Universality: A Theory of Nursing* (1991), which is a full account of her theory with the method; and *Transcultural Nursing: Concepts, Theories, Research and Practices* (2nd edition, 1995). In 1996, Madonna University established the Leininger

S Library Collection and a Reading Room in her honor. She has published more than 200 articles and 45 chapters plus numerous films and research reports focused on transcultural nursing, human care and health phenomena, the future of nursing, and related topics relevant in nursing and anthropology. She serves on eight editorial boards and several referee publications. She is known as one of the most creative, productive, innovative, and futuristic authors in nursing, always providing new and substantive research-based nursing content and with ideas to advance nursing as a discipline and profession.

Leininger has received many awards and honors of her lifetime professional and academic accomplishments. She is listed in *Who's Who of American Women, Who's Who in Health Care, Who's Who in Community Leaders, World's Who's Who of Women in Education, International Who's Who in Community Service, Who's Who in International Women,* and other such listings. Her name appears on the *National Register of Prominent Americans and International Notables, International Women,* and the *National Register of Prominent Community Leaders.* She has received several honorary degrees, such as an L.H.D. from Benedictine College, Ph.D. from the University of Kuopio (Finland), and D.S. from the University of Indiana. In 1976 and 1995 she was recognized for her unique and significant contribution to the American Association of Colleges of Nursing as first full-time president. Leininger received the Russell Sage Outstanding Leadership Award in 1995. Leininger is a Fellow in the American Academy of Nursing, a Fellow of the American Anthropology Society, and a Fellow of the Society for Applied Anthropology. Other affiliations include Sigma Theta Tau, the National Honor Society of Nursing, Delta Kappa Gamma, the National Honorary Society in Education, and the Scandinavian College of Caring Science in Stockholm. She has served as distinguished visiting scholar or lecturer in 85 universities in this country and abroad and was recently visiting professor at six universities in Sweden, Wales, Japan, China, Australia, Finland, and New Zealand. While at Wayne State University, she received the Board of Regents' Distinguished Faculty Awards, Distinguished Research Award, the President's Excellence in Teaching, and the Outstanding Graduate Faculty Mentor Award. Most recently (1996), Madonna University honored her with the dedication of the Leininger Book Collection and a special Leininger Reading Room for her outstanding contributions to nursing and the social sciences and humanities.

THEORETICAL SOURCES

Leininger's theory is derived from the disciplines of anthropology and nursing.[15,21] She has defined transcultural nursing as a major area of nursing that focuses on a comparative study and analysis of different cultures and subcultures in the world with respect to their caring values, expression, and health-illness beliefs and pattern of behavior with the goal to develop a scientific and humanistic knowledge to provide culture-specific and/or culture-universal nursing care practice.[15,21]

Transcultural nursing goes beyond an awareness state to that of using culture care nursing knowledge to practice culturally congruent and responsible care.[15,21] Leininger has stated that in time there will be a new kind of nursing practice that reflects different nursing practices that are culturally defined and grounded and specific to guide nursing care to individuals, families, groups, and institutions. She contends that because culture and care are the broadest and the most holistic means to conceptualize and understand people, this knowledge is central to and imperative to nursing education and practice.[15,21] In addition, she states that transcultural nursing has become one of the most important, relevant, and highly promising areas of formal study, research, and practice because of the multicultural world in which we live.[5,7,21] Leininger predicts that for nursing to be meaningful and relevant to clients and other nurses in the world, transcultural nursing knowledge and competencies will be imperative to guide all nursing decisions and actions for effective and successful outcomes.[15,21,23,24]

Leininger makes a distinction between transcultural nursing and cross-cultural nursing. The former refers to nurses prepared in transcultural nursing who are committed to develop knowledge and practice in transcultural nursing, whereas cross-cultural nursing refers to nurses using applied or medical anthropological concepts, with many nurses not committed to developing transcultural nursing theory and research-based practices.[21] She also identifies that international nursing and transcultural nursing are different. International nursing focuses on nurses functioning between two cultures, and transcultural nursing focuses on several cultures with a comparative theoretical and practice base.[21]

Leininger[9,10,16,21] describes the transcultural nurse as a nurse prepared at the baccalaureate level who is able to apply general transcultural nursing concepts, principles, and practices that are generated by transcultural nurse-specialists. The transcultural nurse-specialist prepared in graduate programs receives in-depth preparation and mentorship in transcultural nursing knowledge and practice. This specialist has acquired competency skills through postbaccalaureate education. "This specialist has studied selected cultures in sufficient depth (values, beliefs, lifeways) and is highly knowledgeable and theoretically based about care, health and environmental factors related to transcultural nursing perspectives."[6:252] The transcultural nurse-specialist serves as an expert field practitioner, teacher, researcher, and/or consultant with respect to select cultures. This individual also values and uses transcultural nursing theory to develop and advance knowledge within the discipline of transcultural nursing, the field Leininger predicts must be the focus of all nursing education and practice.[21]

Leininger[25] holds and promotes a new and different theory from the traditional theory in nursing, which usually defines theory as "a set of logically interrelated concepts, hypotheses propositions which can be tested for the purpose of explaining or predicting an event, phenomenon or situation." Instead, Leininger defines theory as the systematic and creative discovery of knowledge about a domain of interest or a phenomenon that appears important to understand or account for some unknown phenomenon. She believes that nursing theory must take into account the creative discovery about individuals, families, and groups and their caring, values, expressions, beliefs, and actions or practices based on their cultural lifeways to provide effective, satisfying, and culturally congruent nursing care. If nursing practices fail to recognize the cultural care aspects of human needs, there will be signs of less beneficial or efficacious nursing care practices and even evidence of dissatisfaction with nursing services, which limits healing and well-being.[15,19,21]

Leininger developed her Theory of Culture Care Diversity and Universality, which is based on the belief that people of different cultures can inform and are capable of guiding professionals to receive the kind of care they desire or need from others. Because culture is the patterned and valued lifeways of people that influence their decisions and actions, the theory is directed toward nurses to discover and document the world of the client and to use their emic viewpoints, knowledge, and practices, along with appropriate etic (professional knowledge), as bases for making culturally congruent professional actions and decisions.[15,21] Indeed, culture care is the broadest holistic nursing theory because it takes into account the totality and holistic perspective of human life and existence over time, including the social structure factors, world view, cultural history and values, environmental context,[4] language expressions, and folk (generic) and professional patterns. These are some of the critical and essential bases to discover grounded care knowledge as the essence of nursing that can lead to the health and well-being of clients and guide therapeutic nursing practice. The Theory of Culture Care can be inductive and deductive, derived from emic (insider) and etic (outsider) knowledge. Leininger, however, encourages obtaining grounded emic knowledge from the people or the culture because such knowledge is most credible. The theory is not necessarily middle range nor macro theory but must be viewed holistically or with specific domains of interest. Leininger believes the terms middle range and macro are outdated in theory development and uses.[15,21]

USE OF EMPIRICAL EVIDENCE

For more than four decades, Leininger has held that care is the essence of nursing and the dominant, distinctive, and unifying feature of nursing.[2,4,7,15] She states that care is complex, illusive, and often embedded in social structure and other aspects of culture. She holds that there are different forms, expressions, and patterns of care that are diverse, and some are universal.[15]

Leininger favors qualitative ethnomethods, especially ethnonursing, to study care.[8,12] These methods are directed toward discovering the people's "truth," views, beliefs, and patterned lifeways. Ethnoscience is one of the rigorous ethnomethods used in anthropology to discover nursing knowledge. However, in the 1960s, Leininger developed the ethnonursing methods to specifically and systematically study transcultural nursing phenomena. Ethnonursing focuses on the systematic study and classification of nursing care beliefs, values, and practices as cognitively or subjectively known by a designated culture (or cultural representatives) through their local emic people centered language, experiences, beliefs, and value system about actual or potential nursing phenomena such as care, health, and environmental factors.[15,21] Although nursing has used the words "care" and "caring" for more than a century, the definitions and usage have been vague and used as cliches without specific meanings to the client's, or nurse's, culture.[4,5] "Indeed, the concepts about caring have been some of the least understood and studied of all human knowledge and research areas within and outside of nursing."[3:33] With the transcultural culture care theory and ethnonursing method based on emic (insider views) beliefs, one gets close to the discovery of grounded or people-based care because it is primarily data centered from the informants and is not derived from the researcher's etic (outsider views) beliefs and practices. An important purpose of the theory is to document, know, predict, and explain systematically by field-generated data what is diverse and universal about generic and professional care of the cultures being studied within the broad Sunrise Model components. Thus, the purpose of transcultural nursing theory is *to discover* the cultural or people's emic views about care as they know, believe, and practice care and then use this knowledge with appropriate etic professional knowledge to guide care practices. The *goal* of the theory is to provide *culturally congruent and responsible care* that reasonably fits with the client's culture needs, values, beliefs, and lifeways realities.[15,21]

Leininger holds that in-depth and culturally based caring knowledge and practices should uniquely distinguish nursing from the contributions of other disciplines.[5,7] The major reason for studying care theory is that "first, the construct of care appears critical to human growth, development and survival for human beings"[4,5] and from the beginning of human species. The second reason is to explicate and fully understand the cultural knowledge and the roles of caregivers and care recipients in different cultures to provide culturally congruent care. Third, care knowledge is discovered and can be used as essential to promote the healing and well-being of clients and to face death or for the survival of human cultures through time.[4,5,15] Fourth, the nursing profession needs to study systematic care from a broad and holistic cultural perspective to discover the expressions and meanings of care, health, illness, and well-being as nursing knowledge. Leininger finds that care is largely an elusive phenomenon often embedded in cultural lifeways and values.

This knowledge, however, is a sound basis for nurses to guide their practice for culturally congruent care and specific therapeutic ways to maintain health, prevent illness, heal, or to help people face death.[17] A central thesis of the theory is that if the meaning of culture care can be fully grasped, the well-being or health care of individuals, families, and groups can be predicted and culturally congruent care can be provided. Thus care is viewed by Leininger as one of the most powerful constructs and central phenomena of nursing. Such care constructs and patterns, however, must be fully documented, understood, and used so that culturally based care becomes the major guide to transcultural nursing therapy and is used to explain or predict nursing practices.

To date, Leininger has studied several cultures in depth and has studied many cultures with undergraduate and graduate students and faculty by use of mainly qualitative research methods. She has explicated 130 different care constructs in 56 cultures in which each culture has different meanings, cultural experiences, and uses by the people of diverse and some similar cultures.[15,21] A new body of knowledge continues to be discovered by transcultural nurses in the development of transcultural care practices with diverse and similar cultures. In time, Leininger believes that both diverse and universal features of care and health will be documented as the essence of nursing knowledge and practice.

Leininger stated the goal of the care theory is to provide culturally congruent care. She believes nurses must work toward explicating care use and meanings so that culture care, values, beliefs, and lifeways can provide accurate and reliable bases for planning and effectively implementing culture-specific care and to identify any universal or common features about care. She maintains that nurses cannot separate world views, social structure, and cultural beliefs (folk and professional), from health, wellness, illness, or care when working with cultures because these factors are closely linked. Social structure factors such as religion, politics, culture, economics, and kinship are significant forces affecting care and influencing well-being and illness patterns. She also emphasizes the importance of discovering

Major Concepts & Definitions

Leininger has developed many terms relevant to the theory; the major ones are defined here. The reader can study her full theory from her definitive book on the theory.[15:46-49]

1. *Care* (noun) refers to abstract and concrete phenomena related to assisting, supporting, or enabling experiences or behaviors toward or for others with evident or anticipated needs to ameliorate or improve a human condition or lifeway.

2. *Caring* (gerund) refers to actions and activities directed toward assisting, supporting, or enabling another individual or group with evident or anticipated needs to ameliorate or improve a human condition or lifeway, or to face death.

Continued

3. *Culture* refers to the learned, shared, and transmitted values, beliefs, norms, and lifeways of a particular group that guides their thinking, decisions, and actions in patterned ways.

4. *Cultural care* refers to the subjectively and objectively learned and transmitted values, beliefs, and patterned lifeways that assist, support, facilitate, or enable another individual or group to maintain their well-being, health, to improve their human condition and lifeway, or to deal with illness, handicaps, or death.

5. *Cultural care diversity* refers to the variabilities and/or differences in meanings, patterns, values, lifeways, or symbols of care within or between collectivities that are related to assistive, supportive, or enabling human care expressions.

6. *Cultural care universality* refers to the common, similar, or dominant uniform care meanings, patterns, values, lifeways, or symbols that are manifest among many cultures and reflect assistive, supportive, facilitative, or enabling ways to help people. (The term *universality* is not used in an absolute way or as a significant statistical finding.)

7. *Nursing* refers to a learned humanistic and scientific profession and discipline which is focused on human care phenomena and activities in order to assist, support, facilitate, or enable individuals or groups to maintain or regain their well-being (or health) in culturally meaningful and beneficial ways, or to help people face handicaps or death.

8. *Worldview* refers to the way people tend to look out on the world or their universe to form a picture or a value stance about their life or world around them.

9. *Cultural and social structure dimensions* refers to the dynamic patterns and features of interrelated structural and organizational factors of a particular culture (subculture or society) which includes religious, kinship (social), political (and legal), economic, educational, technologic, and cultural values and ethnohistorical factors, and how these factors may be interrelated and function to influence human behavior in different environmental contexts.

10. *Environmental context* refers to the totality of an event, situation, or particular experiences that give meaning to human expressions, interpretations, and social interactions in particular physical, ecological, sociopolitical, and/or cultural settings.

11. *Ethnohistory* refers to those past facts, events, instances, and experiences of individuals, groups, cultures, and institutions that are primarily people-centered (ethno) and that describe, explain, and interpret human lifeways within particular cultural contexts and over short or long periods of time.

12. *Generic (folk or lay) care system* refers to culturally learned and transmitted, indigenous (or traditional), folk (home based) knowledge and skills used to provide assistive, supportive, enabling, or facilitative acts toward or for another individual, group, or institution with evident or anticipated needs to ameliorate or improve a human lifeway or health condition (or well-being), or to deal with handicaps and death situations.

13. *Professional care system(s)* refers to formally taught, learned, and transmitted professional care, health, illness, wellness, and related knowledge and practice skills that prevail in professional institutions usually with multidisciplinary personnel to serve consumers.

14. *Health* refers to a state of well-being that is culturally defined, valued, and practiced, and that reflects the ability of individuals (or groups) to perform their daily role activities in culturally expressed, beneficial, and patterned lifeways.

15. *Cultural care preservation or maintenance* refers to those assistive, supporting, facilitative, or enabling professional actions and decisions that help people of a particular culture to retain and/or preserve relevant care values so that they can maintain their well-being, recover from illness, or face handicaps and/or death.

16. *Cultural care accommodation or negotiation* refers to those assistive, supporting, facilitative, or enabling creative professional actions and decisions that help people of a designated culture to adapt to, or to negotiate with, others for a beneficial or satisfying health outcome with professional care providers.

17. *Cultural care repatterning or restructuring* refers to those assistive, supporting, facilitative, or enabling professional actions and decisions that help clients reorder, change, or greatly modify their lifeways for new, different, and beneficial health care pattern while respecting the clients' cultural values and beliefs and still providing a beneficial or healthier lifeway than before the changes were coestablished with the clients.

18. *Cultural congruent (nursing) care* refers to those cognitively based assistive, supportive, facilitative, or enabling acts or decisions that are tailor made to fit with individual, group, or institutional cultural values, beliefs, and lifeways in order to provide or support meaningful, beneficial, and satisfying health care or well-being services.

generic (folk, local, indigenous) care from the cultures and comparing it with professional care.

Leininger finds that still today cultural blindness, shock, imposition, and ethnocentrism by nurses greatly reduce the quality of care to clients of different cultures.[14,17,21] Moreover, nursing diagnoses and medical diagnoses that are not culturally based and known are serious problems for cultures that lead to unfavorable and sometimes serious outcomes.[13] Providing culturally congruent care is what makes clients satisfied that they received "good care"; it is a powerful healing force for quality health care. Quality care is what clients seek most when they come for services from nurses, and it can only be realized when culturally derived care is known and used.

Major Assumptions

Major assumptions to support Leininger's Culture Care Diversity and Universality Theory are defined below. The definitions were taken from Leininger's definitive book on the theory.[15:44-45]

1. Care is the essence of nursing and a distinct, dominant, central, and unifying focus.
2. Care (caring) is essential for well-being, health, healing, growth, survival, and to face handicaps or death.
3. Culture care is the broadest holistic means to know, explain, interpret, and predict nursing care phenomena to guide nursing care practices.
4. Nursing is a transcultural humanistic and scientific care discipline and profession with the central purpose to serve human beings worldwide.
5. Care (caring) is essential to curing and healing, for there can be no curing without caring.
6. Culture care concepts, meanings, expressions, patterns, processes, and structural forms of care are different (diversity) and similar (towards commonalities or universalities) among all cultures of the world.
7. Every human culture has generic (lay, folk, or indigenous) care knowledge and practices and usually professional care knowledge and practices, which vary transculturally.
8. Cultural care values, beliefs, and practices are influenced by and tend to be embedded in the world view, language, religious (or spiritual),

kinship (social), political (or legal), educational, economic, technological, ethnohistorical, and environmental context of a particular culture.

9. Beneficial, healthy, and satisfying culturally based nursing care contributes to the well-being of individuals, families, groups, and communities within their environmental context.
10. Culturally congruent or beneficial nursing care can occur only when the individual, group, family, community, or culture care values, expressions, or patterns are known and used appropriately and in meaningful ways by the nurse with the people.
11. Culture care differences and similarities between professional caregiver(s) and client (generic) care-receiver(s) exist in any human culture worldwide.
12. Clients who experience nursing care that fails to be reasonably congruent with the client's beliefs, values, and caring lifeways will show signs of cultural conflicts, noncompliance, stresses, and ethical or moral concerns.
13. The qualitative paradigm provides new ways of knowing and different ways to discover epistemic and ontological dimensions of human care transculturally.

Theoretical Assertions

Leininger developed several predictive formulations from her Transcultural Nursing Culture Care Theory as examples to stimulate nursing research. These formulations are based on her ongoing inquiry, research studies, and other anthropological and nursing investigations from mainly qualitative investigations. A major prediction of her theory is that health or well-being can be predicted from the epistemic and ontological dimensions of culture care. Predictive statements have also been formulated on the basis of field studies.

From her many articles and books several predictions, such as the following, have been made by qualitative methods:

1. Identifiable differences in cultural caring values and patterns between and among cultures will lead to major differences in the nursing care expectations and practices.

2. Differences in cultural caring values, norms, and beliefs between technologically dependent and nontechnologically dependent societies will show marked comparative differences.

3. As professional nurses work in strange cultures with different values about nursing care or caring expectations, there will be overt signs of cultural conflicts, clashes, and stresses between the nurse and the client.

4. The greater the evidence of dependence of nursing personnel on technological tasks and activities, the greater the signs of interpersonal distance and fewer client satisfactions.

5. Nursing care interventions that provide culture-specific caring practices to clients will show positive signs of client satisfaction and well-being.

6. From the study and use of cultures, care, beliefs, values, and practices, signs of health or well-being of clients will be discovered.

In *Care: The Essence of Nursing and Health*[5] Leininger identified some theoretical statements, and a few hypotheses, with some added revisions since the book was published in 1984.

1. Intercultural differences in care beliefs, values, and practices will reflect identifiable differences and some commonalities for nursing care practices.

2. Cultures that highly value individualism with independence modes will show signs of self-care practices and values, whereas cultures that do not value individualism and independence will show limited signs of self-care practices and more signs of other-care practices.

3. If there is a close relationship between caregiver's and care receiver's beliefs and practices, client care outcomes will be health promoting and satisfying.

4. Clients from different cultures can identify their caring and noncaring values and beliefs with ethnonursing enablers.

5. The greater the differences between folk or generic care values and professional care values, the greater the signs of cultural conflict and stresses between professional caregivers and clients.

6. Technological caring acts, techniques, and practices differ transculturally and have different outcomes for the health and well-being of clients.

7. The greater the signs of dependency on technology of the nurse, the greater the signs of depersonalized humanistic nursing care to clients.

8. Symbolic forms and ritual functions of nursing care behaviors and practices have different meanings and outcomes in different cultures.

9. Political, religious, economic, kinship, and cultural values and environmental contexts greatly influence cultural practices and the well-being of individuals, families, and groups.

A sample of other predictive statements to be discovered from Leininger's *Transcultural Nursing: Concepts, Theories and Practices* in 1978[3] and 1995[21] includes the following:

1. Cultures that perceived illness to be largely a personal and internal body experience (i.e., caused by physical, genetic, and intrabody stresses) tend to use more technical and physical self-care methods (pills and physical techniques) than do cultures that view illness as cultural beliefs, and extrapersonal and direct cultural experiences.

2. Cultures that strongly emphasize caring values, behaviors, and processes tend to have more females than males in caring roles.

3. Cultures that emphasize curing behaviors and treatment processes tend to have more male curers than female curers.

4. Clients in need of caring services tend to seek first their (local folk or generic healers) caring persons such as family members or friends and only later seek professional caregivers if the folk remedies are not effective, the condition worsens, or death is feared.

5. Ritualized ethnocaring activities that have therapeutic benefits to clients and their families tend to be largely unknown or are less valued by Western professional nurses and physicians.

6. Where there is marked evidence of nurturant caring behaviors in a culture, there will be less need for professional services and curers.

7. Marked differences in generic and professional care practices lead to cultural conflicts and imposition practices.
8. Transculturally prepared nurses can make a major difference in client health care outcomes.
9. Health care reform will be unsuccessful unless cultural values, beliefs, and practices are explicitly known and used.

LOGICAL FORM

Leininger's theory is derived from anthropology and nursing but is reformulated to be transcultural nursing with human care perspective.[21] She developed the ethnonursing nursing research method and has emphasized the importance of studying people from their emic or local knowledge and experiences and later contrasting them with etic (outsider), often nurses', beliefs and practices. Her book *Qualitative Research Methods in Nursing* and related articles provide substantive knowledge about qualitative methods in nursing.[8,15,21]

In her own research, Leininger is skilled in using ethnonursing, ethnography, life histories, life stories, photography, and phenomenological methods that provide a holistic approach to study cultural behavior in diverse environmental contexts. With these qualitative methods, the researcher moves with the people in their daily living activities to grasp their world, and the nurse researcher inductively obtains data of documented descriptive and interpretive accounts from informants through observations and participation or in other ways explicating care as a major challenge within the method. The qualitative approach is important to develop basic and substantive grounded data-based knowledge about cultural care to guide nurses in their work. From the beginning, ethnonursing has been primarily grounded in data from the cultures under study, which is different from grounded theory of Glasser and Strauss.[1]

Leininger has also used the ethnoscience method as a formal and rigorous method to study nursing and human phenomena.[8] Ethnoscience refers to the systematic study of the way of life of a designated cultural group in order to obtain an accurate account of the people's behavior and how they perceive and know their universe."[8] This method involves a logical semantic classifying of data as they reflect the people's views in their words through confirming the credibility of these data with the people. The ethnoscience method provides data that will help nurses understand the meanings of care for whatever phenomena are studied and to explain and predict human behavior within a cultural context.[8] Emic data are largely obtained through ethnoscientific research; the research analyzes both emic and etic data. "An emic analysis reveals the native's or a local culture's way of knowing and classifying their world."[8] An etic analysis searches for common or more universal (outsider) features that may be found in more than one culture. Both emic and etic data are also used in ethnonursing and to discover universal and diverse features. Although other methods of research, such as hypothesis testing and experimental quantitative methods, can be used to study transcultural care, the method of choice depends on the researcher's purposes, the goals of the study, and the phenomena to be studied. Creativity and the willingness of the nurse researcher to use different research methods to discover nursing knowledge are encouraged. However, Leininger holds that qualitative methods are important to establish meanings and accurate cultural knowledge. Quantitative methods have generally been of limited value to study cultures and care. Combining both qualitative and quantitative methods tends to obscure the findings and is a misuse of both paradigms.[15,21]

Leininger developed the Sunrise Model (Fig. 29-1) in the 1970s to depict the essential components of the theory. She has refined the model since the late 1950s, but today the model is definitive and valuable to accurately study the diverse elements or its components of the theory and to make culturally logical clinical assessments. This model and the full theory of cultural care diversity and universality are not addressed here. Only selected ideas are offered to introduce the reader to Leininger's pioneering and creative work of evolving theory through time. The Sunrise Model symbolizes the "rising of the sun (care)."[15,21] The upper half of the circle depicts components of the social structure

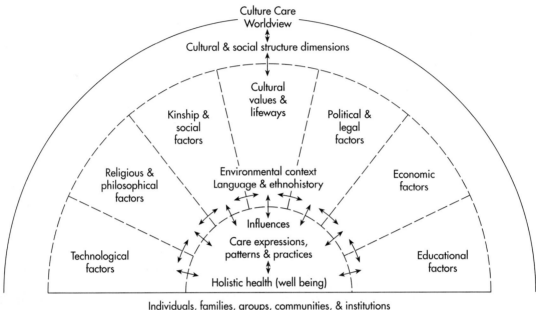

Culture Care
Worldview

Cultural & social structure dimensions

Cultural
values &
lifeways

Kinship &
social
factors

Political &
legal
factors

Religious &
philosophical
factors

Environmental context
Language & ethnohistory

Economic
factors

Influences

Care expressions,
patterns & practices

Technological
factors

Educational
factors

Holistic health (well being)

Individuals, families, groups, communities, & institutions
in
diverse health systems

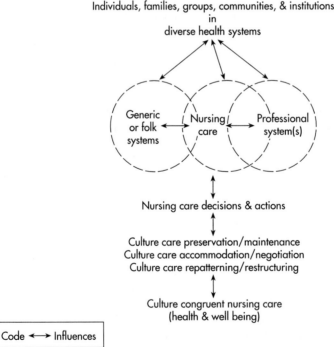

Generic
or folk
systems

Nursing
care

Professional
system(s)

Nursing care decisions & actions

Culture care preservation/maintenance
Culture care accommodation/negotiation
Culture care repatterning/restructuring

Culture congruent nursing care
(health & well being)

Code ◄───► Influences

Fig. **29-1** Leininger's Sunrise Model to depict Theory of Cultural Care Diversity and Universality. *Modified by Madeleine Leininger in personal correspondence of 1996 from Leininger, M.M. (1991). Culture care: Diversity and universality. New York: National League for Nursing, p. 43. Used with permission.*

and world view factors that influence care and health through language, ethnohistory, and environmental context. These factors also influence the folk, professional, and nursing system(s), which are in the middle part of the model. The two halves together form a full sun, which represents the universe that nurses must consider to appreciate human care and health.[15,21] According to Leininger, nursing acts as a bridge between the folk generic and the professional system. Three kinds of nursing care and decisions and actions are predicted in the theory, namely, cultural care preservation and maintenance, cultural care accommodation and/or negotiation, and cultural care repatterning and/or restructuring.[15,21]

The Sunrise Model depicts human beings as inseparable from their cultural background and social structure, worldview, history, and environmental context as a basic tenet of Leininger's theory.[15,21] Gender, race, age, and class are embedded in social structure factors and are studied. Biological, emotional, and other dimensions are studied from a holistic view and not fragmented or separate. Theory generation from this model may occur at multiple levels from the micro range (small-scale specific individuals) or to study groups, families, or communities, or large-scale phenomena such as several cultures. Leininger also describes two phases of generating research knowledge, discovering substantive knowledge (phase 1) to apply the knowledge to practice situations (phase 2).[15,21]

Leininger has also developed a computer software program based on her theory (Leininger-Templin-Thompson Ethnoscript Qualitative Software Program) to assist with detailed analysis of qualitative ethnodata. She has also developed several enablers to study phenomena with four phases of qualitative data analysis. Most important, the qualitative criteria are used to analyze the data; they are (1) credibility, (2) confirmability, (3) meaning in context, (4) saturations, (5) repatterncy, and (6) transferability.[11,15] Quantitative criteria should not be used with qualitative methods because the former have specific criteria to measure data outcomes.

ACCEPTANCE BY THE NURSING COMMUNITY
Practice

Leininger identifies several factors related to the slowness of nurses to recognize and value transcultural nursing and cultural factors in nursing practices and education. First, the theory was conceptualized in the 1950s, when virtually no nurses were prepared in anthropology or cultural knowledge to understand transcultural concepts, models, or her theory. In the early days most nurses had no idea about the nature of anthropology and how anthropological knowledge might contribute to human care and health behaviors or be background knowledge to understand nursing phenomena or problems. Second, although people had long-standing and inherent cultural needs, many clients were reluctant to push health personnel to meet their cultural needs and therefore did not demand that their cultural and social needs be recognized or met.[2,3,21] Third, until the past decade transcultural nursing articles submitted for publication were often rejected because editors did not know, value, or understand the relevance of cultural knowledge to transcultural nursing or as essential to nursing. Fourth, the concept of care was of limited interest to nurses until the late 1970s, when Leininger began promoting the importance of nurses studying human care, obtaining background knowledge in anthropology, and obtaining graduate preparation in transcultural nursing, research, and practice. Fifth, Leininger contends that nursing has tended to remain too ethnocentric and far too involved in following medicine's interest and directions. Sixth, nursing has been slow to make substantive progress in the development of its distinct body of knowledge because many nurses-researchers have been far too dependent on quantitative research methods to get measurable outcomes rather than qualitative data outcomes. The recent acceptance and utilization of qualitative research methods in nursing will provide new insights and knowledge related to nursing and transcultural nursing.[15,21] There is growing interest in using transcultural nursing knowledge, research, and practice by nurses worldwide.

Nurses are now realizing the importance of transcultural nursing, human care, and qualitative methods. Leininger[25] states, "We are entering a new phase of nursing as we value and use transcultural nursing knowledge with a focus on human caring, health and illness behaviors focus. With the migration of many cultural groups and the rise of the consumer cultural identity, and demands in culturally based care, nurses are realizing the need for culturally sensitive and competent practices. Most countries and communities of the world are multicultural today, and so health personnel are expected to understand and respond to clients of diverse and similar cultures. Immigrants and people from unfamiliar cultures expect nurses to respect and respond to values, beliefs, lifeways, and needs. No longer can nurses practice unicultural nursing."

As our world becomes more culturally diverse, nurses will find the urgent need to be prepared to provide culturally competent care. Some nurses are experiencing culture shock, conflict, and clashes as they move from one area to another and from rural to urban communities without transcultural nursing preparation. As cultural conflicts arise, families are less satisfied with nursing and medical services.[15] Nurses who travel and seek employment in foreign lands are experiencing immigrant status. Transcultural nursing education has become imperative for all nurses worldwide.

Certification of transcultural nurses by the Transcultural Nursing Society has provided a major step toward protecting the public from unsafe and culturally incompetent nursing practices.[14] Accordingly, more nurses are seeking transcultural certification to protect themselves and their clients. The *Journal of Transcultural Nursing* has also provided transcultural nurses with research and theoretical perspectives of over 100 cultures worldwide to guide them in their practices.

Education

The inclusion of culture and comparative care in nursing curricula began in 1966 at the University of Colorado, where Leininger was a professor of nursing and anthropology. Awareness of the importance of culture care to nursing gradually began to appear in the late 1960s, but very few nurse-educators were adequately prepared to teach courses on transcultural nursing. Since the world's first master's and doctoral programs in transcultural nursing were approved and implemented in 1977 at the University of Utah, more nurses have been prepared specifically in transcultural nursing. Today, with the heightened public awareness of health care costs, different cultures, and human rights, there is a much greater demand for comprehensive, holistic, and transcultural people care to protect and provide quality-based care and to prevent legal suits related to improper client care. Leininger's[21,23,24] demand for culture-specific care based on theoretical insights has been critical to discover diverse and universal aspects of care. A critical need remains for nurses to be educated in transcultural nursing in undergraduate and graduate programs. There is also a need for well-qualified faculty prepared in transcultural nursing to teach and to guide research in nursing schools within the United States and in other countries.[21,23]

Since 1980, there have been an increasing number of nursing curricula emphasizing transcultural nursing and human care. One of the early programs to focus on care was at Cuestra College in California in the 1970s, in which Dr. McDonald developed an undergraduate nursing program with care as a central curricula theme. Course titles included Caring Concepts I and II, Caring of Families, and Professional Self-Care.[5] In the late 1980s four master's and four doctoral programs in the United States offered transcultural nursing courses, research experiences, and guided field study experiences.[21] Leininger continues to receive numerous requests daily to give courses, lectures, and workshops on human care and transcultural nursing in the United States and other countries. The demand for transcultural nurses far exceeds available faculty, money, and other resources. Therefore in 1996 Leininger put out a call for schools of nursing to offer transcultural programs to meet the worldwide demand from many nurses and cultures.[18,20,23] These nursing programs are urgently needed for practice and preparation for certification of transcultural nurses. They are also needed for research and for worldwide consultation. At this time there are still too few transcultural nursing research funds to study transcultural nursing education and practice. While the societal demand for transcultural nurses is evident, still the educational preparation remains weak and limited for many nurses worldwide. There are still a few graduate nursing programs and faculty members who do not understand transcultural nursing and the Theory of Culture Care and consequently will not permit students to study or research the phenomena, which causes great distress to nursing students.

Research

Many nurses today are using Leininger's Culture Care Theory worldwide. The theory is the only one in nursing focused specifically on culture care and with a research method (ethnonursing) to examine the theory.[15,21] Approximately 100 cultures and subcultures have been studied as of 1995 and more are in progress.[15,21,24] Funds to support transcultural nursing are meager and limited in most societies because biomedical and technical research funds head the priority list. Very few nursing schools receive federal support in the United States for nursing or transcultural nursing research unless they have a quantitative, objective (measurement) focus. Transcultural nurses and other nurses interested in transcultural nursing research are continuing their research despite limited or no funds. Nevertheless, these nurses are leaders in sharing their research at conferences and instructional programs related to transcultural nursing. They also have been instrumental in opening of doors to transcultural nursing in many organizations. Only recently in the 1990s have national and international organizations begun to support transcultural nursing despite societal demands for culturally competent, sensitive, responsible care. Through persistent efforts and exacting competencies of transcultural nurse specialists, progress has been forthcoming. Transcultural nurses have stimulated many nurses to pursue research and to discover some entirely new knowledge in nursing. This knowledge will greatly reshape and transform nursing in the future.

FURTHER DEVELOPMENT

Leininger predicts that all professional nurses in the world must be prepared in transcultural nursing and demonstrate competencies in transcultural nursing.[4,21] Transcultural nursing must become an integral part of education and practice for nurses to be relevant in the twenty-first century. Currently, the demand for prepared transcultural nurses far exceeds the number of nurses, faculty, and clinical specialists in the world. Far more transcultural nurse theorists, researchers, and scholars are urgently needed to continue to develop a new body of transcultural knowledge and to transform nursing education and practice. "By the year 2010 all nurses will need to have a basic knowledge about diverse cultures in the world and an in-depth knowledge of at least two or three cultures."[21,24] Leininger believes transcultural nursing research has already begun to lead to some highly promising and different ways to advance nursing education and practice. All health disciplines, including medicine, pharmacy, social work, etc., will gradually incorporate transcultural health knowledge and practice into their programs of study in the near future. This trend will increase the demand for competent faculty in transcultural health care. Leininger believes that the development of transcultural institutes will be essential to fill the growing need for transcultural nurses prepared to work with other disciplines.[21]

Present and future theories and studies in transcultural nursing will be essential to meet culturally diverse people. The Theory of Culture Care will grow in importance worldwide. Both universal and diverse care knowledge will be extremely important to establish a substantive body of transcultural nursing knowledge and to make nursing a transcultural profession and discipline. Leininger's theory has already gained worldwide interest and use because it is holistic, relevant, and futuristic and deals with specific yet abstract care knowledge. The Sunrise Model remains invaluable as a dominant image and guide to study and assess people of diverse and similar cultural needs.

CRITIQUE
Simplicity

Transcultural nursing theory is really a broad, holistic, comprehensive perspective of human groups, populations, and species. This theory continues to generate many domains of inquiry for nurse researchers to pursue for scientific and humanistic knowledge. The theory challenges nurses to seek both universal and diverse culturally based care phenomena by diverse cultures, the culture of nursing, and the cultures of social unsteadiness worldwide. The theory is truly transcultural and global in scope; it is both complex and practical. It requires transcultural nursing knowledge and appropriate research methods to explicate the phenomena. Leininger's Culture Care Theory is relevant worldwide to help guide nurse researchers in conceptualizing the theory and research approaches and to guide practice. Because of its holistic and comprehensive nature, several concepts and constructs related to social structure, environment, and language are extremely important to discover and obtain culturally based knowledge or knowledge grounded in the people's world. The theory shows multiple interrelationships of concepts and diversity of key concepts and relationships, especially to social structure factors. It requires some basic anthropological knowledge but also considerable transcultural nursing knowledge to be used accurately and scholarly. Once the theory has been fully conceptualized, Leininger finds that undergraduate and graduate nursing students are excited to use the theory and discover how practical, relevant, and useful it is in their work. The use of the Sunrise Model becomes imprinted on their minds as a way of knowing.

Generality

The transcultural nursing theory does demonstrate the criterion of generality because it is a qualitatively oriented theory that is broad, comprehensive, and worldwide in scope. In fact, transcultural nursing theory addresses nursing care from a multicultural and world view perspective. It is useful and applicable to both groups and individuals with the goal of rendering culture-specific nursing care. The broad or generic concepts are well organized and defined for study in specific cultures. The research has led to a vast amount of expert knowledge largely unknown in the past. Many aspects of culture, care, and health, as these factors have an impact on nursing, are being identified. Even more

research is needed for comparative purposes from both culture-specific data and some universal care knowledge. More of the world's cultural groups need to be studied and compared to validate the caring constructs in the future. The theory is most helpful as a guide for the study of any cultures and for the comparative study of several cultures. Findings from the theory are presently being used in client care in a variety of health and community settings worldwide and to transform nursing education and service. It is especially being valued in developing a new and different approach to the traditional community nursing perspective.

Empirical Precision

The transcultural nursing theory is researchable, and qualitative research has been the primary paradigm to discover largely unknown phenomena of care and health in diverse cultures. This qualitative approach differs from the traditional quantitative research method, which renders measurement the goal of research. However, the ethnoscience and ethnonursing research methods are extremely rigorous and linguistically exacting in nature and outcomes. One hundred thirty-five care constructs have been identified and more are being discovered each day along with a wealth of other transcultural nursing knowledge. The important attribute is that accuracy of grounded data derived with the use of ethnomethods or from an emic or people's viewpoint is leading to high credibility, confirmability, and a wealth of empirical data. Ongoing and future research will lead to additional care and health findings as well as implications for ethnonursing practices and education to fit specific cultures and universal features. The qualitative criteria of credibility and confirmability from in-depth studies of informants and their contexts are becoming clearly evident. Unequivocally, a body of transcultural nursing knowledge has been established over the past decade that has a great impact on nursing and many health care systems.[21]

Derivable Consequences

Transcultural nursing theory has important outcomes for nursing. Rendering culture-specific care is a necessary and essential new goal in nursing. It places the transcultural nursing theory central to the domain of nursing knowledge acquisition and use. The theory is highly useful, applicable, and essential to nursing practice, education, and research. The concept of care as the primary focus of nursing and the base of nursing knowledge and practice is long overdue and essential to advance nursing knowledge and practices. Leininger notes that, although nursing has always made claims to the concept of care, rigorous research on care has been limited until the last three decades. Because of its broad and multicultural focus, this theory could well be the means to establish a sound and defensible discipline and profession as well as guiding practice to meet a multicultural world.

CRITICAL THINKING *Activities*

1 Select four research studies reported in the *Journal of Transcultural Nursing* that used Leininger's Culture Care: Diversity and Universality Theory. Each of the studies selected should represent the following: different cultures, research settings, and cultures different from the student's culture.

  a. Analyze each of the studies and identify the relationship of the theory to domain of inquiry, purpose, assumptions, definitions, methods, research design, data analysis, nursing decisions, and conclusions.

  b. Provide evidence that the findings from the studies confirm the findings of the theory in relation to the domain of inquiry, theory tenets, and derivable consequences.

2 Discuss the usefulness of the Culture Care: Diversity and Universality Theory in the twenty-first century to discover nursing knowledge and provide culturally congruent care. Take into consideration the current trends of consumers of health care, cultural diversity factors, and changes in medical and nursing school curricula. Below are some examples of trends and changes you may want to consider in your discussion:

  a. Importance of transcultural nursing knowledge for a growingly diverse world.

  b. An increase of lay support groups to provide information and sharing of experiences and support for patients and/or families experiencing chronic, terminal, or life-threatening illnesses or treatment modalities from diverse and similar (common) cultures.

  c. Use of cultural values, beliefs, health practices, and research knowledge in undergraduate and graduate nursing curricula across the life span.

  d. Inclusion of alternative or generic care in nursing curriculum (e.g., medicine man [healers and curers and herbalists of the Native Americans in the southwest] and use of selected proven Chinese methods for the treatment of chronic diseases).

  e. Use of cultural caring research knowledge as the new and future direction of nursing in the twenty-first century.

  f. Increase in books, audiotapes, and videotapes published on health maintenance, alternative medicine, herbs, vitamins, minerals, and other over-the-counter medications, which demands a transcultural knowledge base.

  g. Spiraling health costs; forced use of health maintenance organizations; lack of health insurance; increased reliance on self-diagnoses, treatment, and care; and increased availability of diagnostic kits such as AIDS testing, glucose monitoring, cholesterol screening, presence of occult blood in the stool, etc.

  h. Problems related to cultural conflicts, stress, pain, and cultural imposition practices.

3 Arrange for several observation and interview experiences at a local university student health center or public health department with people of diverse cultures. Ascertain the following:

a. Identify the cultures represented by the clientele with use of Leininger's theory and the Sunrise Model.

b. What is the cultural mix of the staff (physicians, nurses, social workers, clerical, etc.) of the center or health department? How does the cultural background of the staff differ from that of the clientele?

c. Arrange a conference with the nursing staff and ascertain their culture-based attitudes, values, and beliefs and those that are reflected in the clients using the center/department. Compare and contrast the values, attitudes, and beliefs of the staff with those of the clients. What are the cultural similarities and differences?

d. Arrange an interview with the director of the center/department and ascertain the economic, political, legal, and other factors from Leininger's Sunrise Model that affect the client's utilization of the center/department.

e. Survey the printed materials available in the waiting and examination rooms and classrooms and identify what cultures and languages are depicted by the visual aids, artifacts, and painting.

f. On the basis of data obtained in *a* through *e*, how can the Culture Care: Diversity and Universality Theory assist the organization in providing culturally sensitive and congruent care to the clients using the center/department and increasing the satisfaction with care received?

4 Discuss the type of prerequisite knowledge, experiences, attitudes, and skills needed to effectively utilize the Culture Care: Diversity and Universality theory.

5 Discuss the relevancy of the Culture Care: Diversity and Universality Theory to nurses working in different practice settings and roles.

REFERENCES

1. Glasser, B.G., & Strauss, A.L. (1967). *The discovery of grounded theories: Strategies for qualitative research.* Chicago: Aldine.
2. Leininger, M. (1970). *Nursing and anthropology: Two worlds to blend.* New York: John Wiley & Sons. (Reprinted in 1994 by Greyden Press, Columbus, OH.)
3. Leininger, M. (1978). *Transcultural nursing: Concepts, theories, research, and practice.* New York: John Wiley & Sons. (Reprinted 1994 by Greyden Press, Columbus, OH.)
4. Leininger, M. (1981). *Caring: An essential human need.* Thorofare, NJ: Charles B. Slack. (Reprinted 1988 by Wayne State University Press, Detroit).
5. Leininger, M. (1984). *Care: The essence of nursing and health.* Thorofare, NJ: Charles B. Slack. (Reprinted 1990 by Wayne State University Press, Detroit).
6. Leininger, M. (1984). *Reference sources for transcultural health and nursing.* Thorofare, NJ: Charles B. Slack.
7. Leininger, M. (Ed.) (1988). *Care: Discovery and uses in clinical and community nursing.* Detroit: Wayne State University Press.
8. Leininger, M. (1985). *Qualitative research methods in nursing.* New York: Grune & Stratton.
9. Leininger, M. (1989). Transcultural nurse specialists and generalists: New practitioners in nursing. *Journal of Transcultural Nursing* (1), 4-16.
10. Leininger, M. (1989). Transcultural nurse specialists: Imperative in today's world. *Nursing and Health Care, 10*(5), 250-256.
11. Leininger, M. (Ed.) (1990). *Ethical and moral dimensions of care.* Chapters from conference on the ethics and morality of caring. Detroit: Wayne State University Press.
12. Leininger, M. (1990). Ethnomethods: The philosophic and epistemic bases to explicate transcultural nursing knowledge. *Journal of Transcultural Nursing, 1*(2), 40-51.
13. Leininger, M. (1990). Issues, questions, and concerns related to the nursing diagnosis cultural movement from transcultural nursing perspective. *Journal of Transcultural Nursing, 2*(1), 23-32.
14. Leininger, M. (1991). Becoming aware of types of health practitioners and cultural imposition. *Journal of Transcultural Nursing, 2*(2), 32-39.
15. Leininger, M. (1991). *Culture care diversity and universality: A theory of nursing.* New York: National League for Nursing Press.
16. Leininger, M. (1991). The transcultural nurse specialist: Imperative in today's world. *Perspective in Family and Community Health, 17,* 137-144.

17. Leininger, M. (1994). Quality of life from a transcultural nursing perspective. *Nursing Science Quarterly, 7*(1), 22-28.
18. Leininger, M. (1994). Transcultural nursing education: A worldwide imperative. *Nursing and Health Care, 15*(5), May, 254-257.
19. Leininger, M. (1995). Culture care theory, research and practice. *Nursing Science Quarterly, 9*(20), 71-78.
20. Leininger, M. (1995). Editorial: Teaching transcultural nursing to transform nursing for the 21st century. *Journal of Transcultural Nursing, 6*(2), 2-3.
21. Leininger, M. (1995). *Transcultural nursing: Concepts, theories, research, and practice.* Columbus, OH: McGraw-Hill College Custom Series.
22. Leininger, M. (1996). Academic vitae and communication with contributing author.
23. Leininger, M. (1996). Future directions for transcultural nursing in the 21st century. *International Nursing Review,* November-December.
24. Leininger, M. (1996). Major directions for transcultural nursing: A journey into the 21st century. *Journal of Transcultural Nursing, 7*(2), 37-40.
25. Leininger, M. (1996, Oct. 22). Personal interview.
26. Leininger, M., & Watson, J. (1990). *The caring imperative in education.* New York: National League for Nursing Press.

BIBLIOGRAPHY

Primary sources

Books

Gaut, D., & Leininger, M. (1991). *Caring: The compassionate healer.* New York: National League for Nursing Press.

Hofling, C.F., & Leininger, M. (1960). *Basic psychiatric concepts in nursing.* Philadelphia: JB Lippincott.

Leininger, M. (1970). *Nursing and anthropology: Two worlds to blend.* New York: John Wiley & Sons.

Leininger, M. (1973). *Contemporary issues in mental health nursing.* Boston: Little, Brown.

Leininger, M. (Ed.). (1974). *Health care dimensions* (Vol. 1): *Health care issues.* Philadelphia: F.A. Davis.

Leininger, M. (Ed.). (1975). *Health care dimensions* (Vol. 2): *Barriers and facilitators to quality health care.* Philadelphia: F.A. Davis.

Leininger, M. (Ed.). (1976). *Health care dimensions* (Vol. 3): *Transcultural health care issues and conditions.* Philadelphia: F.A. Davis.

Leininger, M. (Ed.). (1976). *Transcultural nursing care of infants and children.* Salt Lake City: University of Utah College of Nursing.

Leininger, M. (Ed.). (1978). *Transcultural nursing care of the elderly.* Salt Lake City: University of Utah College of Nursing.

Leininger, M. (Ed.). (1978). *Transcultural nursing: Concepts, theories and practices.* New York: John Wiley & Sons.

Leininger, M. (Ed.). (1979). *Transcultural nursing care of the adolescent and middle age adult.* Salt Lake City: University of Utah College of Nursing.

Leininger, M. (Ed.). (1979). *Transcultural nursing: Proceedings from four transcultural nursing conferences.* New York: Masson.

Leininger, M. (Ed.). (1980). *Cultural change, ethics and the nursing care implications.* Salt Lake City: University of Utah College of Nursing.

Leininger, M. (Ed.). (1980). *Transcultural nursing: Teaching, practice, and research.* Salt Lake City: University of Utah College of Nursing.

Leininger, M. (Ed.). (1981). *Caring: An essential human need.* Thorofare, NJ: Charles B. Slack.

Leininger, M. (Ed.). (1984). *Care: The essence of nursing and health.* Thorofare, NJ: Charles B. Slack.

Leininger, M. (1984). *Reference sources for transcultural health & nursing: For teaching curriculum, research, and clinical-field practice.* Thorofare, NJ: Charles B. Slack.

Leininger, M. (Ed.). (1985). *Qualitative research methods in nursing.* New York: Grune & Stratton.

Leininger, M. (Ed.). (1988). *Care: Discovery and uses.* Detroit: Wayne State University Press.

Leininger, M. (Ed.). (1990). *Ethical and moral dimensions of care.* Detroit: Wayne State University Press.

Leininger, M. (1991). *Culture care diversity and universality: A theory of nursing.* New York: National League for Nursing Press.

Leininger, M. (1995). *Transcultural nursing: Concepts, theories, research, and practices.* (2nd Ed.). New York: McGraw-Hill.

Leininger, M., & Watson, J. (Eds.). (1990). *The caring imperative in education.* New York: National League for Nursing.

Leininger, M.M. (Ed.). (1991). *Culture, care, diversity & universality: A theory of nursing.* New York: National League for Nursing (Publication No. 15-2402).

Smith, C.M., Wolf, V.C., & Leininger, M. (Eds.). (1973). *Nursing at the University of Washington, 1973-1975.* Seattle: University of Washington, Office of Publications and Department of Printing.

Book chapters

Leininger, M. (1968). The research critique: Nature, function and art. In M. Batey (Ed.), *Communication nursing research: The research critique* (pp. 20-23). Boulder, CO: Western Interstate Commission on Higher Education.

Leininger, M. (1969). The young child's response to hospitalization: Separation anxiety or lack of mothering care? In M. Batey (Ed.), *Communicating nursing research* (pp. 26-39). Boulder, CO: Western Interstate Commission on Higher Education.

Leininger, M. (1971). Anthropological approach to adaptation: Case studies from nursing. In J. Murphy (Ed.), *Theoretical issues in professional nursing* (pp. 72-102). New York: Appleton-Century-Crofts.

Leininger, M. (1973). The culture concept and its relevance to nursing. In M. Auld & L. Birum (Eds.), *The challenge of nursing: A book of readings* (pp. 39-46). St. Louis: Mosby.

Leininger, M. (1973). Nursing in the context of social and cultural systems. In P. Mitchell (Ed.), *Concepts basic to nursing* (pp. 37-60). New York: McGraw-Hill.

Leininger, M. (1973). Primex. In M. Auld & L. Birum (Eds.), *The challenge of nursing: A book of readings* (pp. 237-242). St. Louis: Mosby.

Leininger, M. (1974, Fall). Humanism, health and cultural values. In *Health care dimensions* (Vol. 1): *Health care issues* (pp. 37-60). Philadelphia: F.A. Davis

Leininger, M. (1975, Spring). Health care delivery systems for tomorrow: Possibilities and guidelines. In *Health Care dimensions* (Vol. 2): *Barriers and facilitators to quality health care* (pp. 83-95). Philadelphia: F.A. Davis.

Leininger, M. (1976). Transcultural nursing: A promising subfield of study for nurse educators and practitioners. In A. Reinhardt (Ed.), *Current practice in family centered community nursing* (pp. 36-50). St. Louis: Mosby.

Leininger, M. (1976, Spring). Conflict and conflict resolutions: Theories and processes relevant to the health professions. In *Health care dimensions* (Vol. 3): *Transcultural health care issues and conditions* (pp. 165-183). Philadelphia: F.A. Davis.

Leininger, M. (1976, Spring). Toward conceptualization of transcultural health care systems: Concepts and a model. In *Health care dimensions* (Vol. 3): *Transcultural health care issues and conditions* (pp. 3-22). Philadelphia: F.A. Davis.

Leininger, M. (1978). Futurology of nursing: Goals and challenges for tomorrow. In N. Chaska (Ed.), *Views through the mist: The nursing profession* (pp. 379-396). New York: McGraw-Hill.

Leininger, M. (1978). Professional, political, and ethnocentric role behaviors and their influence in multidisciplinary health education. In A. Hardy & M. Conway (Ed.), *Role theory: Perspectives for health professionals.* New York: Appleton-Century-Crofts.

Leininger, M. (1981). Transcultural nursing issues for the 1980's. In J. McCloskey & H. Grace (Ed.), *Current issues in nursing.* Boston: Blackwell Scientific Publications.

Leininger, M. (1981). Women's role in society in the 80's. In *Maternal child nursing in the 80's. Nursing perspective: A forum in honor of Katherine Kendall.* College Park, MD: University of Maryland School of Nursing.

Leininger, M. (1983). Intercultural interviews, assessments, and therapy implications. In P. Pederson (Ed.), *Interviews and assessments.* Beverly Hills, CA: Sage.

Leininger, M. (1988). Cultural care and nursing administration. In B. Henry, C. Arndt, M. DiVincenti, & A. Marriner-Tomey (Eds.), *Dimensions of nursing administration.* Boston: Blackwell Scientific Publications.

Leininger, M. (1991). Culture care theory and uses in nursing administration. In *Culture care diversity and universality: A theory of nursing* (pp. 373-390). New York: National League for Nursing.

Leininger, M. (1991). Ethnonursing: A research method with enablers to study the theory of culture care. In *Culture care diversity and universality: A theory of nursing* (pp. 73-118). New York: National League for Nursing.

Leininger, M. (1992). Current issues, problems, and trends to advance qualitative paradigmatic research methods for the future. In *Qualitative health research* (Vol. 2) (pp. 392-415). Newbury Park, CA: Sage.

Leininger, M. (1992). Reflections on Nightingale with a focus on human care theory and leadership. In Nightingale, *Notes on nursing: What it is, and what it is not.* Philadelphia: JB Lippincott.

Leininger, M. (1992). Theory of culture care and uses in clinical and community contexts. In M. Parker (Ed.), *Theories on nursing* (pp. 345-372). New York: National League for Nursing.

Leininger, M. (1992). Transcultural mental health nursing assessment of children and adolescents. In P. West & C. Sieloff Evans (Eds.), *Psychiatric and mental health nursing with children and adolescents* (pp. 53-58). Gaithersburg, MD: Aspen Publications.

Leininger, M. (1993). Culture care theory: The comparative global theory to advance human care nursing knowledge and practice. In D. Gaut (Ed.), *A global agenda for caring* (pp. 3-18). New York: National League for Nursing.

Leininger, M. (1993). Evaluation criteria and critique of qualitative research studies. In J. Morse (Ed.), *Qualitative nursing research: A contemporary dialogue* (pp. 393-414). Newbury Park, CA: Sage.

Journal and other articles

Brenner, P., Boyd, C., Thompson, T.C., Marz, M.S., Buerhaus, P., & Leininger, M.M. (1986). The care symposium: Considerations for nursing administrators. *Journal of Nursing Administration, 16*(1), 25-30.

Gaut, D.A., & Leininger, M.M. (1991). Caring: The compassionate healer. *NLN Publication Center for Human Caring,* No. 15-2401.

Leininger, M. (1961, Oct.). Changes in psychiatric nursing. *Canadian Nurse, 57,* 938-948.

Leininger, M. (1964, June). A Gadsup village experiences its first election. *Journal of Polynesian Society 73,* 29-34.

Leininger, M. (1967, Spring). Nursing care of a patient from another culture: Japanese-American patient. *Nursing Clinics of North America, 2,* 747-762.

Leininger, M. (1967, April). The culture concept and its relevance to nursing. *Journal of Nursing Education, 6,* 27-39.

Leininger, M. (1968, Sept.-Oct.). The research critique: Nature, function, and art. *Nursing Research, 17*(5), 444-449.

Leininger, M. (1968, Nov.). Cultural differences among staff members and the impact on patient care. *Minnesota League for Nursing Bulletin, 16,* 5-9.

Leininger, M. (1968, Nov.). The significance of cultural concepts in nursing. *Minnesota League for Nursing Bulletin, 16,* 3-4.

Leininger, M. (1969, Jan.). Community psychiatric nursing: Trends, issues and problems. *Perspectives in Psychiatric Care, 7,* 10-20.

Leininger, M. (1969, Jan.). Ethnoscience: A new and promising research approach for the health sciences. *Image, 3,* 2-8.

Leininger, M. (1969, Sept. -Oct.). Conference on the nature of science in nursing. Introduction: Nature of science in nursing. *Nursing Research, 18,* 388-389.

Leininger, M. (1970). Some cross-cultural universal and non-universal functions beliefs and practices of food. In J. Dupont (Ed.), *Dimensions of Nutrition* (pp. 153-179). Proceedings of the Colorado Dietetic Association Conference [held in Fort Collins, Colorado, 1969]. Colorado Associated Universities Press, 1970.

Leininger, M. (1970). Witchcraft practices and nursing therapy. *ANA Clinical Conferences* (p. 76). New York: Appleton-Century-Crofts.

Leininger, M. (1971, March). Anthropological issues related to community mental health programs in the United States. *Community Mental Health Journal, 7,* 50-62.

Leininger, M. (1971, Nov.). Dean proposes educational teamwork. *Health Science Review, 1,* 4.

Leininger, M. (1971, Dec.). This I believe . . . about interdisciplinary health education for the future. *Nursing Outlook, 19,* 787-791.

Leininger, M. (1972). Using cultural styles of people: Conflicts and changes in the subculture of nursing. *Psychiatric Nursing Bulletin,* pp. 43-61.

Leininger, M. (1972, July). This I believe . . . about interdisciplinary health education for the future. *AORN Journal,* 16(1), 89-104.

Leininger, M. (1973). Becoming aware of types of health practitioners and cultural imposition. *Speeches presented during the 48th Convention.* American Nurses Association.

Leininger, M. (1973, Winter). Health care delivery systems for tomorrow: Possibilities and guidelines. *Washington State Journal of Nursing, 45,* 10-16.

Leininger, M. (1973, Spring). Witchcraft practices and psychocultural therapy with urban United States families. *Human Organization, 32,* 73-83.

Leininger, M. (1973, March). An open health care system model. *Nursing Outlook, 21,* 171-175.

Leininger, M. (1973, July). Primex: Its origins and significance. *American Journal of Nursing, 73,* 1274-1277.

Leininger, M. (1973, Aug.). Witchcraft practices and psychocultural therapy with U.S. urban families. *Mental Health Digest, 5,* 33-40.

Leininger, M. (1973, Fall). A new model: Working model for future nurse participation and utilization. *Washington State Journal of Nursing, 45,* 7-15.

Leininger, M. (1974). Leadership in nursing: Challenges, concerns, and effect. *The challenge: Rational administration in nursing and health care services,* University of Arizona, pp. 35-53.

Leininger, M. (1974, Spring). Scholars, scholarship and nursing scholarship. *Image, 6,* 1-14.

Leininger, M. (1974, March-April). The leadership crisis in nursing: A critical problem and challenge. *Journal of Nursing Administration, 4,* 28-34.

Leininger, M. (1974, Dec.). Conflict and conflict resolution: Theories and processes relevant to the health professions. *American Nurse, 6,* 17-21.

Leininger, M. (1975, Feb.). Conflict and conflict resolution. *American Journal of Nursing, 75,* 292-296.

Leininger, M. (1975, May). Transcultural nursing presents exciting challenge. *American Nurse, 5,* 4.

Leininger, M. (1976, Feb.). Caring: The essence and central focus of nursing. *American Nurses Foundations, 12,* 2-14.

Leininger, M. (1976, May-June). Doctoral programs for nurses: Trends, questions and projected plans. *Nursing Research, 25,* 201-210.

Leininger, M. (1976, Fall). Two strange health tribes: Gnisrun and Enicidem in the United States. *Human Organization, 35,* 253-261.

Leininger, M. (1977). Cultural diversities of health and nursing care. *Nursing Clinics of North America, 12*(1), 5-18.

Leininger, M. (1977). Roles and directions in nursing and cancer nursing. *Proceedings of the Second National Conference of Cancer Nursing.* American Cancer Society.

Leininger, M. (1977). *Territoriality, power and creative leadership in administrative nursing contexts.* (Publication No. 52-1675:6-18). National League for Nursing.

Leininger, M. (1977, Nov.). Issues in nursing: A learning challenge. *Vital Signs, 2,* 3. (Publication of the Student Nurses' Association, University of Utah.)

Leininger, M. (1978, Spring). Political nursing: Essential for health and educational systems of tomorrow. *Nursing Administration Quarterly, 2*(3), 1-16.

Leininger, M. (1978, March). Changing foci in nursing education: Primary and transcultural care. *Journal of Advanced Nursing, 3*(2), 155-166.

Leininger, M. (1978, March). Nursing in the future: Some brief glimpses (Part I). *Vital Signs, 2,* 7.

Leininger, M. (1978, April). Nursing in the future: Some brief glimpses (Part II). *Vital Signs, 2,* 8.

Leininger, M. (1978, May). Nursing in the future: Some brief glimpses (Part III). *Vital Signs, 2,* 9.

Leininger, M. (1978, Oct.). Transcultural nursing: A new subfield to general nursing and health care knowledge. *Scholarly Lecture Series.* University of Manitoba.

Leininger, M. (1978, Dec.). Creating and maintaining a nursing research support center. *Adelphi Report,* Adelphi University, pp. 35-60.

Leininger, M. (1978, Dec.). Transcultural nursing for tomorrow's nurse. *Imprint, 25*(4), 44-47.

Leininger, M. (1979). Consumer health care needs, nursing leadership and future directions. *Proceedings of the leadership conference.* Seattle: University of Washington, School of Nursing.

Leininger, M. (1979). Principles and guidelines to assist nurses in cross-cultural nursing and health practices. *Hope conference report.* Millwood, VA: International Nursing Project, Hope Health Sciences Education Center.

Leininger, M. (1979, April). Health promotion and maintenance: An old transcultural challenge and a new emphasis for the health professions. Health Promotion: In *Health and Illness, Monograph 4.* Series 1978. Sigma Theta Tau.

Leininger, M. (1979, Oct.). *Sociocultural forces impacting upon health care and the nursing profession.* National Institutes of Health Annual Meeting of Nursing Departments. Washington, DC: National Institutes of Health.

Leininger, M. (1980, Winter). University of Utah nursing clinics. *Western Journal of Nursing Research, 2,* 411.

Leininger, M. (1980, Aug.). Transcultural nursing: A new subfield. *Health Clinics International, 2,* 3-4.

Leininger, M. (1980, Oct.). Caring: A central focus for nursing and health care services. *Nursing and Health Care, 1,* 135-143, 176.

Leininger, M. (1981, Sept.). Transcultural nursing: Its progress and its future. *Nursing and Health Care, 2*(7), 365-371.

Leininger, M. (1982, Jan.). Creativity and challenges for nurse researchers in this economic recession. *Center for Health Research News, 1,* 1. (Publication of the College of Nursing, Wayne State University.)

Leininger, M. (1982, July-Aug.). Woman's role in society in the 1980s. *Issues in Health Care of Women, 3*(4), 203-215.

Leininger, M. (1982, Nov.). Getting to 'Truths' or mastering numbers and research designs. *Center for Health Research News, 1,* 2. (Publication of the College of Nursing, Wayne State University.)

Leininger, M. (1983, March). Creativity and challenges for nurse researchers in this economic recession. *Journal of Nursing Administration, 13,* 21-22.

Leininger, M. (1983, May). Qualitative research methods: A new direction to document and discover nursing knowledge. *Center for Health Research News, 3,* 2. (Publication of the College of Nursing, Wayne State University.)

Leininger, M. (1983, Aug.). Cultural care: An essential goal for nursing and health care. *Journal of Nephrology Nursing, 10,* 11-17.

Leininger, M. (1983, Oct.-Dec.). Community psychiatric nursing in community mental health: Trends, issues, and problems. *Perspective Psychiatric Care, 21*(4), 139-146.

Leininger, M. (1984). Transcultural nursing. *Canadian Nurse, 80*(11), 41-45.

Leininger, M. (1984, March-April). Transcultural nursing: An overview. *Nursing Outlook, 32*(2), 72-73.

Leininger, M. (1985, April). Transcultural care diversity and universality: A theory of nursing. *Nursing and Health Care, 6*(4), 209-212.

Leininger, M. (1985, Feb.). [Translated from 'The Best of Image.' Ethnoscience: A promising research approach to improve nursing practice.] *Kango, 37*(2), 113-123.

Leininger, M. (1986). Care facilitation and resistance factors in the culture of nursing. *Topics in Clinical Nursing, 8*(2), 1-12.

Leininger, M. (1986). Care symposium: Resources on culture (letter). *Journal of Nursing Administration, 16*(6), 35.

Leininger, M. (1986). Caring [reply letter]. *Journal of Nursing Administration, 16*(11), 4.

Leininger, M. (1987). A new generation of nurses discover transcultural nursing [editorial]. *Nursing & Health Care, 8*(5), 263.

Leininger, M. (1987, Summer). Response to "Infant feeding practices of Vietnamese immigrants to the Northwest United States." *Scholarly Inquiry for Nursing Practice, 1*(2), 171-174.

Leininger, M. (1988, Nov.). Leininger's theory of nursing: Cultural care diversity and universality. *Nursing Science Quarterly, 1*(4), 152-160.

Leininger, M. (1992). Transcultural nursing care values, beliefs, and practices of American (USA) gypsies. *Journal of Transcultural Nursing, 4*(1), 17-28.

Leininger, M. (1994). Nursing's agenda of health care reform: Regressive or advanced—discipline status. *Nursing Science Quarterly 7*(2), Special Feature, Summer, 93-94.

Leininger, M. (1994). Reflections: Culturally congruent care: Visible and invisible. *Journal of Transcultural Nursing, 6*(1), 23-25.

Leininger, M. (1995). Culture care theory, research and practice. *Nursing Science Quarterly, 9*(2), 71-78.

Leininger, M. (1995). Founder's focus: Nursing theories and cultures: Fit or misfit? *Journal of Transcultural Nursing, 7*(1), 41-42.

Leininger, M. (1996). Founder's focus: Transcultural nurses and consumers tell their stories. *Journal of Transcultural Nursing, 7*(2), 37-40.

Leininger, M. (1996). Transcultural nursing administration: What is it? *Journal of Transcultural Nursing, 8*(1).

Leininger, M. (1997). Ethnonursing research method: Essential to advance Asian nursing knowledge. Igaku-Soin, Ltd. (Japan), Medical Publishers, Nursing Publishing Department, Special Issue, January, 1997.

Leininger, M., & Cummings, S.H. (1996). Nursing's new paradigm is transcultural nursing: An interview with Madeleine Leininger. *Advanced Practice Nursing Quarterly, 2*(2), 62-70.

Leininger, M., & Shubin, S. (1980, June). Nursing patients from different cultures. *Nursing, 80,* 10.

Leininger, M.M. (1983). Creativity and challenges for nurse researchers in this economic recession part 2. *Nurse Educator, 8*(1), 13-14.

Leininger, M.M. (1984). Qualitative research methods—to document and discover nursing knowledge. *Western Journal of Nursing Research, 6*(2), 151-152.

Leininger, M.M. (1987) Importance and uses of ethnomethods: Ethnography and ethnonursing research. *Recent Advances in Nursing, 17,* 12-36.

Leininger, M.M. (1988). Leininger's theory of nursing: Cultural care diversity and universality. *Nursing Science Quarterly, 1*(4), 152-160.

Leininger, M.M. (1988). Transcultural eating patterns and nutrition: Transcultural nursing and anthropological perspectives. *Holistic Nursing Practice, 3*(1), 16-25.

Leininger, M.M. (1989). The Journal of Transcultural Nursing has become a reality. *Journal of Transcultural Nursing, 1*(1), 1-2.

Leininger, M.M. (1989). The transcultural nurse specialist: Imperative in today's world. *Nursing and Health Care, 10*(5), 250-256.

Leininger, M.M. (1989). Transcultural nurse specialists and generalists: New practitioners in nursing. *Journal of Transcultural Nursing, 1*(1), 4-16.

Leininger, M.M. (1989). Transcultural nursing: Quo vadis (where goeth the field?). *Journal of Transcultural Nursing, 1*(1), 33-45.

Leininger, M.M. (1990). The caring imperative in education. Introduction. Care: The imperative of nursing education and service. *NLN Publication Center for Human Caring, 41-2308,* 1-5.

Leininger, M.M. (1990). Ethnomethods: The philosophic and epistemic bases to explicate transcultural nursing knowledge. *Journal of Transcultural Nursing, 1*(2), 40-51.

Leininger, M.M. (1990). Knowledge about care and caring: State of the art and future developments. Historic and epistemologic dimensions of care and caring with future directions. *ANA Publication, American Academy of Nursing, G-177,* 19-31.

Leininger, M.M. (1990). Issues, questions, and concerns related to the nursing diagnosis cultural movement from a transcultural nursing perspective. *Journal of Transcultural Nursing, 2*(1), 23-32.

Leininger, M.M. (1990). A new and changing decade ahead: Are nurses prepared? *Journal of Transcultural Nursing, 1*(2), 1.

Leininger, M.M. (1990). The significance of cultural concepts in nursing. *Journal of Transcultural Nursing, 2*(1), 52-59.

Leininger, M.M. (1990, Nov.-Dec.). Leininger clarifies transcultural nursing {letter to the editor}. *International Nursing Review,* p. 356.

Leininger, M.M. (1991). Becoming aware of types of health practitioners and cultural imposition. *Journal of Transcultural Nursing, 2*(2), 32-39.

Leininger, M.M. (1991). Leininger's acculturation health care assessment tool for cultural patterns in traditional and non-traditional lifeways. *Journal of Transcultural Nursing, 2*(2), 40-42.

Leininger, M.M. (1991). Second reflection: Comparative care as central to transcultural nursing. *Journal of Transcultural Nursing, 3*(1), 2.

Leininger, M.M. (1991). Transcultural care principles, human rights, and ethical considerations. *Journal of Transcultural Nursing, 3*(1), 21-23.

Leininger, M.M. (1991). Transcultural nursing goals and challenges for 1991 and beyond. *Journal of Transcultural Nursing, 2*(2), 1-2.

Leininger, M.M. (1991). Transcultural nursing: The study and practice field. *Imprint, 38*(2), 55, 57, 59-63.

Leininger, M.M., & Watson, J. (1990). The caring imperative in education. *NLN Publication Center for Human Caring, 41-2308,* 1-297.

McFarland, G., Hall, B., Buckwalter, K., Dumas, R., Haack, M., Leininger, M., McBride, A., McKeon, K., Pender, N., & Tripp-Reimer, T. (1990). Knowledge about care and caring: State of the art and future developments. Group IV: Behavior problems/mental illness/addictions. *ANA Publication, American Academy of Nursing, G-177,* 19-31.

Book prefaces and forewords

Leininger, M. (1972). Introduction. In K. Leahy, M. Cobb, & M. Jones, *Community health nursing.* New York: McGraw-Hill.

Leininger, M. (1972). Introduction. In L. Schwartz & J. Schwartz. *Psychodynamic concepts of patient care.* Englewood Cliffs, NJ: Prentice-Hall.

Leininger, M. (1973, July). Foreword. In M. Disbrow (Ed.), *Meeting consumers' demands for maternity care.* Seattle: University of Washington Press.

Leininger, M. (1974, Fall). Preface. In M. Leininger (Ed.), *Health care issues: Health care dimensions,* Second issue, Philadelphia: F.A. Davis

Leininger, M. (1975, Spring). Preface. In M. Leininger (Ed.), *Transcultural health care issues and conditions: Health care dimensions,* Second issue, Philadelphia: F.A. Davis.

Leininger, M. (1976, Spring). Preface. In M. Leininger (Ed.), *Transcultural health care issues and conditions: Health care dimensions,* Third issue, Philadelphia: F.A. Davis.

Leininger, M. (1978). Foreword. In J. Watson, *Nursing: The philosophy and science of caring.* Boston: Little, Brown.

Leininger, M. (1979) Foreword. In L.S. Bermosk & S.E. Porter, *Women's health and human wholeness.* New York: Appleton-Century-Crofts.

Leininger, M. (1979). Preface. In M. Leininger. (Ed.), *Proceedings of the national transcultural nursing conferences.* New York: Masson.

Leininger, M. (1980). Foreword. *Transcultural nursing: Teaching, research, and practice.* Salt Lake City.

Leininger, M. (1981). Introduction. *Six proceedings of the transcultural nursing conferences in 1976, 1977, 1978, 1979, 1980, 1981.* New York: Masson International Press.

Leininger, M. (1981). Preface. *Caring: An essential human need.* Thorofare, NJ: Charles B. Slack.

Leininger, M. (1981). Preface. *Maternal child nursing in the 80's.* Nursing perspective: A forum in honor of Katherine Kendall. College Park, MD: University of Maryland, School of Nursing.

Leininger, M. (1983). Preface. *Care: The essence of nursing and health.* Thorofare, NJ: Charles B. Slack.

Leininger, M. (1983). Preface. In K. Vestal & C. McKenzie (Eds.), *High risk perinatal nursing*. Philadelphia: WB Saunders.

Leininger, M. (1983). Preface. *Transcultural health and nursing references*. Thorofare, NJ: Charles B. Slack.

Secondary sources

Dissertations

Cameron, C. (1990). *An ethnonursing study of health status of elderly Anglo-Canadian wives providing extended care giving to their disabled husbands*. Detroit: Wayne State University.

Finn, J. (1993). *Professional nurse and generic care giving of child bearing women conceptualized with Leininger's theory of cultural care theory*. Detroit: Wayne State University.

Gates, M. (1988). *Care and care meanings, experiences and orientations of persons dying in hospitals and hospital settings*. Detroit: Wayne State University.

Gelazis, R. (1994). *Lithuanian care: Meanings and experiences with humor using Leininger's cultural care theory*. Detroit: Wayne State University.

Luna, L. (1989). *Care and cultural context of Lebanese Muslims in an urban US community within Leininger's cultural care theory*. Detroit: Wayne State University.

MacNeil, J. (1994). *Cultural care: Meanings, patterns, and expressions for Baganda women as AIDS caregivers within Leininger's theory*. Detroit: Wayne State University.

Miller, J.E. (1996). *Politics and care: A study of Czech Americans within Leininger's theory of culture care diversity and universality*. Detroit: Wayne State University.

Morgan, M. (1994). *African American neonatal care in northern and southern contexts using Leininger's culture care theory*. Detroit: Wayne State University.

Omeri, A.S. (1996). *Transcultural nursing care values, beliefs and practices of Iranian immigrants in New South Wales, Australia*. University of Sydney.

Rosenbaum, J. (1990). *Cultural care, culture health and grief phenomena related to older Greek Canadian widows with Leininger's theory of culture care*. Detroit: Wayne State University.

Spangler, Z. (1991). *Nursing care values and practices of Philippine American and Anglo American nurses*. Detroit: Wayne State University.

Thompson, T. (1990). *A qualitative investigation of rehabilitation nursing care in an inpatient rehabilitation unit using Leininger's theory*. Detroit: Wayne State University.

Villarruel, A. (1993). *Mexican American cultural meanings, expressions: Self-care and dependent care actions associated with experiences of pain*. Detroit: Wayne State University.

Welch, A. (1987). *Concepts of health, illness, caring, aging, and problems of adjustment among elderly Filipinas residing in Hampton Roads, Virginia*. University of Utah.

Wenger, A.F. (1988). *The phenomenon of care of Old Order Amish: A high context culture*. Detroit: Wayne State University.

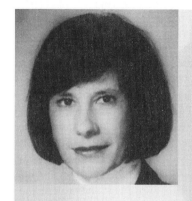

Rosemarie Rizzo Parse

Human Becoming

Kathleen D. Pickrell, Rickard E. Lee, Larry P. Schumacher,
Prudence Twigg

CREDENTIALS AND BACKGROUND OF THE THEORIST

Our lives are composed of situations diverse in richness and magnitude. Much of what adds color to our daily existence slides by us almost unperceived. Other happenings stand out much more sharply and mark our passage through life—educational achievements, employment, close relationships, defining experiences, professional networks, academic networks.

The unfolding of Rosemarie Rizzo Parse's Human Becoming (formerly Man-Living-Health) theory is inseparable from the lesser and greater situations that comprise her life. The idea for the Human Becoming Theory, Parse recalled, "began many years ago when I began to wonder and wander and ask why not? The theory itself . . . surfaced in me in Janusian fashion over the years in interrelationship with oth-

The authors wish to express appreciation to Rosemarie Rizzo Parse for critiquing the original chapter.

ers primarily through my lived experience in nursing."[17:xxiii] Numerous "predecessors, contemporaries, and successors" helped Parse see her idea more clearly.[17:xv] "Yet the theory has only begun to be viewed and enhanced by those who take up the challenge to evolve nursing science to a higher level of complexity and specificity."[17:xiii]

Parse received her nursing education in Pittsburgh. Her master's and doctorate degrees in nursing and higher education were earned at the University of Pittsburgh.

At the time she was developing her theory, Parse was Dean of the School of Nursing at Duquesne University in Pittsburgh. At about this same time—during the 1960s and 1970s—Duquesne was regarded as the center of the existential-phenomenological movement in the United States. Dialogues she had with those in this school of thought (for example, A. van Kaam and A. P. Giorgi) stimulated and focused her thinking.

Currently, Parse is president of Discovery International, Inc., an organization she founded to promote excellence in nursing science. This firm provides consultation services, seminars, and health guidance to individuals, families, and communities. She is also Professor of Graduate Nursing and Niehoff Chair at Marcella Niehoff School of Nursing, Loyola University, Chicago, as well as editor of the scholarly journal *Nursing Science Quarterly.* Her research activities and interests are wide ranging. A partial listing includes lived experiences of hope, laughter, health, aging, quality of life, joy, and sorrow.[20]

THEORETICAL SOURCES

Parse's theoretical sources are a major reason her theory is regarded as unique for nursing.[24:181] By synthesizing the Science of Unitary Human Beings, as developed by Martha E. Rogers, and existential-phenomenological thought, as articulated by Martin Heidegger, Jean-Paul Sartre, and Maurice Merleau-Ponty, Parse pushes nursing toward an unfragmented view of man. Man cannot be reduced to constituent systems or parts and still be understood, she declares. Man is "a living unity."[17:4]

Moreover, Parse challenges the traditional view of nursing as an emerging natural science. Rightly understood, nursing is a human science. The thrust of her approach is clear.

Parse's human science nursing theory is rooted in the belief that humans participate with the universe in the cocreation of health. Essential to the theory is each individual's relationship with the universe, the [coconstitution] of health, the meaning that human beings give to being and becoming, and the human being's freedom to choose alternative ways to becoming.[17:13;19:37-38]

In developing her theory, Parse used Rogers's major principles of helicy, complimentarity (now called *integrality*), and resonancy and her corresponding concepts of energy field, openness, pattern, and organization (Rogers has recently deleted organization) and four-dimensionality. (The reader is referred to the chapter on Rogers's theory for a discussion of these principles and concepts.)

From existential-phenomenological thought, Parse drew the tenets of intentionality and human subjectivity and the corresponding concepts of coconstitution, coexistence, and situated freedom. *Intentionality* "means that in being human man is open, knows, and is present to the world. To be man, then, is to be intentional and to be involved with the world through a fundamental nature of knowing, being present and open."[17:18] Human subjectivity indicates that "man encounters the world and is present to it in a dialectical relationship. Man grows through this relationship, giving meaning to the projects that emerge in the process of becoming. Man coparticipates in the emergence of projects through choosing to live certain values."[17:19] *Coconstitution* "refers to the idea that the meaning emerging in any situation is related to the particular constituents of that situation. . . . Man interrelates with the various views of the world and others and indeed cocreates these views by a personal presence."[17:20]

The term *coexistence* means that "man, an emerging being, is in the world with others. . . . Man knows self in the comprehension of dispersed concrete achievements and through the perceptions of others. Without others one would not know that one is."[18:20] *Situated freedom* indicates that "one participates in choosing the situations in which one finds oneself as well as one's attitude toward the situations."[17:20-21]

Man, therefore, is always choosing. This choosing occurs on two levels: prereflectively and tacitly, and reflectively and explicitly. "In choosing ways of being with situations, one expresses value priorities."[18:21] Our choices, however, "are made without full knowledge of the outcomes yet with full responsibility for the consequences."[17:21]

USE OF EMPIRICAL EVIDENCE

"Nursing does not have practice and research traditions of its own," observed Parse. "Quantitative and qualitative methods of research used to enhance nursing science presently flow from the natural sciences and from the human sciences, respectively."[18:166;21:1-5] Because Parse sees nursing as a human science, she has sought to enhance her theory by using descriptive research methods borrowed from the human sciences. One such method, phenomenology, has become increasingly important in recent years in nursing,[4:31;7:113] psychology,[17] and sociology.[5] Because of its philosophical base, this research method fits well with Parse's theory. It is also congruent with the importance other nurse theorists (e.g., Leininger, Orlando, Patterson and Zderad, Peplau, Travelbee, Watson) have placed on understanding patients' unique perspectives in providing nursing care.[4:34] But phenomenology broadens and deepens the notion of what it means to talk about and study an individual's unique point of view.[6]

MAJOR CONCEPTS & DEFINITIONS

From the assumptions underpinning her theory, Parse drew three thematic elements: meaning, rhythmicity, and cotranscendence. She then deduced the three principles of Human Becoming.

Principle 1: Structuring meaning multidimensionally is cocreating reality through the languaging of valuing and imaging. The essential concepts of this principle are imaging, valuing, and languaging.[17:42-50;18:163-165]

Meaning, the thematic element of Parse's first principle, "arises from the Human Being's interrelationship with the world. It refers to both ultimate meaning and the meaning moments of everyday life."[10:10] Ultimate meaning is our view of life's absolute purpose. It is usually expressed in religious or philosophical language. The meaning moments of everyday life are those common happenings to which we attach varying degrees of significance. We do so through the process of imaging, "the cocreating of reality that, by its very nature, structures the meaning of an experience."[17:42]

Our world view provides the framework for cocreating reality. Valuing "is the Human being's process of confirming cherished beliefs and is reflective of one's world view. This confirming of beliefs is choosing from imaged options and owning the choices."[17:45] Languaging is expressing valued images. It encompasses all modes of self-presentation, including the rhythmical patterns of speech and movement. Our rhythmical patterns of speech and movement reflect our cultural heritage as well.[17:46-50]

Principle 2: Cocreating rhythmical patterns of relating is living the paradoxical unity of revealing-concealing, enabling-limiting while connecting-separating. The essential concepts are revealing-concealing, enabling-limiting, and connecting-separating.[17:50-55;18:163-165]

This principle's thematic element, rhythmicity "is revealed as Human being and universe move toward greater diversity. Rhythmical patterns are cocreated in the human-universe interrelationship and are paradoxes lived all at one."[21:11] Revealing-concealing "is the simultaneous disclosing of some aspects of self and hiding of others."[17:52] When we disclose ourselves to another person, we gain knowledge about ourselves. Yet by moving in one direction, we are limited in another. This is the rhythmical pattern of enabling-limiting. The human "cannot be all possibilities at once, and, in choosing, one is both enabled and limited."[17:53] To move in one direction and not in another involves reordering relationships. "Connecting-separating. . . . can be recognized as man is connecting with one phenomenon and simultaneously separating from others . . . In separating from one phenomenon and dwelling with another, a person integrates thought, becomes more complex, and seeks new unions."[17:53-54]

Principle 3: Cotranscending with the possibles is powering unique ways of originating in the process of transforming. The essential concepts of this principle are powering, originating and transforming.[17:55-67;18:163-165]

Continued

MAJOR CONCEPTS *&* DEFINITIONS—cont'd

Cotranscendence, the thematic element of Parse's third principle, "is the process of reaching out beyond self to the not-yet."[17:12] This process "is powered through origination in transforming."[21:12] Powering "is a continuous rhythmical process incarnating one's intentions and actions in moving toward the possibilities."[17:57] Its rhythm is pushing-resisting, creating a tension, which, when changed, sometimes conflicts. When conflict surfaces, one is faced with new possibilities from which to choose in moving toward the future. Creating unique ways of living is originating. The human originates in mutual energy interchange with the environment. "Powering ways of originating is man distinguishing self from others."[17:60] Transforming is the Human being moving toward greater diversity through living new imaged possibilities and transcending the present. Parse calls transforming "the changing of change, coconstituting anew in a deliberate way."[17:62] Sarter[24:58] views the principles as representing the three aspects of consciousness: knowing, feeling, and willing.

MAJOR ASSUMPTIONS

Parse creatively blended principles, tenets, and concepts from Rogers's Science of Unitary Human Beings and existential-phenomenological thought to craft the assumptions underpinning Human Becoming. Each assumption "connects three specific concepts in a unique way."[17:25] The three concepts Parse unites in each assumption were drawn both from Rogers and from existential phenomenology. This underscores just how firmly Parse's theoretical sources undergird her theory. "To draw upon the work of these theorists, of course, is to build upon a solid foundation and to maintain a bridge to the past necessary in the establishment of any scientific theory."[17:5]

Because Parse treats man, environment, and health as constructs, her assumptions defy classification. (Nursing is not a concept per se; it is the scientific endeavor described by the concepts: it is the discipline itself.) Attempting to force Parse's assumptions into categories labeled man, environment, health, and nursing would wrench them out of context and distort their meaning. Accordingly, Parse's beliefs about these pivotal topics are summarized below, following a listing of the assumptions that underpin the Human Becoming Theory.

Human Becoming: Assumptions With Related Concepts

- The human is coexisting while coconstituting rhythmical patterns with the universe. (Concepts of coconstitution, coexistence, and pattern and organization.)
- The human is an open being, freely choosing meaning in situations and bearing responsibility for decisions. (Concepts of situated freedom, openness, and energy field.)
- The human is a living unity continuously coconstituting patterns of relating. (Concepts of energy field, coconstitution, and pattern and organization.)
- The human is transcending multidimensionally with the possibles. (Concepts of openness, coconstitution, and situated freedom.)
- Becoming is an open process, experienced by the human. (Concepts of openness, coconstitution, and situated freedom.)
- Becoming is a rhythmically coconstituting human-universe process. (Concepts of coconstitution, pattern and organization, and four-dimensionality.)
- Becoming is the human's pattern of relating value priorities. (Concepts of pattern and organization, openness, and situated freedom.)

- Becoming is an intersubjective process of transcending with the possibilities. (Concepts of coexistence, openness, and situated freedom.)
- Becoming is human evolving. (Concepts of coexistence, energy field, and four-dimensionality.)[19:5-6]

Subsequently, Parse synthesized these nine assumptions into the following three:

1. Human becoming is freely choosing personal meaning in situations in the intersubjective process of relating value priorities.
2. Human becoming is cocreating rhythmical patterns of relating in open interchange with the universe.
3. Human becoming is cotranscending multidimensionally with the emerging possibles.[18:161-162;19:6;22:10]

Nursing

By proposing that nursing is a human science, Parse rejects the traditional view of nursing as an emerging natural science. She contends that nursing has paralleled medicine's development, echoing its themes. "Man's participative experience with health situations has been virtually ignored," she declared. "Nursing, rooted in human sciences, focuses on Man as a living unity and Man's qualitative participation with health experiences."[17:4] For nursing to evolve as a distinct discipline, it must move away from its medical model orientation.

Pare strongly affirms nursing's responsibility to society. "The responsibility to society relative to nursing practice is guiding the choosing of possibilities in the changing health process."[17:81] Specifically, "Nursing practice is directed toward illuminating and mobilizing family interrelationships in light of the meaning assigned to health and its possibilities as languaged in the cocreated patterns of relating."[17:82] *Family,* it should be noted, is used by Parse to signify those persons with whom we have close relationships.

Person

Human beings (formerly called Man) are a major reason for nursing's existence. (Another major rea-

son, of course, is health.) This has been the case since the time of Nightingale and the publication of her *Notes on Nursing.*[16] In keeping with this tradition, Parse explicitly discussed human being in her assumptions. Human being is integral to her theory's concepts, principles, theoretical structures, and practice propositions—all of which flow directly from Human Becoming's assumptions. Parse hails Rogers as the first nurse theorist to reject the traditional "totality" paradigm and embrace the "simultaneity" paradigm. The totality paradigm views the human being "as a total, summative organism whose nature is a combination of bio-psycho-social-spiritual features."[18:4] In contrast, the simultaneity paradigm views the human being "as more than and different from the sum of parts, changing mutually and simultaneously with the environment."[18:4]

For Parse, human beings evidence "a pattern of patterns of relating."[17:26] Because we exist in the world with others, we cannot not relate. "When one person encounters another person, rhythmical patterns of relating unfold as words become sentences and are shared with a certain volume at a particular tempo with unique intonation, simultaneously with a certain gaze, gesture, touch, and posture."[17:47-48] In this way, our perceptions of ourselves, others, and our situations emerge. As we live our own life stories and the historical story of our species, we grow more complex and diverse. Living simultaneously in all spheres of time—past, present, and future—we are influenced by our "ancestors, successors, and contemporaries through personal interrelationships, ideas, and future planning."[17:26] They sharpen our sensitivity to life's rhythms—its joys and sorrows, aspirations and disappointments, births, and deaths. We become aware of our mortality and the possible extermination of our species. Art and music heighten our awareness of death: through them we celebrate life and the mystery it holds for us. Human beings, then, experience life as an all-at-once multidimensional experience.

Health

For Parse, health is a lived experience. It is not the absence of disease or a state of well-being, nor can it be placed on a continuum. The human being's "health, then, is not a linear entity that can be interrupted or qualified by terms such as good, bad, more, or less. It is not man adapting to or coping with the environment. Such a description of health dichotomizes and denies man's unitary nature. Unitary man's health is a synthesis of values, a way of living."[17:39] Health occurs as the human being "structures meaning in situations."[17:40] It is a process of being and becoming.

Environment

Human "as a pattern and organization is distinct from the pattern and organization of the environment."[17:26] But humans and the environment (now called universe) are inseparable. Interchanging energy, unfolding together toward greater complexity and diversity, influencing one another's rhythmical patterns of relating, is a construct: Human-Universe. Humans and universe, then, "interchange energy to create what is in the world."[17:27] The human "chooses the meaning given to the situations he creates."[17:27]

THEORETICAL ASSERTIONS

Parse's theoretical structures flow directly from Human Becoming assumptions and principles. Each structure interrelates three concepts (Fig. 30-1). Because the purpose of the theoretical structures is to guide nursing practice and research, Parse invites their validation in these areas. Human Becoming's theoretical structures are:

1. Powering is a way of revealing and concealing imaging.
2. Originating is a manifestation of enabling and limiting valuing.
3. Transforming unfolds in the languaging of connecting and separating.[17:68;18:166]

Other theoretical structures may be derived, Parse noted.

In 1987, Parse expressed her theoretical structures as practice propositions at the next lower level of abstraction. As a practice proposition, the first theoretical structure "can be stated as *struggling to live goals discloses the significance of the situation*"; the second as *"creating anew shows one's cherished beliefs and leads in a directional movement"*; and the third as

Principle 1: Structuring meaning multidimensionally is cocreating reality through the languaging of valuing and imaging.

Principle 2: Cocreating rhythmical patterns of relating is living the paradoxical unity of revealing-concealing and enabling-limiting while connecting-separating.

Principle 3: Cotranscending with the possibles is powering unique ways of originating in the process of transforming.

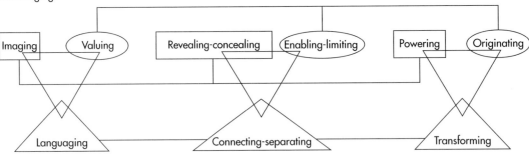

Relationship of the concepts in the squares: *Powering* is a way of *revealing and concealing imaging.*
Relationship of the concepts in the ovals: *Originating* is a manifestation of *enabling and limiting valuing.*
Relationship of the concepts in the triangles: *Transforming* unfolds in the *languaging of connecting and separating.*

Fig. **30-1** Relationship of principles, concepts, and theoretical structures of Theory of Human Becoming. *From Parse, R.R. (1981). Man-living-health: A theory of nursing. New York: John Wiley & Sons, p. 69.*

"changing views emerge in speaking and moving with others."[18:169-171] Parse cautions, however, that "the details of nursing practice can only be specified in the context of particular nurse-person and nurse-group situations."[18:170]

LOGICAL FORM

The inductive-deductive process was central to the creation of Human Becoming. The theory originated from Parse's lived experiences in nursing practice. She deductively crafted major components of Human Becoming from Rogers's Science of Unitary Human Beings and existential-phenomenological thought—along with her intuitive sense—Parse methodically derived Human Becoming's assumptions, concepts, principles, theoretical structures, and propositions. Each assumption interrelates three foundational concepts, each principle three of Human Becoming's concepts, and each theoretical structure a concept from each principle.

ACCEPTANCE BY THE NURSING COMMUNITY

Practice

Human Becoming presents an implicit guide for practice. Parse feels that nursing based on Human Becoming is quite unlike nursing based on other models.[19:81] Winkler observed, "Basing care planning on the client's perspective of health and her/his care would encourage innovation in activities designated nursing, and acceptance of unique self-care activities."[27:292]

In the original presentation of her theory, Parse discussed in detail a family situation and its implications from the perspective of her theory.[17:82-89] In the example, she viewed nursing practice as an "intersubjective participation in guiding [the family] in the choosing of possibles in the changing health process."[17:89]

Unlike some more established models, Human Becoming has not been used extensively in practice. Its practice methodology is evolving. Butler used the theory to change the health situation of a family facing the loss of its central figure after major neurosurgery.[3] Papers on the theory's applicability to prac-

tice have been presented in the United States and Canada.[9-12] Mitchell used Parse's theory to guide care for an elderly woman.[15] In a replication of a study done by Parse in 1987, Santopinto[23] is studying the difference Parse's theory makes in a practice setting.

Education

Parse writes for an audience composed of graduate students in nursing, faculty in schools of nursing, and nursing administrators in university and major health care settings. Her unwavering focus, however, is on master's and doctoral students—nursing's emerging scholars. They will be the ones most likely to share or adopt her perspective and conduct much of the research needed to develop her theory further. They will also use her model for curriculum development as they gain faculty rank.

In *Man-Living-Health: A Theory of Nursing*, Parse presented a sample master's-in-nursing curriculum that incorporated the assumptions, principles, concepts, and theoretical structures of Man-Living-Health.[17:96-112] She outlined in detail this process-based curriculum, including course descriptions and course sequencing. Two courses in nursing theory are listed as focal courses in the curriculum, indicating the importance Parse attaches to theory and its development.

Research

Human Becoming has been validated by research. Six studies using qualitative methodologies—descriptive, phenomenological, and ethnographic—have been published.[21] In addition to validating Parse's theory, these studies complemented each other. The authors explained the complementarity thus:

> The qualitative approach offers the researcher the opportunity to study the emergence of patterns in the whole configuration of Man's lived experiences. It is an approach in which the researcher explicitly participates in uncovering the meaning of these experiences as humanly lived.[21:3]

Human Becoming has embedded in it countless research questions. A research method specifically designed to investigate these questions is evolving.[18:172-178] The advantage of this theory-derived research method is the congruence of the approach with the belief system. Any theory—including this one—must be learned in detail before it can be used in research. This takes time. The qualitative research studies needed to develop the theory are another time-consuming process. Once completed, research may take up to 2 years before it is published. To broaden the theory's "circle of contagiousnesss,"[14:158] Parse has conducted several programs in which results of research studies related to her theory have been presented. A number of master's theses have been completed using Parse's theory.[20] Doctoral dissertations are beginning to be written using Human Becoming. For instance, Beauchamp is investigating the concept of power, specifically the decision by those who test positive for the human immunodeficiency virus antibody to seek treatment.[2] He is being assisted in this research by Marchette.[13] Postdoctoral studies are in progress as well. Smith is investigating the lived experience of struggling through the difficulty of unemployment.[25] Liehr and Flores are studying the human experience of "living on the edge." Participants in the study are persons who have suffered at least one cardiac arrest. To understand cocreating living on the edge, the study has been expanded to include participants' spouses.[8] These studies are an important indication that more research related to Human Becoming will be forthcoming.

FURTHER DEVELOPMENT

We can anticipate Human Becoming's continuing evolution. Ongoing research is expected to refine concepts, clarify interrelationships, and lead to higher levels of theory development. As schools of nursing adopt and teach Human Becoming, nurses can be expected to use it more in practice. As nurses use the theory in practice to guide patients through the changing health process, its usefulness will be more fully appreciated by society.

Unfortunately, many nurses avoid exploring this theory because of its very abstract language and philosophical base. Those who shun attempting to learn it forget that effort and discipline are required to move from "a state of understanding less to one of understanding more."[1:8] Parse, Coyne, and Smith reframed this belief specifically for nursing when they wrote:

> Learning the theory in scientific disciplines requires formal study, a reverence for quiet contemplation, and creative synthesis. Neither [Man-Living-Health] nor the methodologies presented in this work can be learned quickly. The nature of the content compels the learner to abide with the conceptualizations and study the movements in discourse required by scholars who aspire to research and theory development in nursing.[21:191]

CRITIQUE

Human Becoming is an abstract and complex theory. It is a theory—and not a model—because its concepts and interrelationships have received empirical validation.

Simplicity

In keeping with the theoretical discourse, Human Becoming's major concepts are defined by Parse in highly abstract and philosophical terms. Parse's use of quotations and references in *Man-Living-Health: A Theory of Nursing* rounded out the concepts and rendered them more understandable. The examples Parse cited were clear and simple. However, a first-time reader might be tempted to dismiss them as too simple to convey the complexity inherent in her theory. To do so, though, would be a mistake; lingering with her examples and drawing them out are more beneficial. Parse's principles, theoretical structures, and practice propositions clearly set forth the interrelationships she sees operating in the world. Consistent with the expectations we have of any scientific theory, Human Becoming has the potential to describe, explain, and predict.

Generality

Human Becoming's conceptualization is broad in scope and applicable to individuals, families, or communities in change or crisis. To say, as Winkler[27:289] did, that Parse ignores biological manifestations is to miss her point: Human Becoming is about the unity of man's lived experience. It is facile to talk about the biological manifestations of a physical condition and not talk about it phenomenologically. For example, when discussing chronic pain, Turk, Holzman, and Kerns[26:446] stated that "a psychologically based treatment, or any treatment, must consider the patient's perspective and the phenomenology of chronic pain in developing and implementing a therapeutic regimen." The same can be said about diabetes, asthma, or cardiovascular disease—in children and adults. Because Human Becoming addresses the lived experience of health, it is at the cutting edge of health care.

Empirical Precision

Parse defines Human Becoming's concepts denotatively and at the philosophical level of discourse. Although the concepts are highly abstract and theoretical, they can be observed in situations nurses encounter daily. But without study many nurses will not see what is going on around them. For this reason Parse's theory is exciting: it fires the imagination because it enables us to see anew. Linking it and research and practice will help us "better understand how Man chooses and bears responsibility for the rhythmical patterns of personal health."[22:201]

Derivable Consequences

Parse allies nursing and the human sciences. This is in sharp contrast to most theories of nursing, which mirror medical science. With consumers more aware of strategies for promoting their health and demanding a greater voice in its management, Parse's emphasis on Human's participation in and responsibility for health is timely. Societal questions about the quality of life in chronic, terminal, and marginal conditions suggest the potential Parse's theory has for meeting nursing's responsibility to society by addressing these questions. "Parse's model," predicted Phillips, "will contribute to a transformation of the knowledge base of nursing and the practice of nursing from a unitary perspective. The Human Becoming model provides new hope that there will be greater focus in the future of [sic] the meaning and quality of life and health that transcends the disease orientation; it will deal with improved quality of life for all people as perceived by them."[22:201-202]

The future of Human Becoming lies in demystifying the language, developing middle-range testable theory and, most important, convincing nurses to replace the scientific method with the humanistic method.

CRITICAL THINKING *Activities*

1 Mrs. Brown, a 48-year-old woman, is diagnosed with breast cancer. She has not told her daughter about her diagnosis because she is afraid of the daughter's response. Use Parse's concepts to uncover the meaning of this situation for Mrs. Brown and show how you will help her move beyond her fear.

2 Mr. Smith, an 88-year-old man, has been in the hospital for several days. Although he is alert, the nursing staff reports that he "fidgets," "seems extremely nervous," and "calls out to his wife." Several of his nurses have asked the physician to prescribe a tranquilizer. Use Parse's concepts to discuss Mr. Smith's behavior and his feelings about the hospitalization.

REFERENCES

1. Adler, M.J., & Van Doren, C. (1972). *How to read a book.* New York: Touchstone Books.
2. Beauchamp, C.J. (1988, May). Personal communication.
3. Butler, M.J. (1988). Family transformation: Parse's theory in practice. *Nursing Science Quarterly, 1*(2), 68-74.
4. Cohen, M.Z. (1987). A historical overview of the phenomenological movement. *Image, 19*(1), 31-34.
5. Giddens, A. (1976). *New rules of sociological method.* New York: Basic Books.
6. Jennings, J.L. (1986). Husserl revisited: The forgotten distinction between psychology and phenomenology. *American Psychologist, 41,* 1231-1240.
7. Knaack, P. (1984). Phenomenological research. *Western Journal of Nursing Research, 6*(1), 107-114.
8. Liehr, P. (1988, July). Personal communication.

9. Magan, S.J. (1983, Oct. 15; 1984, Jan. 28; 1985, Aug. 22-23). *Mobilizing energies in the structuring of meaning of changing health patterns.* Paper presented at Nursing Science Symposium, Pittsburgh, PA; Dayton, OH; Nurse Theorist Conference, Edmonton, Alberta.

10. Magan, S.J. (1984, Sept. 22). *Shifting rhythms in changing health patterns.* Paper presented at Nursing Science Symposium, Pittsburgh, PA.

11. Magan, S.J. (1986, May). *The lived experience of hopefulness: A phenomenological study.* Cassette Recording No. DII-301. Louisville, KY: Meetings International.

12. Magan, S.J. (1986, May). *The lived experience of hopefulness: A phenomenological study.* Paper presented at Discovery International Incorporated's Nursing Science Symposium, Pittsburgh, PA.

13. Marchette, L. (1988, July). Personal communication.

14. Meleis, A.I. (1985). *Theoretical nursing: Development and progress.* Philadelphia: Lippincott.

15. Mitchell, G. (1986). Utilizing Parse's theory of Man-Living-Health in Mrs. M's neighborhood. *Perspectives, 10*(4), 5-7.

16. Nightingale, F. (1969). *Notes on nursing.* New York: Dove Publications. (Originally published in 1860.)

17. Parse, R.R. (1981). *Man-Living-Health: A theory of nursing.* New York: John Wiley & Sons.

18. Parse, R.R. (Ed.). (1987). *Nursing science: Major paradigms, theories, and critiques.* Philadelphia: Saunders.

19. Parse, R.R. (Ed.). (1995). *Illuminations: The human becoming theory in practice and research.* New York: National League for Nursing.

20. Parse, R.R. (1996, June). Personal communication.

21. Parse, R.R., Coyne, A.B., & Smith, M.J. (Eds.) (1985). *Nursing research: Qualitative methods.* Bowie, MD: Brady Communications.

22. Phillips, J.R. (1987). A critique of Parse's Man-Living-Health theory. In R.R. Parse (Ed.), *Nursing science: Major paradigms, theories, and critiques* (pp. 181-204). Philadelphia: Saunders.

23. Santopinto, M.D.A. (1988, March). Personal communication.

24. Sarter, B. (1988). Philosophical sources of nursing theory. *Nursing Science Quarterly, 1*(2), 52-59.

25. Smith, M. (1988, April; 1988, July). *The lived experience of struggling through difficulty for persons who are unemployed.* Paper presented at Sigma Theta Tau—Delta Xi Research Day, Kent State University, Kent, OH; Wayne State University School of Nursing Summer Research Symposium, Detroit.

26. Turk, D.C., Holzman, A.D., & Kerns, R.D. (1986). Chronic pain. In K.A. Holroyd & T.L. Creer (Eds.), *Self-management of chronic disease: Handbook of clinical interventions and research* (pp. 441-472). Orlando: Academic Press.

27. Winkler, S.J. (1983). Parse's theory of nursing. In J. Fitzpatrick & A. Whall (Eds.), *Conceptual models of nursing: Analysis and application* (pp. 275-294). Bowie, MD: Robert J. Brady.

BIBLIOGRAPHY

Primary sources

Books

Parse, R.R. (1974). *Nursing fundamentals.* Flushing, NY: Medical Examination.

Parse, R.R. (1981). *Man-living-health: A theory of nursing.* New York: John Wiley & Sons.

Parse, R.R. (1987). *Nursing science: Major paradigms, theories, and critiques.* Philadelphia: Saunders.

Parse, R.R. (1995). *Illuminations: The human becoming theory in practice and research.* New York: National League for Nursing.

Parse, R.R., Coyne, A.B., & Smith, M.J. (1985). *Nursing research: Qualitative methods.* Bowie, MD: Robert J. Brady.

Doctoral dissertation

Parse, R.R. (1969). An instructional model for the teaching of nursing, interrelating objectives and media. (Doctoral dissertation, University of Pittsburgh.) *Dissertation Abstracts International, 31*, 180A.

Book chapters

Parse, R.R. (1978). Rights of medical patients. In C. Fisher, *Client participation in human services.* New Brunswick, NJ: Transaction.

Parse, R.R. (1981). Caring from a human science perspective. In M.M. Leininger (Ed.), *Caring: An essential human need.* Thorofare, NJ: Charles B. Slack.

Parse, R.R. (1988). Parse's Man-living-health model and administration of nursing services. In B. Henry, C. Arndt, M. DiVencenti, & A. Marriner-Tomey (Eds.), *Dimensions of nursing administration: Theory, research, education, and practice.* Cambridge, MA: Blackwell Scientific Publications.

Parse, R.R. (1989). Man-living-health: A theory of nursing. In Riehl-Sisca, J.P., *Conceptual models for nursing practice.* Norwalk, CT: Appleton & Lange.

Parse, R.R. (1989). The phenomenological research method: Its value for management science. In B. Henry, C. Arndt, M. DiVencenti, & A. Marriner-Tomey (Ed.), *Dimensions of nursing administration: Theory, research, education, and practice.* Cambridge, MA: Blackwell Scientific Publications.

Parse, R.R. (1991). Parse's theory of human becoming. In I.E. Goertzen (Ed.), *Differentiating nursing practice: Into the twenty-first century* (pp. 51-53). Kansas City, MO: American Academy of Nursing.

Parse, R.R. (1993). Parse's human becoming theory: Its research and practice implications. In M.E. Parker (Ed.), *Patterns of nursing theories in practice.* New York: National League for Nursing Press.

Journal articles

Parse, R.R. (1967, Aug.). The advantages of the ADN program. *Journal of Nursing Education, 6*, 15.

Parse, R.R. (1990). Parse's research methodology with an illustration of the lived experience of hope. *Nursing Science Quarterly, 3,* 9-17.

Parse, R.R. (1991). Phenomenology and nursing. *Japanese Journal of Nursing, 17*(2), 261-269.

Parse, R.R. (1992). Human becoming: Parse's theory of nursing. *Nursing Science Quarterly, 5,* 35-42.

Parse, R.R. (1992). Nursing knowledge for the 21st century: An international commitment. *Nursing Science Quarterly, 5,* 8-12.

Parse, R.R. (1993). The experience of laughter: A phenomenological study. *Nursing Science Quarterly, 6,* 39-43.

Parse, R.R. (1994). Laughing and health: A study using Parse's research method. *Nursing Science Quarterly, 7,* 55-64.

Parse, R.R. (1994). Quality of life: Sciencing and living the art of human becoming. *Nursing Science Quarterly, 7,* 16-21.

Parse, R.R. (1995). Mensh(werden)-leben-gesundheit: Die pflegetheorie von Parse [Man-living-health: Parse's theory of nursing]. In M. Mischo-Kelling & K. Wittneben (Eds.), *Pflegebildung und pflegetheorien.* Munchen: Urban & Schwarzenberg.

Parse, R.R. (1996, Spring). Building knowledge through qualitative research: The road less traveled. *Nursing Science Quarterly, 9*(1), 10-6 (65 ref).

Editorials

Parse, R.R. (1988). Beginnings . . . the knowledge of a discipline. *Nursing Science Quarterly, 1,* 1-2.

Parse, R.R. (1988). Creating traditions: The art of putting it together. *Nursing Science Quarterly, 1,* 45.

Parse, R.R. (1988). The mainstream of science: Framing the issue. *Nursing Science Quarterly, 1,* 93.

Parse, R.R. (1988). Scholarly dialogue: The fire of refinement. *Nursing Science Quarterly, 1,* 141.

Parse, R.R. (1989). Essentials for practicing the art of nursing. *Nursing Science Quarterly, 2,* 111.

Parse, R.R. (1989). Making more out of less . . . publishing the same manuscript in more than one journal. *Nursing Science Quarterly, 2,* 155.

Parse, R.R. (1989). Martha E. Rogers: A birthday celebration. *Nursing Science Quarterly, 2,* 55.

Parse, R.R. (1989). Qualitative research: Publishing and funding. *Nursing Science Quarterly, 2,* 1-2.

Parse, R.R. (1990). Nurse theorist conference comes to Japan. *Japanese Journal of Nursing Research, 23*(3).

Parse, R.R. (1990). Nursing theory-based practice. *Nursing Science Quarterly, 3,* 53.

Parse, R.R. (1990). Promotion and preventions: Two distinct cosmologies. *Nursing Science Quarterly, 3,* 101.

Parse, R.R. (1990). A time for reflection and projection. *Nursing Science Quarterly, 3,* 143.

Parse, R.R. (1991). Electronic publishing: Beyond browsing. *Nursing Science Quarterly, 4,* 1.

Parse, R.R. (1991). Growing the discipline of nursing. *Nursing Science Quarterly, 4,* 139.

Parse, R.R. (1991). Mysteries of health and healing: Two perspectives. *Nursing Science Quarterly, 4,* 93.

Parse, R.R. (1991). The right soil, the right stuff. *Nursing Science Quarterly, 4,* 47.

Parse, R.R. (1992). Moving beyond the barrier reef. *Nursing Science Quarterly, 5,* 97.

Parse, R.R. (1992). The performing art of nursing. *Nursing Science Quarterly, 5,* 147.

Parse, R.R. (1992). The unsung shapers of nursing science. *Nursing Science Quarterly, 5,* 47.

Parse, R.R. (1993). Cartoons: Glimpsing paradoxical moments. *Nursing Science Quarterly, 6,* 1.

Parse, R.R. (1993). Critical appraisal: Risking to challenge. *Nursing Science Quarterly, 6,* 163.

Parse, R.R. (1993). Nursing and medicine: Two different disciplines. *Nursing Science Quarterly, 6,* 109.

Parse, R.R. (1993). Plant now; reap later. *Nursing Science Quarterly, 6,* 55.

Parse, R.R. (1993). Scholarly dialogue: Theory guides research and practice. *Nursing Science Quarterly, 6,* 12.

Parse, R.R. (1994). Charley Potatoes or mashed potatoes? *Nursing Science Quarterly, 7,* 97.

Parse, R.R. (1994). Martha E. Rogers: Her voice will not be silenced. *Nursing Science Quarterly, 7,* 47.

Parse, R.R. (1994). Scholarship: Three essential processes. *Nursing Science Quarterly, 7,* 143.

Parse, R.R. (1995). Building the realm of nursing knowledge. *Nursing Science Quarterly, 8,* 51.

Parse, R.R. (1995). Nursing theories and frameworks: The essence of advanced practice nursing. *Nursing Science Quarterly, 8,* 1.

Parse, R.R. (1995, Winter). Again: what is nursing? *Nursing Science Quarterly, 8*(4), 143 (12 ref).

Parse, R.R. (1996, Spring). Hear ye, hear ye, novice and seasoned authors! *Nursing Science Quarterly, 9*(1), 1.

Unpublished manuscripts

Parse, R.R. (1984). *Man-living-health in practice.* Unpublished manuscript.

Parse, R.R. (1986). *An emerging methodology for the Man-living health theory.* Unpublished manuscript.

Parse, R.R. (1991). *Man-living health: Theory, research and practice.* Paper presented at Kyoto, Japan.

Parse, R.R. (1991). *Nursing frameworks as guides to practice.* Keynote address at Third South Florida Nurse Theorist Conference, Cedars Medical Center, Miami, FL.

Parse, R.R. (1991). *Nursing knowledge for the 21st century: An international commitment.* Keynote address at Discovery International, Inc., Biennial Nurse Theorist Conference, Tokyo, Japan.

Parse, R.R. (1991). *Parse in question and answer.* Discovery International, Inc., Biennial Nurse Theorist Conference, Tokyo, Japan.

Parse, R.R. (1991). *Parse's theory.* Paper presented at Discovery International, Inc., Biennial Nurse Theorist Conference, Tokyo, Japan.

Parse, R.R. (1991). *Phenomenology as a way of living.* Paper presented at Interpersonal Relationships Society, Tokyo, Japan.

Parse, R.R. (1991). *Theory and research as tools for practice.* Paper presented at University of Michigan, School of Nursing, Centennial Celebration, Ann Arbor, MI.

Parse, R.R. (1992). Immersion weekend on Parse's human becoming theory with Parse Interest Group, Killington, VT.

Parse, R.R. (1992). *Nursing knowledge-based practice: An ethical commitment.* Paper presented at European Nursing Congress 1992, Amsterdam, The Netherlands.

Parse, R.R. (1993). *Critique of critical phenomena of nursing science suggested by O'Brien, Reed, and Stevenson.* Proceedings of the 1993 Annual Forum on Doctoral Nursing Education: A Call for Substance: Preparing Leaders for Global Health (pp. 71-81). St. Paul, MN: University of Minnesota School of Nursing.

Parse, R.R. (1993). *The human becoming theory in practice: A research study at Royal Ottawa Hospital.* Presented at Ottawa, Ontario, Canada.

Parse, R.R. (1993). *The human becoming theory in practice and research.* Paper presented at Geneva, Switzerland.

Parse, R.R. (1993). *The human becoming theory: Its research and practice methodologies.* Paper presented at University of Illinois, Chicago, IL.

Parse, R.R. (1993). *True presence in languaging without words.* Presented at Immersion Weekend of International Consortium of Parse Scholars, McHenry, MD.

Parse, R.R. (1994). *Critique of the unitary field pattern profile portrait research method.* Paper presented at the 5th Annual Rogerian Conference at New York University, New York.

Parse, R.R. (1994). *Facing the mystery of being in true presence.* Presented at Immersion Weekend of International Consortium of Parse Scholars, Niagara-on-the-Lake, Ontario, Canada.

Parse, R.R. (1994). *Human becoming theory.* Paper presented at the O'Connor Chair for Nursing Lecture Series, Hartwick College, Oneonta, NY.

Parse, R.R. (1994). *The human becoming theory in practice.* Paper presented at International Congress, Aarau, Switzerland.

Parse, R.R. (1994). *Human becoming theory in practice and research* (workshop). Padua, Italy.

Parse, R.R. (1994). *Knowledge building through qualitative research.* Paper presented at the Second Annual International Qualitative Nursing Research Colloquium, Loyola University, Chicago.

Parse, R.R. (1994). *Quality of life: Ethics and values.* Presented at National Council for International Health Conference, Arlington, VA.

Parse, R.R. Nursing theory-guided practice. *Journal of Pediatric Oncology.* In press.

Parse, R.R. *The language of nursing knowledge: Saying what we mean.* Submitted for publication.

Cassette recordings

Parse, R.R. (Speaker). (1985). *Presentation at nurse theorist conference.* Cassette Recording No. DII-105. Louisville, KY: Meetings International.

Parse, R.R. (Speaker). (1986). *An emerging research methodology unique to nursing.* Cassette Recording No. DII-303. Louisville, KY: Meetings International.

Parse, R.R. (Speaker). (1986). *The ethnographic method.* Cassette Recording No. DII-204. Louisville, KY: Meetings International.

Parse, R.R. (Speaker). (1986). *The phenomenological method.* Cassette Recording No. DII-202. Louisville, KY: Meetings International.

Parse, R.R. (Speaker). (1986). *Quantitative and qualitative methods in nursing research.* Cassette Recording No. DII-201. Louisville, KY: Meetings International.

Parse, R.R. (Speaker). (1987). *Parse's theory.* Cassette Recording No. DII-403. Louisville, KY: Meetings International.

Parse, R.R. (Speaker). (1987). *Small group C.* Cassette Recording No. DII-411. Louisville, KY: Meetings International.

Parse, R.R. (Speaker). (1989). *Health as a personal commitment in Parse's theory.* Cassette Recording No. DII-503. Louisville, KY: Meetings International.

Parse, R.R. (Speaker). (1990). *Parse's research and practice methodologies.* Cassette Recording No. DII-601. Louisville, KY: Meetings International.

Parse, R.R. (Speaker). (1993). *Quality of life and human becoming.* Cassette Recording No. DII-701. Louisville, KY: Veranda Communications.

Parse, R.R., Cody, W.K., Beauchamp, C.J., Smith, M.C., Menke, E.M., Mitchell, G.J., & Santopinto, M.D.A. (Speakers). (1990). *Panel discussion/retrospective and evaluation.* Cassette Recording No. DII-605. Louisville, KY: Meetings International.

Parse, R.R., Leininger, M.M., Rogers, M.E., Peplau, H.E., & King, I.M. (Speakers). (1993). *Nursing and the next millennium* [panel discussion with the theorists]. Cassette Recording No. DII-708. Louisville, KY: Veranda Communications.

Parse, R.R., Meleis, A.I., Newman, B.M., Rogers, M.E., Pender, N.J., & King, I.M. (Speakers). (1989). *Panel discussion with theorists.* Cassette Recording No. DII-507. Louisville, KY: Meetings International.

Parse, R.R., Orem, D.E., Roy, C., King, I.M., Rogers, M.E., & Peplau, H.E. (Speakers). (1985). *Panel discussion with nurse theorists.* Cassette Recording No. DII-112. Louisville, KY: Meetings International.

Parse, R.R., & Phillips, J.R. (Speakers). (1985). *Parse's Man-living-health theory of nursing.* Cassette Recording No. DII-109. Louisville, KY: Meetings International.

Parse, R.R., Sklar, M., & Smith, M.J. (Speakers). (1986). *Panel discussion.* Cassette Recording No. DII-305. Louisville, KY: Meetings International.

Videotape recordings

Parse, R.R. (1985). *Presentation at nurse theorist conference.* Videotape Recording No. DII-V-105. Louisville, KY: Meetings International.

Parse, R.R. (Speaker).(1987). *Parse's theory.* Videotape Recording No. DII-V-403. Louisville, KY: Meetings International.

Parse, R.R. (Speaker). (1989). *Health as a personal commitment in Parse's theory.* Videotape Recording No. DII-V-503. Louisville, KY: Meetings International.

Parse, R.R. (Speaker). (1990). *A portrait in excellence.* Helene Fuld Health Trust. Oakland, CA: Studio Three Production.

Parse, R.R. (Speaker). (1993). *Quality of life and human becoming.* Videotape Recording No. DII-V-701. Louisville, KY: Veranda Communications.

Parse R.R., Leininger, M.M., Rogers, M.E., Peplau, H., & King, I.M. (Speakers). (1993). *Nursing and the next millennium* [panel discussion with the theorists]. Videotape Recording No. DII-V-708. Louisville, KY: Veranda Communications.

Parse, R.R., Meleis, A.I., Neuman, B.M., Rogers, M.E., Pender, N.J., & King, I.M. (Speakers). (1989). *Panel discussion with theorists.* Videotape Recording No. DII-V-507. Louisville, KY: Meetings International.

Parse, R.R., Orem, D.E., Roy, C., King, I.M., Rogers, M.E., & Peplau, H.E. (Speakers). (1985). *Panel discussion with nurse theorists.* Videotape Recording No. DII-V-112. Louisville, KY: Meetings International.

Parse, R.R., Peplau, H.E., King, I.M., Roy, C., Rogers, M.E., Watson, J., & Leininger, M. (Speakers). (1987). *Panel discussion with theorists.* Videotape Recording No. DII-V-408. Louisville, KY: Meetings International.

Book reviews

Parse, R.R. (1975). Nursing fundamentals. *Australian Nurses Journal, 5,* 37, August 1975.

Parse, R.R. (1981). Man-living-health: A theory of nursing. *International Journal of Rehabilitation Research, 4,* 449, 1981. *Western Journal of Nursing Research, 5,* 105-106, Winter 1982.

Parse, R.R. (1986). Nursing research: Qualitative methods. *Research in Nursing and Health, 9,* 360-361, 1986.

Parse, R.R. (1990). Health: A personal commitment. *Nursing Science Quarterly, 3,* 136-140.

Secondary sources

Book reviews

Jacobs-Kramer, M.K., Levine, M.E., & Menke, E.M. (1988). Three perspectives on a scholarly work [review of *Nursing science: Major paradigms, theories, and critiques*]. *Nursing Science Quarterly, 1,* 182-186.

Limandri, B.J. (1982). [Review of *Man-living-health: A theory of nursing*]. *Western Journal of Nursing Research, 4*(1), 105-106.

Rawnsley, M.M. (1988). Quest for quality: A comparative review [Review of *Nursing research: Qualitative methods*]. *Nursing Science Quarterly, 1,* 40-41.

Books

Chinn, P.L., & Kramer, M.K. (1995). *Theory and nursing: A systematic approach* (4th ed.). St. Louis: Mosby.

Fawcett, J. (1993). *Analysis and evaluation of nursing theories.* Philadelphia: F.A. Davis.

Fitzpatrick, J.J., & Whall, A.L. (1989). *Conceptual models of nursing: Analysis and application* (2nd ed.). Norwalk, CT: Appleton & Lange.

George, J. (1990). *Nursing theories: The base for professional nursing practice* (3rd ed.). New York: Prentice Hall.

Meleis, A.I. (1985). *Theoretical nursing: Development and progress.* Philadelphia: Lippincott.

Book chapters

Cowling, P.L. (1989). Parse's theory of nursing. In J.J. Fitzpatrick & A.L. Whall (Eds.), *Conceptual models of nursing: Analysis and application* (pp. 385-400). Norwalk, CT: Appleton & Lange.

Hickman, J.S. (1990). Rosemarie Rizzo Parse. In J.B. George (Ed.), *Nursing theories: The base for professional nursing practice* (3rd ed.) (pp. 311-332). Norwalk, CT: Appleton & Lange.

Lee, R.E., & Schumacher, L.P. (1989). Rosemarie Rizzo Parse: Man-living-health. In A. Marriner-Tomey (Ed.), *Nurse theorists and their work* (2nd ed.) (pp. 174-186). St. Louis, MO: Mosby.

Mitchell, G.J. (1991). Distinguishing practice with Parse's theory. In I.E. Goertzen (Ed.), *Differentiating nursing practice: Into the twenty-first century* (pp. 55-58). Kansas City, MO: American Academy of Nursing.

Mitchell, G.J. (1993). Parse's theory in practice. In M.E. Parker (Ed.), *Patterns of nursing theories in practice.* New York: National League for Nursing Press.

Phillips, J. (1987). A critique of Parse's man-living-health theory. In R. Parse (Ed.), *Nursing science: Major paradigms, theories, and critiques* (pp. 181-204). Philadelphia: Saunders.

Pugliese, L. (1989). The theory of man-living-health: An analysis. In J.P. Riehl-Sisca (Ed.), *Conceptual models for nursing practice.* (3rd ed.) (pp. 259-266). Norwalk, CT: Appleton & Lange.

Smith, M.J. (1989). Research and practice application related to man-living-health. In J.P. Riehl-Sisca (Ed.), *Conceptual models for nursing practice.* (3rd ed.) (pp. 267-276). Norwalk, CT: Appleton & Lange.

Winkler, S.J. (1983). Parse's theory of nursing. In J.J. Fitzpatrick & A.L. Whall (Eds.), *Conceptual models of nursing: Analysis and application.* Bowie, MD: Robert J. Brady.

Directories and biographical sources

Sigma Theta Tau. (1987). *Directory of nurse researchers* (2nd ed.). Indianapolis: Author.

Journal articles

Butler, M.J. (1988). Family transformation: Parse's theory in practice. *Nursing Science Quarterly, 1*(2), 68-74.

Butler, M.J., & Snodgrass, F.G. (1991). Beyond abuse: Parse's theory in practice. *Nursing Science Quarterly, 4*(2), 76-82.

Kleffel, D. (1991). Rethinking the environment as a domain of nursing knowledge. *Advances in Nursing Science, 14*, 40-51.

Martin, M.L., Forchuk, C., Santopinto, M., & Butcher, H.K. (1992). Alternative approaches to nursing practice: Application of Peplau, Rogers, and Parse. *Nursing Science Quarterly, 5*, 80-85.

Mitchell, G. (1986). Utilizing Parse's theory of man-living-health in Mrs. M's neighborhood. Perspectives, 10(4), 5-7.

Mitchell, G.J. (1988). Man-living-health: The theory in practice. *Nursing Science Quarterly, 1*(3), 120-127.

Mitchell, G.J. (1990). The lived experience of taking life day-by-day in later life: Research guided by Parse's emergent method. *Nursing Science Quarterly, 3*(1), 29-36.

Mitchell, G.J. (1990). Struggling in change: From the traditional approach to Parse's theory-based practice. *Nursing Science Quarterly, 3*(4), 170-176.

Mitchell, G.J. (1991). Nursing diagnosis: An ethical analysis. *IMAGE: Journal of Nursing Scholarship, 23*, 99-103.

Mitchell, G.J. (1994). Discipline-specific inquiry: The hermeneutics of theory-guided nursing research. *Nursing Outlook, 42*(5), 224-228.

Mitchell, G.J., & Pilkington, B. (1990). Theoretical approaches in nursing practice: A comparison of Roy and Parse. *Nursing Science Quarterly, 3*(2), 81-87.

Nagle, L.M., & Mitchell, G.J. (1991). Theoretic diversity: Evolving paradigmatic issues in research and practice. *Advances in Nursing Science, 14*, 17-25.

Newman, M.A., Sime, A.M., & Corcoran-Perry, S.A. (1991). The focus of the discipline of nursing. *Advances in Nursing Science, 14*, 1-6.

Profile: Rosemarie Rizzo Parse (1991). *The Japanese Journal of Nursing, 55*(8), 744.

Randell, B.P. (1992). Nursing theory: The 21st century. *Nursing Science Quarterly, 5*, 176-185.

Ray, M.A. (1990). Critical reflective analysis of Parse's and Newman's research methodologies. *Nursing Science Quarterly, 3*(1), 44-46.

Santapinto, M.D.A. (1989). The relentless drive to be ever thinner: A study using the phenomenological method. *Nursing Science Quarterly, 2*(1), 29-36.

Sarter, B. (1988). Philosophical sources of nursing theory. *Nursing Science Quarterly, 1*(2), 52-59.

Smith, M.C., & Hudepohl, J.H. (1988). Analysis and evaluation of Parse's theory of man-living-health. *Canadian Journal of Nursing Research, 20*(4), 43-58.

Takahashi, T. (1992). Perspective on nursing knowledge. *Nursing Science Quarterly, 5*, 86-91.

Unpublished manuscripts

Magan, S.J. (1983, Oct. 15; 1984, Jan. 28; 1985, Aug. 22-23). *Mobilizing energies in the structuring of meaning of changing health patterns.* Paper presented at Nursing Science Symposium, Pittsburgh, PA; Dayton, OH; Nurse Theorist Conference, Edmonton, Alberta.

Magan, S.J. (1984, Sept. 22). *Shifting rhythms in changing health patterns.* Paper presented at Nursing Science Symposium, Pittsburgh, PA.

Mitchell, G. (1987, Nov.). *Man-living-health in practice with the elderly.* Paper presented at Gerontological Society meeting, Washington, DC.

Mitchell, G. (1988, July). *Man-living-health in practice.* Paper presented at Wayne State University Summer Research Symposium, Detroit.

Santopinto, M.D.A. (1987, May; 1988, Feb.). *A phenomenological study of the relentless drive to be ever thinner.* Paper presented at the annual convention of the Registered Nurse Association, Ontario, Canada; First Interamerican Symposium of Qualitative Nursing Research, São Paolo, Brazil.

Smith, M. (1988, April; 1988, July). *The lived experience of struggling through difficulty for persons who are unemployed.* Paper presented at Sigma Theta Tau—Delta Xi Research Day, Kent State University, Kent, Ohio; Wayne State University School of Nursing Summer Research Symposium, Detroit.

Cassette recordings

Magan, S.J. (Speaker). (1986). *The lived experience of hopefulness: A phenomenological study.* Cassette Recording No. DII-301. Louisville, KY: Meetings International.

Sklar, M. (Speaker). (1986). *The experience of living in a three generational family constellation: A case study.* Cassette Recording No. DII-302. Louisville, KY: Meetings International.

Smith, M.J. (Speaker). (1986). *The experience of being confined: A study using the emerging method.* Cassette Recording No. DII-304. Louisville, KY: Meetings International.

Smith, M. (Moderator). (1986). *Panel discussion of research related to man-living-health: Evaluation.* Cassette Recording No. DII-305. Louisville, KY: Meetings International.

Authors citing Parse's works

Banonis, B.C. (1989). The lived experience of recovering from addiction: A phenomenological study. *Nursing Science Quarterly, 2*, 37-43.

Batra, C. (1987). Nursing theory for undergraduates. *Nursing Outlook, 35*(4), 189-192.

Boyd, C.O. (1989). Dialogue on a research issue: Phenomenological research in nursing—response. *Nursing Science Quarterly, 2*, 16-19.

Boyd, C.O. (1990). Critical appraisal of developing nursing research methods. *Nursing Science Quarterly, 3*, 42-43.

Campbell, J. (1986). A survivor group for battered women. *Advances in Nursing Science, 8*(2), 13-20.

Cody, W.K. (1991). Grieving a personal loss. *Nursing Science Quarterly, 4*, 61-68.

Cody, W.K. (1991). Multidimensionality: Its meaning and significance. *Nursing Science Quarterly, 4*, 140-141.

Cody, W.K. (1995). The lived experience of grieving for families living with AIDS: Family-centered research using Parse's method. In R.R. Parse, *Illuminations: The human becoming theory in practice and research*. New York: National League for Nursing.

Cody, W.K. (1995). Of life immense in passion, pulse, and power: Dialoguing with Whitman and Parse, A hermeneutic study. In R.R. Parse, *Illuminations: The human becoming theory in practice and research*. New York: National League for Nursing.

Cody, W.K., & Mitchell, G.J. (1992). Parse's theory as a model for practice: The cutting edge. *Advances in Nursing Science, 15*(2), 52-65.

Cohen, M.Z. (1987). A historical overview of the phenomenological movement. *Image, 19*(1), 31-34.

Costello-Nickitas, D.M. (1994). Choosing life goals: A phenomenological study. *Nursing Science Quarterly, 7*, 87-92.

Counts, M.M., & Boyle, J.S. (1987). Nursing, health, and policy within a community context. *Advances in Nursing Science, 9*(3), 12-23.

Cull-Wilby, B.L., & Pepin, J.I. (1987). Toward a coexistence of paradigms in nursing knowledge development. *Journal of Advanced Nursing, 12*(4), 515-521.

Daly, J. (1995). The lived experience of suffering. In R.R. Parse, *Illuminations: The human becoming theory in practice and research*. New York: National League for Nursing. In press.

DeFeo, D.J. (1990). Change: A central concern in nursing. *Nursing Science Quarterly, 3*, 88-94.

Duffy, M.E. (1986). Qualitative research: An approach whose time has come. *Nursing and Health Care, 7*(5), 237-239.

Dzurec, I.C. (1989). Necessity for and evolution of multiple paradigms for nursing research: A post-structural perspective. *Advances in Nursing Science, 11*(4), 69-77.

Forrest, D. (1989). The experience of caring. *Journal of Advanced Nursing, 14*, 815-823.

Futrell, M., Wondolowski, C., & Mitchell, G.J. (1994). Aging in the oldest old living in Scotland: A phenomenological study. *Nursing Science Quarterly, 6*, 189-194.

Gortner, S.R., & Schultz, P.R. (1988). Approaches to nursing science methods. *Image, 20*(1), 22-24.

Haase, J.E. (1987). Components of courage in chronically ill adolescents: A phenomenological study. *Advances in Nursing Science, 9*(2), 64-80.

Heine, C. (1991). Development of gerontological nursing theory: Applying man-living-health theory of nursing. *Nursing & Health Care, 12*, 184-188.

Hinds, P.S. (1990). Further assessment of a method to estimate reliability and validity of qualitative research findings. *Journal of Advanced Nursing, 15*, 430-435.

Holmes, C.A. (1989). Health care and the quality of life: A review. *Journal of Advanced Nursing, 14*, 833-839.

Holmes, C.A. (1990). Alternatives to natural science foundations for nursing. *International Journal of Nursing Studies, 27*, 187-198.

Jameton, A. (1989). Ethical inquiry and the concept of research. *Advances in Nursing Science, 11*(3), 11-24.

Jonas, C.M. (1992). The meaning of being an elder in Nepal. *Nursing Science Quarterly, 5*, 171, 175.

Jonas, C.M. (1995). Evaluation of the human becoming theory in family practice. In R.R. Parse, *Illuminations: The human becoming theory in practice and research*. New York: National League for Nursing.

Kelley, L.S. (1991). Struggling with going along when you do not believe. *Nursing Science Quarterly, 4*, 123-129.

Kidd, P., & Morrison, E.F. (1988). The progression of knowledge in nursing: A search for meaning. *IMAGE: Journal of Nursing Scholarship, 20*(4), 222-224.

Liehr, P.R. (1989). The core of true presence: A loving center. *Nursing Science Quarterly, 2*, 7-8.

Malinski, V.M. (1990). Three perspectives on a scholarly issue. *Nursing Science Quarterly, 3*, 49-50.

Mattice, M. (1991). Parse's theory of nursing in practice: A manager's perspective. *Canadian Journal of Nursing Administration, 4*(1), 11-13.

Mattice, M., & Mitchell, G.J. (1990). Caring for confused elders. *Canadian Nurse, 86*(11), 16-18.

McKenna, H.P. (1989). The selection by ward managers of an appropriate nursing model for long-stay psychiatric patient care. *Journal of Advanced Nursing, 14*, 762-775.

McMahon, S. (1991). The quest for synthesis: Human-companion animal relationships and nursing theories. *Holistic Nursing Practice, 5*(2), 1-5.

Mitchell, G.J. (1990). Struggling in change: From the traditional approach to Parse's theory-based practice. *Nursing Science Quarterly 3*(4), 170-176.

Mitchell, G.J. (1991). Diagnosis: Clarifying or obscuring the nature of nursing. *Nursing Science Quarterly, 4*, 52-53.

Mitchell, G.J. (1991). Nursing diagnosis: An ethical analysis. *IMAGE: Journal of Nursing Scholarship, 23*(2), 99-103.

Mitchell, G.J. (1992). Is nursing pot-bound? *Nursing Science Quarterly, 5*, 152-153.

Mitchell, G.J. (1992). Parse's theory and the multidisciplinary team: Clarifying scientific values. *Nursing Science Quarterly, 5*, 104-106.

Mitchell, G.J. (1993). Living paradox in Parse's theory. *Nursing Science Quarterly, 6*, 44-51.

Mitchell, G.J. (1993). Time and a waning moon: Seniors describe the meaning to later life. *Canadian Journal of Nursing Research, 25*(1), 51-66.

Mitchell, G.J. (1994). The meaning of being a senior: A phenomenological study and interpretation with Parse's theory of nursing. *Nursing Science Quarterly, 7*, 70-79.

Mitchell, G.J. (1995). Evaluation of the human becoming theory in practice in an acute care setting. In R.R. Parse, *Illuminations: The human becoming theory in practice and research*. New York: National League for Nursing.

Mitchell, G.J. (1995). The lived experience of restriction-freedom in later life. In R.R. Parse, *Illuminations: The human becoming theory in practice and research*. New York: National League for Nursing.

Mitchell, G.J., & Cody, W.K. (1992). Nursing knowledge and human science: Ontological and epistemological considerations. *Nursing Science Quarterly, 5*, 54-61.

Mitchell, G.J., & Copplestone, C. (1990). Applying Parse's theory to perioperative nursing: A nontraditional approach. *AORN Journal, 51*(3), 787-798.

Mitchell, G.J., & Heidt, P. (1994). The lived experience of wanting to help another. *Nursing Science Quarterly, 7*, 119-127.

Mitchell, G.J., & Santopinto, M.D.A. (1988). An alternative to nursing diagnosis. *Canadian Nurse, 84*(10), 25-28.

Mitchell, G.J., & Santopinto, M.D.A. (1988). The expanded role nurse: A dissenting viewpoint. *Canadian Journal of Nursing Administration, 4*(1), 8-14.

Moch, S.D., & Diemert, C.A. (1987). Health promotion within the nursing environment. *Nursing Administration Quarterly, 11*(3), 9-12.

Moch, S.D. (1989). Health within illness: Conceptual evolution and practice possibilities. *Advances in Nursing Science, 11*(4), 23-31.

Moch, S.D. (1990). Health within the experience of breast cancer. *Journal of Advanced Nursing, 15*, 1426-1435.

Moody, L. (1990). *Advancing nursing science through research* (Vols. 1 & 2). Newbury Park, CA: Sage.

Munhall, P.L. (1989). Philosophical ponderings on qualitative research methods in nursing. *Nursing Science Quarterly, 2*, 20-27.

Myers, S.T. (1989). Guidelines for integration of quantitative and qualitative approaches. *Nursing Research, 38*, 299-301.

Nokes, K.M., & Carver, K. (1991). The meaning of living with AIDS: A study using Parse's theory of man-living-health. *Nursing Science Quarterly, 4*, 175-179.

Onega, L.L. (1991). A theoretical framework for psychiatric nursing practice. *Journal of Advanced Nursing, 16*, 68-73.

Pearson, B.D. (1987). Pain control: An experiment with imagery. *Geriatric Nursing, 8*(1), 28-30.

Perry, J. (1985). Has the discipline of nursing developed to the stage where nurses do think nursing? *Journal of Advanced Nursing, 10*(1), 31-37.

Phillips, J.R. (1989). Qualitative research: A process of discovery. *Nursing Science Quarterly, 2*, 5-6.

Phillips, J.R. (1990). Guest editorial: New methods of research: Beyond the shadows of nursing science. *Nursing Science Quarterly, 3*, 1-2.

Pilkington, F.B. (1993). The lived experience of grieving the loss of an important other. *Nursing Science Quarterly, 6*, 130-139.

Quiquero, A., Knights, D., & Meo, C.O. (1991). Theory as a guide to practice: Staff nurses choose Parse's theory. *Canadian Journal of Nursing Administration, 4*(1), 14-16.

Rasmusson, D.L., Jonas, C.M., & Mitchell, G.J. (1991). The eye of the beholder: Applying Parse's theory with homeless individuals. *Clinical Nurse Specialist Journal, 5*(3), 139-143.

Ray, M.A. (1987). Technological caring: A new model in critical care. *Dimensions of Critical Care Nursing, 6*(3), 166-173.

Ray, M.A. (1990). Critical reflective analysis of Parse's and Newman's research methodologies. *Nursing Science Quarterly, 3*, 44-46.

Reed, P.G. (1986). Religiousness among terminally ill and healthy adults. *Research in Nursing and Health, 9*(1), 35-41.

Reed, P.G. (1987). Constructing a conceptual framework for psychosocial nursing. *Journal of Psychosocial Nursing and Mental Health Services, 25*(2), 24-28.

Ruffingrahal, M.A. (1985). Qualitative methods in community analysis. *Public Health Nursing, 2*(3), 130-137.

Samarel, N. (1989). Caring for the living and dying: A study of role transition. *International Journal of Nursing Studies, 26*, 313-326.

Santopinto, M.D. (1989). The relentless drive to be ever thinner: A study using the phenomenological method. *Nursing Science Quarterly, 2*, 29-36.

Santopinto, M.D.A., & Smith, M.C. Evaluation of the human becoming theory in practice with adults and children. In R.R. Parse, *Illuminations: The human becoming theory in practice and research*. New York: National League for Nursing. In Press.

Sarter, B. (1987). Evolutionary idealism: A philosophical foundation for holistic nursing theory. *Advances in Nursing Science, 9*(2), 1-9.

Simmons, S.J. (1989). Health: A concept analysis. *International Journal of Nursing Studies, 26*, 155-161.

Smith, M.C. (1990). Nursing's unique focus on health promotion. *Nursing Science Quarterly, 3*, 105-106.

Smith, M.C. (1990). Pattern in nursing practice. *Nursing Science Quarterly, 3*, 57-59.

Smith, M.C. (1990). Struggling through a difficult time for unemployed persons. *Nursing Science Quarterly, 3*, 18-28.

Smith, M.C. (1991). Existential-phenomenological foundations in nursing: A discussion of differences. *Nursing Science Quarterly, 4*, 5-6.

Smith, M.J. (1984). Transformation: A key to shaping nursing. *Image, 16*(1), 28-30.

Smith, M.J. (1989). Research and practice application related to man-living-health. In J. Riehl-Sisca (Ed.), *Conceptual models for nursing practice* (3rd ed.) (pp. 267-276). Norwalk, CT: Appleton & Lange.

Thompson, J.L. (1985). Practical discourse in nursing: Going beyond empiricism and historicism. *Advances in Nursing Science, 7*(4), 59-71.

Uys, L.R. (1987). Foundational studies in nursing. *Journal of Advanced Nursing, 12*(3), 275-280.

Watson, J. (1990). Caring knowledge and informed moral passion. *Advances in Nursing Science, 13*(1), 15-24.

Wondolowski, C., & Davis, D.K. (1988). The lived experience of aging in the oldest old: A phenomenological study. *American Journal of Psychoanalysis, 48*, 261-270.

Wondolowski, C., & Davis, D.K. (1991). The lived experience of health in the oldest old: A phenomenological study. *Nursing Science Quarterly, 4*, 113-118.

Woods, N.F. (1988). Being healthy: Women's images. *Advances in Nursing Science, 11*(1), 36-46.

Yeo, M. (1989). Integration of nursing theory and nursing ethics. *Advances in Nursing Science, 11*(3), 33-42.

Other sources

Atran, S. (1981). Natural classification. *Social Science Information, 20*(1), 37-91.

Bargagliotti, L.A. (1983). Researchmanship: The scientific method and phenomenology. *Western Journal of Nursing Research, 5*(4), 409-411.

Benner, P. (1985). Quality of life: A phenomenological perspective on explanation, prediction, and understanding in nursing science. *Advances in Nursing Science, 8*(1), 1-14.

Bullington, J., & Karlsson, G. (1984). Introduction to phenomenological psychological research. *Scandinavian Journal of Psychology, 25*(1), 51-63.

Davis, A.J. (1973). The phenomenological approach in nursing research. In E. A. Garrison (Ed.), *Doctoral preparation for nurses with emphasis on the psychiatric field* (pp. 213-228). San Francisco: University of California Press.

Evaneshko, V., & Kay, M.A. (1982). The ethnoscience research technique. *Western Journal of Nursing Research, 4*(1), 49-64.

Giorgi, A.P. (1983). Concerning the possibility of phenomenological psychological research. *Journal of Phenomenological Psychology, 14*(2), 129-169.

Giorgi, A.P. (1984). Towards a new paradigm for psychology. *Studies in the Social Sciences, 23*, 9-28.

Griffin, A.P. (1983). A philosophical analysis of caring in nursing. *Journal of Advanced Nursing Science, 8*(4), 289-295.

Heidegger, M. (1962). *Being and time.* New York: Harper & Row.

Heidegger, M. (1972). *On time and being.* New York: Harper & Row.

Jennings, J.L. (1986). Husserl revisited: The forgotten distinction between psychology and phenomenology. *American Psychologist, 41*, 1231-1240.

Knaack, P. (1984). Phenomenological research. *Western Journal of Nursing Research 6*(1), 107-114.

Merleau-Ponty, M. (1956). What is phenomenology? *Cross Currents, 6*, 59-70.

Merleau-Ponty, M. (1963). *The structure of behavior.* Boston: Beacon Press.

Merleau-Ponty, M. (1973). *The prose of the world.* Evanston, IL: Northwestern University Press.

Merleau-Ponty, M. (1974). *Phenomenology of perception.* New York: Humanities Press.

Oiler, C. (1982). The phenomenological approach in nursing research. *Nursing Research, 31*(3), 178-181.

Payne, L. (1983). Health: A basic concept in nursing theory. *Journal of Advanced Nursing Science, 8*(5), 393-395.

Polanyi, M. (1958). *Personal knowledge.* Chicago: University of Chicago Press.

Reed, P.G. (1983). Implications of the life-span developmental framework for well-being in adulthood and aging. *Advances in Nursing Science, 6*(1), 18-25.

Rogers, M.E. (1961). *Educational revolution in nursing.* New York: Macmillan.

Rogers, M.E. (1970). *An introduction to the theoretical basis of nursing.* Philadelphia: F.A. Davis.

Rogers, M.E. (1980). Nursing : A science of unitary man. In J.P. Riehl & C. Roy (Eds.), *Conceptual models for nursing practice* (2nd ed.) (pp. 329-337). New York: Appleton-Century-Crofts.

Sartre, J.P. (1963). *Search for a method.* New York: Alfred A. Knopf.

Sartre, J.P. (1964). *Nausea.* New York: New Dimensions.

Sartre, J.P. (1966). *Being and nothing.* New York: Washington Square.

Schneider, K.J. (1986). Encountering and integrating Kierkegaard's absolute paradox. *Journal of Humanistic Psychology, 26*(3), 62-80.

Stern, P. (1980, Feb.). Grounded theory methodology. *Image, 12*, 20-23.

Stevens, B.J. (1984). *Nursing theory: Analysis, application, evaluation.* Boston: Little, Brown.

Unpublished manuscripts

Beauchamp, C.J. (1990). *The lived experience of struggling with making a decision in a critical life situation.* Paper presented at Discovery International, Inc., Nursing Science Seminar, Research and Practice Related to Parse's Theory of Nursing, Cincinnati, OH.

Cody, W.K. (1990). *The lived experience of grieving a personal loss.* Paper presented at Discovery International, Inc., Nursing Science Seminar, Research and Practice Related to Parse's Theory of Nursing, Cincinnati, OH.

Cody, W.K. (1990). *The lived experience of grieving a personal loss.* Paper presented at University of California, Los Angeles, National Nursing Theory Conference, Los Angeles.

Cody, W.K. (1990). *Parse's theory in practice with a grieving family.* Paper presented at Sigma Theta Tau, Alpha Phi Chapter, Annual Research Day, Hunter-Bellevue School of Nursing, City University of New York.

Jonas, C. (1989). *The lived experience of being an elder in Nepal.* Research study presented at the World Congress on Gerontology, Acapulco, Mexico.

Jonas, C. (1989). *Parse's theory in practice with older people.* Paper presented at St. Michael's Hospital, Toronto, Canada.

Jonas, C. (1989). *Parse's theory: Research and practice.* Paper presented at the University of Toronto, School of Nursing, Canada.

Jonas, C. (1990). *Practicing Parse's theory with groups of individuals in the community.* Paper presented at The Queen Elizabeth Hospital, Toronto, Ontario.

Kelley, L.S. (1989). *The lived experience of "struggling with going along in a situation you do not believe in": Using the man-living-health methodology.* Paper presented at conference sponsored by Barry University School of Nursing Honor Society, Sigma Theta Tau, Beta Tau Chapter, University of Miami, and South Florida Nursing Research Society.

Kelley, L.S. (1990). *The lived experience of "struggling with going along in a situation you do not believe in": Using the man-living-health methodology.* Paper presented at University of California, Los Angeles, National Nursing Theory Conference, Los Angeles.

Liehr, P.R. (1988, December). *A study of the experience of "living on the edge."* Research study presented at the Southern Council on Collegiate Education for Nursing, Atlanta.

Mattice, M. (1990). *Evaluating Parse's theory in practice.* Paper presented at the Queen Elizabeth Hospital, Toronto, Ontario.

Menke, E.M. (1990). *Critique of the research studies and the research methodology.* Paper presented at Discovery International, Inc., Nursing Science Seminar, Research and Practice Related to Parse's Theory of Nursing, Cincinnati, OH.

Misselwitz, S.K. (1989). *A phenomenological study of getting through the day for women who are homeless.* Research study presented at conference sponsored by Barry University School of Nursing Honor Society, Sigma Theta Tau, Beta Tau Chapter, University of Miami, and South Florida Nursing Research Society.

Mitchell, G.J. (1990). *A dialogue with nurse theorists: A basis for differentiating nursing practice—Parse in practice.* Paper presented at American Academy of Nursing Conference, Charleston, SC.

Mitchell, G.J. (1990). *An evaluation study of Parse's theory of nursing in an acute care setting.* Conducted and presented study at St. Michael's Hospital, Nursing Department, Toronto, Canada.

Mitchell, G.J. (1990). *From traditional nursing to Parse's theory.* Paper presented at the Queen Elizabeth Hospital, Toronto, Ontario.

Mitchell, G.J. (1990). *Nursing practice guided by Parse's theory.* Paper presented at North Shore Medical Center, Miami, FL.

Mitchell, G.J. (1990). *Parse in practice.* Paper presented at University of California, Los Angeles, National Nursing Theory Conference, Los Angeles.

Mitchell, G.J. (1990). *Parse's theory as a guide to practice.* Paper presented at Discovery International, Inc., Nursing Science Seminar, Research and Practice Related to Parse's Theory of Nursing, Cincinnati, OH.

Pilkington, B. (1990). *Research guided by Parse's theory.* Paper presented at the Queen Elizabeth Hospital, Toronto, Ontario.

Santopinto, M.D.A. (1987). *Parse's theory of nursing as a base for innovative practice.* Paper presented at Hamilton Psychiatric Hospital, Hamilton, Ontario.

Santopinto, M.D.A. (1988). *Close encounters of the theoretical kind: Three theory-based approaches.* Paper presented at Tenth Southeastern Conference of Specialists in Psychiatric-Mental Health Nursing, Asheville, NC.

Santopinto, M.D.A. (1988). *A qualitative evaluation study of Parse's theory in practice: What happens when theory is implemented?* Research study presented at Eighth Annual SC-CEN Research Conference, Emory University, Atlanta, Georgia.

Santopinto, M.D.A. (1988). *A test of Parse's theory in a gerontological setting: An evaluation study.* Research study presented at Ryerson Theory Congress, Toronto, Ontario.

Santopinto, M.D.A. (1989). *An emergent methodology study of caring about self for individuals who exercise relentlessly.* Research study presented at the Scientific Sessions of the Sigma Theta Tau Research Conference, Taipei, Taiwan.

Santopinto, M.D.A. (1989). *An evaluation study of Parse's practice methodology in a chronic care setting.* Research study presented at 19th Quadrennial Congress of the International Council of Nurses, Seoul, Korea.

Santopinto, M.D.A. (1990). *An evaluation of Parse's theory.* Paper presented at University of California, Los Angeles, National Nursing Theory Conference, Los Angeles.

Santopinto, M.D.A. (1990). *An evaluation study of Parse's theory in practice.* Paper presented at Discovery International, Inc., Nursing Science Seminar, Research and Practice Related to Parse's Theory of Nursing, Cincinnati, OH.

Santopinto, M.D.A. (1990). *An evaluation study of Parse's theory in practice in a chronic long-term setting.* Paper presented at Battle Creek Veterans Administration Medical Center Conference, Kalamazoo, MI.

Smith, M.C. (1990). *The lived experience of hope in families of critically ill persons.* Paper presented at University of California, Los Angeles, National Nursing Theory Conference, Los Angeles.

Smith, M.C. (1990). *Speculation on Parse in nursing education.* Paper presented at the Queen Elizabeth Hospital, Toronto, Ontario.

Cassette recordings

Beauchamp, C.J. (Speaker). (1990). *The lived experience of struggling with making a decision in a critical life situation.* Cassette Recording No. DII-602. Louisville, KY: Meetings International.

Cody, W.K. (Speaker). (1990). *The lived experience of grieving a personal loss.* Cassette Recording No. DII-602. Louisville, KY: Meetings International.

Menke, E.M. (Speaker). (1990). *Critique of the research studies and the research methodology.* Cassette Recording No. DII-603. Louisville, KY: Meetings International.

Menke, E.M. (Moderator). (1990). *Panel discussion/retrospective and evaluation.* Cassette Recording No. DII-605. Louisville, KY: Meetings International.

Mitchell, G.J. (Speaker). (1990). *Parse's theory as a guide to practice.* Cassette Recording No. DII-604. Louisville, KY: Meetings International.

Santopinto, M.D.A. (Speaker). (1990). *An evaluation study of Parse's theory in practice.* Cassette Recording No. DII-604. Louisville, KY: Meetings International.

Smith, M.C. (Speaker). (1990). *The lived experience of struggling through difficult times.* Cassette Recording No. DII-603. Louisville, KY: Meetings International.

Theses and dissertations

Beauchamp, C. (1990). *The lived experience of struggling with making a decision in a critical life situation.* Unpublished doctoral dissertation, University of Miami.

Brunsman, C.S. (1988). *A phenomenological study of the lived experience of hope in families with chronically ill children.* Unpublished master's thesis, Michigan State University.

Cody, W.K. (1989). *Grieving a personal loss: A preliminary investigation of Parse's man-living-health methodology.* Unpublished master's thesis, Hunter College, City University of New York.

Cody, W.K. (1992). *The meaning of grieving for families living with AIDS.* Doctoral dissertation, University of South Carolina. (University Microfilms International No. 9307924)

Dowling, T.C. (1987). *Sharing who you really are with another: A phenomenological inquiry.* Unpublished master's thesis, Hunter College, City University of New York.

Huckshorn, K.A. (1988). *The lived experience of creating a new way of being.* Unpublished master's thesis, Florida State University.

Mitchell, G.J. (1992). *Exploring the paradoxical experience of restriction-freedom in later life: Parse's theory-guided research.* Unpublished doctoral dissertation, University of South Carolina.

Nickitas, D.M. (1989). *The lived experience of choosing among life goals: A phenomenological study.* Unpublished doctoral dissertation, Adelphi University.

Petras, E.M. (1986). *The lived experience of sharing a painful moment with someone close: A phenomenological study.* Unpublished master's thesis, Hunter College, City University of New York.

Santopinto, M.D.A. (1987). *The relentless drive to be ever thinner: A phenomenological study.* Unpublished master's thesis, University of Western Ontario.

Sklar, M.B. (1985). *Qualitative investigation of the health patterns lived in an intergenerational family lifestyle.* Unpublished master's thesis, Hunter College, City University of New York.

Tambini, D. (1993). *Attentive presence: A phenomenological study.* Unpublished master's thesis, Hunter College, City University of New York.

Miscellaneous

Arndt, M.J. (1995). Parse's theory of human becoming in practice with hospitalized adolescents. *Nursing Science Quarterly, 8,* 86-90.

Baumann, S.L. (1995). Two views of homeless children's art: Psychoanalysis and Parse's human becoming theory. *Nursing Science Quarterly, 8,* 65-70.

Cody, W.K. (1995). Intersubjectivity: Nursing's contribution to the explication of its postmodern meaning. *Nursing Science Quarterly, 8,* 52-54.

Cody, W.K. (1995). The meaning of grieving for families living with AIDS. *Nursing Science Quarterly, 8,* 127-132.

Davis, D.K., & Cannava, E. (1995). The meaning of retirement for communally-living retired performing artists. *Nursing Science Quarterly, 8,* 57.

Kelley, L. (1995). Parse's theory in practice with a group in the community. *Nursing Science Quarterly, 8,* 127-132.

Mitchell, G.J. (1995). Intimacy in the nurse-person process. *Nursing Science Quarterly, 8,* 102-103.

Mitchell, G.J. (1995). Letters to the editor. *Nursing Outlook, 43,* 190.

Mitchell, G.J. (1995). Nursing diagnosis: An obstacle of caring ways. In A. Boykin (Ed.), *Power, politics & public policy: A matter of caring* (pp. 11-23). New York: National League for Nursing Press Publication No. 14-2684.

Mitchell, G.J. (1995). Reflection: The key to breaking with tradition. *Nursing Science Quarterly, 8,* 57.

Rendon, D.C., Sales, R., Leal, I., & Pique, J. (1995). The lived experience of aging in community-dwelling elders in Valencia, Spain: A phenomenological study. *Nursing Science Quarterly, 8*(4), 152, 157.

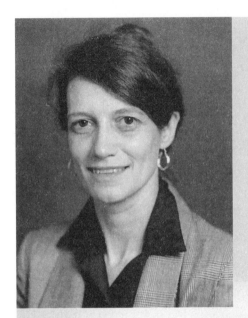

Joyce J. Fitzpatrick

Life Perspective Rhythm Model

Phyllis MacDonald du Mont, Sr. Judith E. Alexander, Sarah J. Beckman, Patricia Chapman-Boyce, Sydney Coleman-Ehmke, Cheryl A. Hailway, Rhonda G. Justus, Rosalyn A. Pung, Cathy R. Smith

CREDENTIALS AND BACKGROUND OF THE THEORIST

Joyce J. Fitzpatrick was born May 4, 1944. She received her B.S.N. in 1966 from Georgetown University in Washington, D.C., and her M.S. in psychiatric-mental health from The Ohio State University in

The authors wish to express appreciation to Dr. Joyce J. Fitzpatrick for critiquing the original chapter.

Columbus in 1967. She took post-master's courses in Community Health at Ohio State (1971 to 1972). Fitzpatrick received a Ph.D. in nursing from New York University in 1975. In 1987, she attended Harvard University's Institute for Educational Management. She completed the Case Western Reserve University Executive MBA Program in the 1990s.[11]

Fitzpatrick has held many positions, including staff nurse, public health nurse, instructor, and the director of training for suicide prevention, all in Columbus, Ohio. She has served as an assistant professor at New York University. She then became an associate professor at Wayne State University, where she later held the positions of Chairperson for the Department of Nursing Systems and Director of the Center for Health Research. In addition, Fitzpatrick has been a visiting professor at Rutgers University, College of Nursing. In 1982 she became Professor and Dean of Nursing at Case Western University and Administrative Associate at University Hospitals of Cleveland. Since 1988, she has held the Elizabeth Brooks Ford Professor of Nursing chair.

Since 1974, Fitzpatrick has been a consultant to academic institutions in the areas of faculty development, research, program development (at both the master's and doctoral levels) and in the design of conceptual frameworks. These institutions have included Columbia University, Indiana University, Michigan State University, Ohio State University, Rutgers University, University of Kansas, University of South Carolina, University of Tennessee at Memphis, University of Virginia, Vanderbilt University, and Wright State University.

Fitzpatrick has also been a consultant in the nonacademic sector. This work has included such diverse projects as developing a computerized nursing information system for Hospital Corporation of America, Nashville, Tennessee; staff development work at a psychiatric facility in Toronto, Canada; and consultant to the Director of Nursing Affairs for the American Medical Association.[11]

The recipient of numerous awards and honoraries, in 1994 Fitzpatrick was recognized as a Distinguished Scholar in Residence by the Institute of Medicine, the American Academy of Nurses, and the American Nurses Foundation. On six occasions, her books have received the *American Journal of Nursing's* Book of the Year award.

Fitzpatrick is actively involved in building a community of nurse scholars and delineating the field of inquiry for nursing knowledge. She has an extensive program of research and has received research grants totaling more than $4 million.[11] She is a prolific writer and presenter with many articles, editorials, book chapters, textbooks, conferences, and work-

shops to her credit. She has been the editor of *Applied Nursing Research* since 1987.

THEORETICAL SOURCES FOR THEORY DEVELOPMENT

Fitzpatrick constructed her theory on the basis of concepts and principles of Martha Rogers. In the Life Perspective Rhythm Model, she incorporated the Rogerian concepts of helicy (change manifested as nonrepeating rhythmicities), resonancy (identification of human and environmental fields as wave patterns and organizations in continuous change), and complementarity (the mutual, continuous interaction between human and environmental fields).[21,22] From the biological sciences, Fitzpatrick drew on theories of biological and circadian rhythms. She specifically cited the theoretical work of Haus[15] and Luce.[17] She noted, however, that "conceptualizations underlying these works are contiguous rather than comparable and exact in reference to human rhythms."[9:299] Her clinical work with persons experiencing illness or institutionalization or confronting death led her to explore crisis theories. The work of Caplan on crisis theory has been explicitly cited by Fitzpatrick[8:23-24; 9:310] as an influence.

USE OF EMPIRICAL EVIDENCE

An early (1975) empirical investigation of the subjective experience of temporal patterns by Fitzpatrick raised questions about how to measure temporal patterns without implying a linear view of time and health.[9] Fitzpatrick described the need to "directly attend to the multidimensional nature of human experience."[9:297] This concern led to the design of studies to explore temporal and motor patterns in persons experiencing a specific environmental condition (hospitalization or institutionalization) contrasted with persons not in crisis (well and in the community). The results revealed nonrepeating rhythmic patterns related to time and made manifest in an environment-person interaction best characterized as a crisis. Fitzpatrick proposed the Life Perspective Rhythm Model on the basis of these results, clinical observations, and a Rogerian perspective.[9]

MAJOR CONCEPTS & DEFINITIONS

The major concepts in this model include *nursing, person, environment, and health.* The definition of *crisis* is also needed to comprehend the theory. Fitzpatrick stated, "The meaning attached to life, the basic understanding of human existence, is a central concern of nursing."[9:301] She described *nursing* as a profession and a science. "Nursing interventions can be focused on enhancing the developmental process towards health so that individuals may be led to develop their potential as human beings."[9:301] She suggested that the focus of nursing science should be to elucidate the relationships "among basic concepts of person and health and the further delineation of the indices of holistic human functioning."[9:301] *Person* is seen as an open system, a unified whole in continuous mutual interaction with the *environment.* Thus, the person and environment are integral with one another. The person-environment interaction is manifested in patterns. "Human development is understood to proceed rhythmically."[9:300] There are both overall life patterns (toward increasing complexity and rapidity) and "patterns within patterns or rhythms within an overall life rhythm."[9:300-301] The rhythm of life is manifested through crises (both developmental and situational). *Crises* are defined as the "rhythmic peaks"[9:296] in the development of a person. Crises are time limited and represent both a threat to the person's integrity and an opportunity for growth.

Health is viewed as a human dimension under continuous development, a heightened awareness of the meaningfulness of life.[9:306] Health, humanness, and the meaning attached to life are all interwoven into Fitzpatrick's definition of health. Because the heightened awareness of the meaning of life is a dimension of health that can transcend death, it can be identified as the core, essential quality of health as discussed in the Life Perspective Rhythm Model.

MAJOR ASSUMPTIONS

Fitzpatrick repeats the five basic assumptions proposed by Rogers in her theory of unitary man:

1. Man is a unified whole possessing his own integrity and manifesting characteristics that are more than and different from the sum of his parts.
2. Man and environment are open systems, continually exchanging matter and energy with each other.
3. The life process evolves irreversibly and unidirectionally along the space-time continuum.
4. Pattern and organization identify man and reflect his innovative wholeness.
5. Man is characterized by the capacity for abstraction and imagery, language and thought, sensation and emotion.[9:300]

In addition, there are other assumptions and principles, both explicit and implicit, in the theory. These include:

1. The meaning attached to life is essential to maintain life and enhance health.[9:295]
2. Human development proceeds rhythmically.[9:300]
3. The rhythms of life are revealed by crises (peak waveforms).[9:300]
4. The rhythms of life become progressively more rapid.[9:300]
5. Human development occurs in the context of continuous person-environment interaction.[9:300]
6. Health is a basic human dimension related to the meaningfulness attached to life.[9:301]
7. Health is a continuously developing human characteristic.[9:301]

THEORETICAL ASSERTIONS

"The Life Perspective Rhythm Model is a developmental model that proposes that the process of human development is characterized by rhythms."[9:300] The person is an open system in continuous mutual interaction with the environment. Human development proceeds rhythmically, and patterns can be perceived. These patterns are indices of human holistic functioning. Four basic patterns have been identified: temporal patterns, motion patterns, perceptual patterns, and consciousness patterns. Over a lifetime, there is a trend toward increasing rapidity with respect to the temporal pattern. (The overall patterns related to other indices have not been characterized.) However, within that overall pattern there may be situational or developmental events that are manifested by time-limited changes in wave patterns[8] (these are described as peaks or troughs and correspond to crises). Fitzpatrick described these as "rhythms within an overall life rhythm."[9:300]

Health is a basic human dimension manifested in a heightened awareness of the meaning attached to life. Thus, even in the process of dying, health can be enhanced. Health undergoes continuous development. "The meaning attached to life, the basic understanding of human existence, is a central concern of nursing as science and profession."[9:301] The goal of nursing interventions is to enhance "the developmental process towards health so that individuals will be led to develop their potential as human beings."[9:301]

LOGICAL FORM

Fitzpatrick developed the Life Perspective Rhythm Model with use of a deductive logical approach; that is, the author uses empirical findings to support a proposed developmental model. This proposed model was based on a synthesis of Rogerian concepts, theories of rhythmicity (from biology), and Caplan's crisis theory (from psychiatry). The assumptions and definitions of Rogerian science have widespread acceptance within nursing. Fitzpatrick emphasized the dimension of rhythmicity as described in Rogers's concept of helicy. The integration of insights from the study of crisis theory resulted in her idea regarding the pivotal nature of rhythmic peaks. This concept was a logical extension of the wave pattern dimension of Rogers's concept of reso-

nancy. The developmental aspects of her theory are consistent both with Rogerian science and biological science. The theoretical derivation of her model is logical and free of obvious contradictions.

The concepts of health, person, environment, nursing, and nursing interventions are each described in Fitzpatrick's model. She further asserted that persons would manifest temporal, motion, consciousness, and perceptual patterns. Pressler[18:308] adapted Rogers's Slinky model to depict the essential concepts and their relationships in diagrammatic form (Fig. 31-1).

The concepts of person, nursing, and nursing activity are reasonable and clear. Although there is no in-depth description of the concept of environment, Fitzpatrick described it as an open system in continuous interaction with human beings. She also depicted the environment as exhibiting patterns and rhythms (light and dark; seasons).

It is not clear why the four patterns of human functioning were chosen. Fitzpatrick[9:300] noted these to be consistent with the rhythmic correlates developed by Rogers. An equally logical argument could be made for considering perception to be a dimension of consciousness. Pressler observed that Margaret Newman has proposed that consciousness includes the perceptual, temporal, and motion patterns.[18,19] Within Fitzpatrick's model, this could be an example of a "pattern within a pattern" but requires further clarification. There is also the question of why there are no additional rhythmic patterns, such as emotion or mood patterns. Clarification of the boundaries and relationships among these pattern manifestations would enhance efforts to develop research strategies to operationalize these concepts.

Fitzpatrick has not clearly and logically defined the concept of health. In the model, the description of health is intimately linked to life, awareness of the meaningfulness of life, humanness, and development. The meanings attached to life are described as essential to maintain life. In addition, it is implied that health may be defined as the absence of disease, the quality of life, and optimum wellness. Furthermore, there is no description of how this formulation of health could be applied to infants, demented individuals, and persons with personality or thought

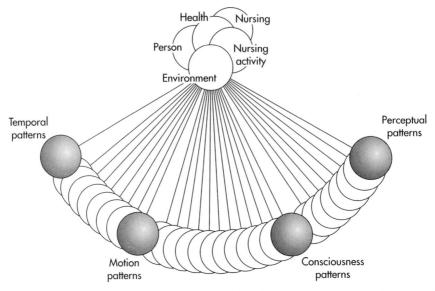

Fig. **31-1** Relationships within Life Perspective Model. *From Pressler, J.L. (1983). Fitzpatrick's rhythm model: Analysis for nursing science. In J.J. Fitzpatrick & A. Whall, Conceptual models of nursing: Analysis and application. Bowie, MD: Robert J. Brady.*

disorders. A comprehensive definition of health would avoid logical problems created by endorsing divergent definitions of health.

ACCEPTANCE BY THE NURSING COMMUNITY

Practice

This model has not been adopted as a framework to guide overall nursing practice. Specific nursing interventions have been supported by empirical evidence gathered in studies of rhythmicities based on Fitzpatrick's work. These include reminiscence therapy, rocking, reality orientation, and music therapy.[10]

Education

Although Fitzpatrick has incorporated the model into her graduate level theory and research course, it has not been adopted by any other schools as a framework for teaching. The theory is potentially adaptable to such use.

Research

Fitzpatrick and her colleagues[5-7,12,13] have conducted several studies of temporal patterns; however, there has been no similar program of study regarding the motion of pattern, perceptual pattern, or consciousness pattern.[18,19] Several of Fitzpatrick's doctoral students[1,2,14,20] have advanced the development of her theory by conducting research exploring concepts derived from her theory. These have included studies exploring health, life perspective, suicide, and gerontology.

Criddle[4] cited Fitzpatrick in the integration of findings from a phenomenological study of healing. In their 1995 study of the relationship between creativity and health among adolescents, Yarchenski and Mahon[23] found support for the model in that the relationship between rhythmicity and health merged developmentally (during late adolescence as opposed to early adolescence). Keane[16] found that purpose in life was a significant predictor of current life satisfaction among cancer patients.

FURTHER DEVELOPMENT

The Life Perspective Rhythm Model is in an early stage of development. Clarification of the multiple definitions given to health and of the relationship of perceptual patterns to consciousness patterns is needed. Researchers exploring the temporal patterns and motion patterns dimensions of the theory have encountered difficulties operationalizing these concepts. Research designs using methodologies that could allow exploration of multidimensional, nonlinear processes must be developed if the theory is to advance. The continued use of the model by researchers and theorists indicates both interest and promise. The long-term impact of the model on nursing science is, as yet, uncertain.

CRITIQUE
Clarity

Fitzpatrick consistently follows theoretical form by stating a hypothesis and listing assumptions. Assumptions and principles are plainly identified. However, the central concept of health is somewhat unclear.

Simplicity

This model is holistic and complex. It is difficult to comprehend the complicated interrelationships among health, nursing, person, environment, and nursing interventions in respect to the temporal, motion, consciousness, and perceptual patterns. This complexity makes operationalization of concepts challenging. This obstacle may impede research applications.

Generality

Although the theory does not restrict application to specific populations, most of the empirical research with the model has been done with the elderly or with clients termed death involved (suicidal or terminally ill). Research with participants from all life stages is needed. The utility of the theory in applications involving persons with immature or disordered thought processes is unclear.

Empirical Precision

Fitzpatrick and her colleagues have found some preliminary success evaluating several of the relationships presented in the model. Review of the current literature reveals that only a few other educators, researchers, or students are actively involved in the process of empirically testing relationships proposed in this model. Interested researchers are encouraged to become more involved in efforts to advance the model.

Derivable Consequences

The derivable consequences connect the theory with achievable nursing outcomes. The possible applications and usefulness of this developing model have not yet been demonstrated. The research to date and the development of support for holistic nursing interventions is promising, warranting further work and development. Further development of the model could broaden our understanding of nursing as a human science and move nursing closer to holistic nursing practice.[3:133-143]

CRITICAL THINKING *Activities*

1 Some nursing researchers have suggested that only qualitative methods can be used to investigate holistic human phenomenon.

   a. From the perspective of the Life Perspective Rhythm Model, discuss some of the potential problems in using quantitative methodology.

   b. Do you think that this model would allow you to make predictions about pattern characteristics that could be statistically tested?

2 You have a client who is a married 36-year-old mother of two teenage children. She has just been told that she has chronic fatigue syndrome.

   a. Discuss how this might be manifested in her temporal, perceptual, consciousness, and motion patterns.

b. How could you explore the meaning of her symptoms with her?

c. What would it look like if her health were enhanced?

3 You are participating in a team conference about a 48-year-old HIV-positive client. He has been feeling good. He has known about his HIV status for 15 months. He has an excellent support system. His current problem is weight gain, which threatens his borderline blood pressure.

a. How would his temporal, perceptual, consciousness, or motions patterns have an impact on his weight?

b. What sorts of interventions might help him become aware of his rhythmic patterns as they relate to his health?

c. How could you propose to lead him toward a repatterning that might enhance his health? Be sure to address the meaningfulness he attaches to life.

4 Rhythmic waveforms are most apparent during situational or developmental crises. A person's sense of the meaningfulness of life is often manifested as a sense of purpose. For each of the following persons, discuss the possible effects on the indices of human functioning (temporal, motion, perceptual, and consciousness patterns). From the perspective of Fitzpatrick's model, describe two nursing goals for each person.

a. A new, first-time mother of a healthy term baby.

b. A 55-year-old "graduate" of a cardiac rehabilitation program who has "lost" his disability benefits. (He no longer meets criteria for disability.)

c. A father who has just learned that his 19-year-old son has schizophrenia.

d. A 30-year-old woman experiencing an exacerbation of multiple sclerosis.

e. A 14-year-old boy who has just started to shave.

REFERENCES

1. Ashford, P.A. (1981). *Temporal experience of individuals in a suicidal crisis.* Unpublished master's research project, Wayne State University.
2. Ashworth, P.E. (1980). *Health status perception in middlescence I and middlescence II.* Unpublished master's research project, Wayne State University.
3. Chinn, P.L., & Jacobs, M.K. (1983). Theory and nursing: A systematic approach. St. Louis: Mosby.
4. Criddle, L. (1993). Healing from surgery: A phenomenological study. *Image: Journal of Nursing Scholarship, 25*(3), 208-213.
5. Downs, F.S., & Fitzpatrick, J.J. (1984). Preliminary investigation of the reliability and validity of a tool for the assessment of body position and motor activity. In F.S. Downs (Ed.), *A sourcebook of nursing research* (3rd ed). Philadelphia: F.A. Davis (Reprinted from *Nursing Research* [1976], *25*, 404-408.)
6. Fitzpatrick, J.J. (1978). Aging and institutionalization as determinants of temporal and motor phenomena. *Image, 10,* 24.
7. Fitzpatrick, J.J. (1980). Patients' perception of time: Current research. *International Nursing Review, 27*(5), 143-153, 160.
8. Fitzpatrick, J.J. (1982). The crisis perspective: Relationship to nursing. In J.J. Fitzpatrick, et al. (Eds.), *Nursing models and their psychiatric mental health applications.* Bowie, MD: Robert J. Brady.
9. Fitzpatrick, J.J. (1983). A life perspective rhythm model. In J.J. Fitzpatrick & A.L. Whall (Eds.), *Conceptual models of nursing: Analysis and application.* Bowie, MD: Robert J. Brady.
10. Fitzpatrick, J.J. (1983). Techniques of gerontological counseling. In S. Lego (Ed.), *Lippincott manual of psychiatric nursing.* Philadelphia: Lippincott.
11. Fitzpatrick, J.J. (1996). Curriculum vitae.
12. Fitzpatrick, J.J., & Donovan, M.J. (1978, July). Temporal experience and motor behavior among the aging. *Research in Nursing and Health, 1,* 60-68.
13. Fitzpatrick, J.J., Donovan, M.J., & Johnson, R.L. (1980). Experience of time during the crisis of cancer. *Cancer Nursing, 3*(3), 191-194.
14. Floyd, J.A. (1982). *Hospitalization, sleep-wake patterns, and circadian type of psychiatric patients.* Unpublished doctoral dissertation, Wayne State University.
15. Haus, E. (1964). Periodicity in response and susceptibility to environmental stimuli. *Annals of the New York Academy of Science, 107,* 361-373.
16. Keane, S.M. (1991). *Gynecological cancer as crisis: Predictors of adjustment.* Unpublished doctoral dissertation, Case Western Reserve University.

17. Luce, G.G. (1970). *Biological rhythms in psychiatry and medicine.* National Institute of Mental Health, U.S. Department of Health Education, and Welfare, Washington, DC.

18. Pressler, J.L. (1983). Fitzpatrick's rhythm model: Analysis for nursing science. In J. Fitzpatrick & A. Whall, *Conceptual models of nursing: Analysis and application.* Bowie, MD: Robert J. Brady.

19. Pressler, J.L. (1989). Fitzpatrick's rhythm model: A second look. In J. Fitzpatrick & A. Whall, (1989), *Conceptual models of nursing: Analysis and application* (2nd ed.). Norwalk, CT: Appleton & Lange.

20. Reed, P.G. (1982). *Religious perspective, death perspective, and well-being among death-involved and non-death-involved individuals.* Unpublished doctoral dissertation, Wayne State University.

21. Roger, M.E. (1970). *An introduction to the theoretical basis of nursing.* Philadelphia: F.A. Davis.

22. Rogers, M.E. (1980). Nursing: A science of unitary man. In J.P. Riehl & C. Roy (Eds.), *Conceptual models for nursing practice* (2nd ed.). New York: Appleton-Century.

23. Yarchenski, A., & Mahon, N.E. (1995). Rogers' pattern manifestations and health in adolescents. *Western Journal of Nursing, 17*(4), 383-397.

BIBLIOGRAPHY

Primary sources

Books

Abraham, I.L., Nadzam, D.M., & Fitzpatrick, J.J. (Eds.). (1989). *Statistics and quantitative methods in nursing: Issues and strategies for research and education.* Philadelphia: Saunders.

Fitzpatrick, J.J., & Martinson, I. (Eds.). (1996). *Selected writings of Rosemary Ellis: In search of the meaning of nursing science.* New York: Springer.

Fitzpatrick, J.J., & Norbeck, J. (Eds.). (1996). *Annual review of nursing research* (Vol. 14). New York: Springer.

Fitzpatrick, J.J., & Norbeck, J. (Eds.). (1997). *Annual review of nursing research* (Vol. 15). New York: Springer.

Fitzpatrick, J.J., & Stevenson, J.S. (Eds.). (1993). *Annual review of nursing research* (Vol. 11). New York: Springer.

Fitzpatrick, J.J., & Stevenson, J. (Eds.) (1995). *Annual review of nursing research* (Vol. 13). New York: Springer.

Fitzpatrick, J.J., Stevenson, J., & Polis, N. (Eds.). (1994). *Annual review of nursing research* (Vol. 12). New York: Springer.

Fitzpatrick, J.J., Stevenson, J.S. & Polis, N.S. (Eds.). (1994). *Nursing research and its utilization.* New York: Springer.

Fitzpatrick, J.J., & Taunton, R.L. (Eds.). (1987). *Annual review of nursing research* (Vol. 5). New York: Springer.

Fitzpatrick, J.J., Taunton, R.L., & Beneliol, J.Q. (1988). *Annual review of nursing research* (Vol. 6). New York: Springer.

Fitzpatrick, J.J., Taunton, R.L., & Beneliol, J.Q. (1989). *Annual review of nursing research* (Vol. 7). New York: Springer.

Fitzpatrick, J.J., Taunton, R.L., & Beneliol, J.Q. (1990). *Annual review of nursing research* (Vol. 8). New York: Springer.

Fitzpatrick, J.J., Taunton, R.L., & Beneliol, J.Q. (1992). *Annual review of nursing research* (Vol. 10). New York: Springer.

Fitzpatrick, J.J., Taunton, R.L., & Jacox, A. (1991). *Annual review of nursing research* (Vol. 9). New York: Springer.

Fitzpatrick, J.J., & Whall, A.L. (1983). *Conceptual models of nursing: Analysis and application.* Bowie, MD: Robert J. Brady.

Fitzpatrick, J.J., & Whall, A.L. (1989). *Conceptual models of nursing: Analysis and application* (2nd ed.). Norwalk, CT: Appleton & Lange.

Fitzpatrick, J.J., & Whall, A.L. (1996). *Conceptual models of nursing: Analysis and application* (3rd ed.). Norwalk, CT: Appleton & Lange.

Fitzpatrick, J.J., Whall, A.L., Johnston, R.L, & Floyd, J.A. (1982). *Nursing models and their psychiatric mental health applications.* Bowie, MD: R.J. Brady.

Werley, H.H., & Fitzpatrick, J.J. (Eds.). (1984). *Annual review of nursing research* (Vol. 1). New York: Springer.

Werley, H.H., & Fitzpatrick, J.J. (Eds.). (1984). *Annual review of nursing research* (Vol. 2). New York: Springer.

Werley, H.H., & Fitzpatrick, J.J. (Eds.). (1985). *Annual review of nursing research* (Vol. 3). New York: Springer.

Werley, H.H., & Fitzpatrick, J.J., Taunton, R.L. (Eds.). (1986). *Annual review of nursing research* (Vol. 4). New York: Springer.

Books under review or contract

Fitzpatrick, J.J. (Ed.). *Annual review of nursing research* (Vol. 16). New York: Springer.

Fitzpatrick, J.J. *Encyclopedia of nursing research.* New York: Springer.

Fitzpatrick, J.J., & Stevenson, J.S. (Eds.), *Annual review of nursing research* (Vols. 11-13). New York: Springer.

Fitzpatrick, J.J., Taunton, R.L., & Jacox, A. (Eds.), *Annual review of nursing research* (Vols. 9-10). New York: Springer.

Shamian, J., Cowling, W.R. III, & Fitzpatrick, J.J. *Advanced critical analysis of nursing management theories.* Book prospectus, in review.

Shamian, J., & Fitzpatrick, J.J. *Advanced critical analysis of nursing management theories.* Book prospectus, in review.

Chapters and proceedings

Abraham, I.L, & Fitzpatrick, J.J. (1986). Expert systems for nursing practice: Developing and implementing decision-support technology in nursing. In B. DuGas, G. Hefferman, M. Light, A. O'Connor, H. Oglivie, & E. Zwarts (Eds.), *Proceedings of the National Symposium on Computer Applications for Nursing.* Ottawa, Canada: University of Ottawa.

Abraham, I.L., & Fitzpatrick, J.J. (1986). Research environments in nursing: Rationale and requirements for computing. *Proceedings of the Ninth Annual Symposium on Computer Applications in Medical Care.* Silver Springs, MD: IEEE Computer Society.

Abraham, I.L., & Fitzpatrick, J.J. (1987). Knowing for nursing practice: Patterns of knowledge and their emulation in expert systems. In W.W. Stead (Ed.), *Proceedings of the Eleventh Annual Symposium on Computer Applications in Medical Care* (pp. 88-92). Silver Springs, MD: IEEE Computer Society.

Abraham, I.L., Fitzpatrick, J.J. (1990). On the scientific and technical requirements for computing resources. In V.K. Saba, K. Rieder, & D. Pocklington (Eds.), *A review of computer technology in nursing.* Berlin: Springer Verlag.

Abraham, I.L., Fitzpatrick, J.J., & Jewell, J.A. (1988). The Artificial Intelligence in Nursing Project: Developing advanced technology for expert care. In K. Hanna (Ed.), *Clinical judgment and decision-making: The future with nursing diagnosis.* New York: John Wiley & Sons.

Abraham, I.L., Nadzam, D.M., & Fitzpatrick, J.J. (1986). Statistics and quantitative methods in nursing: Overview of a recent invitational conference. *Bulletin on Teaching of Statistics in the Health Sciences* (pp. 1-4). American Statistical Association, No. 41, Winter.

Abraham, I.L., Nadzam, D.M., & Fitzpatrick, J.J. (Eds.). (1989). Statistics in nursing curricula. In I.L. Abraham, D.M. Nadzam, & J.J. Fitzpatrick (Eds.), *Statistics and quantitative methods in nursing: Issues and strategies for research and education.* Philadelphia: Saunders.

Adams-Davis, K., & Fitzpatrick, J.J. (1995). The nursing health center: A model of public/private partnership for health care delivery. In B. Murphy (Ed.), *Nursing centers: The time is now.* New York: National League for Nursing. Publication No. 41-2629.

Downs, F.S., & Fitzpatrick, J.J. (1984). Preliminary investigation of the reliability and validity of a tool for the assessment of body position and motor activity. In F.S. Downs (Ed.), *A source book of nursing research* (3rd ed.). Philadelphia: F.A. Davis. (Reprinted from *Nursing Research,* 1976, *25,* 404-408.)

Fitzpatrick, J.J. (1976). Repatterning alcoholic behaviors: Nursing strategies. In J. Chodil (Ed.), *Proceedings of the 8th Annual Clinical Sessions.* New York: New York University.

Fitzpatrick, J.J. (1982). The crisis perspective: Relationship to nursing. In J.J. Fitzpatrick, et al., *Nursing models and their psychiatric mental health applications.* Bowie, MD: Robert J. Brady.

Fitzpatrick, J.J. (1982). The path of nursing, the path of science? In V. Engle, *Proceedings of the Fourth Annual Research Symposium of the Michigan Sigma Theta Tau Consortium.* Indianapolis: Sigma Theta Tau.

Fitzpatrick, J.J. (1983). Integrating the domains of nursing. In *Proceedings of the 1982 Forum on Doctoral Education in Nursing.* Cleveland, OH: Case Western Reserve University.

Fitzpatrick, J.J. (1983). In J.J. Fitzpatrick & A.L. Whall (Eds.), *Conceptual models of nursing: Analysis and application.* Bowie, MD: Robert J. Brady. Chapter 1 Overview of nursing models and nursing theories (Whall), Chapter 17 A life perspective rhythm model, Chapter 19 Nursing models: Summary and future projections (Whall), Comparison chart of nursing models (Whall).

Fitzpatrick, J.J. (1983). Techniques of gerontological counseling. In S. Lego (Ed.), *Lippincott manual of psychiatric nursing.* Philadelphia: Lippincott.

Fitzpatrick, J.J. (1984). Gerontological counseling. In S. Lego (Ed.), *The American handbook of psychiatric nursing* (pp. 357-363). Philadelphia: Lippincott.

Fitzpatrick, J.J. (1984). Reaction to the debate: The research doctorate and the professional doctorate. In *The 1984 National Forum on Doctoral Education in Nursing Proceedings: Epistemological strategies in nursing.* Denver, CO: University of Colorado School of Nursing.

Fitzpatrick, J.J. (1985). Reaction to Fagin: Institutionalizing faculty practice. In *Proceedings of the Second National Conference on Faculty Practice.* Kansas City, MO, American Academy of Nursing. (Ed.), *Proceedings of doctoral programs in nursing: Consensus for quality, August, 1984.* Washington, DC: American Association of Colleges of Nursing.

Fitzpatrick, J.J. (1985). Response to institutionalizing practice: Historical and future perspectives. In K.E. Barnard & G.R. Smith (Eds.), *Faculty practice in action, Second Annual Symposium on Nursing Faculty Practice* (pp. 28-30). Kansas City, MO: American Academy of Nursing.

Fitzpatrick, J.J. (1985). Response to manpower in nursing homes: Implications for research. In M.S. Harper & B. Lebowitz (Eds.), *Mental illness in nursing homes: Agenda for research* (pp. 281-305). Rockville, MD: National Institute of Mental Health.

Fitzpatrick, J.J. (1987). Etiology: Conceptual concerns. *Proceedings of the 1986 North American Nursing Diagnosis Association (NANDA) Conference.*

Fitzpatrick, J.J. (1987). In V. Malinski (Ed.), *Explorations in Martha Rogers' science of unitary human beings.* East Norwalk, CT: Appleton-Century-Crofts. Chapter 1 Introduction to Rogers' science of unitary human beings, Chapter 6 Critique: Relationship between the perception of the speed of time and the process of dying (Rawnsley), Chapter 7 Critique: Relationship of time experience, creativity traits, differentiation, and human field motion (Ference), Chapter 8 Critique: Relationship between hyperactivity in children and perception of short wavelength light (Malinski), Chapter 9 Critique: Relationship between visible lightwaves and the experience of pain (McDonald), Chapter 10 Critique: Relationship of mystical experience, differentiation, and creativity in college students (Cowling), Chapter 11 Critique: Relationship of creativity, actualization, and empathy in unitary human development (Raile-Alligood), Chapter 12 Critique: Relationship between imposed motion and human field motion in elderly individuals living in nursing homes (Gueldner), Chapter 13 Critique: Investigation of the principle of helicy: The relationship of human field motion and power (Barrett).

Fitzpatrick, J.J. (1987). Nursing. In A.J. Goldstein (Ed.), *Peterson's accounting to zoology.* Princeton, NJ: Peterson's Guides.

Fitzpatrick, J.J. (1987). Nursing education. *Peterson's annual guides to graduate study, book 3. Graduate programs in the biological, agricultural, and health sciences 1987* (21st ed.). Princeton, NJ: Peterson's Guides.

Fitzpatrick, J.J. (1987). Philosophical approach: Empiricism. In *Proceedings of the Fourth Nursing Science Colloquium* (pp. 19-30). Boston: Boston University.

Fitzpatrick, J.J. (1988). Nursing: How do we know; what do we do; and how can we enhance nursing knowledge and practice. In *Proceedings of Nursing and Computers, Third International Symposium on Nursing Use of Computers and Information Science* (pp. 58-65). St. Louis: Mosby.

Fitzpatrick, J.J. (1988). Toward a nursing minimum data set: Group 1 Review and summary. In H.H. Werley & N.L. Lange (Eds.), *Nursing minimum data set.* New York: Springer.

Fitzpatrick, J.J. (1989). Conceptual basis for the organization and advancement of nursing knowledge: Nursing diagnosis/taxonomy. In N.L. Chaska (Ed.), *Proceedings of the 1989 Forum on Doctoral Education in Nursing.* Indianapolis: Indiana University.

Fitzpatrick, J.J. (1989). In J.J. Fitzpatrick & A.L. Whall (Eds.), *Conceptual models of nursing: Analysis and application.* Norwalk, CT: Appleton & Lange. Chapter 3 Guidelines for analysis of nursing conceptual models (Whall), Chapter 26 A life perspective rhythm model, Chapter 28 The empirical approach to the development of nursing science, Appendix: Comparison chart of nursing models (Whall).

Fitzpatrick, J.J. (1990). Inquiry in nursing: Issues on consistency and integration. In *Proceedings of the First and Second Rosemary Ellis Scholars Retreat,* Cleveland: Case Western Reserve University School of Nursing.

Fitzpatrick, J.J. (1991). Positioning nursing to meet its destiny. In I.A. Gunn (Ed.), *Proceedings of the National Conference on Prescriptive Authority.* Clemson, SC: Clemson University.

Fitzpatrick, J.J. (1991). Taxonomy II: Definitions and development. In RM Carroll-Johnson (Ed.), *Classification of nursing diagnoses. Proceedings of the Ninth Conference.* Philadelphia: Lippincott.

Fitzpatrick, J.J. (1991). The translation of NANDA Taxonomy I into ICD Code. In RM Carroll-Johnson (Ed.), *Classification of nursing diagnoses. Proceedings of the Ninth Conference.* Philadelphia: Lippincott.

Fitzpatrick, J.J. (1994). Funding for nursing research through NIMH and the private sector. In J.J. Fitzpatrick, J.S. Stevenson, & N.S. Polis (Eds.), *Nursing research and its utilization.* New York: Springer.

Fitzpatrick, J.J. (1994). Rogers' contribution to the development of nursing as a science. In V.M. Malinski & E.M. Barret (Eds.), *Martha E. Rogers: Her life and her work* (pp. 322-329). Philadelphia: F.A. Davis.

Fitzpatrick, J.J. (1996). Chapter 26 A life perspective rhythm model, Chapter 28 The empirical approach to the development of nursing science. In J.J. Fitzpatrick & A.L. Whall (Eds.), *Conceptual models of nursing: Analysis and application.* (3rd ed.). Norwalk, CT: Appleton & Lange.

Fitzpatrick, J.J. (1996). Mentoring for international educational program development. In C. Vance & R. Olson (Eds.), *The mentor connection in nursing.*

Fitzpatrick, J.J. (1996). Nursing theory and metatheory. In J. Fawcette & I. King (Eds.), *The language of nursing theory and metatheory.*

Fitzpatrick, J.J., Abraham, I.L. (1987). Contractual community relationships for research. *Issues in Higher Education, Proceedings of Academic Chairpersons: Organizational Structure, Change, and Development, 25,* 107-110.

Fitzpatrick, J.J., & Abraham, I.L. (1987). Developing collegial relationships through scholarship. In W.E. Cashin & A. Noma (Eds.), *Proceedings of the Third Annual Conference on Academic Chairpersons: Unraveling the paradox, 20,* 105-108. Orlando: Center for Faculty Evaluation and Development.

Fitzpatrick, J.J., Abraham, I.L, & Nadzam, D.M. (1989). Statistics and quantitative methods in nursing summarized: Issues and strategies for the future. In I.L. Abraham, D.M. Nadzam, & J.J. Fitzpatrick (Eds.), *Statistics and quantitative methods in nursing: Issues and strategies for research and education.* Philadelphia: Saunders.

Fitzpatrick, J.J., & Anderson, G.C. (1986). Group summary: Setting the agenda for the year 2000: Knowledge development in nursing. *Proceedings of the AAN Annual Meeting and Scientific Session.* Kansas City, MO: American Academy of Nursing.

Fitzpatrick, J.J., & Donovan, M.J. (1986). Interpretations of life and death: Relationships to health. *Proceedings of the Twelfth World Conference on Health Education.* Dublin, Ireland: International Health Educator's Association.

Fitzpatrick, J.J., & Holloran, E.J. (1985). Proactivating a collaborative service education climate. In *MAIN Proceedings: Thriving or surviving? Managing pro-active environments for nursing* (pp. 29-41). Indianapolis: Midwest Alliance in Nursing.

Fitzpatrick, J.J., & Modly, D.M. (1990). The first doctor of nursing (ND) program. In N.L. Chaska (Ed.), *The nursing profession: Turning points* (pp. 93-99). St. Louis: Mosby.

Fitzpatrick, J.J., & Simpson, R.L. (1989). Proposed model of coding of patient nurse data. In B. Barber, D. Cao, D. Qin, & G. Wagner (Eds.), *Medinfo 89: Proceedings of the Sixth International Conference on Medical Informatics.* New York: NHC.

Fitzpatrick, J.J., & Whall, A.L. (1983). Nursing models: Summary and future projections. In J.J. Fitzpatrick & A.L. Whall (Eds.), *Conceptual models of nursing: Analysis and application.* Bowie, MD: Robert J. Brady.

Fitzpatrick, J.J., & Whall, A.L. (1983). Overview of nursing models and nursing theories. In J.J. Fitzpatrick & A.L. Whall (Eds.), *Conceptual models of nursing: Analysis and application.* Bowie, MD: Robert J. Brady.

Jewell, J.A., Abraham, I.L., & Fitzpatrick, J.J. (1989). The Laboratory for AI Research in Nursing: Initial equipment configuration. *Proceedings of the American Association for Medical Systems and Informatics.*

Johnston, R.L., & Fitzpatrick, J.J. (1982). Relevance of psychiatric mental health nursing theories to nursing models. In J.J. Fitzpatrick, et al., *Nursing models and their psychiatric mental health applications*. Bowie, MD: Robert J. Brady.

Kerr, M.E., & Fitzpatrick, J.J. (1990). Qualitative research methodologies: Synthesis and recommendations. In *Monograph of the Invitational Conference on Research Methods for Validating Nursing Diagnosis*. St. Louis: North American Nursing Diagnosis Association.

Kirk, L.W., Abraham, I.L., Jane, L.H., & Fitzpatrick, J.J. (1986). Comprehensive computerization of a school of nursing: Planning aspects and system description. In R. Salamon, B. Blum, & M. Jorgenson (Eds.), *Medinfo 86*, (Vol. 2). Amsterdam: North-Holland/Elsevier.

Nadzam, D.M., Fitzpatrick, J.J., & Abraham, I.L. (1989). Statistics, quantitative methods, and the discipline of nursing. In I.L. Abraham, D.M. Nadzam, & J.J. Fitzpatrick (Eds.), *Statistics and quantitative methods in nursing: Issues and strategies for research and education*. Philadelphia: Saunders.

Roy, C., Rogers, M.E., Fitzpatrick, J.J., Newman, M.A., & Orem, D.E. (1981). Theoretical framework for classification of nursing diagnosis: Panel discussion. In M.J. Kim & D. Moritz (Eds.), *Classifications of nursing diagnosis: Proceedings of the third and fourth national conferences*. New York: McGraw-Hill.

Journal articles

Abraham, I.L, Fitzpatrick, J.J., & Jane, L.H. (1986). Computers in critical care nursing: Yet another technology? *Dimensions of Critical Care Nursing, 5*, 325-326.

Anderson, R.M., Thurkettle, M.A., & Fitzpatrick, J.J. (1985). The new breed! *Nursing Success Today, 2*(3), 4-8.

Brennan, P.F., & Fitzpatrick, J.J. (1993). On the essential integration of nursing and informatics. *AACN Clinical Issues in Critical Care Nursing, 3*(4), 797-803.

Briody, M.E., Carpenito, L.J., Jones, D.T., & Fitzpatrick, J.J (1992). Toward further understanding of nursing diagnosis: An interpretation. *Nursing Diagnosis, 3*(3), 124-128.

Clochesy, J.M., Daly, B.J., Idemoto, B.K., Steel, J., & Fitzpatrick, J.J. (1994). Preparing advanced practice nurses for acute care. *American Journal of Critical Care, 3*(4), 255-259.

Downs, F.S., & Fitzpatrick, J.J. (1976, Nov.-Dec.). Preliminary investigation of the reliability and validity of a tool for the assessment of body position and motor activity. *Nursing Research 25*, 404-408.

Fitzpatrick, J. (1970). Learning is . . . *Capital, 54*, 7-9.

Fitzpatrick, J. (1978). Aging and institutionalization as determinants of temporal and motor phenomena. *Image, 10*, 24.

Fitzpatrick, J.J. (1980, Sept.-Oct.). Patients' perceptions of time: Current research. *International Nursing Review, 27*(5), 143-153, 160.

Fitzpatrick, J.J. (1983). Suicidology and suicide prevention: Historical perspectives from the nursing literature. *Journal of Psychosocial Nursing and Mental Health Service, 21*(5), 20-28.

Fitzpatrick, J.J. (1984, Sept.-Oct.). Customizing reusable stoma plates. *Journal of Enterostomal Therapy, 11*, 196-198.

Fitzpatrick, J.J. (1985). Endowed chairs in nursing: State of the art. *Journal of Professional Nursing, 1*(3), 145-147.

Fitzpatrick, J.J. (1987). Professional doctorate as entry into clinical practice. In *Perspectives in Nursing 1987-1989* (pp. 53-56). New York: National League for Nursing.

Fitzpatrick, J.J. (1987). Use of existing nursing models. *Journal of Gerontological Nursing, 13*(9), 8-9.

Fitzpatrick, J.J. (1988). The clinical nurse-midwife as scientist. *Journal of Nurse Midwifery, 33*(1), 37-39.

Fitzpatrick, J.J. (1988). GN theory based on Rogers' conceptual model. *Journal of Gerontological Nursing, 14*(9), 14-16.

Fitzpatrick, J.J. (1988). Nursing: How can we enhance nursing knowledge and practice. *Nursing and Health Care, 9*, 517-521.

Fitzpatrick, J.J. (1989). Endowed chairs in nursing: A 1988 update. *Journal of Professional Nursing, 5*, 23-24.

Fitzpatrick, J.J. (1989). Towards new visions of nursing. *Ireland Nursing Forum and Health Services*, 31-35.

Fitzpatrick, J.J. (1990). Conceptual basis for the organization and advancement of nursing knowledge: Nursing diagnosis/taxonomy. *Nursing Diagnoses, 1*, 17-21.

Fitzpatrick, J.J. (1996). Twelve principles of successful fund raising. *Nursing Leadership Forum, 2*, 4-7.

Fitzpatrick, J.J., & Abraham, I.L. (1987). Contractual community relationships for research. *Issues in Higher Education, 25*, 107-110.

Fitzpatrick, J.J., & Abraham, I.L. (1987). Toward the socialization of scholars and scientists. *Nurse Educator, 12*, 23-25.

Fitzpatrick, J.J., Abraham, I.L., & Pressler, J.L. (1989). Developing scientific relationships through leadership. *Nurse Educator, 14*, 6-7.

Fitzpatrick, J.J., & Behrman, R.E. (1985). The university and the hospital: Old friends, new allies. *Nursing and Health Care, 6*, 383-384.

Fitzpatrick, J.J., Boyle, K.K., & Anderson, R.M. (1986). Evaluation of the doctor of nursing (ND) program: Preliminary findings. *Journal of Professional Nursing, 2*(6), 365-372.

Fitzpatrick, J.J., & Donovan, M.J. (1978, July). Temporal experience and motor behavior among the aging. *Research in Nursing and Health, 1*, 60-68.

Fitzpatrick, J.J., & Donovan, M.J. (1979, May-June). A follow-up study of the reliability and validity of the motor activity rating scale. *Nursing Research, 28*, 179-181.

Fitzpatrick, J.J., Donovan, M.J., & Johnston, R.L. (1980). Experience of time during the crisis of cancer. *Cancer Nursing, 3*(3), 191-194.

Fitzpatrick, J.J., & Evans, B. (1989). Honorary doctorates awarded to nurses: A 51 year review. *Journal of Professional Nursing, 5*(3), 159-163.

Fitzpatrick, J.J., Halloran, E.J., & Algase, D.L. (1987). An experiment in nursing revisited. *Nursing Outlook, 35*(1), 29-33.

Fitzpatrick, J.J., Kerr, M., Saba, V.K., Hoskins, L.M., Hurley, M., Mills, W., Rottkamp, B., & Warren, J.J. (1989). NANDA taxonomy I: Proposed ICD-CM 10 Version. *Applied Nursing Research, 2,* 90-91.

Fitzpatrick, J.J., Kerr, M.E., Saba, V.K., Hoskins, L.M., Hurley, M.E., Mills, W.C., Rottkamp, B.C., Warren, J.J., & Carpenito, L.J. (1989). Translating nursing diagnosis into ICD code. *American Journal of Nursing, 89,* 493-495.

Fitzpatrick, J.J., & Macaluso, J. (1985, Oct.). Shadow positioning technique: A method for post-mortem identification. *Journal of Forensic Science, 30,* 1226-1229.

Fitzpatrick, J.J., & Reed, P.G. (1980). Stress in the crisis experience: Nursing interventions. *Occupational Health Nursing, 28*(12), 19-21.

Fitzpatrick, J.J., & Renner, E.A. (1991). Research development. *Nurse Educator, 16,* 31, 35.

Fitzpatrick, J.J., & Whall, A.L. (1984). Points of view: Should nursing models be used in psychiatric nursing practice? *Journal of Psychosocial Nursing, 22*(6), 44-45.

Fitzpatrick, J.J., & Whall, A.L. (1984, June). Should nursing models be used in psychiatric nursing practice? *Journal of Psychosocial Nursing and Mental Health Services, 222,* 44-45.

Fitzpatrick, J.J., & Wohlford, N. (1991). MSN is the appropriate academic credential for nurse anesthetists . . . point/counterpoint. *Nurse Anesthesia, 2*(4), 160-164.

Fitzpatrick, J.J., Wykle, M.L., & Morris, D.L. (1990). Collaboration in care and research. *Archives of Psychiatric Nursing, 6,* 53-61.

Fitzpatrick, J.J., & Zanotti, R. (1995). Nursing diagnosis internationally. *Nursing Diagnosis, 6,* 42-47.

Flagherty, G.G., & Fitzpatrick, J.J. (1978, Nov.-Dec.). Use of a relaxation technique to increase comfort level of postoperative patients: A preliminary study. *Nursing Research, 27,* 352-355.

Goldberg, W.G., & Fitzpatrick, J.J. (1980, Nov.-Dec.). Movement therapy with the aged. *Nursing Research, 29,* 339-346.

Horowitz, B., Fitzpatrick, J.J., & Flaherty, G. (1984). Relaxation techniques to relieve pain in postoperative open heart surgery patients: A clinical study. *Dimensions of Critical Care Nursing Journal, 3*(6), 364-371.

Kerr, M., Hoskins, L.M., Fitzpatrick, J.J., Warren, J.J., Avant, K.C., Hurley, M., Luney, M., Mills, W.C., & Rottkamp, B.C. (1993). Taxonomic validation: An overview. *Nursing Diagnosis, 4*(1), 6-14.

Kiley, M., Halloran, E.J., Weston, J.L., Ozbolt, J.G., Werleg, H.H., Gordon, M., Giovennetti, P., Thompson, J.D., Simpson, R.L., Ziedstorff, R.D., Fitzpatrick, J.J., Davis, H.S., Cook, M., & Grier, M. (1983). Computerized nursing information systems (NIS). *Nursing Management, 14*(7), 26-29.

Pacini, C.M., & Fitzpatrick, J.J. (1982). Sleep patterns of hospitalized aged individuals. *Journal of Gerontological Nursing, 8*(6), 327-332.

Pressler, J.L., & Fitzpatrick, J.J. (1988). Rosemary Ellis: Contributions of Rosemary Ellis to Knowledge Development for Nursing. *Image, 20*(1), 28-30.

Roberts, B.L., & Fitzpatrick, J.J. (1983, March). Improving balance: Therapy of movement. *Journal of Gerontological Nursing, 9*(3), 150-156.

Roslaniec, A., & Fitzpatrick, J.J. (1979, Dec.). Changes in mental status in older adults with four days of hospitalization. *Research in Nursing and Health, 2,* 177-187.

Steele, J.E., Wagner, A.D., Adams-Davis, K.M., & Fitzpatrick, J.J. (1994). Planning a community nursing center. *International Nursing Review, 41,* 151-154.

Study Group on Nursing Information Systems (1983). Special report. Computerized nursing information systems: An urgent need. *Research in Nursing and Health, 6,* 101-105.

Wilson, L.M., & Fitzpatrick, J.J. (1984). Dialectic thinking as a means of understanding systems-in-development: Relevance to Rogers' principles. *Advances in Nursing Science, 6*(2), 24-41.

Zanotti, R., & Fitzpatrick, J. (1993). Nursing care and decision support tools. *Information Technology in Nursing, 5,* 5-7.

Thesis

Fitzpatrick, J.J. (1967). *A study of staff nurses' perceptions of the importance of selected nursing activities in carrying out their nursing role.* Unpublished master's thesis, Ohio State University.

Dissertation

Fitzpatrick, J.J. (1975). *An investigation of the relationship between temporal orientation, temporal extension, and time perception.* Unpublished doctoral dissertation, New York University.

Abstracts, book reviews, editorials

Downs, F.S., & Fitzpatrick, J.J. (1977). Preliminary investigation of the reliability and validity of a tool for the assessment of body position and motor activity. *Psychological Abstracts.* Washington, DC: American Psychological Association (Research abstract).

Fitzpatrick, J. (1978). Temporal experiences among hospitalized individuals: A pilot study. In R. Williams & C. Wrotny (Eds.), *Health promotion: In health and illness: Proceedings of the First Annual Research Symposium of the Michigan Sigma Theta Tau Consortium.* Indianapolis: Sigma Theta Tau (Abstract).

Fitzpatrick, J. (1980). Identity crisis resolved. *Center for Health Research NEWS, 2*(1), 1.

Fitzpatrick, J. (1980). Review of *Nursing theory: Analysis, application, evaluation* by Barbara J. Stevens. *Nursing Research, 29,* 114.

Fitzpatrick, J. (1980). Time is relevant. *Center for Health Research NEWS, 1*(2), 1.

Fitzpatrick, J. (1980). Why a newsletter? *Center for Health Research NEWS, 1*(1), 1.

Fitzpatrick, J.J. (1980). Abstract: Hospitalization as a crisis: An exploration of temporal experiences, in WICHE proceedings, *Communicating Nursing Research Directions for the 1980s, 13,* 48 (Abstract).

Fitzpatrick, J. (1981). Answer 2 to research replication: Questions and answers. *Western Journal of Nursing Research, 3,* 96-97.

Fitzpatrick, J. (1981). Is nursing the science of health? *Center for Health Research NEWS, 2*(2), 1.

Fitzpatrick, J. (1981). Review of *The many faces of suicide: Indirect self-destructive behavior* by N.L. Farberow (Ed.). *Nursing Outlook, 29,* 435.

Fitzpatrick, J. (1981). Toward the future . . . *Center for Health Research NEWS, 2*(3), 1.

Fitzpatrick, J.J. (1975). *An investigation of the relationship between temporal orientation, temporal extension, and time perception.* Unpublished doctoral dissertation. New York University (Abstract).

Fitzpatrick, J. (1982). Review of *Readings on the research process in nursing* by D.J. Fox & I.R. Leeser (Eds.). *Nursing Research, 31,* 158.

Fitzpatrick, J.J. (1981 to 1985). Message from the chairperson. *CNR Council of Nurse Researchers Newsletter.* Kansas City, MO: American Nurses Association.

Fitzpatrick, J.J. (1982). Preface in *Creating research environments for the 1980s (MNRS).* Indianapolis: Midwest Alliance in Nursing.

Fitzpatrick, J.J. (1983). Review of *Suicide intervention for nurses* by M. Miller (Ed.), *Journal of Psychosocial Nursing, 21*(2), 39.

Fitzpatrick, J.J. (1984). Why research? (Editorial). *Nursing Success Today, 1*(4), 3.

Fitzpatrick, J.J. (1987). Visions of nursing. *Nurse Educator, 12*(2), 7-8.

Fitzpatrick, J.J. (1988). Harmonic convergence (Editorial). *Applied Nursing Research, 1*(1), 1.

Fitzpatrick, J.J. (1988). Images of nurses (Editorial). *Applied Nursing Research, 1*(2), 53.

Fitzpatrick, J.J. (1988). The joys and triumphs of clinical researchers (Editorial). *Applied Nursing Research, 1*(3), 107-108.

Fitzpatrick, J.J. (1989). Caring and quality care: Process and outcome (Editorial). *Applied Nursing Research, 2*(4), 149.

Fitzpatrick, J.J. (1989). The lone researcher (Editorial). *Applied Nursing Research, 2*(1), 1.

Fitzpatrick, J.J. (1989). Room at the top (Editorial). *Applied Nursing Research, 2*(2), 63.

Fitzpatrick, J.J. (1989). Some of my best friends are . . . (Editorial). *Applied Nursing Research, 2*(3), 107.

Fitzpatrick, J.J. (1990). Applied nursing research (Editorial). *Applied Nursing Research, 3*(4), 139.

Fitzpatrick, J.J. (1990). The culture of nursing (Editorial). *Applied Nursing Research, 4*(1), 1.

Fitzpatrick, J.J. (1990). The power of the written word (Editorial). *Applied Nursing Research, 3*(1), 1.

Fitzpatrick, J.J. (1990). Symbols of nursing (Editorial). *Applied Nursing Research 4,*(2), 139.

Fitzpatrick, J.J. (1990). Where is the other applied nursing research? (Editorial). *Applied Nursing Research, 3*(2), 47.

Fitzpatrick, J.J. (1990). Your editor is your friend (Editorial). *Applied Nursing Research, 3*(3), 89.

Fitzpatrick, J.J. (1991). Little science (Editorial). *Applied Nursing Research, 4*(4), 151.

Fitzpatrick, J.J. (1991). The politics of research (Editorial). *Applied Nursing Research, 4*(3), 99.

Fitzpatrick, J.J. (1992). Caring words (Editorial). *Applied Nursing Research, 5*(1), 1.

Fitzpatrick, J.J. (1992). How to behave at a research meeting (Editorial). *Applied Nursing Research, 5*(2), 57-58.

Fitzpatrick, J.J. (1992). Weaving the web of community relations. (Editorial). *Applied Nursing Research, 5*(3), 109-110.

Fitzpatrick, J.J. (1993). Celebrations: five years and Index Medicus. (Editorial). *Applied Nursing Research, 6*(3), 105.

Fitzpatrick, J.J. (1993). The named nurse . . . a primary nurse in our language and nursing culture (Editorial). *Applied Nursing Research, 6*(1), 1.

Fitzpatrick, J.J. (1993). The reformers are coming (Editorial). *Applied Nursing Research, 6*(2), 53.

Fitzpatrick, J.J. (1993). The warming of global nursing (Editorial). *Applied Nursing Research, 6*(4), 145.

Fitzpatrick, J.J. (1994). A call to words (Editorial). *Applied Nursing Research, 7*(1), 1.

Fitzpatrick, J.J. (1994). A health care system built on greed (Editorial). *Applied Nursing Research, 7*(3), 111.

Fitzpatrick, J.J. (1994). Thank you, nurse (Editorial). *Applied Nursing Research, 7*(2), 51.

Fitzpatrick, J.J. (1995). The making of a manuscript (Editorial). *Applied Nursing Research, 8*(1), 1-2.

Fitzpatrick, J.J. (1995). We've come a long way: A 1995 report of endowed chairs in nursing (Editorial). *Journal of Professional Nursing, 11*(6), 320-324.

Fitzpatrick, J.J. (1995). When primary care is politically correct (Editorial). *Applied Nursing Research, 8*(2), 55.

Fitzpatrick, J.J. (1995). Where has all the caring gone? (Editorial). *Applied Nursing Research, 8*(4), 155.

Fitzpatrick, J.J. (1996). Every nurse should be a patient, every researcher should be a subject (Editorial). *Applied Nursing Research, 9*(1), 1.

Fitzpatrick, J.J., & Boyle, K.K. (1987). Evaluation of graduates of the doctor of nursing (ND) program. *Proceedings of the 11th Annual Midwest Nursing Research Society Conference* (Abstract).

Fitzpatrick, J.J., Donovan, M.J., & Johnston, R. (1979). Temporal experiences among terminally ill cancer patients: An exploratory study. *Proceedings of the Second Annual Research Symposium, Michigan Sigma Theta Tau Consortium* (Abstract). Indianapolis: Sigma Theta Tau.

Fitzpatrick, J.J., Donovan, M.J., & Johnston, R.L. (1985). Adult developmental stage, depression and the experience of time (Abstract). *Gerontologist, 25,* 128-129.

Fitzpatrick, J.J., & Hott, J.R. (October, 1987). Preface. *Proceedings of the American Nurses Association Council of Nurse Researchers International Conference*, pp. 1-3.

Fitzpatrick, J.J., Johnston, R.L., & Donovan, M.J. (1980). Hospitalization as a crisis: Relation to temporal experience, in WICHE proceedings (Abstract). *Communicating Nursing Research Directions for the 1980's, 13,* 48.

Fitzpatrick, J.J., Reed, P.G., Donovan, M.J., & Zurakowski, T. (1983). Programmatic research on suicide: A nursing perspective (Abstract). *Proceedings of the American Association of Suicidology Annual Meeting,* New York.

Fitzpatrick, J.J., & Zanotti, R. (1994). Martha Rogers (Obituary). *International Nursing Review, 41*(3), 74.

Fitzpatrick, J.J., & Zanotti, R. (1994). On the shoulders of giants . . . (Editorial). *Applied Nursing Research, 7*(4), 163-164.

Johnston, R.L., Fitzpatrick, J.J., & Donovan, M.J. (1982). Developmental stage: Relationship to the experience of time (Abstract). *Nursing Research, 31,* 120.

Reed, P.G., et al. (1982). Suicidal crisis: Relationship to the experience of time (Abstract). *Nursing Research, 31,* 122.

See, E.M., Fitzpatrick, J.J., & Halloran, E.J. (1987). An organizational model for faculty practice. *Proceedings of the 1986 MAIN Seventh Annual Fall Workshop* (Abstract). Overland Park, KS.

Sills, G.M., & Fitzpatrick, J.J. (1979). Women: Psychotropic drug use and eclectic relaxation therapy (Abstract). In *Nursing Research: Synopses of selected clinical studies.* Kansas City: American Nurses' Association.

Werley, H.H., & Fitzpatrick, J.J. (1986). Annual review of nursing research: A valuable research tool. *Proceedings of the 1986 International Nursing Research Conference* (Abstract). Edmonton, Alberta, Canada.

Correspondence

Fitzpatrick, Joyce (1984). Personal correspondence.

Fitzpatrick, J.J. (1992). Personal correspondence.

Interview

Fitzpatrick, J.J. (1984, March 22). Telephone interview.

Fitzpatrick, J.J. (1985). Telephone interviews.

Fitzpatrick, J.J. (1988). Telephone interviews.

Bulletins

Abraham, I.L, Nadzam, D.M., & Fitzpatrick, J.J. (1986). Statistics and quantitative methods in nursing: Overview of a recent invitational conference. *Bulletin on Teaching of Statistics in the Health Sciences,* pp. 1-4. American Statistical Association, No. 41, Winter.

Fitzpatrick, J.J. (1987). *The ND program: Integration of past and future.* Cleveland, OH: Frances Payne Bolton School of Nursing.

Secondary sources
Book reviews

Fitzpatrick, J.J., Whall, A.L., & Johnston, R.L. (1982). *Nursing models and their psychiatric mental health applications. American Journal of Nursing, 1,* 10-103, January 1983. *Nursing Outlook, 3,* 148, May-June 1983. *Research in Nursing and Health, 1,* 41, March 1983.

Chapters

Beckman, S.J., Chapman-Boyce, P., Coleman-Ehmke, S., Hailway, C.A., Justus, R.G., Pung, R.A., & Smith, C.R. (1989). Joyce J. Fitzpatrick life perspective model. In A. Marriner-Tomey (Ed.), *Nursing theorists and their work* (2nd ed.) (pp. 420-431). St. Louis: Mosby.

Beckman, S.J., Chapman-Boyce, P., Coleman-Ehmke, S., Hailway, C.A., & Pung, R.A. (1986). Joyce J. Fitzpatrick life perspective model. In A. Marriner (Ed.), *Nursing theorists and their work* (pp. 361-368). St. Louis: Mosby.

Pressler, J.L. (1983). Fitzpatrick's rhythm model: Analysis for nursing science. In J. Fitzpatrick & A. Whall, *Conceptual models of nursing: Analysis and application.* Bowie, MD: Robert J. Brady.

Pressler, J.L. (1989). Fitzpatrick's rhythm model: A second look. In J. Fitzpatrick & A. Whall (Eds.), *Conceptual models of nursing: Analysis and application.* Norwalk, CT: Appleton & Lange.

Biographical sources

Fitzpatrick, J.J. (1980, Aug.). *Directory of nurses with doctoral degrees* (Vol. 1). Kansas City: American Nurses Association.

Fitzpatrick, J.J. (1984, Jan.). *The national faculty directory* (Vol. 1). Detroit: Gale Research.

Other sources

Caplan, G. (1961). *An approach to community mental health.* New York: Grune & Stratton.

Caplan, G. (1964). *Principles of preventive psychiatry.* New York: Basic Books.

Chinn, P.L., & Kramer, M.K. (1995). *Theory and nursing: A systematic approach* (4th ed.). St. Louis: Mosby.

Flaco, S.M., & Lobo, M.L. (1980). Martha Rogers. In Nursing Theories Conference Group, J.B. George, Chairperson, *Nursing theories: The base for professional nursing practice.* Englewood Cliffs, NJ: Prentice-Hall.

Haus, E. (1978). Perspectives on nursing theory. *Advances in Nursing Science, 1,* 37-48.

Lachmann, F.M. (1985). On transience and the sense of temporal continuity. *Continuing Psychiatry, 21,* 193.

Luce, G.G. (1970). *Biological rhythms in psychiatry and medicine.* National Institute of Mental Health. Washington, DC: U.S. Department of Health, Education, and Welfare.

Rogers, M.E. (1967). *The theoretical basis of nursing* . Philadelphia: F.A. Davis.

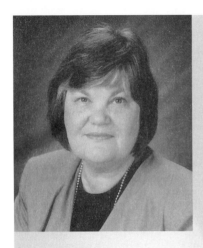

CHAPTER

32

Margaret A. Newman

Model of Health

Snehlata Desai, M. Jan Keffer, DeAnn M. Hensley,
Kimberly A. Kilgore-Keever, Jill Vass Langfitt, LaPhyllis Peterson

CREDENTIALS AND BACKGROUND OF THE THEORIST

Margaret A. Newman was born on October 10, 1933,[47:588] in Memphis, Tennessee. She earned her first bachelor's degree in home economics and English from Baylor University in Waco, Texas, in 1954 and her second in nursing from the University of Tennessee in Memphis in 1962.

Newman received her master's degree in medical-surgical nursing and teaching from the University of California, San Francisco, in 1964. She earned her Ph.D. in nursing science and rehabilitation nursing from New York University in New York City in 1971.

The authors wish to express appreciation to Dr. Margaret A. Newman for critiquing the chapter and Sudha Patel for assistance.

Newman progressed through the academic ranks at the University of Tennessee, New York University, and Pennsylvania State University and was a professor at the University of Minnesota in Minneapolis. In addition, she has been the director of nursing for the Clinical Research Center at the University of Tennessee, the acting director of the Ph.D. program in the Division of Nursing at New York University, and Professor-in-Charge of the Graduate Program and Research at Pennsylvania State University.

Newman was admitted to the American Academy of Nursing in 1976. She received the Outstanding Alumnus Award from the University of Tennessee College of Nursing in Memphis in 1975, the Distinguished Alumnus Award from the Division of Nursing at New York University in 1984, and was admitted in 1988 to the Hall of Fame at the University of Mississippi School of Nursing.[30] She was a Latin American Teaching Fellow in 1976 and 1977 and an *American Journal of Nursing* Scholar in 1979. She was Distinguished Faculty at the Seventh International Conference on Human Functioning at Wichita, Kansas, in 1983, and received the Distinguished Alumnus Award from the Division of Nursing at New York University in 1984, and is listed in *Who's Who in American Women,* and *Who's Who in America.*[50] Newman was included in 1990 as one of the featured nursing theorists in the videotape series sponsored by Helene Fuld Health Trust.[30] She was a Distinguished Resident at Westminster College, Salt Lake City, Utah, in 1991 and received the Distinguished Scholar in Nursing, New York University Division of Nursing, in 1992, the Sigma Theta Tau Founders Elizabeth McWilliams Miller Award for Excellence in Research in 1993, and the Nurse Scholar Award at Saint Xavier University School of Nursing in 1994.[36]

In 1985, as a Traveling Research Fellow, Newman conducted workshops in four locations throughout New Zealand.[26] At the University of Tampere, Finland, in 1985 Newman was the major speaker for a week-long conference on the Theory of Consciousness as it related to nursing.[26] Newman has presented many papers on topics pertaining to her Theory of Health as expanding consciousness. She published *Theory Development in Nursing* in 1979, *Health as Expanding Consciousness* in 1986 and 1994, and *A Developing Discipline* in 1995. *A Developing Discipline* is a collection of Margaret Newman's life work.[19,21] She has written numerous articles in journals and book chapters. In 1986 she did a case study analysis of practice in three sites within the Minneapolis–St. Paul area in which she discussed the background of the health care system, findings within each site, and conclusions concerning the changes necessary for hospital nursing practice.[38] From 1986 to 1997, Dr. Newman has investigated sequential patterns of persons with heart disease and cancer.[41] Her more recent publications reflect her passion for integration of nursing theory, practice, and research. Her evolving viewpoints on trends in philosophy of nursing, analysis of theoretical models of nursing practice, and nursing research are noteworthy.[32,33]

During 1989 and 1990, Dr. Newman was the principal investigator of a project that explored the theory and structure of a professional model of nursing practice. This research was conducted at Carondelet St. Mary's Community Hospitals and Health Centers in Tucson, Arizona.[29,40] In addition to her research and teaching, Dr. Newman is sought for consultation with regard to expanding her theory of health from over 40 states and Australia, Brazil, Canada, Finland, Germany, Japan, New Zealand, and the United Kingdom.[31]

Newman has served on several editorial boards, including *Nursing Research, Western Journal of Nursing Research, Nursing and Health Care, Advances in Nursing Science,* and *Nursing Science Quarterly.*[31] She participates as a member of the nurse-theorist task force since 1978 with the North American Nursing Diagnosis Association (NANDA).

RELATIONSHIP TO METAPARADIGM CONCEPTS

Nursing's major assumptions of nursing, person, health, and environment are not addressed explicitly in the Theory of Health. In the following paragraphs implicit definitions from Newman's work were used to discuss the four nursing components.

Nursing's metaparadigm concepts of nursing, person, health, and environment were not explicitly defined in the 1986 book *(Health as Expanding Consciousness).* Newman has described in her article in *Nursing Science Quarterly* her understanding of the concepts.[28]

Nursing

Nursing is seen as providing a partner in the process of expanding consciousness. The nurse can connect with the person when new rules are sought.[28]

The nurse is the facilitator who helps an individual, family, or community focus on his or her pattern.[23:73] The nursing process is one of pattern recognition. Newman utilized the assessment framework developed by the nurse-theorist group of NANDA to assist the nurse in pattern identification. The dimensions of the assessment framework—exchanging, communicating, relating, valuing, choosing, moving, perceiving, feeling, and knowing—are considered manifestations of the unitary pattern.[23:73]

"Pattern recognition comes from within the observer."[25:38] The nurse perceives the patterns of the set of data or sequence of events, and the pattern of the individual changes with the new information. The process of pattern recognition first involves an attempt to view the pattern of a person as "sequential patterns over time."[25:38] Data from interviews of "healthy" adults could be grouped into sequential patterns. A follow-up interview is then conducted to share the investigator's findings with the subjects. The nurse can use this process to identify the current pattern of an individual to establish a plan of care.[25]

Person

Throughout Newman's work the terms *client, patient, person, individual,* and *pattern* are used interchangeably. Person is defined as "consciousness." Persons as individuals are identified by their individual patterns of consciousness.[23:33]

Environment

Environment is not explicitly defined, but is described as being the larger whole, that which is beyond the consciousness of the individual. The pattern of consciousness that is the person interacts within the pattern of consciousness that is the family and within the pattern of community interactions.[23:32] A major assumption is that "consciousness is coextensive in the universe and resides in all matter."[23:33]

Newman identifies interactions between person and environment as a key process that creates unique configuration for each individual. Patterns of person-environment evolve to higher levels of consciousness for the self. The assumption is that all matter in the universe-environment possesses consciousness, but at different levels. Interpretation of Newman's view clarifies that it is the interaction pattern of a person with the environment. Disease in human energy field is an indicator of a unique pattern of person-environment interaction (Fig. 32-1).

Health

Health is the major concept of Newman's Theory of Expanding Consciousness. A fusion of disease and nondisease creates a synthesis that is regarded as health.[18:56] Because disease and nondisease are each reflections of the larger whole, a new concept is formed: pattern of the whole.[23:12] Newman stated that the "essence of the emerging paradigm of health is pattern recognition."[23:13] Health and the evolving pattern of consciousness are the same.[28]

THEORETICAL SOURCES

Central to Newman's assumptions was the philosopher Hegel's "dialectical process of the fusion of opposites."[19:56] Newman used many fields of inquiry as sources for theory development. The rationale for drawing broad conclusions from the use of a limited number of concepts came from Capra, a physicist. Capra held that many phenomena can be explained in terms of a few. Newman[19:59] drew from Capra in general, and Bentov in particular, for her position on the importance of health expansion of consciousness. Newman credited "Dorothy Johnson, during my undergraduate studies, and Martha Rogers, in a more extensive way, during my graduate study as those nurse theorists most influential on my thinking."[21]

Bohm's Theory of Implicate Order supports Newman's postulate that disease is a manifestation of the pattern of health. Newman stated she began to comprehend "the underlying, unseen pattern that manifests itself in varying forms, including disease, and the interconnectedness and omnipresence of all that there is.[21] Young's Theory of Human Evolution pinpointed for Newman the role of pattern recognition and "was the impetus for . . . efforts to integrate the basic concepts of my theory—movement, space, time, and consciousness—into a dynamic portrayal of life and health."[21] Moss's experience of love as the highest level of consciousness "provided affirmation and elaboration of my intuition regarding the nature of health."[21] Ilya Prigogine, a chemist and winner of the Nobel Prize for his Theory of Dissipative Structures, described the pattern of harmony and disharmony as part of a rhythmic process. Newman incorporated Prigogine's theory.[30]

USE OF EMPIRICAL EVIDENCE

Evidence for the Theory of Health emanated from Newman's early personal family experiences. Her

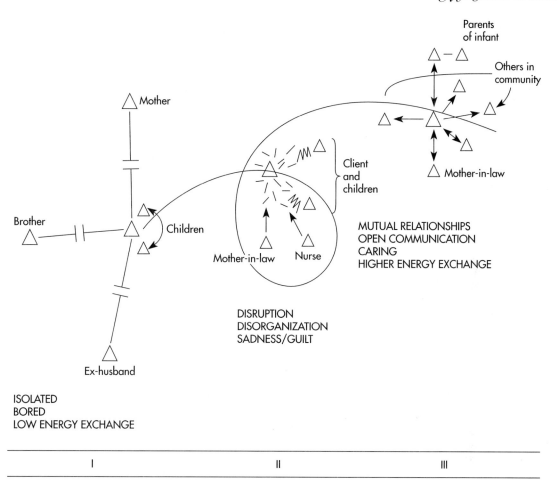

Fig. **32-1** Sequential patterns of person-environment relationships. *From Newman, M.A. (1987). Nursing's emerging paradigm: The diagnosis of pattern. In A.M. McLane (Ed.),* Classification of nursing diagnoses: Proceedings of the Seventh Conference. *St. Louis: Mosby, p. 56. Reprinted with permission.*

mother's struggle with amyotrophic lateral sclerosis, a chronic illness, and her dependence on Newman, then a young college graduate, sparked an interest in nursing. From that experience evolved the idea that "illness reflected the life patterns of the person and that what was needed was the recognition of that pattern and acceptance of it for what it meant to that person."[21]

Throughout Newman's writing, terms are used such as *call to nursing,*[21] *growing conscience-like feeling,*[21] *fear,*[21] *power,*[21] *meaning of life and health,*[21] *belief of life after death,*[21] *rituals of health,*[21] and *love.*[21] The terms provide a clue concerning Newman's en-

deavors to make logical a disturbing life experience. The life experience triggered her beginning maturation toward theory development in nursing. Within her philosophical framework, Newman began to develop a synthesis of disease-nondisease—health as recognition of the total patterning of a person.

Research has been conducted on the theoretical sources used.[24] In 1979, Newman[19:23] wrote that "in order for nursing research to have meaning in terms of theory development, it must (1) have as its purpose the testing of theory, (2) make explicit the theoretical framework upon which the testing relies, and

Major Concepts & Definitions

Health Health encompasses disease and non-disease. Health can be regarded as the evolving pattern of the person and the environment.[31:13] Health is viewed as a process of "developing awareness of self and environment together with increasing ability to perceive alternatives and respond in a variety of ways."[18] Health is viewed as the "pattern of the whole" of a person.[23:12] Health is described as including "disease as a meaningful manifestation of the pattern of the whole and is based on the premise that life is an ongoing process of expanding consciousness."[29]

Using Hegel's dialectical fusion of opposites, Newman explains how the concept disease fuses with its opposite, nondisease, or absence of disease, to create a new concept, health. She explains that this new paradigm of health is relational and is "patterned, emergent, unpredictable, unitary, intuitive, and innovative"; whereas the traditional paradigm is linear, causal, predictive, dichotomous, rational, and controlling. However, she appeals to take the characteristics of old paradigm of health as special cases of new holistic paradigm to find patterns and new meaning. To her, health and the evolving pattern of consciousness are the same. The essence of the emerging paradigm of health is recognition of pattern. Newman sees the life process as a progression toward higher levels of consciousness.[33,34]

Pattern Pattern is what identifies an individual as a particular person. Examples of explicit manifestations of the underlying pattern of a person would be the genetic pattern that contains information that directs our becoming, the voice pattern, the movement pattern.[23] Characteristics of pattern include movement, diversity, and rhythm. Pattern is "somehow intimately involved in energy exchange and transformation."[23]

In *Health as Expanding Consciousness*, Newman developed pattern as a major concept that was used to understand the individual as a whole being. Newman described a paradigm shift that was oc-curring in the field of health care. The shift was from treatment of symptoms of a disease to the search for patterns. Newman stated that the patterns of interaction of person-environment constitute health.[23] Embedded within the concepts of movement, time, and space is the idea that an event such as a disease occurrence is part of a larger process.

"By interacting with the event, no matter how destructive the force might seem to be, its energy augments our own and enhances our power in the situation. In order to see this, it is necessary to grasp the pattern of the whole."[23]

Consciousness *Consciousness* is defined as the "informational capacity of the system: the ability of the system to interact with its environment."[23] In 1978 three correlates of consciousness (time, movement, space) were cited as explanations for the changing pattern of the whole and major concepts in the theory of health.

The life process was seen as a progression toward higher levels of consciousness.[16] "The expansion of consciousness is what life, and therefore health, is all about."[16] Newman referred to the time sense as a factor altered in the changing level of consciousness. Thus the perception of time was seen as an indicator of man's health status.[16]

Bentov defined absolute consciousness as "a state in which contrasting concepts become reconciled and fused. Movement and rest fuse into one."[1:67] The last stage of absolute consciousness is equated with love, where all opposites are reconciled and all experiences are accepted equally and unconditionally (e.g., love and hate, pain and pleasure, disease and nondisease).

Reed concurs that Newman's theory "describes the phase of evolutionary development at which the person moves beyond a focus on self as limited by time, and space and physical concerns."[43] To Newman, transcendence is a process through which the person reaches the highest level of consciousness.

MAJOR CONCEPTS & DEFINITIONS—cont'd

Movement "Movement is the means whereby one perceives reality and, therefore, is a means of becoming aware of self."[21:165] Newman[18:23] emphasized that "movement through space is integral to the development of a concept of time in man and is utilized by man as a measure of time." She maintained that "movement brings about change, without which there is no manifest reality."[19:61] To further explain this concept Newman[16:1] used the example of "the person restricted in his mobility by structural or psychological pathology [who] must adapt to an altered rate of movement."

Time and space Time and space have a complementary relationship.[19:61] "The concept of space is inextricably linked to the concept of time. . . . When one's life space is decreased, as by either physical or social immobility, one's time is increased."[16:61]

Time in Newman's model includes a sense of time perspective, that is, orientation to past, present, and future, but it centers primarily on time as perceived duration. Perceived duration is used synonymously with subjective time as defined by Bentov.[18:290-291] Newman used Bentov's conceptualization of time as an index of consciousness to demonstrate expanding consciousness across life span.

---

(3) reexamine the theoretical underpinnings in light of the findings." She believes that if health is considered an individual personal process, future research should focus on longitudinal studies to explore changes and similarities in personal meaning and patterns.

MAJOR ASSUMPTIONS

The foundation for Newman's assumptions[19:56] is her definition of health, which is grounded in Rogers's 1970 model for nursing that focuses on wholeness, person-environment, life process, pattern/organization, and man's capacity for the higher, complex processes of the mind.[19:57] From this, Newman[19:57-58] developed the following assumptions:

1. Health encompasses conditions heretofore described as illness, or in medical terms, pathology.
2. These "pathological" conditions can be considered a manifestation of the total pattern of the individual.
3. The pattern of the individual that eventually manifests itself as pathology is primary and exists prior to structural or functional changes.
4. Removal of the pathology in itself will not change the pattern of the individual.
5. If becoming "ill" is the only way an individual's

pattern can manifest itself, then that is health for that person.
6. Health is the expansion of consciousness.

Newman's implicit assumptions about human nature include being (1) different from the sum of the parts, (2) an open energy system, (3) having continuous interconnectedness with open system of universe-environment, and (4) continuously engaged in evolving their own pattern of the whole.

Newman developed her central premise and assumption, "Health is the expansion of consciousness."[16:58] The "process of unfolding consciousness will occur regardless of what we as nurses do. We can, however, assist clients in getting in touch with what is going on, and in that way facilitate the process."[23]

THEORETICAL ASSERTIONS

In *Theory Development in Nursing,* Newman delineated the relationships between movement, space, time, and consciousness. "Time and space have a complementary relationship."[19:60;21:165] Newman gave examples of this relationship at the macrocosmic, microcosmic, and humanistic (everyday) levels. She stated that at the humanistic level "the highly mobile individual lives in a world of expanded space and compartmentalized time. When one's life space is decreased, as by either physical or social immobility, one's time is increased."[19:61]

"Movement is a means whereby space and time become a reality."[19:60;21:165] Man is in a constant state of motion and is constantly changing. This occurs both internally, at the cellular level, and externally through body movement and interaction with the environment. This movement through time and space is what gives man his unique perception of reality. Movement brings change and enables the individual to experience the world around him.[19:61-63]

"Movement is a reflection of consciousness."[19:60;21:165] Movement not only is the means of experiencing reality, but it is also the means by which one expresses his thoughts and feelings about the reality he experiences. An individual conveys his awareness of self through the movement involved in language, posture, and body movement.[19:62] "The rhythm and pattern which are reflected in movement are an indication of the internal organization of the person and his perception of the world. Movement provides a means of communication beyond that which language can convey."[19:62]

"Time is a function of movement."[14:165;19:60] This assertion is supported by Newman's previous studies regarding the experience of time as related to movement and gait tempo.[17] Newman's research shows that the slower one walks, the less subjective time one experiences. When compared with clock time, however, time seems to "fly." Although the individual who is moving quickly subjectively feels he is "beating the clock," he finds when checking a clock that time seems to be dragging.[16:1;19:63]

"Time is a measure of consciousness."[19:60] This assertion was first proposed in 1977 by Bentov, who measured consciousness with a ratio of subjective to objective time. Newman applied this measure of consciousness to the subjective and objective data compiled in her research. She found that the consciousness index increased with age. Some of her most recent research has also supported the finding of increasing consciousness with age.[20:293] Newman[16:64] cited this evidence as support for her position that the life process evolves toward consciousness expansion. "However, certain moods, such as depression, may be accompanied by a diminished sense of time."[39:139]

Excellent examples were used by Newman to illustrate the centrality of space-time, one of which is included here.[23:56]

Mrs. V. made repeated attempts to *move* away from husband and to *move* into an educational program to become more independent. She felt she had no *space* for herself, and she tried to distance herself (*space*) from her husband. She felt she had no *time* for leisure (self), was overworked, and was constantly meeting other people's needs. She was submissive to the demands and criticism of her husband.

Newman stated that the crucial task "is to be able to see the concepts of movement-space-time in relation to each other, all at once, as patterns of evolving consciousness."[23:48]

In *Health as Expanding Consciousness*, Newman drew heavily on the theoretical work of Young's *The Reflexive Universe: Evolution of Consciousness.* "The central theme of Young's theory is that a self, or a universe, is of the same nature. The essential nature is undefinable, but the beginning and the end are characterized by complete freedom, unrestricted choice."[23:43]

Newman established a corollary between her model of health as expanding consciousness and Young's conception of the evolution of human beings (Fig. 32-2).

We come into being from a state of potential consciousness, are bound in time, find our identity in space, and through movement learn the "law" of the way things work and make choices that ultimately take us beyond space and time to a state of absolute consciousness.[23:46]

Since beginning the development of her theory, Newman moved from the "restrictions in movement-space-time" to an "awareness that extend[ed] beyond the physical self."[23:46] She assumed that the awareness corresponded to the "inward, self-generated reformation that Young [spoke] of as the turning point of the process."[23:46] "Progression to the sixth state (timelessness) involves increasing freedom from time."[23:46] Finally, the last stage is absolute consciousness, "which had been equated with love."[23:47]

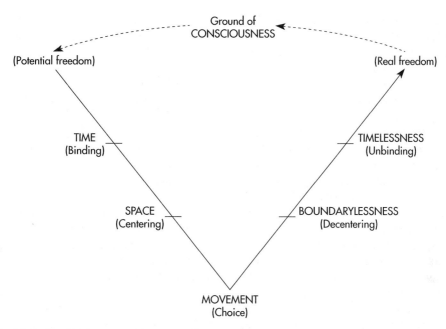

Fig. **32-2** Parallel between Newman's Theory of Expanding Consciousness and Young's stages of human evolution. *From Newman, M.A. (1990). Newman's theory of health as praxis. Nursing Science Quarterly, 1(3), 37-41. Reprinted with permission.*

LOGICAL FORM

In the early development of the theory, Newman utilized both inductive and deductive logic. Inductive logic is based on observing particular instances and then relating those instances to form a whole. Newman's Theory Development was derived from her earlier research on time perception and gait tempo. Time and movement, along with space and consciousness, are subsequently used as central components in her conceptual framework. These concepts help explain "the phenomena of the life process and therefore of health."[19:59]

While Newman started with a rational, empirical approach that was both inductive and deductive, she found it restrictive, and little by little she relinquished some of the experimental control. Her work evolved to a more interactive, integrative approach that continued to be objective and controlled. When that still did not work, she gave up the research paradigm with its objectivity and control and allowed the principles

of her theoretical paradigm to guide her research. Then she began to see the core of pattern and process as nursing practice. She saw the evolving pattern as meaning in process that required an approach of mutual process, not just objective observation. Patterns showed that expanding consciousness was related to quality and connectedness of relationships. The nurse-researcher's creative presence was important to the participant's insight. Newman concludes that it is in living a theory that we experience it. She labels her research hermeneutic dialectic because it is interpretative and uses logical examination of ideas.[26]

ACCEPTANCE BY THE NURSING COMMUNITY
Practice

In Newman's view, the responsibility of professional nursing practice is "to establish a primary relationship with the client for the purpose of identifying health care needs and facilitating the client's action potential and decision-making ability."[33:12] Communication and collaboration with other nurses, associates, and health care professionals are essential. Maintenance of a direct, ongoing relationship so long as nursing consultation and services are required is the structure of the practice. Such primary care providers focusing directly and completely relates to her view of the role of professional nursing, which Newman refers to as nursing clinician/case manager, which is the sine qua non of the integrative model.[33:12]

Relating her theory of health as expanding consciousness, and acknowledging the contemporary and radical shift in philosophy of nursing that views health as a unitary human field dynamic embedded in a larger unitary field, Newman believes that "the goal of nursing is not to make people well, or to prevent their getting sick, but to assist people to utilize the power that is within them as they evolve toward higher levels of consciousness."[19:67] She states that the task of nursing is not to try to change the pattern of another person but to recognize it as information that depicts the whole and relate to it as it unfolds.[34:13] Nursing is providing a partner in the process of expanding consciousness. The nurse's role is to connect with the person when new rules are sought. Thus, the nurse is viewed as a facilitator who assists the clients-individuals, families, or community to focus on recognizing and accepting their own patterns.

At first, Newman's Model of Health was useful in the practice of nursing because it contained concepts used by the nursing profession. Movement and time are an intrinsic part of nursing intervention such as range-of-motion and ambulation.[24] During the 1980s, Doberneck[2] used Newman's model to work with caregivers of chronically ill people. Doberneck believed Newman's model addressed issues intrinsic to caring that other theories omit, such as unconditionally being with another person and noncommitment to specific predetermined outcomes.[2]

Also during the 1980s, Marchione used Newman's model to investigate and report the meaning of disabling events in families. She presented a case study in which an additional person became part of the nuclear family for an extended period of time. The addition was a disruptive event for the family and created disturbances in time, space, movement, and consciousness. Analysis of the case study of the family suggested that Newman's work with patterns could be utilized to understand family interactions.[11]

Kalb applied Newman's Theory of Health in the clinical management of pregnant women hospitalized for complications of maternal-fetal health. The pregnant woman is the conduit through which care can be delivered to the unborn child; therefore, she becomes the choice maker for the care of the child.[7]

Gustafson found that practice as a parish nurse supported Newman's Theory of Health as demonstration of pattern recognition. Patient needs were based on effective communication and quality nursing decisions and actions by the development of pattern recognition.[6]

More recently, Endo has studied pattern recognition as nursing intervention with adults with cancer.[3] Quinn's reconceptualization of therapeutic touch describes a shared consciousness.[42] Litchfield describes the patterning of nurse-client relationships in families with frequent illnesses and hospitalization of toddlers.[10] Schubert viewed the nurse-client relationship as progressing from trusting through joining to bonding.[47] Lamb and Stempel[9] describe the role of the nurse as an insider-expert. Newman, Lamb, and Michaels describe the role of the nurse case manager at St. Mary's as emanating from a philosophical/theoretical base agreeing with the unitary-transformative paradigm and exemplifying an integrated stage of professional nursing.[40]

From the inception of Newman's theory in 1971 until the present, numerous nurse-practitioners/scientists have used the theory either to incorporate the concepts in their nursing practice or to test the theory empirically.

Newman[23] did not advocate one model as the sole basis for curriculum. Rather, students should have the opportunity to study various approaches to health and nursing and to choose what is relevant to them in their practice and research.

Newman has consulted with faculty and students from numerous universities. Graduate students at various institutions conduct research based on her theory.

Newman's Theory of Pattern Recognition provides the basis for the process of nurse-client interaction. Newman suggested that the task in intervention is pattern recognition accomplished by the health professional becoming "aware of the pattern of the other person by sensing into her/his/*own* pattern."[28] Newman suggested that the professional should focus on the pattern of the other person, in effect acting like the "reference beam in a hologram."[23:73] The holographic model of intervention is described by "imagining the emanating waves that appear when two pebbles are thrown into water. As the waves radiate . . . they meet and interact . . . [forming] an interference pattern"[23:70] (Fig. 32-3).

Newman stated that a new role is needed for the nurse to function in the paradigm of the evolving consciousness of the whole. "Nurses need to be free to relate to patients in an ongoing partnership that is not limited to a particular place or time."[23:89] Nursing education would revolve around the "concept of pattern: pattern as substance, pattern as process, and pattern as method."[23:89] Education by this method would enable nursing to be an important resource for the continued development of health care. Newman stated that nursing is at the intersection of the focus of the health care industry; thus, "nursing is in position to bring about the fluctuation within the system that will shift the system to a new higher order of functioning."[23:90]

Examining pragmatic adequacy of Newman's theory in relation to nursing education reveals that teaching the research method associated with the theory also teaches the students a practice method that is congruent with the theory. Newman sees the theory, the practice, and the research as a process rather than a separate domain of nursing discipline. Teaching the Theory of Health as expanding consciousness would necessitate a shift in thinking from the existing view of health to a newer and synthesized view that accepts disease as a manifestation of health. Not only that, learning to let go of the professional's control and respecting the client's choices are an integral part of practice within this framework. Students and practicing nurses who plan to use Newman's theory will face personal transformation in learning to recognize pattern by being participant-observer of phenomena related to health. Thus, one's personal experience will be the core of not just teaching and practice but research as well. Newman explains that the nurse would need to sense into her own pattern as an indication of the nurse-client interacting pattern.[33,34]

Research

Research has a dual role: to test theory and establish a scientific knowledge base from which to practice professional nursing. In addition to Newman, several researchers have undertaken research about time, space, or movement. Newman and Gaudiano focused on the occurrence of depression in the elderly.[39] Mentzer and Schorr used Newman's Model of Duration of time as an index to consciousness in a study of institutionalized elderly.[13]

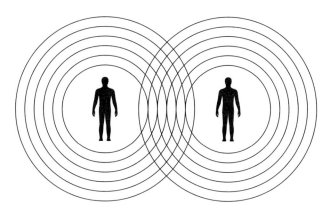

Fig. **32-3** Interaction pattern of two persons—a holographic model of intervention.
From Newman, M. (1986). Health as expanding consciousness. *St. Louis: Mosby, p. 71.*

Fryback's dissertation revealed that persons with acquired immunodeficiency syndrome/human immunodeficiency syndrome infection did describe health within physical, health promotion, and spiritual domain and thus was congruent with Newman's theory.[5] Others investigating health as expanding consciousness include Smith with rural African-American women,[48] Yamashita with Japanese family caregivers,[51] and Endo with Japanese women diagnosed with ovarian cancer.[3] Newman states that her research over time assisted not just clients who participated but also her and fellow researchers in gaining a better understanding of self as a nurse-researcher and understanding the limitations of previous methods used.

Newman stated that research should center around "participatory investigations in which subjects (clients) are our partners, our coresearchers, in our search for health patterns."[23:94] This method of inquiry is called *cooperative inquiry* or *interactive, integrative participation*. Newman moved her research method toward this coinvestigatory method in recent research involving a community investigation.[23:95] Newman investigated a method to describe pattern as unfolding and evolving over time.[27,28] She utilized the method of interviewing a subject in different time frames to establish a pattern for that subject.[25] Newman stated that during the development of a methodology to test the theory of health "sharing our (researcher's) perception of the person's pattern with the person was meaningful to the participants and stimulated new insights in our own lives."[30:37] The process made a difference in the researchers' lives as well as the participants' lives. Newman asserted that the research process was also nursing practice. "And it was fun."[30:37] More recently, she has stipulated a protocol for the research and has labeled it "hermeneutic dialectic."

FURTHER DEVELOPMENT

Newman reported that operationalization of the model of health as expanding consciousness has been approached in two ways: (1) by research methods designed to describe and test the relationships between the major concepts of movement, time, space, and consciousness and (2) by attempts to describe evolving patterns of consciousness in terms of the integration of movement-space-time.[23:48] Schorr and others have studied relationships between key concepts.

Health patterns in 60 aging women were investigated using the Theory of Health as the theoretical framework. The phenomenon of powerlessness was assumed to be operative for the subjects but was rejected in favor of high levels of perceived situational control or powerfulness. The results supported Newman's model of health as expanding consciousness.[44]

Schorr and Schroeder[45,46] studied differences in consciousness with regard to time and movement, with results supporting the concept of expanding consciousness.[46] In another study by Schorr and Schroeder, relationships among type A behavior, temporal orientation, and death anxiety were examined as manifestations of consciousness, with mixed results.[45]

Newman's work stresses concept of pattern recognition, of "grasping the whole in order for the parts to be meaningful."[18:36] A number of studies that address research within the Newman theoretical framework have been conducted. Moch[14] described the experiences of 20 women with breast cancer. Through pattern analyses of the person environment based on the NANDA taxonomy I dimensions, themes developed that were consistent with health as expanding consciousness.

Newman and Moch[41] studied the life patterns of 11 clients in a cardiac rehabilitation center. The objectives of the study were to "describe the individual patterns of interaction of persons with coronary heart disease, to discern similarities and differences among the individual patterns, and to interpret these findings in terms of the conceptual congruence of the overall pattern with the theory of health as expanding consciousness."[41:161] The results identified similar patterns of emerging consciousness for the participants, thus supporting the Theory of Health.

More recent studies of pattern include Endo,[3] Litchfield,[10] Newman and Moch,[41] Smith,[48] and Yamashita.[51]

Newman's work has evolved from the testing of time, movement, and consciousness through identification of sequential patterns of person-environment to recognition of the integrality of nurse-client dialogue in the client's evolving insight and actions. Once again, the original concepts of movement-time-space are seen as dimensions in the unitary patterns of consciousness as the theory development continues.

CRITIQUE

Clarity

Semantic clarity is evident in the definitions, descriptions, and dimensions of the concepts of the theory. Clarity is needed regarding movement as a concept or dimension.

Simplicity

In Newman's *Theory Development in Nursing,* the concepts of movement, time, space, and consciousness with the five resulting relationship statements represented the evolution of the theory at that time. In *Health as Expanding Consciousness,* pattern became a major concept included for the purpose of understanding consciousness. Simplicity was sacrificed when pattern of the whole was used to describe the Theory of Health. The theory is unitary in terms of pattern.

The deeper meaning of the Theory of Health as expanding consciousness is complex. The theory as a whole must be understood—not the isolated concepts. If one wanted to use a positivist approach, Newman's original propositions would serve as guides for hypothesis development. However, researchers who have tried that have concluded that that approach is inadequate to study the theory. As Newman has advocated in the 1994 edition of her book, the holistic approach of the hermeneutic dialectic method is consistent with the theory and requires a high level of understanding of the theory on the part of the researcher to extend the theory in praxis research.[37]

Generality

The concepts in Newman's theory are broad in scope because they all relate to health. This renders her the-ory generalizable. The broad scope provides a focus for future theory development.

Empirical Precision

In the early stages of development aspects of the theory have been operationalized and tested within a traditional scientific mode. However, quantitative methods are inadequate in capturing the dynamic, changing nature of this model. A hermeneutic dialectic approach is being developed for a full explication of its meaning and application.

Derivable Consequences

The focus of Newman's Theory of Health as Expanding Consciousness provides an evolving guide for all health-related disciplines. In the quest for understanding the phenomenon of health, this unique view of health challenges us to make a difference in nursing practice by the application of this theory.

CRITICAL THINKING *Activities*

1 What is the world view of nursing? What is the nurse-scientist view of nursing?

2 How does that world view dictate or direct knowledge development for nursing?

3 What dictates the change in paradigms of health, health care practice, and nursing practice? Examine Newman's view about it.

4 How is the process of "health as expanding consciousness" different from the process of self-actualization? Compare and contrast the characteristics of both processes/phenomena.

5 Where and how does Newman accept or depart from the Rogerian "unitary man" theory?

6 How does Newman relate her Theory of Health with contemporary and future nursing practice, education, and research?

7 How do you agree or disagree with her claims and explanations regarding relatedness

of her theory with the pragmatic expectations of the nursing profession?

REFERENCES

1. Bentov, I. (1977). *Stalking the wild pendulum.* New York: E.P. Dutton.
2. Doberneck, B. (1985). Graduate student at Pennsylvania State University. Telephone interview.
3. Endo, E. (1996). *Pattern recognition as a nursing intervention with adults with cancer.* Doctoral dissertation, University of Minnesota.
4. Engle, V. (1986). The relationship of movement and time to older adults' functional health. *Research in Nursing and Health, 9,* 123-129.
5. Fryback, P.B. (1991). Perceptions of health by persons with a terminal disease: Implications for nursing. *Dissertation Abstracts International, 52,* 1951B.
6. Gustafson, W. (1990). Application of Newman's theory of health: Pattern recognition as nursing practice. In M. Parker (Ed.), *Nursing theories in practice* (pp. 141-161). New York: National League for Nursing.
7. Kalb, K.A. (1990). The gift: Applying Newman's theory of health in nursing practice. In M. Parker (Ed.), *Nursing theories in practice* (pp. 163-186). New York: National League for Nursing.
8. Kim, H.S. (1983). *The nature of theoretical thinking in nursing.* Norwalk, CT: Appleton-Century-Crofts.
9. Lamb, G.S., & Stempel, J.E. (1994). Nurse case management from the client's view: Growing as insider-expert. *Nursing Outlook, 42,* 7-13.
10. Litchfield, M.C. (1993). The process of health patterning in families with young children who have been repeatedly hospitalized. Master's thesis, University of Minnesota.
11. Marchione, J. (1985). Associate professor, University of Akron. Telephone interview.
12. Marchione, J.M. (1986). Pattern as methodology for assessing family health: Newman's theory of health. In P. Winstead-Fry (Ed.), *Case studies in nursing theory.* New York: National League for Nursing.
13. Mentzer, C., & Schorr, J.A. (1986). Perceived situational control and perceived duration of time: Expressions of life patterns. *Advances in Nursing Science, 9*(1), 13-20.
14. Moch, S.D. (1990). Health within the experience of breast cancer. *Journal of Advanced Nursing, 15,* 1426-1435.
15. Moss, R. (1981). *The I that is we.* Millbrae, CA: Celestial Arts.
16. Newman, M.A. (1971). *An investigation of the relationship between gait tempo and time perception.* Unpublished doctoral dissertation, New York University.
17. Newman, M.A. (1972). Time estimation in relation to gait tempo. *Perceptual and Motor Skills, 34,* 359-366.
18. Newman, M.A. (1978). *Second Annual Nurse Educator's Conference.* Held in New York City, December 4-6, 1978. (Audiotape).
19. Newman, M.A. (1979). *Theory development in nursing.* Philadelphia: F.A. Davis.
20. Newman, M.A. (1982, Sept.-Oct.). Time as an index of expanding consciousness with age. *Nursing Research, 31,* 290-293.
21. Newman, M.A. (1983). Newman's health theory. In I.W. Clements & F.B. Roberts, *Family health: A theoretical approach to nursing care.* New York: John Wiley & Sons.
22. Newman, M.A. (1985). Telephone interview.
23. Newman, M.A. (1986). *Health as expanding consciousness.* St. Louis: Mosby.
24. Newman, M.A. (1987). Aging as increasing complexity. *Journal of Gerontological Nursing, 13*(9), 16-18.
25. Newman, M.A. (1987). Patterning. In M. Duffy & N.J. Pender (Eds.), *Conceptual issues in health promotion, a report of proceedings of a Wingspread conference,* Racine, WI, April 13-15, 1987. Indianapolis: Sigma Theta Tau.
26. Newman, M.A. (1988). Personal correspondence.
27. Newman, M.A. (1989). The spirit of nursing. *Holistic Nursing Practice, 3*(3), 1-6.
28. Newman, M.A. (1990). Newman's theory of health as praxis. *Nursing Science Quarterly, 3,* 37-41.
29. Newman, M.A. (1990). Shifting to higher consciousness. In M. Parker (Ed.), *Nursing theories in practice* (pp. 129-139). New York: National League for Nursing.
30. Newman, M.A. (1991). Health conceptualizations. In J.J. Fitzpatrick, R.L. Taunton, & A.K. Jacox (Eds.), *Annual review of nursing research* (Vol. 9). New York: Springer.
31. Newman, M.A. (1992). Curriculum vitae.
32. Newman, M.A. (1992). Nightingale's vision of nursing theory and health. In Nightingale, F., *Notes on nursing: What it is, and what it is not* (Commemorative edition, pp. 44-47). Philadelphia: Lippincott. (Original work published in 1958.)
33. Newman, M.A. (1994). *Health as expanding consciousness.* New York: National League for Nursing Press.
34. Newman, M.A. (1995). *A developing discipline: Selected works of Margaret Newman.* New York: National League for Nursing Press.
35. Newman, M.A. (1996). Curriculum vitae.
36. Newman, M.A. (1996). Personal correspondence.
37. Newman, M.A. (1996). Telephone interviews.
38. Newman, M.A., & Autio, S. (1986). *Nursing in a prospective payment system health care environment.* Minneapolis: University of Minnesota.
39. Newman, M.A., & Guadiano, J.K. (1984). Depression as an explanation for decreased subjective time in the elderly. *Nursing Research, 33,* 137-139.
40. Newman, M.A., Lamb, G.S., & Michaels, C. (1991). Nurse case management: The coming together of theory and practice. *Nursing & Health Care, 12*(8), 404-408.
41. Newman, M.A., & Moch, S.D. (1991). Life patterns of persons with coronary heart disease. *Nursing Science Quarterly, 4,* 161-167.

42. Quinn, J.F. (1992). Holding sacred space: The nurse as healing environment. *Holistic Nursing Practice, 6*(4), 26-36.

43. Reed, P.G. (1996, Spring). Transcendence: Formulating nursing perspectives. *Nursing Science Quarterly, 9*(1), 2-4.

44. Schorr, J.A., Farnham, R.C., & Ervin, S.M. (1991). Health patterns in aging women as expanding consciousness. *Advances in Nursing Science, 13*(4), 52-63.

45. Schorr, J.A., & Schroeder, C.A. (1989). Consciousness as a dissipative structure: An extension of the Newman model. *Nursing Science Quarterly, 2*, 183-193.

46. Schorr, J.A., & Schroeder, C.A. (1991). Movement and time: Exertion and perceived duration. *Nursing Science Quarterly, 4*, 104-112.

47. Schubert, P.E. (1989). *Mutual connectedness: Holistic nursing practice under varying conditions of intimacy.* Doctoral dissertation, University of California, San Francisco.

48. Smith, C.A. (1995). The lived experience of staying healthy in rural African American families. *Nursing Science Quarterly, 8*(1), 17-21.

49. Who's who of American women. (1983-1984). Chicago: Marquis.

50. Whyte, L.L. (1974). *The universe of experience.* New York: Harper & Row.

51. Yamashita, M. (1995). *Family coping with mental illness: An application of Newman's research as praxis.* Paper presented at the Midwest Nursing Research Society 19th Annual Conference, Kansas City, MO.

BIBLIOGRAPHY

Primary sources

Books

Downs, F.S., & Newman, M.A. (Eds.). (1973). *A source book of nursing research.* Philadelphia: F.A. Davis.

Downs, F.S., & Newman, M.A. (Eds.). (1977). *A source book of nursing research.* Philadelphia: F.A. Davis.

Newman, M.A. (1979). *Theory development in nursing.* Philadelphia: F.A. Davis. (Japanese rights assigned to Gendasha Publishing Company, Tokyo, 1986.)

Newman, M.A. (1986). *Health as expanding consciousness.* St. Louis: Mosby. (Japanese translation, 1995; Korean translation, 1996.)

Newman, M.A. (1994). *Health as expanding consciousness* (2nd ed.). New York: National League for Nursing Press.

Newman, M.A. (1995). *A developing discipline: Selected work of Margaret Newman.* New York: National League for Nursing Press.

Newman, M.A., & Autio, S. (1986). *Nursing in a prospective payment system health care environment.* Minneapolis: University of Minnesota.

Book chapters

Downs, F.S., & Newman, M.A. (1977). Elements of a research critique. In F.S. Downs & M.A. Newman (Eds.), *A source book of nursing research* (2nd ed.) (pp. 1-12). Philadelphia: F.A. Davis.

Field, L., & Newman, M.A. (1982). Clinical application of the unitary man framework: Case study analysis. In M.J. Kim & D.A. Morita (Eds.), *Classification of nursing diagnosis* (pp. 249-263). New York: McGraw-Hill.

Newman, M.A. (1973). Identifying patient needs in short-span nurse-patient relationships. In M.E. Auld & L.H. Birum (Eds.), *The challenge of nursing* (pp. 98-103). St. Louis: Mosby.

Newman, M.A. (1981). The meaning of health. In G.E. Laskar (Ed.), *Applied systems research and cybernetics:* Vol. 4. *Systems research in health care, biocybernetics and ecology* (pp. 1739-1743). New York: Pergamon.

Newman, M.A. (1983). The continuing revolution: A history of nursing science. In N.L. Chaska (Ed.), *The nursing profession: A time to speak* (pp. 385-393). New York: McGraw-Hill.

Newman, M.A. (1983). Health as expanding consciousness. In *Proceedings of Seventh International Conference on Human Functioning.* Wichita, KS: Biomedical Synergistics Institute.

Newman, M.A. (1983). Newman's health theory. In I. Clements & F. Roberts (Eds.), *Family health: A theoretical approach to nursing care* (pp. 161-175). New York: John Wiley & Sons.

Newman, M.A. (1983). Nursing's theoretical evolution. In T. A. Duespohol (Ed.), *Nursing in transition* (pp. 15-24). Rockville, MD: Aspen Systems.

Newman, M.A. (1986). Nursing's theoretical evolution. In L.H. Nicoll (Ed.), *Perspectives on nursing theory* (pp. 72-78). Boston: Little, Brown.

Newman, M.A. (1987). Nursing's emerging paradigm: The diagnosis of pattern. In A.M. McLane (Ed.), *Classification of nursing diagnoses,* Proceedings of the Seventh Conference, North American Nursing Diagnosis Association (pp. 53-60). St. Louis: Mosby.

Newman, M.A. (1987). Patterning. In M. Duffy & N.J. Pender (Eds.), *Conceptual issues in health promotion: A report of proceedings of a Wingspread conference,* Racine, WI: Indianapolis: Sigma Theta Tau.

Newman, M.A. (1990). Nursing paradigms and realities. In N.L. Chaska (Ed.), *The nursing profession: Turning points* (pp. 230-235). St. Louis: Mosby.

Newman, M.A. (1990). Professionalism: Myth or reality. In N.L. Chaska (Ed.), *The nursing profession: Turning points* (pp. 49-52). St. Louis: Mosby.

Newman, M.A. (1990). Shifting to higher consciousness. In M. Parker (Ed.), *Nursing theories in practice* (pp. 129-139). New York: National League for Nursing.

Newman, M.A. (1992). Nightingale's vision of nursing theory and health. In F. Nightingale, *Notes on nursing: What it is, and what it is not* (Commemorative edition, pp. 44-47). Philadelphia: Lippincott. (Original work published in 1958.)

Newman, M.A. (1996). Prevailing paradigms in nursing. In J.W. Kenney (Ed.), *Philosophical and theoretical perspectives for advanced nursing practice* (pp. 302-307). Sudbury, MA: Jones and Bartlett.

Newman, M.A. (1996). Theory of the nurse-client partnership. In E. Cohen (Ed.), *Nurse case management in the 21st century* (pp. 119-123). St. Louis: Mosby.

Newman, M.A., Sime, A.M., & Corcoran-Perry, S.A. (1996). The focus of the discipline of nursing. In J.W. Kenney (Ed.), *Philosophical and theoretical perspectives for advanced nursing practice* (pp. 297-301). Sudbury, MA: Jones and Bartlett.

Roy, C., Rogers, M.E., Fitzpatrick, J.J., Newman, M., & Orem, D.E. (1982). Nursing diagnosis and nursing theory. In M.J. Kim & D.A. Moritz (Eds.), *Classification of nursing diagnosis* (pp. 215-231). New York: McGraw-Hill.

Journal articles

Allender, C.D., Egan, E.C., & Newman, M.A. (1995). An instrument for measuring differentiated nursing practice. *Nursing Management 26*(4), 42-44.

Butrin, J., & Newman, M.A. (1986). Health promotion in Zaire: Time perspective and cerebral hemispheric dominance as relevant factors. *Public Health Nursing, 3*(3), 183-191.

Lamendola, F., & Newman, M.A. (1994). The paradox of HIV/AIDS as expanding consciousness. *Advances in Nursing Science, 16*(3), 13-21.

Newman, M.A. (1966). Identifying and meeting patients' needs in short-span nurse-patient relationships. *Nursing Forum, 5,* 76-86.

Newman, M.A. (1972). Time estimation in relation to gait tempo. *Perceptual and Motor Skills, 34,* 359-366.

Newman, M.A. (1972, July). Nursing's theoretical evolution. *Nursing Outlook, 20,* 449-453.

Newman, M.A. (1975, Nov.). The professional doctorate in nursing: A position paper. *Nursing Outlook, 23,* 704-706.

Newman, M.A. (1976, Aug.). Movement, tempo, and the experience of time. *Nursing Research, 25,* 273-279.

Newman, M.A. (1982, Sept.-Oct.). Time as an index of expanding consciousness with age. *Nursing Research, 31,* 290-293.

Newman, M.A. (1982, Oct.). What differentiates clinical research? *Image, 14,* 86-88.

Newman, M.A. (1983). Editorial. *Advances in Nursing Science, 5,* x-xi.

Newman, M.A. (1984, Dec.). Nursing diagnosis: Looking at the whole. *American Journal of Nursing, 84*(12), 1496-1499.

Newman, M.A. (1984). {Review of *Annual review of nursing research,* Vol. I, 1983}. *American Journal of Nursing, 84,* 1437-1438.

Newman, M.A. (1987). Aging as increasing complexity. *Journal of Gerontological Nursing, 13*(9), 16-18.

Newman, M.A. (1987). Commentary: Perception of time among Japanese inpatients. *Western Journal of Nursing Research, 9*(3), 299-300.

Newman, M.A. (1989). The spirit of nursing. *Holistic Nursing Practice, 3*(3), 1-6.

Newman, M.A. (1990). Newman's theory of health as praxis. *Nursing Science Quarterly, 3,* 37-41.

Newman, M.A. (1990). Toward an integrative model of professional practice. *Journal of Professional Nursing, 6,* 167-173.

Newman, M.A. (1991). Commentary: Research as practice. *Nursing Science Quarterly, 4*(3), 100-101.

Newman, M.A. (1991). Health conceptualizations. *Annual Review of Nursing Research, 9,* 221-243.

Newman, M.A. (1991). Health conceptualizations. In Fitzpatrick, J.J., Taunton, R.L, & Jacox, A.K. (Eds.), *Annual Review of Nursing Research* (Vol. 9). New York: Springer.

Newman, M.A. (1991). Life patterns of persons with coronary heart disease. *Nursing Science Quarterly, 4*(4), 161-167.

Newman, M.A. (1992). Prevailing paradigms in nursing. *Nursing Outlook, 40*(1), 10-13, 32.

Newman, M.A. (1994). Into the 21st century. *Nursing Science Quarterly, 7*(1), 44-46.

Newman, M.A. (1994). Theory for nursing practice. *Nursing Science Quarterly, 7*(4), 153-157.

Newman, M.A., & Gaudiano, J.K. (1984, May-June). Depression as an explanation for decreased subjective time in the elderly. *Nursing Research, 33,* 137-139.

Newman, M.A., Lamb, G.S., & Michaels, C. (1991). Nurse case management: The coming together of theory and practice. *Nursing & Health Care, 12*(8), 404-408.

Newman, M.A., & Moch, S.D. (1991). Life patterns of persons with coronary heart disease. *Nursing Science Quarterly, 4,* 161-167.

Newman, M.A., & O'Brien, R.A. (1978, Feb.). Experiencing the research process via computer simulation. *Image, 10,* 5-9.

Newman, M.A., Sime, A.M., & Corcoran-Perry, S.A. (1991). The focus of the discipline of nursing. *Advances in Nursing Science, 14*(1), 1-6.

Portonova, M., Young, E., & Newman, M.A. (1984). Elderly women's attitudes toward sexual activity among their peers. *Health Care for Women, International, 5*(5/6), 289-298.

Dissertation

Newman, M.A. (1971). An investigation of the relationship between gait tempo and time perception. Unpublished doctoral dissertation, New York University, School of Education.

Reports

Newman, M.A. (1977). Nursing course content in doctoral education. *Proceedings of National Conference on Doctoral Education in Nursing.* Philadelphia: University of Pennsylvania.

Newman, M.A. (1982). What differentiates clinical research? *Proceedings of the Second Phyllis J. Verhonick Nursing Research Course.* Washington, DC: Nursing Research Service, Walter Reed Army Medical Center.

Newman, M.A. (1984). Health as expanding consciousness. *Proceedings of the Third Phyllis J. Verhonick Nursing Research Course.* Washington, DC: Nursing Research Service, Walter Reed Army Medical Center.

Newman, M.A. (1985). Health as expanding consciousness. *Proceedings of Ninth National Forum of Doctoral Education in Nursing.* Birmingham, AL: University of Alabama School of Nursing.

Newman, M.A. (1991). [Review of Barrett, E.A.M. (Ed.), *Visions of Rogers' science-based nursing*]. *Nursing Science Quarterly, 4*(1), 41-42.

Newman, M.A. (1991). [Review of Lowenberg, J.S., *Caring and responsibility: The crossroads between holistic practice and traditional medicine.*] *Journal of Professional Nursing, 7*(5), 319-320.

Newman, M., & Autio, S. (1986). Nursing in the world of DRGs and prospective payment. *CURA Reporter* (Published by University of Minnesota Center for Urban and Regional Affairs), *16*(5), 1-7.

Newman, M.A., & Gaudiano, J.K. (1983). Depression as an explanation for decreased subjective time in the elderly. In M.C. Smith (Ed.), *Proceedings of the Second Annual Research Conference of the Southern Council on Collegiate Education in Nursing.*

Newman, M.A., Tompkins, E.S., Isenberg, M.A., Fitzpatrick, J.J., & Scott, D.W. (1980). Movement, time and consciousness: Parameters of health (Symposium). *Proceedings of Western Society for Research in Nursing Research, 13,* 45-49.

Audiotapes

Newman, M.A. (1978, Dec. 4-6). Paper presented at Second Annual Conference, New York City. Tapes available from Teach 'em Inc., 160 E. Illinois Street, Chicago, IL 60611.

Newman, M.A. (1984, May). Paper presented at Nursing Theory Conference, Boyle, Letourneau Conference, Edmonton, Canada. Tapes available from Ed Kennedy, Kennedy Recording, R.R. 5, Edmonton, Alberta, Canada T5P 4B7 (403-470-0013).

Videotape

Margaret Newman, nurse theorists: Portraits of excellence (1990). Produced by Helene Fuld Health Trust. A Studio Three Production. Oakland, CA.

Correspondence

Newman, M.A. (1984). Personal correspondence.
Newman, M.A. (1985). Personal correspondence.
Newman, M.A. (1988). Personal correspondence.
Newman, M.A. (1992). Personal correspondence.
Newman, M.A. (1996). Personal correspondence.

Interview

Newman, M.A. (1985). Telephone interview.
Newman, M.A. (1996). Telephone interview.

Secondary sources

Book reviews

Newman, M.A. (1980). *Theory development in nursing.*
  Continuing Education in Nursing, 2, 8+, Nov.-Dec. 1979.
  Nursing Administration Quarterly, 4, 81-82, Spring, 1980.
  Nursing Leadership, 3, 38, March, 1980.
  Nursing Research, 29, 311, Sept.-Oct., 1980.
  Western Journal of Nursing Research, 2, 250-251, Spring, 1980.

Newman, M.A. (1994). *Health as expanding consciousness.*
  Journal of Advanced Nursing, 21(2), February 1992.
  Image: Journal of Nursing Scholarship, 27(2), Summer, 1995.

Books

Chinn, P.L., & Kramer, M.K. (1995). *Theory and nursing: A systematic approach* (4th ed.). St. Louis: Mosby.

Fawcett, J. (1993). *Analysis and evaluation of nursing theories.* Philadelphia: F.A. Davis.

Kim, H.S. (1983). *The nature of theoretical thinking in nursing.* Norwalk, CT: Appleton-Century-Crofts.

Marchione, J. (1993). *Margaret Newman: Health as expanding consciousness.* Newbury Park, CA: Sage.

Meleis, A.J. (1991). *Theoretical nursing: Development and progress* (2nd ed.). Philadelphia: Lippincott.

Who's who of American women (1983-1985). Chicago: Marquis Who's Who.

Who's who in America. (1996).

Book chapters

Burd, C. (1985). Appendix D. Newman's nursing theory of health. In B.W. Duldt & K. Geffin, *Theoretical perspectives for nursing.* Boston: Little, Brown.

Chinn, P.L. (1983). Nursing theory development: Where we have been and where we are going. In N.L. Chaska (Ed.), *The nursing profession: A time to speak.* New York: McGraw-Hill.

Engle, V. (1983). Newman's model of health. In J.J. Fitzpatrick & A.L. Whall (Eds.), *Conceptual models of nursing: Analysis and application* (pp. 263-273). Bowie, MD: Robert J. Brady.

George, J.B. (1990). Other extant theory. In J.B. George (Ed.), *Nursing theories* (3rd ed.) (pp. 373-379). Norwalk, CT: Appleton & Lange.

Gustafson, W. (1990). Application of Newman's theory of health: Pattern recognition as nursing practice. In M. Parker (Ed.), *Nursing theories in practice* (pp. 141-161). New York: National League for Nursing.

Hichman, J.S. (1995). An introduction to nursing theory. In George, J.B. (1995, 4th ed.). *Nursing theories. The base for professional nursing practice* (pp. 1-12). Norwalk, CT: Appleton & Lange.

Kalb, K.A. (1990). The gift: Applying Newman's theory of health in nursing practice. In M. Parker (Ed.), *Nursing theories in practice* (pp. 163-186). New York: National League for Nursing.

Marchione, J.M. (1986). Pattern as methodology for assessing family health: Newman's theory of health. In P. Winstead-Fry (Ed.), *Case studies in nursing theory.* New York: National League for Nursing.

Journal articles

Batra, C. (1987). Nursing theory for undergraduates. *Nursing Outlook, 35*(4), 189-192.

Bramlett, M.H., Gueldner, S.H., & Sowell, R.L. (1990). Consumer-centric advocacy: Its connection to nursing frameworks. *Nursing Science Quarterly, 3,* 156-161.

Boyd, C.O. (1990). Critical appraisal of developing nursing research methods. *Nursing Science Quarterly, 3,* 42-43.

Cull-Wilby, B.L., & Pepin, J.I. (1987). Towards a coexistence of paradigms in nursing knowledge development. *Journal of Advanced Nursing, 12,* 515-521.

DeGrott, H.A., Ferketich, S.L., & Larson, P.J. (1987). Theory development in a non-university service setting. *Journal of Nursing Administration, 17*(4), 38-44.

Doherty, W.J. (1985). Family interventions in health care. *Family Relations, 34,* 129-137.

Engle, V.F. (1984, Oct.). Newman's conceptual framework and the measurement of older adults' health. *Advances in Nursing Science, 7*(1), 24-36.

Engle, V.F. (1986). The relationship of movement and time to older adults' functional health. *Research in Nursing and Health, 9,* 123-129.

Engle, V.F., & Graney, M.J. (1985-86). Self-assessed and functional health of older women. *International Journal of Aging and Human Development, 22*(4), 301-313.

Gulick, E.E., & Bugg, A. (1992). Holistic health patterning in multiple sclerosis. *Research in Nursing and Health, 15,* 175-185.

Gupta, S., & Cummings, L.L. (1986). Perceived speed of time and task affect. *Perceptual and Motor Skills, 63,* 971-980.

Jennings, B.M. (1987). Nursing theory development: Successes and challenges. *Journal of Advanced Nursing, 12,* 63-69.

Keene, L. (1985). Nursing as a partnership. *New Zealand Nursing Journal, 78*(12), 10-11.

Meleis, A.I. (1990). Being and becoming healthy: The core of nursing knowledge. *Nursing Science Quarterly, 3,* 107-114.

Mentzer, C.A., & Schorr, J.A. (1986). Perceived situational control and perceived duration of time: Expressions of life patterns. *Advances in Nursing Science, 9*(1), 12-20.

Mitchell, G.J., & Cody, W.K. (1992). Nursing knowledge and human science: Ontological and epistemological considerations. *Nursing Science Quarterly, 5,* 54-61.

Moccia, P. (1985). A further investigation of "dialectical thinking as a means of understanding systems-in-development: Relevance to Rogers's principles." *Advances in Nursing Science, 7*(4), 33-38.

Moch, S.D. (1990). Health within the experience of breast cancer. *Journal of Advanced Nursing, 15,* 1426-1435.

Peplau, H.E. (1988). The art and science of nursing: Similarities, differences, and relations. *Nursing Science Quarterly, 1*(1), 8-15.

Pridham, K.F., & Hansen, M.F. (1985). Nursing and medicine: Complementary modes of thought and action. *Public Health Nursing, 2*(4), 195-201.

Ray, M.A. (1990). Critical reflective analysis of Parse's and Newman's research methodologies. *Nursing Science Quarterly, 3,* 44-46.

Reed, P.G. (1986). Developmental resources and depression in the elderly. *Nursing Research, 35*(6), 368-374.

Rosenbaum, J.N. (1986). Comparison of two theorists on care: Orem and Leininger. *Journal of Advanced Nursing, 11,* 409-419.

Roy, C. (1979, March-April). Relating nursing theory to education: A new era. *Nurse Educator, 29,* 16-21.

Sanders, S.A. (1986). Development of a tool to measure subjective time experience. *Nursing Research, 35*(3), 178-182.

Sarter, B. (1987). Evolutionary idealism: A philosophical foundation for holistic nursing theory. *Advances in Nursing Science, 9*(2), 1-9.

Sarter, B. (1988). Philosophical sources of nursing theory. *Nursing Science Quarterly, 1,* 52-60.

Schorr, J.A., Farnham, R.C., & Ervin, S.M. (1991). Health patterns in aging women as expanding consciousness. *Advances in Nursing Science, 13*(4), 52-63.

Schorr, J.A., & Schroeder, C.A. (1989). Consciousness as a dissipative structure: An extension of the Newman model. *Nursing Science Quarterly, 2,* 183-193.

Schorr, J.A., & Schroeder, C.A. (1991). Movement and time: Exertion and perceived duration. *Nursing Science Quarterly, 4,* 104-112.

Shah, S.K., Harasymiw, S.J., & Stahl, P.L. (1986). Stroke rehabilitation: Outcome based on Brunnstrom recovery stages. *Occupational Therapy Journal of Research, 6*(6), 365-376.

Silva, M.C. (1986). Research testing nursing theory: State of the art. *Advances in Nursing Science, 9*(1), 1-11.

Silva, M.C., & Rothbart, D. (1984). An analysis of changing trends in philosophies of science on nursing theory development and testing. *Advances in Nursing Science, 6,* 1-13.

Smith, M.J. (1984). Temporal experience and bed rest: Replication and refinement. *Nursing Research, 33*(5), 298-302.

Tompkins, E. (1980, Nov.-Dec.). Effect of restricted mobility and dominance in perceived duration. *Nursing Research, 29*(6), 333-338.

Whall, A.L. (1986). The family as the unit of care in nursing: A historical review. *Public Health Nursing, 3*(4), 240-249.

News releases

Brown, N.M. (1983, Nov.). The body is not a machine. *Research/Penn State 4*(4), 19-20.

M.A. Newman appointed as full tenured professor at University of Minnesota School of Nursing (1984, March). *Nursing Outlook, 32,* 2.

Abstract

Newman, M.A. (1981). Relationship of age to perceived duration. *Abstracts of ANF funded research 1979-1980*. Kansas City: American Nurses' Foundation.

Dissertations

Brenner, P.S. (1987). Temporal perspective, professional identity, and perceived well-being. *Dissertation Abstracts International, 47,* 4821B.

Burritt, J.E. (1988). The effects of perceived social support on the relationship between job stress and job satisfaction and job performance among registered nurses employed in acute care facilities. *Dissertation Abstracts International, 49,* 2123B.

Butrin, J.E. (1990). The experience of culturally diverse nurse-client encounters. *Dissertation Abstracts International, 51,* 2815B.

Capers, C.F. (1987). Perceptions of problematic behavior as held by lay black adults and registered nurses. *Dissertation Abstracts International, 47,* 4467B.

Collins, A.S. (1992). Effects of positional changes on selected physiological and psychological measurements in clients with atrial fibrillation. *Dissertation Abstracts International, 53,* 200B.

DeBrun, K.T. (1989). An investigation of the relationships among standing, sitting, recumbent postures, judgment of time duration and preferred personal space in adult females. *Dissertation Abstracts International, 50,* 122B.

Endo, E. (1996). *Pattern recognition as a nursing intervention with adults with cancer.* Ph.D. dissertation, University of Minnesota.

Engle, V.F. (1981). A study of the relationship between self-assessment of health, function, personal tempo, and time perception in elderly women. *Dissertation Abstracts International, 42,* 967B.

Flannery, J.C. (1988). Validity and reliability of levels of cognitive functioning assessment scale for adults with closed head injuries. *Dissertation Abstracts International, 48,* 3248B.

Fryback, P.B. (1991). Perceptions of health by persons with a terminal disease: Implications for nursing. *Dissertation Abstracts International, 52,* 1951B.

Fulton, B.J. (1993). Evaluation of the effectiveness of the Neuman systems model as a theoretical framework for baccalaureate nursing programs. *Dissertation Abstracts International, 53,* 5641B.

Goble, D.S. (1991). A curriculum framework for the prevention of child sexual abuse. *Dissertation Abstracts International, 52,* 2004A.

Harbin, P.D.O. (1990). A Q-analysis of the stressors of adult female nursing students enrolled in baccalaureate schools of nursing. *Dissertation Abstracts International, 50,* 3919B.

Heaman, D.J. (1992). Perceived stressors and coping strategies of parents with developmentally disabled children. *Dissertation Abstracts International, 52,* 6316B.

Jonsdottir, H. (1995). *Life patterns of people with chronic obstructive pulmonary disease: isolation and being close in.* Ph.D. dissertation, University of Minnesota.

Kelley, F.J. (1990). Spatial temporal experiences and self-assessed health in the older adult. *Dissertation Abstracts International, 51,* 1194B.

Lancaster, D.R.N. (1992). Coping with appraised threat of breast cancer: Primary prevention coping behaviors utilized by women at increased risk. *Dissertation Abstracts International, 53,* 202B.

Leners, D.W. (1990). The deep connection: an echo of transpersonal caring. *Dissertation Abstracts International, 51,* 2818B.

McDaniel, G.M.S. (1990). The effects of two methods of dangling on heart rate and blood pressure in postoperative abdominal hysterectomy patients. *Dissertation Abstracts International, 50,* 3923B.

Moch, S.D. (1989). Health in illness: Experiences with breast cancer. *Dissertation Abstracts International, 50,* 497B.

Moody, N.B. (1991). Selected demographic variables, organizational characteristics, role orientation, and job satisfaction among nurse faculty. *Dissertation Abstracts International, 52,* 1356B.

Norman, S.E. (1991). The relationship between hardiness and sleep disturbances in HIV-infected men. *Dissertation Abstracts International, 51,* 4780B.

Norris, E.W. (1990). Physiologic response to exercise in clients with mitral valve prolapse syndrome. *Dissertation Abstracts International, 50,* 5549B.

Noveletsky-Rosenthal, H.T. (1996). *Pattern recognition in older adults living with chronic illness.* Ph.D. dissertation, Boston College.

Page, G. (1989). An exploration of the relationship between daily patterning and weight loss maintenance. *Dissertation Abstracts International, 50,* 497B.

Peoples, L.T. (1991). The relationship between selected client, provider, and agency variables and the utilization of home care services. *Dissertation Abstracts International, 51,* 3782B.

Poole, V.L. (1992). Pregnancy wantedness, attitude toward pregnancy, and use of alcohol, tobacco, and street drugs during pregnancy. *Dissertation Abstracts International, 52,* 5193B.

Pothiban, L. (1993). Risk factor prevalence, risk status, and perceived risk for coronary heart disease among Thai elderly. *Dissertation Abstracts International, 54,* 1337B.

Rowe, M.L. (1990). The relationship of commitment and social support to the life satisfaction of caregivers to patients with Alzheimer's disease. *Dissertation Abstracts International, 51,* 1747B.

Rowles, C.J. (1993). The relationship of selected personal and organizational variables and the tenure of directors of nursing in nursing homes. *Dissertation Abstracts International, 53,* 4593B.

Schlosser, S.P. (1985). The effect of anticipatory guidance on mood state in primiparas experiencing unplanned cesarean delivery (metropolitan area, Southeast). *Dissertation Abstracts International, 46,* 2627B.

Schmitt, N.A. (1992). Caregiving couples: The experience of giving and receiving social support. *Dissertation Abstracts International, 52,* 5761B.

Sipple, J.E.A. (1989). A model for curriculum change based on retrospective analysis. *Dissertation Abstracts International, 50,* 1927A.

Smith, C.T. (1990). The lived experience of staying healthy in rural black families. *Dissertation Abstracts International, 50,* 3925B.

Smith, S.K. (1995). *Women's experiences of victimizing sexualization.* Ph.D. dissertation, University of Minnesota.

Tennyson, M.G. (1992). Becoming pregnant: Perceptions of black adolescents. *Dissertation Abstracts International, 52,* 5196B.

Terhaar, M.F. (1989). The influence of physiologic stability, behavioral stability and family stability on the preterm infant's length of stay in the neonatal intensive care unit. *Dissertation Abstracts International, 50,* 1328B.

Vincent, J.L.M. (1988). A Q analysis of the stressors of fathers with an infant in an intensive care unit. *Dissertation Abstracts International, 49,* 3111B.

Watson, L.A. (1991). Comparison of the effects of usual, support, and informational nursing interventions on the extent to which families of critically ill patients perceived their needs were met. *Dissertation Abstracts International, 52,* 2999B.

Webb, C.A. (1988). A cross-sectional study of hope, physical status, cognitions and meaning and purpose of pre- and post-retirement adults. *Dissertation Abstracts International, 49,* 1922A.

Whately, J.H. (1989). Effects of health locus of control and social network on risk-taking in adolescents. *Dissertation Abstracts International, 50,* 129B.

Theses

Allender, C. (1993). *An instrument to measure Newman's trilevel model of differentiated nursing practice.* Master's thesis, University of Minnesota.

Anderson, R.R. (1992). Indicators of nutritional status as a predictor of pressure ulcer development in the critically ill adults. *Masters Abstracts International, 30,* 92.

Averill, J.B. (1989). The impact of primary prevention as an intervention strategy. *Masters Abstracts International, 27,* 89.

Baskin-Nedzelski, J. (1992). Job stressors among visiting nurses. *Masters Abstracts International, 30,* 79.

Bessenghini, C. (1990). Stressful life events and angina in individuals undergoing exercise stress testing. *Masters Abstracts International, 28,* 569.

Blount, K.R. (1989). The relationship between the parents' and five to six-year-old child's perception of life events as stressors within the Neuman health care system framework. *Masters Abstracts International, 27,* 487.

Burgess, Y. (1988). An investigation of the relationships among systolic blood pressure, rate of speech, and perceived duration of time. *Masters Abstracts International, 27,* 373.

Butrin, J. (1983). *Differences in time perspective and hemisphericity between educated and noneducated Zairians.* Master's thesis, Pennsylvania State University.

Elgar, S.J. (1992). The influence of companion animals on perceived social support and perceived stress among family caregivers. *Masters Abstracts International, 30,* 732.

Fields, W.L. (1988). The effects of the 12-hour shift on fatigue and critical thinking performance in critical care nurses. *Masters Abstracts International, 26,* 237.

Finney, G.A.H. (1990). Spiritual needs of patients. *Masters Abstracts International, 28,* 272.

Goldstein, L.A. (1988). Needs of spouses of hospitalized cancer patients. *Masters Abstracts International, 26,* 105.

Griscabage, D. (1982). *Relationships among state anxiety time estimation, body movement, and repression-sensitization in preoperative patients.* Master's thesis, Pennsylvania State University.

Harper, B. (1993). Nurses' beliefs about social support and the effect of nursing care on the cardiac clients' attitudes in reducing cardiac risk status. *Masters Abstracts International, 31,* 273.

Haskill, K.M. (1988). Sources of occupational stress of the community health nurse. *Masters Abstracts International, 26,* 106.

Jonsdottir, H. (1988). *Health patterns of clients with chronic obstructive pulmonary disease.* Unpublished master's thesis, University of Minnesota.

Kuhn, M.E. (1989). Comparison of health beliefs of adolescents with diabetes and those of their mothers. *Masters Abstracts International, 28,* 412.

Litchfield, M.C. (1993). *The process of health patterning in families with young children who have been repeatedly hospitalized.* Master's thesis, University of Minnesota.

Morris, D.C. (1991). Occupational stress among home care first line managers. *Masters Abstracts International, 29,* 443.

Murphy, N.G. (1990). Factors associated with breastfeeding success and failure: A systematic integrative review (infant nutrition). *Masters Abstracts International, 28,* 275.

Petock, A.M. (1991). Decubitus ulcers and physiological stressors. *Masters Abstracts International, 29,* 267.

Pollard, M. (1981). *Emotional expressiveness in cancer and noncancer patients.* Master's thesis, Pennsylvania State University.

Pollock, D. (1983). *The relationship of sleep deprivation to cerebral hemisphericity and temporal orientation.* Master's thesis, Pennsylvania State University.

Sammarco, C.C.A. (1990). The study of stressors of the operating room nurse versus those of the intensive care unit nurse. *Masters Abstracts International, 28,* 276.

Scarpino, L.L. (1988). Family caregivers' perceptions associated with the chemotherapy treatment setting for the oncology client. *Masters Abstracts International, 26,* 424.

Sullivan, M.M. (1991). Comparisons of job satisfaction scores of school nurses with job satisfaction normative scores of hospital nurses. *Masters Abstracts International, 20,* 652.

Terhaar, N.C. (1989). Blood sugar and cognition patterns in the elderly. *Masters Abstracts International, 28,* 116.

Wilkey, S.F. (1990). The effects of an eight-hour continuing education course on the death anxiety levels of registered nurses. *Masters Abstracts International, 28,* 480.

Zack, C. (1983). *Hospitalized patients' personal space preferences in relation to female and male nurses.* Master's thesis, Pennsylvania State University.

Other

Acton, H.B. (1967). George Wilhelm Freidrich Hegel 1770-1831. In *The encyclopedia of philosophy* (Vols. 3 & 4). New York: Macmillan & Free Press.

Barnard, R. (1973). *Field-dependent-independence and selected motor abilities.* Unpublished doctoral dissertation, New York University.

Bentov, I. (1977). *Stalking the wild pendulum.* New York: E.P. Dutton.

Bentov, I. (1978, Nov. 17-20). *The mechanics of consciousness.* Paper presented at the symposium on New Dimensions of Consciousness, sponsored by Sufi Order in the West. New York.

Bohm, D. (1980). Wholeness and the implicate order. London: Routledge and Kegan Paul.

Capra, F. (1975). *The tao of physics.* Boulder, CO: Thambhala Publications.

Chapman, J. (1978). The relationship between auditory stimulation and gross motor activity of short-gestation infants. *Research in Nursing and Health, 1,* 29-36.

de Chardin, T. (1971). *Activation of energy.* New York: Harcourt, Brace, & Jovanovich.

Downs, F., & Fitzpatrick, J. (1976). Preliminary investigation of the reliability and validity of a tool for the assessment of body position and motor activity. *Nursing Research, 25,* 404-408.

Engle, V. (1981). *A study of the relationship between self-assessment of health, function, personal tempo and time perception in elderly women.* Unpublished doctoral dissertation, Wayne State University.

Fitzpatrick, J., & Donovan, M. (1978). Temporal experience and motor behavior among the aging. *Research in Nursing and Health, 1,* 60-68.

Gendlin, E.T. (1978). *Focusing.* New York: Everest.

Goldberg, W., & Fitzpatrick, J. (1980). Movement therapy and the aged. *Nursing Research, 29,* 339-346.

Marcuse, H. (1954). *Reason and revolution: Hegel and the rise of social theory* (2nd ed.). New York: Beacon.

Moss, R. (1981). *The I that is we.* Millbrae, CA: Celestial Arts.

Prigogine, I. (1976). Order through fluctuation: Self-organization and social system. In E. Jantsch, & C.H. Waddington (Eds.), *Evolution and consciousness* (pp. 93-133). Reading, MA: Addison-Wesley.

Prigogine, I., Allen, P.M., & Herman, R. (1977). Long term trends and the evolution of complexity. In E. Laszlo & J. Bierman (Eds.), *Goals in a global community: The original background papers for goals for mankind* (Vol. 1) (pp. 1-63). New York: Pergamon.

Reed, P.G. (1996, Spring). Transcendence: Formulating nursing perspectives. *Nursing Science Quarterly, 9*(1), 2-4.

Rogers, M.E. (1970). *An introduction to the theoretical basis of nursing.* Philadelphia: F.A. Davis.

Rogers, M.E. (1980). Nursing, a science of unitary man. In J.P. Riehl & C. Roy, *Conceptual models for nursing practice.* New York: Appleton-Century-Crofts.

Smith, M. (1979). Duration experience for bed-confined subjects: A replication and refinement. *Nursing Research, 28,* 139-144.

Tompkins, E. (1980). Effect of restricted mobility and dominance in perceived duration. *Nursing Research, 29,* 333-338.

Whyte, L.L. (1974). *The universe of experience.* New York: Harper & Row.

Young, A.M. (1976). *The reflexive universe: Evolution of consciousness.* San Francisco: Robert Briggs.

Interviews

Doberneck, B. (1985). Graduate student at Pennsylvania State University. Telephone interview.

Marchione, J. (1985). Associate professor at University of Akron. Telephone interview.

Evelyn Adam

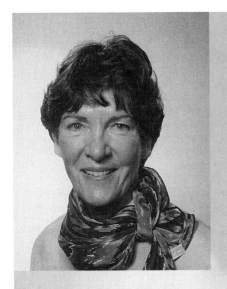

Conceptual Model for Nursing

Linda S. Harbour, Terri Creekmur, Janet DeFelice, Marilyn Sue Doub,
Anne Hodel, Ann Marriner Tomey, Cheryl Y. Petty

CREDENTIALS AND BACKGROUND OF THE THEORIST

Evelyn Adam was born April 9, 1929, in Lanark, Ontario, Canada. She graduated from Hotel Dieu Hospital in Kingston, Ontario, in 1950 with a Diploma in Nursing. She received a B.Sc. degree in 1966 from the University of Montreal and an M.N. degree from the University of California, Los Angeles, in 1971. There she met Dorothy Johnson, who she feels has

The authors wish to express appreciation to Evelyn Adam for editing the chapter.

"definitely been the most important influence" on her professional life.[6]

In 1979 she published her first book, *Être Infirmière* (third edition, 1991) and in 1980 wrote the English version of *To Be a Nurse* (second edition, 1991). Since then, her book has been translated into Dutch (1981), Spanish (1982), Italian (1989), Portuguese (1993), and Japanese (1996). Adam authored several chapters and was coeditor of *La personne âgée et ses besoins: Interventions infirmières*. This book, published in 1996, presents the nursing care of the aged based on Virginia Henderson's model for nursing care. Adam has also written numerous articles on conceptual models for nursing and has coauthored several others. Professional journals publishing her articles include *Infirmière Canadienne, Canadian Nurse, Journal of Advanced Nursing, Nursing Papers: Perspectives in Nursing,* and *Journal of Nursing Education.*

Adam has been a visiting professor at several universities. She has functioned as a resource person and speaker for various professional corporations, clinical and educational settings, and national and international conventions. From 1983 to 1989 she was a member of the review board for *Nursing Papers.* She taught at both undergraduate and graduate levels at the Faculty of Nursing of the University of Montreal. She was faculty secretary from 1982 until her retirement in 1989, at which time the university named her professor emeritus. She has been in *Who's Who in the World* since its eighth edition (1987/1988). In 1992, Laval University (Quebec City) awarded her an honorary doctorate. In 1995, the Order of Nurses of Quebec awarded her its highest distinction, the Order of Merit, in recognition of her important contributions to nursing. She continues to write and also does consulting work.

Although nursing care of the elderly is a recent professional interest, promoting conceptual models for nursing has predominated since 1970. She strongly feels that "nursing practice, education, and research must be based on an explicit frame of reference specific to nursing."[6]

Adam's work makes an important distinction between a conceptual model and a theory. "A [conceptual] model is usually based on, or derives from, a theory. . . . A model, emerging from a theory, may become the basis for a new theory."[1:40] "A conceptual model, for whatever discipline, is not reality; it is a mental image of reality or a way of conceptualizing reality. A conceptual model *for* nursing is therefore a conception *of* nursing."[4:42]

Adam[5,6] accepts Roy and Roberts' definition[11:5] of a theory as "a system of interrelated propositions used to describe, predict, explain, understand, and control a part of the empirical world."

Therefore a theory is useful to more than one discipline. A conceptual model for a discipline is useful only to that particular discipline. Adam[7] believes, "The day may come when nursing theory will be as

useful to related disciplines as existing theories, developed in other fields, are today useful to nursing."

Adam[2:5] writes that "a conceptual model is an abstraction, a way of looking at something, an invention of the mind."

> A conceptual model for a discipline is a very broad perspective, a global way of looking at a discipline. Most of the conceptual models for nursing that we know have come from two sources: one, a theory, chosen by the author, and the other, her professional experience.[6]

A conceptual model is the precursor of a theory. The model specifies the discipline's focus of inquiry, identifies those phenomena of particular interest to nursing, and provides a broad perspective for nursing research, practice, and education. The study of phenomena that concern nursing, that is, nursing research, may lead to theories that will describe, explain, or predict those phenomena. Such theories will not be theories of *nursing* but theories *of the phenomena* that are nursing's focus of inquiry.[5:12]

Many nurses are unable to communicate clearly and explicitly their conception of the service they offer to society. Adam contends this is not because they do not have a conception of nursing but because their conceptual base is not clear. If the nurse's mental image of nursing is vague or blurred, it will therefore be difficult to put into words. The nurse will then be unable to articulate his or her particular role in health care and may well find that professional activities are based on a perspective borrowed from another discipline.

Adam[1:41] states that "a model indicates the goal of our [nursing] profession—an ideal and limited goal, because it gives us direction for nursing practice, nursing education, and nursing research." Nurses who have a clear, concise conceptual base specific to nursing will be able to identify areas for theory development, prepare future practitioners of nursing, and demonstrate in their own practice nursing's contribution to health care. In this way health care will improve and the nursing profession will grow.

Although it is not necessary for every nurse to adopt the same conceptual model, it is essential that every nurse have a concise and explicit framework on which to base his or her work. The conceptual model is "the conceptual departure point" for teaching, research or nursing care. Speaking figuratively, Adam places the conceptual model in the nurse's occipital lobe, known also as the visual lobe. The nurse uses a great deal of scientific knowledge as well as experience, intuition, and creativity. In drawing on this knowledge, the nurse is guided by the conceptual model, that is, the mental image of nursing.[7]

The abstraction that is the conceptual model is linked to the reality that is nursing practice through the nursing process.[2] The data we collect depend on our conceptual base. The way we interpret the data, the plan we develop, the nursing action we choose, and the evaluation of our intervention also depend on our model. The number of steps in the nursing process is not significant because the difference is the conceptual base.[6]

In addition to the conceptual model and the nursing process, the nurse must also establish with the client what will be perceived to be a helping relationship. Adam considers this perhaps the most important component of being a nurse. It is the climate of empathy, warmth, mutual respect, caring, and acceptance that determines the effectiveness of nursing care.[2:50;7]

Adam feels that three components constitute nursing practice: the client, the nurse (with his or her conceptual model as a base for the nursing process), and the relationship between the client and the nurse. She has created a pictorial representation of nursing practice in her books (Fig. 33-1).[2:43;2:55;7]

Adam insists that the helping relationship and the systematic process (which nurses have, perhaps wrongly, labeled the "nursing" process) are important to all health professionals. Nursing fits into the whole of health care as an integral component of the interdisciplinary health team. Each discipline makes a unique contribution to the promotion and preservation of health and to the prevention of health problems. Although some services overlap within this interdisciplinary health team, each discipline is present because of its distinct and specific contribution to health.

This relationship can be illustrated with a schematic flower (Fig. 33-2). Each petal represents a distinct health discipline: nursing, medicine, physical therapy, speech therapy, or nutrition, for example. The center of the flower indicates the shared

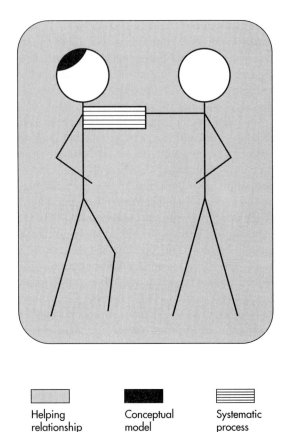

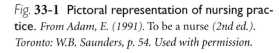

Fig. **33-1** **Pictoral representation of nursing practice.** *From Adam, E. (1991).* To be a nurse *(2nd ed.). Toronto: W.B. Saunders, p. 54. Used with permission.*

functions. A part of each petal is separate and distinct from the others, and the largest part of each petal represents the unique contribution of each discipline. Our conceptual model clarifies and makes explicit nursing's "petal."

Nurses currently have several conceptual models from which to choose. The decision to adopt one of the conceptual models for (not *of*) nursing is often made by considering the eventual evaluation of that particular model. Adam insists that conceptual models must be evaluated by criteria different from those used to evaluate theories. She quotes the three criteria established by Dorothy Johnson[10]:

1. *Social significance.* Clients would be asked whether the service (nursing) was significant to their health.

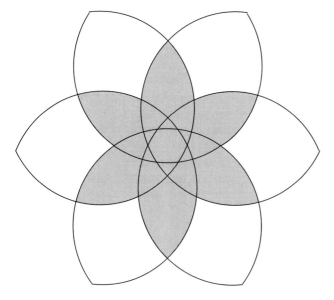

Fig. **33-2** Interdisciplinary health team illustrated with schematic flower. *From Adam, E. (1991).* To be a nurse *(2nd ed.). Toronto: W.B. Saunders. Used with permission.*

2. *Social congruence.* Clients would be asked whether the service (nursing) was congruent with their expectations.
3. *Social utility.* Nurses would be asked whether the conceptual model provided useful direction for education, practice, and research.

Such criteria are extrinsic to the model itself. However, for these criteria to be used, the conceptual model in question must already have been adopted in practice, education, and research settings. A vicious cycle may develop because some nurses may hesitate to adopt a model until it has been evaluated and it cannot be evaluated until it has been adopted.*

Adam recognizes that a model can be evaluated intrinsically for clarity, logic, and other criteria that will help nurses choose one model rather than another. However, the social decisions (extrinsic criteria) constitute the definitive evaluation of the conceptual base of a service profession.[3,9]

Adam's conviction that every nurse should have a conceptual base specific to nursing rather than one borrowed from another discipline has led her to publish many articles and books, to speak at professional meetings, and to teach courses on this subject. She feels that the existing models are often viewed as being too abstract or too complex and therefore beyond the understanding of many nurses. Adam published *Être Infirmière* and *To Be a Nurse* to help nurses understand the writings of Virginia Henderson. She accomplished this by placing Henderson's concept of nursing within the structure of a conceptual model and by developing and refining the subconcepts identified by Henderson.

This chapter evaluates the conceptual model Adam developed in her book. The model is not a theory, but it does suggest areas for theory development.

SUMMARY OF THE CONCEPTUAL MODEL FOR NURSING

In *To Be a Nurse,* Adam explains the essential elements of a conceptual model as presented by Dorothy Johnson. She then develops Virginia Henderson's concepts within the structure of a conceptual model.*

Assumptions

The assumptions that form the theoretical foundation of Virginia Henderson's vision of nursing are drawn in

---

*References 3:11; 4:44; 5:16-18; 7.

*The following summary material is reprinted with permission from Adam, E. (1980). *To Be a Nurse.* Philadelphia: WB Saunders, pp 13-15.

part from the works of Edward Thorndike, an American psychologist, and in part from Henderson's experience in rehabilitation. There are three assumptions:

1. Every individual strives for and desires independence.
2. Every individual is a complex whole, made up of fundamental needs.
3. When a need is not satisfied, it follows that the individual is not complete, whole, or independent.

Values

Virginia Henderson's conception of nursing is also composed of three beliefs:

1. The nurse has a unique function, although she shares certain functions with other professionals.
2. When the nurse takes over the physician's role, she delegates her primary function to inadequately prepared personnel.
3. Society wants and expects this service (nursing) from the nurse and no other worker is as able, or willing, to give it.

Major Units

The following are major units of Henderson's model[2:13-15;9]:

1. The goal of nursing is to maintain or restore the client's independence in the satisfaction of his fundamental needs.
2. The client or beneficiary of the nurse's service is a whole being made up of 14 fundamental needs:
   a. Breathe normally.
   b. Eat and drink adequately.
   c. Eliminate body wastes.
   d. Move and maintain desirable postures.
   e. Sleep and rest.
   f. Select suitable clothes—dress and undress.
   g. Maintain body temperature within normal range [by adjusting clothing and modifying the environment].
   h. Keep the body clean and well groomed and protect the integument.

i. Avoid dangers in the environment and avoid injuring others.
   j. Communicate with others in expressing emotions, needs, fears, or opinions.
   k. Worship according to one's faith.
   l. Work in such a way that there is a sense of accomplishment.
   m. Play or participate in various forms of recreation.
   n. Learn, discover, or satisfy the curiosity that leads to normal development and health, and use the available health facilities.
3. The role of the nurse is a complementary-supplementary one.
4. The source of difficulty or the probable origin of those problems known as nursing problems is an insufficiency of either knowledge, will, and/or strength.
5. The intervention: the focus, or center of attention of the nurse's action is the client's resources (knowledge, will, and strength).
6. The desired consequences are need satisfaction, independence in need satisfaction, or in some cases a peaceful death.

THEORETICAL SOURCES

Adam[6] says she chose to work with Henderson's concept of nursing for two reasons. First, she felt that Henderson's work was "partly known but badly known," that is, incompletely known or understood, although many nurses were acquainted with it. She hoped that her own publications would contribute to the recognition of Henderson's work as a useful conceptual base for nursing practice, research, and education. In addition, she felt that Henderson's work was more immediately accessible than other works were, because the language was already familiar to nurses. Adam[6] "is not saying that Henderson's frame of reference is any better, or more useful, or more significant or more congruent than others. Such an evaluation has not yet been done . . . but it seems more immediately accessible."

Adam's concern for the need of an explicit conceptual model for nursing was developed when she was a student of Dorothy Johnson. It was also through Johnson that Adam became familiar with the structure of a conceptual model: assumptions, values, and major units. Adam[6;10:7-15] believes Johnson was the first nurse to avail herself of that structure, which was already being used in fields such as sociology, psychology, and mathematics.

USE OF EMPIRICAL EVIDENCE

In choosing Virginia Henderson's writings as the basis of the conceptual model, Adam accepted the scientific principles on which Henderson based her work. The chapter on Virginia Henderson discusses the contribution of Claude Bernard's principle of physiological balance and Abraham Maslow's hierarchy of needs. Because Adam did not change the basic content but merely developed it further, this empirical foundation also is unchanged.

In the previous section of this chapter the source of the structure (assumptions, values, and six major units) was identified as sociology, mathematics, and other sciences. This structure has been extensively used in several sciences so it has good reliability.

MAJOR CONCEPTS & DEFINITIONS*

Assessment Tool Instrument that the professional uses in collecting information about the beneficiary, the nursing history tool, the data collection tool.

Assumption The theoretical or scientific basis of a conceptual model, the premises that support the major units of the model.

Beneficiary The second major unit of a conceptual model; the person or group of persons toward whom the professional directs her activities; the client; the patient.

Change A substitution of one thing in place of another, an alteration.

Collection of Data The first step of the nursing process, the collecting of information about the client, the client's nursing history.

Concept An idea, a mental image, a generalization formed and developed in the mind.

Conception A way of conceptualizing a reality, an invention of the mind, a mental image. Depending on its level of abstraction, a conception may be a philosophy, a theory, or a conceptual model.

Conceptual Model An abstraction or a way of conceptualizing a reality; a theoretical frame of reference sufficiently explicit so as to provide direction for a particular discipline; a conception made up of assumptions, values, and major units.

Conceptual Model for Nursing A mental representation, concept, or conception of nursing that is sufficiently complete and explicit so as to provide direction for all fields of activity of the nursing profession.

Consequences The sixth major unit of a conceptual model, the results of the professional's efforts to attain the ideal and limited goal.

Goal of the Profession The first major unit of a conceptual model, the end that the members of the profession strive to achieve.

Helping Relationship The interaction between the beneficiary (the helpee) and the professional (the helper) that aids the helpee to live more fully; the interpersonal exchange in which the helper illustrates such facilitating qualities as empathy, respect, and others.

Intervention The fifth major unit of a conceptual model, the focus and modes of the professional's intervention. (In the context of the nursing process, the intervention is the fourth step [implementation of the plan of action or the nursing action itself.])

*Reprinted with permission from Adam, E. (1980). *To Be a Nurse.* Philadelphia: W.B. Saunders, pp 116-118.

Continued

MAJOR CONCEPTS & DEFINITIONS—cont'd

Intervention Focus Part of the fifth major unit of a model; the focus, or center, of the professional's attention at the moment he intervenes with a client.

Intervention Modes Part of the fifth major unit, the means or ways of intervening at the professional's disposal.

Major Units The six essential components of a complete and explicit conception.

Need A requirement, a necessity.

Need, Fundamental A requirement common to all human beings, well or ill.

Need, Individual A specific, particular, or personal requirement that derives from a fundamental need.

Nursing Care Plan A written plan of action, the written communication that comes from the second and third steps of the nursing process, a plan to be followed, a projection of what is to be done.

Nursing Process A methodical, systematic way of proceeding toward an action; a dynamic and logical method; a five-step process.

Practice One of the three fields of activity of a service profession (the other two being education and research), the field of activity of the administrator and the practitioner of the service.

Problem A difficulty to be reduced or removed.

Problem-Solving Method The scientific process of solving problems, the systematic manner of proceeding used to solve problems.

Role The third major unit of a conceptual model, the part played by the professional, the societal function of the professional.

Source of Difficulty The fourth major unit of a conceptual model, the probable origin of the client difficulty with which the professional is prepared to cope.

Values The value system underlying a conceptual model.

MAJOR ASSUMPTIONS

In developing Henderson's work into a conceptual model, Adam[2:14;9] described the goal of nursing as maintaining or restoring the client's independence in the satisfaction of the 14 fundamental needs. The nurse plays a complementary-supplementary role, complementing and supplementing the client's resources (strength, knowledge, and will).

The nurse has a unique province, although she shares certain functions with other health professionals. Society wants and expects the nurse to provide her unique service. In this model, the person is portrayed as a complex whole, made up of 14 fundamental needs and the resources to satisfy them. Each need has biological, physiological, psychosociocultural dimensions. When a need is not satisfied, the person is not complete, whole, or independent. The nurse's client may also be a family or a group.[3:97-100] The concept of environment is specifically addressed in only one of the fundamental needs. However, environment is implicit in all the fundamental needs because the sociocultural dimension is integral to each need.

Health is not defined separately in *To Be a Nurse*. But Adam uses this term in discussing the goal of nursing. She says, "The goal of nursing is to maintain or to restore the client's independence in the satisfaction of his fundamental needs. This goal, congruent with the goal common to the entire health team, makes clear the nurse's specific contribution to the preservation and improvement of health."[2:14] Because an entirely satisfactory definition of health is still a subject of debate, it behooves each health discipline to make explicit its particular contribution to health.[3:95]

THEORETICAL ASSERTIONS

In the description of the conceptual model's major units, the relationships among the basic concepts can be seen in the elements Adam has labeled beliefs and values. She feels these constitute the *why* of the model and must be shared by all who use the model. Values are not subject to the criteria of *truths* but must reflect the values of the larger society nursing wishes to serve.

1. "The nurse has a unique function, although she shares certain functions with other professionals."[2:13] The nurse must have a conceptual model to have a distinct professional identity and to assert herself as a colleague of the other health team members.
2. "When the nurse takes over the physician's role, she delegates her primary function to inadequately prepared personnel."[2:13] The nurse who strives to assume the physician's role will relinquish the nurse's role to some other care provider who may not have the skills and the knowledge base required for nursing.
3. "Society wants and expects this service (nursing) from the nurse and no other worker is as able, or willing to give it."[2:14] Nursing owes its existence to the fact that it fulfills a societal need, as does any service profession.

LOGICAL FORM

Adam has used the structure of a conceptual model that was useful in various other sciences before being introduced into nursing. The essential elements of a model for a helping or service profession follow.

Assumptions

The assumptions are "the suppositions that are taken for granted by those who wish to use the model; they are the 'how' of the model, its foundation."[2:6]

Beliefs and Values

The beliefs and values "constitute the 'why' of the model and are not subject to the criteria of truth." They must "reflect the value system of the larger society that the profession wishes to serve" and "be shared by the members of the profession who wish to use the model."[2:7]

Major Units

The major units "are the 'what' of the conceptual model." They "make clear what nursing is in any setting and at any time."[2:7]

Ideal and limited goal. The ideal and limited goal of the profession is "*ideal* because it represents the ideal that all members of the profession would like to achieve and *limited* because it delineates the parameters of the profession."[2:7]

Beneficiary. The beneficiary of the professional service is "that person or group of persons toward whom the professional directs his attention." "The nurse must have a clear mental image of her client—whether he is well or ill."[2:8]

Role of the professional. The role of the professional is "the role in society played by the members of the discipline."[2:8]

Source of difficulty of the beneficiary. The source of difficulty of the beneficiary "refers to the probable origin of the client's difficulty; one with professional, because of his education and experience, is prepared to cope."[3:8] "The probable origin of those client problems which the nurse is prepared to solve must be made explicit."[2:9]

Intervention

Intervention focus. The focus or center of the intervention is "the focus of the professional's attention at the moment he intervenes with the client. The patient or beneficiary is perceived as an extremely complex individual; however, within that complexity only one aspect can receive all the professional's attention at any given moment. . . . No one person can do everything at the same time."[2:9]

Intervention modes. The modes of intervention "are the means the professional has at his disposal to intervene. . . . A conceptual model for nursing will indicate what means are at the nurse's disposal when she intervenes as a health professional."[2:9]

Consequences. The consequences "are the desired results of the professional activities and must be congruent with the ideal goal."[2:10]

Adam has developed Henderson's concept of nursing into a conceptual model for nursing by placing Henderson's writings in the structure of a model.

She has supplied the logical form that was less apparent in Henderson's work. Through the logical form of the resulting conceptual model, clear direction is provided to nursing practitioners, educators, and researchers.

Through the use of the structure that comprises a conceptual model and Henderson's writings, it may be said that Adam used the deductive form of logical reasoning.

ACCEPTANCE BY THE NURSING COMMUNITY

Practice

Basing practice on this conceptual model, the nurse is seen in a complementary-supplementary role, and the goal is client independence in the satisfaction of his needs. The model serves as a guide for using the nursing process and the problem-solving method. Guided by the 14 fundamental needs, the practitioner, in whatever setting, will assess the independence of the client in need satisfaction. The nurse will then identify the client's specific needs, determine the source of difficulty, and plan the intervention to complement client strength, will, or knowledge. After the care is given, it is evaluated in reference to the client's objectives—have the specific needs been satisfied and has the client's independence been increased? A *nursing problem*—a client's health problem requiring a nurse's intervention—is a dependency problem in need satisfaction.[2:40] A *nursing diagnosis* is a specific need that is unsatisfied because of insufficient strength, will, or knowledge. Criteria for identifying specific needs have been developed.[2:73] According to Adam, the nurse "carries out the social mission of contributing to the public's improved health by working toward greater client independence."[2:66]

Education

Adam discusses the educational objectives and goals and the program content in *To Be a Nurse*. She states, "Following Henderson's concept of nursing, the nursing curriculum is planned to prepare a health worker capable of maintaining and restoring the client's independence in the satisfaction of his fundamental needs."[2:57] With this concept, a student learns the complementary-supplementary role. Adam divides the program into official and unofficial content, both of equal importance. Unofficial content "covers everything that is learned in an educational program without being taught."[2:58] Official content "is formally recognized and actually taught."[2:58] Official content is further divided into nursing and nonnursing.

According to Henderson's frame of reference, nursing content includes:

1. The goal of nursing, which is to preserve or reestablish the client's independence in the satisfaction of his basic needs.
2. The detailed description of the 14 fundamental needs, each with its biological, physiological, psychological, social, and cultural dimensions.
3. The individual variations in fundamental needs.
4. The various problems of dependence originating from a lack of strength, will, or knowledge.
5. The explanation of the complementary-supplementary role.
6. The description of the various needs of intervention.
7. The study of the desired consequences: continued or increased independence and, in certain circumstances, a peaceful death.
8. The study of the systematic process and the problem-solving method as applied to nursing.[2:58-59]

Essential subject matters, regardless of the conceptual model for nursing, are "the helping relationship, . . . the concept of health, . . . and the history of nursing."[2:59]

The theoretical courses, in the nonnursing content, include anatomy, physiology, pathology, psychology, sociology, and anthropology. In relation to Henderson's model, the first three relate to the biophysiological dimension and the last three to the psychosociocultural aspect of the fundamental needs.

Subject matter derived from the conceptual model's assumptions is "the concepts of independence and dependence; the concepts of universal and individual human needs, hierarchy of human needs, and need satisfaction; and the concept of wholeness."[2:60]

The practical aspect of nursing content consists of technical procedures and clinical experiences. Techniques are important in the complementary-supplementary role because the nurse is assisting the client in those activities that cannot be completed because of insufficient strength, will, or knowledge. Techniques help pursue the goal of client independence in the satisfaction of his needs. Adam[2:62] feels that "the goal of clinical experiences is to provide the student with opportunities to help a client recover his independence in the satisfaction of his basic needs."

Although the level of education may increase, the model remains the conceptual base. Baccalaureate students' formal education will help them identify complex and subtle specific needs, find new ways of complementing and supplementing, and form and continue a helping relationship. Master's level students learn to be specialists in independence nursing or in the teaching and administration of independence nursing. Doctoral students may use the concept of independence in need satisfaction as a basis of research for theory development.

Research

Adam posed 12 questions from the conceptual model for research development. These include:

1. How can client independence be measured?
2. How can his degree of dependence be quantified?
3. What dependency problems are solved by what nursing interventions?
4. At what point must the intervention be discontinued if independence is to be promoted?
5. How can certain interventions be made more easily acceptable?
6. How can the nurse determine how much intervention is enough?
7. What dependency problems are most often encountered among selected groups—e.g.,

cancer patients, the aged, the mentally confused?
8. How does pain, anxiety, etc., affect independence?
9. How can linguistic barriers be overcome?
10. How can the nurse help certain ethnic or socioeconomic groups to be independent?
11. How can the nurse increase client participation in health care?
12. Is the conceptual model socially useful, significant, and congruent?[2:66-67]

Adam[5] states that various clinical and educational settings in Canada are at varying stages of basing nursing care and teaching on Henderson's model and that the research for a small number of master's theses has been based on this model. Correspondence received from Canada, the United States, and abroad indicates her books have received very favorable reviews.

FURTHER DEVELOPMENT

Although no empirical evidence has been collected for theories deriving from this model, Adam believes that the model could be the basis for theory development.[8:9] As with other conceptual models for nursing, this one specifies nursing's focus of inquiry. From Henderson's conceptual departure point of independence in need satisfaction, descriptive and experimental studies could be carried out to result in the identification of descriptive terms peculiar to the concept under scrutiny. The identification of descriptive terms is the first step in theory development. Possible developments might be a theory of need satisfaction or a theory of complementing knowledge or of supplementing motivation in specific client populations. Such theories would not be theories of nursing, but theories of the phenomena that concern nursing.[5]

"Nurse theorists will of course look at phenomena that interest other disciplines as well. They must, however, study them from a nursing perspective if they want to develop nursing theory."[8:9] "For example, if pain were studied from Henderson's perspective, it would be examined as a phenomenon that interferes with client independence in need satisfaction."[8:10]

In a letter of February 16, 1988, Evelyn Adam states, "Some Ontario colleges and clinical settings are showing increasing interest in basing their practice and teaching on Henderson's model as I presented it. It is still popular in Quebec and in the Atlantic provinces. Graduate students often quote it as their conceptual departure point, i.e., to justify their research project. They seldom seek to develop it."

CRITIQUE

Simplicity

The essential elements listed by Adam give the appearance of a simple conceptual model. However, on closer inspection, we find that the number of subconcepts produces a complex picture. The interrelatedness of the components necessary for the care of the whole client also adds to the complexity of the model. The concepts presented are clearly defined and easy to follow.

Generality

The assumptions, values, and major units involve nursing and clients in all aspects of society. They are not limited to age, medical diagnosis, or health care setting. Each of the 14 basic needs has biophysiological and psychosociocultural aspects.

Empirical Precision

Although testing of the model is unavailable at this time, it appears to have the potential for a high degree of empirical precision. This is related to its reality base and designated subconcepts.

Derivable Consequences

Because of the empirically based concepts and broad scope, the model is potentially applicable to nursing practice, education, and research.

CONCLUSION

Adam's work in developing the conceptual model is unique in that she has taken Henderson's previously existing concept of nursing and presented it within the previously existing structure of a model. The result is something more than the sum of the two. It is a complete, concise, explicit conceptual model. Adam then clarified the interrelatedness of the model, the process, and the client-nurse relationship. Making a clear distinction between model and theory, Adam explained the impact of the model on nursing research, practice, and education.

Adam[6] states that "the adoption of a conceptual model will not solve all of nursing's problems." A conceptual model makes explicit nursing's particular contribution to health care and provides nurses with a professional identity and a conceptual point of departure.

It would seem that every nurse who adopts a concise and explicit conceptual model is a potential nursing theorist. A nurse who is able to articulate the scope of nursing practice would be more likely to identify areas for nursing theory development and nursing research. Imagine that the majority of nurses have an explicit conceptual model, that is, a conceptual departure point for theory development, and are able and willing to provide written documentation that would become the basis for empirical evidence. This opens the door to a marked increase in nursing theory and knowledge.

CRITICAL THINKING *Activities*

1 Adam states that all nurses have a conceptual model for nursing practice, but it is often "blurred" and difficult to communicate. From the perspective that the nurse needs a clear conceptual model of nursing as a basis for the nursing process, identify components of the theorist's development of Virginia Henderson's concept of nursing that you could utilize in implementing the nursing process.

2 Analyze the components of Henderson's model as developed by Adam and identify those, if any, that you think are significant in clarifying nursing's unique contribution to health care. State the rationale for your response.

3 Review Adam's three theoretical assertions (beliefs/values). Do you think that these theoretical assertions reflect values of today's society that nursing serves?

4 Analyze your practice from the perspective of Adam's development of Henderson's concept of nursing. Is this conceptual model appropriate for adoption, implementation, and evaluation in your practice? State the rationale for your response.

REFERENCES

1. Adam, E. (1975, Sept.). A conceptual model for nursing. *Canadian Nurse, 71,* 40-41.
2. Adam, E. (1980). *To be a nurse.* Philadelphia: Saunders.
3. Adam, E. (1983). *Être infirmière* (2nd ed.). Montréal: Editions HRW Ltée.
4. Adam, E. (1983). Frontiers of nursing in the 21st century: Development of models and theories on the concept of nursing. *Journal of Advanced Nursing, 8,* 41-45.
5. Adam, E. (1983). Modèles conceptuels. *Nursing Papers: Perspectives in Nursing, 15*(2), 10-21.
6. Adam, E. (1984, Dec. 4). Personal interview.
7. Adam, E. (1985, April). Toward more clarity in terminology—frameworks, theories and models. *Journal of Nursing Education 24*(4), 151-155.
8. Adam, E. (1987). Nursing theory: What it is and what it is not. *Nursing Papers: Perspectives in Nursing, 19*(2), 5-14.
9. Adam, E. (1996, Nov. 1). Telephone interview.
10. Johnson, D. (1974, Sept.-Oct.). Development of theory: A requisite for nursing as a primary health profession. *Nursing Research, 23*(5), 372-377.
11. Roy, C., & Roberts, S.L. (1981). *Theory construction in nursing: An adaptation model.* Englewood Cliffs, NJ: Prentice-Hall.

BIBLIOGRAPHY

Primary sources

Books

Adam, E. (1979). *Être infirmière.* Montréal: Editions HRW Ltee.
Adam, E. (1980). *To be a nurse.* Philadelphia: Saunders.
Adam, E. (1981). *To be a nurse.* (Dutch translation). Holland: De Tÿdstroom.
Adam, E. (1982). *To be a nurse.* (Spanish translation). Madrid: Editora Inportecnica.

Adam, E. (1983). *Être infirmière* (2nd ed.). Montréal: Editions HRW Ltée.
Adam, E. (1991). *Être infirmière* (3rd ed.). Montréal: Êtudes Vivantes.
Adam, E. (1991). *To be a nurse* (2nd ed.). Toronto: Saunders.
Adam, E. (1992). *To be a nurse.* (Italian translation). Milan: Catholic University of Milan.
Adam, E. (1993). *To be a nurse.* (Portuguese translation). Lisbon: Instituto Piaget.
Adam, E. (1996). *To be a nurse.* (Japanese translation). Tokyo: Igaku-Shoin.
Lauzon, S., & Adam, E. (Eds.). (1996). *La personne âgée et ses besoins: Interventions infirmières.* Montreal: Editions du Renouveau Pédagogique.

Book chapters

Adam, E. (1983). Development of models and theories on the concept of nursing. In *Health care for all: Challenge for nursing* (17th quadrennial Congress, ICN 1981). Geneva: ICN.
Adam, E. (1983). The shape of the nursing world to come: The nursing process. In *Health care for all: Challenge for nursing,* (17th quadrennial Congress, ICN 1981). Geneva: ICN.
Adam, E. (1984). Modèles conceptuels. In M. McGee (Ed.), *Theoretical pluralism in nursing science.* Ottawa: University of Ottawa Press.
Adam, E. (1990). Levels of abstraction in nursing content development. In *Proceedings of the First and Second Rosemary Ellis Scholars' Retreat* (pp. 229-261). Cleveland, OH: Case Western Reserve University.
Adam, E. (1992). Contemporary conceptualizations of nursing. In J.F. Kikuchi & H. Simmons (Eds.) *Philosophic inquiry in nursing* (pp. 55-63). Newbury Park, CA: Sage.

Journal articles

Adam, E. (1975, Sept.). A conceptual model for nursing. *Canadian Nurse, 71*(9), 40-41.
Adam, E. (1975, Sept.). Un modèle conceptuel: à quoi bon? *L'infirmière Canadienne, 19*(9), 22-23.
Adam, E. (1981, Sept.). CNA's standards for nursing practice: An interpretation. *Canadian Nurse, 77*(8), 32-33.
Adam, E. (1981, Sept.). Les normes de la pratique infirmière de l'A.I.I.C.: Une interprétation. *L'Infirmière Canadienne, 23*(9), 28-29.
Adam, E. (1983). Frontiers of nursing in the 21st century: Development of models and theories on the concept of nursing. *Journal of Advanced Nursing, 8,* 41-45.
Adam, E. (1983). Modèles conceptuels. *Nursing Papers: Perspectives in Nursing, 15*(2), 10-21.
Adam, E. (1984). Questions et réponses relatives au schème conceptuel de Virginia Henderson. *L'Infirmière Canadienne, 26*(3), 27-31.
Adam, E. (1985, April). Toward more clarity in terminology: Frameworks, theories, and models. *Journal of Nursing Education, 24*(4), 151-155.

Adam, E. (1987). Nursing theory: What it is and what it is not. *Nursing Papers: Perspectives in Nursing, 19*(2), 5-14.

Guyonnet, M., Adam, E. (1992). L'infirmière dans l'equipe pluridisciplinaire. *Canadian Nurse/L'infirmière canadienne, 88*(10), 41-44.

Reports

Adam, E. (1980). Implementing the curriculum based on a nursing model. In *Back to basics* (pp. 22-28). Ottawa: A.I.I.C.

Adam, E., et al. (1980). *Normes de la pratique infirmière.* Ottawa: A.I.I.C.

Adam, E. (1980). Programmes s'inspirant d'un modèle nursing. In *Retour aux sources* (pp. 27-33). Ottawa: A.I.I.C.

Adam, E., et al. (1980). *Standards for nursing practice.* Ottawa: A.I.I.C.

Adam, E. (1981). The case for a conceptual model. In *Proceedings from Nursing Explorations 1980,* School of Nursing, McGill University.

Adam, E. (1981). L'application d'un model conceptuel au programme de'ètudes collegial. Dans *Rapport du-Colloque des Techniques infirmières Partie I* (pp. 49-55). *Gouvernement du Québec.*

Adam, E. (1981). Leadership in nursing: The case for a conceptual model. In *Report of Annual Meeting,* (pp. 1-15). CAUSN, Western Region, University of Saskatchewan. Saskatoon, Saskatchewan.

Correspondence

Adam, E. (1984, Oct. 2). Personal correspondence.

Adam, E. (1984, Nov. 1). Telephone interview.

Adam, E. (1984, Nov. 4). Telephone interview.

Adam, E. (1984, Nov. 6). Personal correspondence.

Adam, E. (1984, Nov. 12). Telephone interview.

Adam, E. (1984, Nov. 26). Telephone interview.

Adam, E. (1984, Dec. 4). Personal interview (Videotape).

Adam, E. (1988, Feb. 16). Personal correspondence.

Adam, E. (1988, April 2). Telephone interview.

Adam, E. (1993). Personal correspondence.

Secondary sources

Books

Chinn, P., & Kramer, M. (1995). *Theory and nursing: A systematic approach* (4th ed.). St. Louis: Mosby.

Henderson, V. (1966). *The nature of nursing.* New York: Macmillan.

Journal articles

Henderson, V. (1964). The nature of nursing. *American Journal of Nursing, 64,* 62-68.

Henderson, V. (1982). The nursing process: Is the title right? *Journal of Advanced Nursing, 7,* 103-109.

Winkler, J. (1983). Conceptual models (a response to "Modèles conceptuels," by E. Adam). *Nursing Papers: Perspectives in nursing, 15*(4), 69-70.

Book reviews

Adam, E. (1979). *Être infirmière.*
   Infirmière Canadienne, 21, 46, April 1979.
   Infirmière Canadienne, 21, 10, June 1979.
   Revue de l'infirmière (Paris) 6, 75, June 1979.
   Revue de l'infirmière (Paris), 8, 8-9, October 1979.
   Infirmière enseiqnante (Paris), 10, 11, February 1980.
   Le Devoir (daily newspaper, Montreal), March 19, 1979.

Adam, E. (1980). *To be a nurse.*
   Canadian Nurse, 77, 50, March 1981.
   Nursing Times, 77, 1041, June 1981.
   Australian Nurses Journal, 11, 28, October 1981.
   Continuing Education in Nursing, 12, 39, November-December 1981.

Other

Riehl, J.P., & Roy, C. (1974). *Conceptual models for nursing practice.* New York: Appleton-Century-Crofts.

Riehl, J.P., & Roy, C. (1980). *Conceptual models for nursing practice* (2nd ed.) New York: Appleton-Century-Crofts.

Roy, C., & Roberts, S.L. (1981). *Theory construction in nursing: An adaptation model.* Englewood Cliffs, NJ: Prentice-Hall.

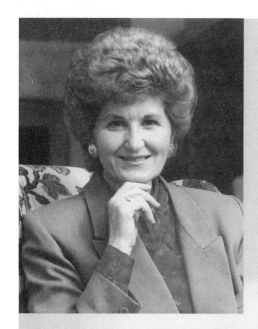

Nola J. Pender

The Health Promotion Model

Lucy Anne Tillett

CREDENTIALS AND BACKGROUND OF THE THEORIST

Nola J. Pender made an early commitment to the profession of nursing when, at the age of 7 years, she observed the nursing care given to her hospitalized aunt. This desire to give care to others developed through experience and education to a belief that the goal of nursing was to help people care for themselves. Dr. Pender has made an impact on knowledge

The author appreciates the critique of the original chapter by Nola J. Pender.

about the promotion of health through her research, teaching, presentations, and writings.

Pender was born in 1941 in Lansing, Michigan, the only child of parents who were strong supporters of education for women. This family encouragement for her goal of becoming a registered nurse led her to attend the School of Nursing at West Suburban Hospital in Oak Park, Illinois. This school was chosen for its ties with Wheaton College and its strong Christian foundation. She received her nursing diploma in 1962 and began working on a medical-surgical unit in a Michigan hospital.

In 1964 Pender completed her B.S.N. at Michigan State University in East Lansing. She credits Helen Penhale, the assistant to the dean, for helping to streamline her program and foster her options for further education. As was common in the 1960s, Pender changed her major from nursing as she pursued her graduate degrees. She earned her M.A. in human growth and development from Michigan State University in 1965. Her Ph.D. in psychology and education was completed in 1969 at Northwestern University in Evanston, Illinois. Dr. Pender's dissertation investigated developmental changes in encoding processes of short-term memory in children.[5:4283-A]

At the time of earning her Ph.D., Pender notes a shift in her thinking toward defining the goal of nursing care as the optimal health of the individual. A series of conversations with Dr. Beverly McElmurry at Northern Illinois University and reading *High-Level Wellness* inspired her to look at health and nursing in a broader way.[4] Her marriage to Albert Pender, an associate professor of business and economics who has collaborated with his wife in writing about the economics of health care, and the birth of a son and daughter, provided personal influence in the desire to learn more about optimizing human health.

In 1975 Dr. Pender published "A Conceptual Model for Preventive Health Behavior,"[6:385-390] which was a basis for studying how individuals made decisions about their own health care in a nursing context. This article identified factors that were found to influence decision making and actions of individuals in preventing disease. In 1982 the first edition of the text *Health Promotion in Nursing Practice* was published with the concept of promoting optimal health superseding disease prevention. The health promotion model made its first appearance in that edition and appears in revision in the 1987 edition of the book.[7] The third edition, in 1996, presented the latest revision of the health promotion model.[8]

A 6-year study funded by the National Institutes of Health was conducted at Northern Illinois University in DeKalb by Pender's colleagues Susan Walker, Ed.D., Karen Sechrist, Ph.D., and Marilyn Frank-Stromborg, Ed.D. The study tested the validity of the health promotion model.[10] An instrument, the Health Promoting Lifestyle Profile, was developed by the research team to study the health promoting behavior of working adults, older adults, cardiac rehabilitation patients, and ambulatory cancer clients.[12] Published results from these studies support the health promotion model,[12] which Pender refers to as a model "in evolution."[11]

Nola Pender has provided important leadership in the development of nursing research in the United States. Her work in support of the National Center for Nursing Research in the National Institutes of Health was instrumental to its formation in 1981. She has promoted scholarly activity in nursing through her involvement with Sigma Theta Tau, the Midwest Nursing Research Society, and the Council of Nurse Researchers of the American Nurses Association. Inducted as a Fellow of the American Academy of Nursing in 1981, she served as President of the Academy from 1991 until 1993. As director of the Center for Nursing Research at the University of Michigan School of Nursing since 1990, she is heavily involved in building nursing research. A child/adolescent health behavior research center initiated in 1991 at the University of Michigan represents Dr. Pender's hopes to continue to study and influence the health-promoting behaviors of individuals by understanding how these behaviors are first established in youth.[11] Dr. Pender has published numerous articles on exercise, behavior change, and relaxation training as aspects of health promotion. She is recognized as an expert and serves frequently as a speaker and consultant on these topics.

THEORETICAL SOURCES

The health promotion model (Fig. 34-1) has its base in the social learning theory of Albert Bandura,[2] which postulates the importance of cognitive processes in the changing of behavior. Fishbein's theory of reasoned action, which asserts that behavior is a function of personal attitudes and social norms,[1] is also important to the model's development. The Health Promotion Model is similar in construction[3] to the Health Belief Model but is not limited to explaining disease prevention behavior and expands to encompass behaviors for enhancing health. Dr. Pen-

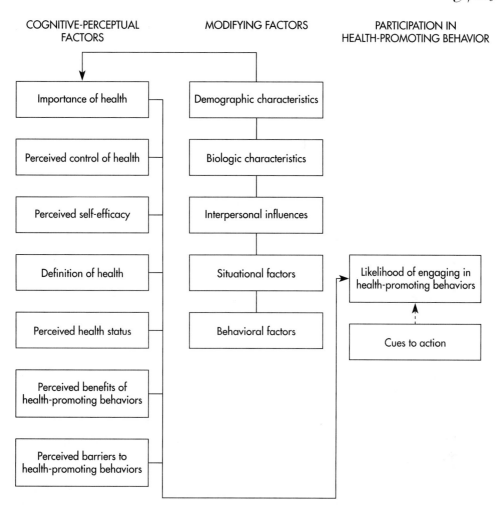

COGNITIVE-PERCEPTUAL FACTORS

MODIFYING FACTORS

PARTICIPATION IN HEALTH-PROMOTING BEHAVIOR

Importance of health

Perceived control of health

Perceived self-efficacy

Definition of health

Perceived health status

Perceived benefits of health-promoting behaviors

Perceived barriers to health-promoting behaviors

Demographic characteristics

Biologic characteristics

Interpersonal influences

Situational factors

Behavioral factors

Likelihood of engaging in health-promoting behaviors

Cues to action

Fig. **34-1 Health Promotion Model.** *From Pender, N.J. (1987).* Health promotion in nursing practice *(2nd ed.). New York: Appleton & Lange, p. 58. Used with permission.*

der's background in human development, experimental psychology, and education accounts for this foundation of social psychology and learning theory for her Health Promotion Model.

USE OF EMPIRICAL EVIDENCE

The Health Promotion Model in its 1987 form identified cognitive perceptual factors in the individual that are modified by situational, personal, and interpersonal characteristics to result in the participation in health-promoting behaviors in the presence of a

cue to action. The identified proposed factors were determined by extensive review of health behavior research.[7:60-66] The 1996 revision of the model (Fig. 34-2) adds three new variables that serve to influence the individual to engage in health-promoting behaviors: activity-related affect, commitment to a plan of action, and immediate competing demand and preferences. The Health Promotion Model serves the function of identifying concepts relevant to health-promoting behaviors and integrating research findings in such a way as to facilitate the generation of testable hypotheses.

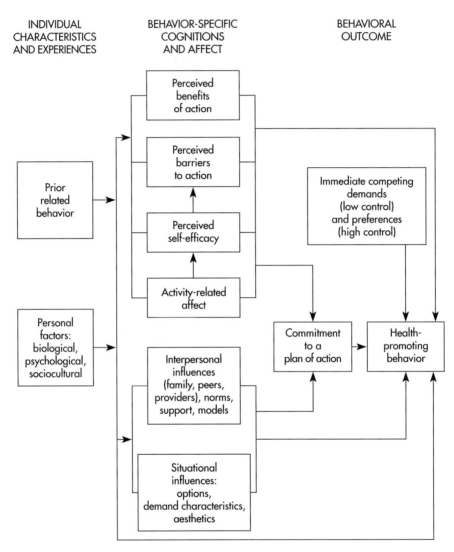

INDIVIDUAL
CHARACTERISTICS
AND EXPERIENCES

BEHAVIOR-SPECIFIC
COGNITIONS
AND AFFECT

BEHAVIORAL
OUTCOME

Perceived
benefits
of action

Perceived
barriers
to action

Prior
related
behavior

Perceived
self-efficacy

Immediate competing
demands
(low control)
and preferences
(high control)

Activity-related
affect

Personal
factors:
biological,
psychological,
sociocultural

Commitment
to a
plan of action

Health-
promoting
behavior

Interpersonal
influences
(family, peers,
providers), norms,
support, models

Situational
influences:
options,
demand characteristics,
aesthetics

Fig. **34-2** **Revised Health Promotion Model.** *From Pender, N.J. (1996).* Health promotion in nursing practice *(3rd ed.). Stamford, CT: Appleton & Lange, p. 67. Used with permission.*

Major Concepts & Definitions

The following are cognitive-perceptual factors, defined as "primary motivational mechanisms"[7] for the activities related to health promotion:

1. *Importance of health.* Individuals who value health highly are more likely to seek it.
2. *Perceived control of health.* The individual's perception of his own ability to change his health can motivate his desire for health.
3. *Perceived self-efficacy.* The individual's strong belief that a behavior is possible can influence the occurrence of that behavior.
4. *Definition of health.* The individual's definition of what health means, ranging from absence of disease to high-level well-being, can influence what behavior changes will be attempted.
5. *Perceived health status.* The current state of feeling well or feeling ill can determine the likelihood that health-promoting behaviors will be initiated.
6. *Perceived benefits of behaviors.* Individuals may be more inclined to begin or continue health-promoting behaviors if the benefits to such behaviors are considered high.
7. *Perceived barriers to health-promoting behaviors.* The individual's belief that an activity or behavior is difficult or unavailable may influence his intention to engage in it.

Modifying factors such as age, gender, education, income, body weight, family patterns of health care behaviors, and expectations of significant others also play roles in the determination of health care behaviors. These modifying factors are seen as having indirect influence on behavior, with the cognitive-perceptual factors bearing directly on behaviors.

The revised health promotion model identifies these additional concepts[8]:

1. *Prior related behavior* is a behavioral factor having direct and indirect effects. It is consistent with the focus on perceived self-efficacy[2] that future behavior is influenced by success or failure with prior attempts at similar acts.
2. *Activity-related affect* consists of the subjective positive or negative feelings associated with a particular behavior that directly influence the performance of the behavior and indirectly influence it by enhancing self-efficacy.
3. *Commitment to a plan of action* includes the concept of intention with a planned strategy that causes the intention to be formalized into a commitment to oneself or another.
4. *Immediate competing demands and preferences* refine the concepts of "benefits and barriers" by viewing these alternatives to planned behavior that occur just before the intended activity.

   Competing demands refer to conflicts over which the individual has low control, such as a crying child when it is exercise time. Competing preferences are alternate behaviors with high personal control, such as the choice of ice cream over an apple as a snack because it is a favorite flavor.

MAJOR ASSUMPTIONS

Health is seen as a positive high-level state. The individual is assumed to have a drive toward health. The individual's definition of health for himself has more importance than a general denotative statement about health. Pender reviews major health views from medicine, nursing, psychology, and sociology.

The person is the individual and the focus of the model. Each person is uniquely expressed by his or her own pattern of cognitive-perceptual and modifying factors. Pender does not propose the model as explanatory for aggregates.

THEORETICAL ASSERTIONS

The model represents the interrelationships between cognitive-perceptual factors and modifying factors influencing the occurrence of health-promoting behaviors as this knowledge emerged from research findings. Specific theoretical assertions are not indicated by Pender.

LOGICAL FORM

The Health Promotion Model has been formulated through induction by use of existing research to form a pattern of knowledge. Middle-range theories have commonly been built through this approach. The Health Promotion Model is a conceptual model that was formulated with the goal of integrating what is known about health-promoting behavior to generate questions for further testing. This model provides a framework for seeing more clearly how the results of previous research fit together and also how concepts can be manipulated for further study.

ACCEPTANCE BY THE NURSING COMMUNITY
Practice

The concept of health promotion is a popular one in practice. Wellness as a nursing specialty has exploded in the past decade. Personal responsibility for health care is the cornerstone of every plan for health care reform in the United States. The financial, human, and environmental cost to society for individuals who do not engage in health prevention and promotion has been high. Understanding how consumers can be motivated to attain personal health has social relevance that will be of increasing importance to planners of health care delivery and those who provide the care. *Health Promotion in Nursing Practice* has proved to be a primary resource in the addition of health promotion to the practice of nursing.

Education

The use of the health promotion model has not been established in nursing education. Health promotion is a new emphasis that is currently placed behind illness care as clinical education is taking place in acute care settings.[9]

Research

The Health Promotion Model is primarily a tool for research. Dozens of research reports have been published that use the model and the Health Promoting Lifestyle Profile. The model has implications for application by emphasizing the importance of individual assessment of the factors believed to influence health behavior changes.

FURTHER DEVELOPMENT

The model continues to be refined and tested for its power to explain the relationships among the factors believed to influence health behavior changes. Dr. Pender plans further testing with populations across the life span, and aggregates, to determine the model's validity and expand the usefulness of the evolving model.

CRITIQUE
Simplicity

The Health Promotion Model is simple to understand. Its language is clear and accessible to nurses. The relationships among the various factors in each set are linked, but the relationships require further clarification. The sets of factors, as being direct or indirect influences, are clearly set out in a visually simple diagram that shows their association. Factors are seen as independent, but the sets have an interactive effect that results in action.

Generality

The model is middle range in scope. It is highly generalizable to adult populations. The research used to derive the model was based on male, female, young, old, well, and ill samples. Applicability of the model to children aged 10 to 16 years is currently being tested.

Empirical Precision

The model has been supported through testing by Pender and others as a framework for explaining health promotion. The Health Promoting Lifestyle Profile has emerged as an instrument to assess health-promoting behaviors.[12]

Derivable Consequences

Dr. Pender has identified health promotion as a goal for the twenty-first century, just as disease prevention was a task of the twentieth century. The model can potentially influence the interaction between the nurse and the consumer. Pender has responded to the political, social, and personal environment of her time to clarify nursing's role in delivering health-promotion services to persons of all ages.

CRITICAL THINKING *Activities*

1 Choose one health-promoting behavior in which you do not engage. Identify your own factors, as defined in the Health Promotion Model, that contribute to your decision not to participate. Include immediate competing alternatives.

2 Analyze the factors present in your life that contribute to your participation in any health-promoting activity in which you currently engage. Place each factor under the appropriate label from the Health Promotion Model.

3 Prepare your own description of wellness. Ask three friends, three family members, and three co-workers to describe what wellness means to them. Compare the descriptions given by individuals with different ages and backgrounds. How are they alike? Is "absence of disease" more prominent than positive, active statements of health?

4 Consider the changes made in health care delivery in the last century related to advances in disease prevention and cure. What changes can you predict for the nurse of 2050 if health promotion becomes the primary focus of health care? Include the potential locations for the work of nursing to be done, possible new tools, and how the shift in emphasis would affect the demand for nurses.

REFERENCES

1. Azjen, I, & Fishbein, M. (1980). *Understanding attitudes and predicting social behaviors.* Englewood Cliffs, NJ: Prentice-Hall.
2. Bandura, A. (1977). Self-efficacy: Toward a unifying theory of behavioral change. *Psychology Review, 84*(2), 191-215.
3. Becker, M.H. (1974). *The health belief model and personal behavior.* Thorofare, NJ: Charles B. Slack.
4. Dunn, H.L. (1961). *High-level wellness.* Arlington, VA: Beatty.
5. Pender, N.J. (1970). A developmental study of conceptual, semantic differential, and acoustical dimensions as encoding categories in short-term memory. *Dissertation Abstracts International, Section A, 30*(10), 4283.
6. Pender, N.J. (1975). A conceptual model for preventive health behavior. *Nursing Outlook, 23*(6):385-390.
7. Pender, N.J. (1987). *Health promotion in nursing practice* (2nd ed.). New York: Appleton & Lange.
8. Pender, N.J. (1996). *Health promotion in nursing practice* (3rd ed.). Stamford, CT: Appleton & Lange.
9. Pender, N.J., Baraukas, V.H., Hayman, L., Rice, V.H., & Anderson, E.T. (1992). Health promotion and disease prevention: Toward excellence in nursing practice and education. *Nursing Outlook, 40*(3), 106-120.
10. Pender, N.J., Walker, S.N., Sechrist, K.R., & Stromborg, M.F. (1988). Development and testing of the health promotion model. *Cardiovascular Nursing, 24*(6), 41-43.
11. Personal interview. March 16, 1992.
12. Walker, S.N., Sechrist, K.R., & Pender, N.J. (1987). The health-promoting lifestyle profile: Development and psychometric characteristics. *Nursing Research, 36*(2), 76-80.

BIBLIOGRAPHY

Primary sources

Books

Pender, N.J. (1982). *Health promotion in nursing practice.* New York: Appleton-Century-Crofts.

Pender, N.J. (1987). *Health promotion in nursing practice* (2nd ed.). New York: Appleton & Lange.

Pender, N.J. (1996). *Health promotion in nursing practice* (3rd ed.). Stamford, CT: Appleton & Lange.

Book chapters

Pender, N.J. (1984). Health promotion and illness prevention. In H. Werley & J. Fitzpatrick (Eds.), *Annual review of nursing research* (pp. 83-105). New York: Springer.

Pender, N.J. (1985). Self modification. In G. Bulechek & J. McCloskey (Eds.), *Interventions: Treatments for nursing diagnosis* (pp. 80-91): Philadelphia: Saunders.

Pender, N.J. (1986). Health promotion: Implementing strategies. In B. Logan & C. Dawkins (Eds.), *Family-centered nursing in the community* (pp. 295-334). Menlo Park, CA: Addison-Wesley.

Pender, N.J. (1987). Health and health promotion: The conceptual dilemmas. In *Conceptual issues in health promotion: The Wingspread conference* (pp. 7-23). Indianapolis: Sigma Theta Tau International.

Pender, N.J. (1989). Languaging a health perspective for NANDA taxonomy on research and theory. In R.M. Carroll-Johnson (Ed.), *Classification of nursing diagnoses* (pp. 31-36). Philadelphia: Lippincott.

Pender, N.J. (1989). The pursuit of happiness, stress, and health. In S. Wald (Ed.), *Community health nursing: issues and topics* (pp. 145-175). Englewood Cliffs, NJ: Prentice-Hall.

Pender, N.J., & Sallis, J. (1995). Exercise counseling by health professionals. In R. Dishman (Ed.), *Exercise adherence* (2nd ed.), Champaign, IL: Human Kinetics.

Journal articles

Brimmer, P.F., Skoner, M., Pender, N.J., Williams, C.A., Fleming, J.W., & Werley, H.H. (1983). Nurses with doctoral degrees: Education and employment characteristics. *Research in Nursing and Health, 6,* 157-165.

Garcia, A.W., Broda, M.A., Frenn, M., Coviak, C., Pender, N.J., & Ronis, D.L. (1995). Gender and developmental differences in exercise beliefs among youth and prediction of their exercise behavior. *Journal of School Health, 65*(6), 213-219.

Pender, N.J. (1967). The debate as a teaching and learning tool. *Nursing Outlook, 15,* 42-43.

Pender, N.J. (1970). A developmental study of conceptual, semantic differential, and acoustical dimensions as encoding categories in short term memory. *Dissertation Abstracts International, Section A, 30*(10), 4283.

Pender, N.J. (1971). Students who choose nursing: Are they success oriented? *Nursing Forum, 16*(1), 64-71.

Pender, N.J. (1974). Patient identification of health information received during hospitalization. *Nursing Research, 23*(3), 262-267.

Pender, N.J. (1975). A conceptual model for preventive health behavior. *Nursing Outlook, 23*(6), 385-390.

Pender, N.J. (1984). Physiologic responses of clients with essential hypertension to progressive muscle relaxation training. *Research in Nursing and Health, 7,* 197-203.

Pender, N.J. (1985). Effects of progressive muscle relaxation training on anxiety and health locus of control among hypertensive adults. *Research in Nursing and Health, 8,* 67-72.

Pender, N.J. (1987). Interview: James Michael McGinnis, MD, MPP. *Family and Community Health, 10*(2), 59-65.

Pender, N.J. (1988). Research agenda: Identifying research ideas and priorities. *American Journal of Health Promotion, 2*(4), 42-51.

Pender, N.J. (1988). Research agenda: The influences of health policy on an evolving research agenda. *American Journal of Health Promotion, 2*(3), 51-54.

Pender, N.J. (1990). Expressing health through lifestyle patterns. *Nursing Science Quarterly, 3*(3), 115-122.

Pender, N.J. (1990). Research agenda: A revised research agenda model. *American Journal of Health Promotion, 4*(3), 220-222.

Pender, N.J., Barkaukas, V.H., Hayman, L., Rice, V.H., & Anderson, E.T. (1992). Health promotion and disease prevention: Toward excellence in nursing practice and education. *Nursing Outlook, 40*(3), 106-120.

Pender, N.J., & Pender, A.R. (1980). Illness prevention and health promotion services provided by nurse practitioners: Predicting potential consumers. *American Journal of Public Health, 70*(8), 798-803.

Pender, N.J., & Pender, A.R. (1986). Attitudes, subjective norms, and intentions to engage in health behaviors. *Nursing Research, 35*(1), 15-18.

Pender, N.J., Sechrist, K.R., Stromborg, M., & Walker, S.N. (1987). Collaboration in developing a research program grant. *Image, 19*(2), 75-77.

Pender, N.J., Smith, L.C., & Vernof, J.A. (1987). Building better workers. *AAOHN Journal, 35*(9), 386-390.

Pender, N.J., Walker, S.N., Sechrist, K.R., & Stromborg, M.F. (1988). Development and testing of the health promotion model. *Cardiovascular Nursing, 24*(6), 41-43.

Pender, N.J., Walker, S.N., Stromborg, M.F., & Sechrist, K.R. (1990). Predicting health promoting lifestyles in the workplace. *Nursing Research, 39*(6), 326-332.

Sechrist, K.R., Walker, S.N., & Pender, N.J. (1987). Development and psychometric evaluation of the exercise benefits/barriers scale. *Research in Nursing and Health, 10,* 357-365.

Stromborg, M.F., Pender, N.J., Walker, S.N., & Sechrist, K.R. (1990). Determinants of health-promoting lifestyle in ambulatory cancer patients. *Social Science and Medicine, 31*(10), 1159-1168.

Walker, S.N., Ken, M.J., Pender, N.J., & Sechrist, K.R. (1990). A Spanish language version of the health promoting lifestyle profile. *Nursing Research, 39*(5), 268-273.

Walker, S.N., Sechrist, K.R., & Pender, N.J. (1987). The health-promoting lifestyle profile: Development and psychometric characteristics. *Nursing Research, 36*(2), 76-81.

Walker, S.N., Volkan, K., Sechrist, K.R., & Pender, N.J. (1988). Health-promoting life styles of older adults: Comparisons with young and middle-aged adults, correlates and patterns. *Advances in Nursing Science, 11*(1), 76-90.

Secondary sources

Dissertations

Barnett, F.C. (1989). The relationship of selected cognitive-perceptual factors to health-promoting behaviors of adolescents. University of Texas, Austin.

Fehir, J.S. (1988). Self-rated health status, self-efficacy, motivation, and selected demographics as determinants of health-promoting lifestyle behavior in men 35 to 64 years old: A nursing investigation. University of Texas, Austin.

Hudak, J.W. (1988). A comparative study of the health beliefs and health-promoting behaviors of normal weight and overweight male Army personnel. Catholic University of America.

Kerr, M.J. (1994). Factors related to Mexican-American workers' use of hearing protection. University of Michigan.

Index